Neural Stem Cells
in
Health and Disease

Neural Stem Cells
in
Health and Disease

Editor

Ashok K. Shetty

Institute for Regenerative Medicine
Texas A&M Health Science Center College of Medicine, USA

World Scientific

NEW JERSEY · LONDON · SINGAPORE · BEIJING · SHANGHAI · HONG KONG · TAIPEI · CHENNAI · TOKYO

Published by

World Scientific Publishing Co. Pte. Ltd.

5 Toh Tuck Link, Singapore 596224

USA office: 27 Warren Street, Suite 401-402, Hackensack, NJ 07601

UK office: 57 Shelton Street, Covent Garden, London WC2H 9HE

Library of Congress Cataloging-in-Publication Data
Neural stem cells in health and diseases / [edited by] Ashok K. Shetty.
    p. ; cm.
  Includes bibliographical references and index.
  ISBN 978-9814623179 (hardcover : alk. paper)
  I. Shetty, Ashok K., editor.
  [DNLM: 1. Neural Stem Cells--physiology. 2. Neurodegenerative Diseases--therapy.
3. Stem Cell Transplantation. WL 102.3]
  QP363.5
  612.6'4018--dc23
                                    2015015461

British Library Cataloguing-in-Publication Data
A catalogue record for this book is available from the British Library.

COVER ART CREDIT
Cover Art designed by:
Ms. Adrian Bates, Research Assistant, Institute for Regenerative Medicine,
Texas A&M HSC College of Medicine, Temple, TX 76502

Typeset by Stallion Press
Email: enquiries@stallionpress.com

Contents

About the Editor

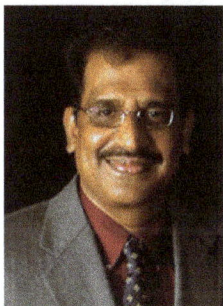

Dr. Ashok K. Shetty is Director of Neurosciences at the Institute for Regenerative Medicine and Professor in the Department of Molecular and Cellular Medicine, Texas A&M Health Science Center College of Medicine, Temple, Texas, USA. Dr. Shetty is also Research Career Scientist at the Olin E. Teague Veterans' Affairs Medical Center, Central Texas Veterans Healthcare System in Temple, Texas, USA. Dr. Shetty received his Masters degree in human anatomy from the Kasturba Medical College Manipal, of Mysore University in 1983. He obtained his Ph.D. degree in Neuroscience from the All India Institute of Medical Sciences, New Delhi in 1990. Following his postdoctoral research work at Montana State University and Duke University, Dr. Shetty joined the Division of Neurosurgery (Department of Surgery) at the Duke University Medical Center as an Assistant Professor in 1995. He became an Associate Professor in 1999 and held the position of Professor from 2004 to 2011. Dr. Shetty joined the faculty at Texas A&M University Health Science Center in July 2011.

Dr. Shetty is currently Charter Member of the NIH Study Section, Developmental Brain Disorders (Brain Disorders and Clinical Neuroscience IRG). Previously, Dr. Shetty served as Charter Member of the NIH Study Section CNNT (Brain Disorders and Clinical Neuroscience ZRG1, 2004–2008) and as member of over 25 other study section panels of the NIH, study section panels of Congressionally Directed Medical Research Program of the Department of Defense, Maryland State Stem Cell Research Fund and New York State Stem Cell Research Fund. He has also served as reviewer of grant applications for over 12 international funding agencies from Germany, France, England, Israel, India, Singapore and Italy. Dr. Shetty is currently Co-Chief Editor of the journal *Aging and Disease,* and Associate Editor of journals, *Frontiers in Epilepsy, Molecular and Cellular Epilepsy and Neurogenesis.* Dr. Shetty also serves as an Editorial Board Member of many international journals, which include *Stem Cells, Aging Cell, Stem Cells International, Current Aging Science, Frontiers in Neurogenesis, Frontiers in Aging Neuroscience, Frontiers in Neuropharmacology* and *Frontiers in Cellular Biochemistry.* Dr. Shetty has authored 112 publications and his work has appeared in a number of top-class journals including *Molecular Psychiatry, Neuropsychopharmacology, Journal of Neuroscience, Stem Cells, Aging Cell, Progress in Neurobiology, Neurotherapeutics, Pharmacology and Therapeutics, Neurobiology of Aging, Neurobiology of Disease, Neuroscience & Biobehavioral Reviews, Stem Cells Translational Medicine, Experimental Neurology and Scientific Reports.* Dr. Shetty has received over 5,700 citations for his published research articles. As per the Essential Science Indicators of Thompson Reuters, Dr. Shetty is among the top 1% of scientists worldwide in the field of Neuroscience and Behavior, in terms of citations received for articles published over ten-year periods.

Dr. Shetty has received research grant awards from the National Institute of Neurological Disorders and Stroke (NINDS), National Institute for Aging (NIA) and National Center for Complementary and Alternative Medicine (NCCAM) of National Institutes of Health, peer reviewed medical research program (PRMRP) grants from the Department of Defense (DOD), and Merit Review Awards from the Department of Veterans Affairs (DVA). Dr. Shetty's current research is focused on developing clinically applicable strategies that enhance brain function after injury, disease or aging, which include the following: (1) Elucidating mechanisms by which transplanted neuronal precursors, neural stem cells or inhibitory interneuron progenitors promote brain repair and ease spontaneous seizures, cognitive dysfunction and depression in prototypes of status epilepticus, temporal lobe epilepsy and traumatic brain injury. The donor cells derived from brain tissues as well as human-induced pluripotent stem cells are employed. (2) Studying mechanisms of brain dysfunction in prototypes of Gulf War Illness and developing treatment strategies to ease cognitive and mood impairments in Gulf War Illness. (3) Developing approaches to improve hippocampus neurogenesis, and memory and mood function in aging and neurological diseases via stimulation of endogenous neural stem/progenitor cells. (4) Analyzing promising neuroprotective compounds and drugs for their usefulness to block chronic epilepsy development after an initial precipitating injury such as status epilepticus or traumatic brain injury including mild traumatic brain injury induced by blast shock waves.

Contributing Authors

Ashok K. Shetty, Ph.D.
Professor and Director of Neurosciences
Institute for Regenerative Medicine and Department of Molecular and Cellular Medicine
Texas A&M Health Science Center College of Medicine
Research Career Scientist, Central Texas Veterans Health Care System
5701 Airport Road, Module C, Temple Texas 76502, USA
E-mail: shetty@medicine.tamhsc.edu

J. Martin Wojtowicz, Ph.D.
Professor and Graduate Co-Coordinator
Department of Physiology
University of Toronto
Medical Sciences Building
1 King's College Circle
Toronto, ON, M5S 1A8, Canada
Email: martin.wojtowicz@utoronto.ca

Yao Fang Tan
Department of Physiology
University of Toronto
Medical Sciences Building
1 King's College Circle
Toronto, ON, M5S 1A8, Canada

Matthew B. Eastman
Department of Physiology and Neurobiology
University of Connecticut
75 N. Eagleville Road, Unit 3156
Storrs, CT 06269-3156, USA

Rebecca L. Acabchuk
Department of Physiology and Neurobiology
University of Connecticut
75 N. Eagleville Road, Unit 3156
Storrs, CT 06269-3156, USA

Joanne C. Conover, Ph.D.
Associate Professor
Department of Physiology and Neurobiology
University of Connecticut
75 N. Eagleville Road, Unit 3156
Storrs, CT 06269-3156, USA
Email: joanne.conover@uconn.edu

Lalitha Madhavan, M.D., Ph.D.
Assistant Professor
Department of Neurology and Evelyn F. McKnight Brain Institute
University of Arizona
1501, N Campbell Ave
Tucson, AZ 85724, USA
Email: lmadhavan@email.arizona.edu

Lauren S. Y. Wood
M.D. Candidate
Department of Neurology
Stanford University School of Medicine
265 Campus Dr., SIM1, G3077
Stanford, CA 94305, USA
E-mail: lswood@stanford.edu

Michelle Monje, M.D., Ph.D.
Assistant Professor
Department of Neurology
Stanford University School of Medicine
265 Campus Dr., SIM1, G3077
Stanford, CA 94305, USA
Email: mmonje@stanford.edu

Kunlin Jin, M.D., Ph.D.
Professor
Department of Pharmacology and Neuroscience
University of North Texas Health Science Center
Fort Worth, Texas 76107, USA
Email: Kunlin.Jin@unthsc.edu

Bethany E. Hosford
Neuroscience Ph.D. Candidate
Department of Anesthesia
Cincinnati Children's Hospital Medical Center
3333 Burnet Ave, ML 2001
Cincinnati, OH 45229-3039, USA
E-mail: bethany.hosford@cchmc.org

Steve C. Danzer, Ph.D.
Associate Professor
Department of Anesthesia
Cincinnati Children's Hospital Medical Center
3333 Burnet Ave, ML 2001
Cincinnati, OH 45229-3039, USA
Email: Steve.Danzer@cchmc.org

Aminul I. Ahmed, M.A., M.B./Ph.D.
Clinical Lecturer in Neurosurgery
Clinical Neurosciences
University of Southampton
Southampton General Hospital

Tremona Road
Southampton, SO16 6YD, UK
Email: A.Ahmed@soton.ac.uk

William P. Gray
Professor of Neurosurgery
Director HCRW BRAIN Unit
Neuroscience and Mental Health Research Institute
School of Medicine, Cardiff University
Institute of Psychological Medicine and Clinical Neurosciences
Cardiff, UK
E-mail: GrayWP@cf.ac.uk

Orly Lazarov, Ph.D.
Associate Professor
Department of Anatomy and Cell Biology
University of Illinois at Chicago
Chicago, IL, USA
E-mail: olazarov@uic.edu

Jennifer L. Wagner
Department of Pharmaceutical Sciences
University of Kentucky
789 S. Limestone, BPC 473
Lexington, KY 40536-0596, USA

Emily A. Barton
Department of Psychology
University of Houston
126 Heyne Building, Room 231D
Houston, TX 77204-5022, USA

Chelsea R. Geil
Department of Pharmaceutical Sciences
University of Kentucky
789 S. Limestone, BPC 473
Lexington, KY 40536-0596, USA

J. Leigh Leasure
Department of Psychology
University of Houston
126 Heyne Building, Room 231D
Houston, TX 77204-5022, USA

Kimberly Nixon, Ph.D.
Associate Professor
Department of Pharmaceutical Sciences
University of Kentucky
789 S. Limestone, BPC 473
Lexington, KY 40536-0596, USA
E-mail: kim-nixon@uky.edu

Chitra D. Mandyam, Ph.D.
Associate Professor
Committee on the Neurobiology of Addictive Disorders
The Scripps Research Institute
10550 North Torrey
Pines Road, SP30-2400
La Jolla, CA 92037, USA
Email: cmandyam@scripps.edu

Fang Liu, Ph.D.
Division of Neurotoxicology
National Center for Toxicological Research (NCTR)
Food and Drug Administration (FDA)
3900 NCTR Road, HFT-132
Jefferson, AR 72079, USA
E-mail: Fang.Liu@fda.hhs.gov

Merle G. Paule, Ph.D.
Division of Neurotoxicology
National Center for Toxicological Research (NCTR)
Food and Drug Administration (FDA)
3900 NCTR Road, HFT-132, USA
Jefferson, AR 72079

Tucker A. Patterson, Ph.D.
Division of Neurotoxicology
National Center for Toxicological Research (NCTR)
Food and Drug Administration (FDA)
3900 NCTR Road, HFT-132
Jefferson, AR 72079, USA

Cheng Wang, Ph.D.
Division of Neurotoxicology
National Center for Toxicological Research (NCTR)
Food and Drug Administration (FDA)
3900 NCTR Road, HFT-132
Jefferson, AR 72079, USA

William Slikker, Jr., Ph.D.
Office of the Director
National Center for Toxicological Research
U.S. Food & Drug Administration
3900 NCTR Road
Jefferson, AR 72079-9502, USA
E-mail: William.Slikker@fda.hhs.gov

Derek K. Smith
Department of Molecular Biology
Hamon Center for Regenerative Science and Medicine
UT Southwestern Medical Center
6000 Harry Hines Boulevard
Dallas, Texas 75390, USA
Email: Derek.Smith@UTSouthwestern.edu

Wenze Niu
Department of Molecular Biology
Hamon Center for Regenerative Science and Medicine
UT Southwestern Medical Center
6000 Harry Hines Boulevard
Dallas, Texas 75390, USA
Email: Wenze.Niu@UTSouthwestern.edu

Chun-Li Zhang, Ph.D.
Associate Professor
Department of Molecular Biology
Hamon Center for Regenerative Science and Medicine
UT Southwestern Medical Center
6000 Harry Hines Blvd
Dallas, Texas 75390, USA
Email: Chun-Li.Zhang@UTSouthwestern.edu

Marcel M. Daadi, Ph.D.
Associate Scientist & Director,
   Stem Cells & Regenerative Medicine
Southwest National Primate Research Center
Texas Biomedical Research Institute
Adjunct Associate Professor
Department of Cellular & Structural Biology
Department of Radiology, Medical School
UT Health Science Center at San Antonio
San Antonio, Texas 78227, USA
Phone: 210-258-9210
Email: mdaadi@txbiomed.org

Ike dela Peña
Center of Excellence for Aging and Brain Repair
Department of Neurosurgery and Brain Repair
University of South Florida College of Medicine
12901 Bruce B. Downs Blvd. MDC 78
Tampa, FL 33612, USA

Alesia Antoine
Center of Excellence for Aging and Brain Repair
Department of Neurosurgery and Brain Repair
University of South Florida College of Medicine
12901 Bruce B. Downs Blvd. MDC 78
Tampa, FL 33612, USA

Stephanny Reyes
Center of Excellence for Aging and Brain Repair
Department of Neurosurgery and Brain Repair
University of South Florida College of Medicine
12901 Bruce B. Downs Blvd. MDC 78
Tampa, FL 33612, USA

Diana Hernandez
Center of Excellence for Aging and Brain Repair
Department of Neurosurgery and Brain Repair
University of South Florida College of Medicine
12901 Bruce B. Downs Blvd. MDC 78
Tampa, FL 33612, USA

Sandra Acosta
Center of Excellence for Aging and Brain Repair
Department of Neurosurgery and Brain Repair
University of South Florida College of Medicine
12901 Bruce B. Downs Blvd. MDC 78
Tampa, FL 33612, USA

Mibel Pabon
Center of Excellence for Aging and Brain Repair
Department of Neurosurgery and Brain Repair
University of South Florida College of Medicine
12901 Bruce B. Downs Blvd. MDC 78
Tampa, FL 33612, USA

Naoki Tajiri
Center of Excellence for Aging and Brain Repair
Department of Neurosurgery and Brain Repair
University of South Florida College of Medicine
12901 Bruce B. Downs Blvd. MDC 78
Tampa, FL 33612, USA

Yuji Kaneko
Center of Excellence for Aging and Brain Repair
Department of Neurosurgery and Brain Repair
University of South Florida College of Medicine
12901 Bruce B. Downs Blvd. MDC 78
Tampa, FL 33612, USA

Cesar V. Borlongan, Ph.D.
Professor and Director
Center of Excellence for Aging and Brain Repair
Department of Neurosurgery and Brain Repair
University of South Florida College of Medicine
12901 Bruce B. Downs Blvd. MDC 78
Tampa, FL 33612, USA
Email: cborlong@health.usf.edu

Bharathi Hattiangady, Ph.D.
Assistant Professor
Institute for Regenerative Medicine and Department of Molecular
  and Cellular Medicine
Texas A&M Health Science Center College of Medicine
Research Service, Olin E. Teague Veterans' Medical Center,
Central Texas Veterans Health Care System
Temple, Texas 76502, USA
E-mail: hattiangady@medicine.tamhsc.edu

Samuel E. Marsh
Department of Neurobiology & Behavior
Sue & Bill Gross Stem Cell Research Center
Institute for Memory Impairments and Neurological Disorders
University of California
Irvine 845 Health Sciences Rd
3200 Gross Hall
Irvine, CA 92697-9016, USA

Mathew Blurton-Jones, Ph.D.
Assistant Professor
Department of Neurobiology & Behavior
Sue & Bill Gross Stem Cell Research Center
Institute for Memory Impairments
  and Neurological Disorders
University of California
Irvine 845 Health Sciences Rd
3200 Gross Hall
Irvine, CA 92697-9016, USA
Email: mblurton@uci.edu

Christopher J. Haas
Drexel University College of Medicine
Department of Neurobiology & Anatomy
Philadelphia, PA 19129, USA

Joseph F. Bonner
University of California, Irvine
Reeve-Irvine Research Center
Irvine, CA 92697, USA

George Ghobrial
Thomas Jefferson University Hospital
Department of Neurosurgery
Philadelphia, PA 19107, USA

Itzhak Fischer, Ph.D.
Professor and Chair
Drexel University College of Medicine
Department of Neurobiology & Anatomy
Philadelphia, PA 19129, USA
E-mail: ifischer@drexelmed.edu

Mohan C. Vemuri, Ph.D.
Director, Cell Biology at Thermo Fisher Scientific
Thermo Fisher Scientific
7335 Executive Way
Frederick, MD 21704, USA
Email: mohan.vemuri@thermofisher.com

Mahendra S. Rao, M.D., Ph.D.
Director, NIH Intramural Center for Regenerative Medicine
  (NIH-CRM)
National Institutes of Health
Bethesda, Maryland, USA
Current address: CSO at Mahendra Rao LLC
Q therapeutics, Salt Lake City, Utah, USA
E-mail: mrao1234@verizon.net

Introduction

Neural Stem Cells in Health and Disease

Ashok K. Shetty

Neural stem cells (NSCs) are self-renewing, multipotent cells found in both the developing and adult central nervous system (CNS) (Gage and Temple, 2013). During development, NSCs generate the vast majority of cells making up the CNS including: neurons, astrocytes and oligodendrocytes. The primitive NSCs are a subclass of radial glial cells (Noctor *et al.*, 2001), which continually produce more restricted neuronal and glial progenitors that are recognized as transit amplifying (or intermediate) progenitors (Englund *et al.*, 2005). These cells exhibit limited self-renewal and proliferative activity compared to NSCs and hence supply differentiated progeny (Davis and Temple, 1994; Gage and Temple, 2013). When the CNS is created with the necessary numbers and types of progenitors and differentiated cells, proliferating NSCs in the majority of CNS regions undergo diminution in number, either owing to terminal differentiation or acquisition of a quiescent state.

In the postnatal and adult periods, NSCs or their progenitors proficient for producing neurons are confined to only a few regions of the CNS known as neurogenic regions. The resident NSCs in these regions proliferate and generate neurons and glia all through life, a phenomenon now referred to as *adult neurogenesis* which entered into the limelight through wide-ranging research during the last two decades. This finding has overthrown one of the principal

1

doctrines concerning the mammalian brain that neurons were generated in entirety during development and hence are not restored when they perish due to disease or injury. Although the notion of cell division and neuronal differentiation occurring in the postnatal and adult brain has been around since the 1960s (Altman and Das, 1965, Altman, 1969; Kaplan and Hinds, 1977; Goldman and Nottebohm, 1983), an inspiring discovery — both neurons and astrocytes can be produced in culture from cells isolated from the adult mammalian brain (Reynolds and Weiss, 1992) — in the early nineties elicited massive awareness for studying NSCs and neurogenesis in the adult brain in both normal and disease states.

NSCs in Neurogenic Regions of the Adult Brain

Many studies have now lucidly ascertained the manifestation of proliferating NSCs and neurogenesis throughout life in two distinct regions of the adult mammalian brain: the subventricular zone (SVZ) covering the walls of forebrain lateral ventricles and the subgranular zone (SGZ) of the dentate gyrus (DG) in the hippocampal formation (Ihrie and Alvarez-Buylla, 2011; Yao *et al.*, 2012). Analogous to NSCs in the developing CNS, NSCs in the adult brain exhibit ability for proliferation, self-renewal and generation all three major CNS cell types (Ihrie and Alvarez-Buylla, 2011; Ming and Song, 2011). In the SVZ, proliferation of NSCs and/or intermediate progenitors generates a pool of neuroblasts, which migrate into the olfactory bulb through a channel called the rostral migratory stream (RMS, Ihrie and Alvarez-Buylla, 2011). There, they undergo differentiation and maturation into olfactory bulb interneurons. In the SGZ of the DG, proliferation of NSCs and intermediate progenitors generate mostly new neurons and some glia. Newly generated neurons then migrate into the granule cell layer (GCL), where they mature as dentate granule cells. These new granule cells then establish afferent connectivity with axons from the entorhinal cortex, and efferent connectivity with CA3 pyramidal neurons (Yao *et al.*, 2012). Both SVZ and SGZ are also active in the adult human brain. The human SGZ generates new granule cells for the DG as in rodents (Eriksson *et al.*, 1998; Spalding *et al.*, 2013). On the other hand, the human SVZ appears to contribute new neurons mostly to the striatum (Ernst *et al.*, 2014). This is in sharp contrast to the SVZ of rodents, which generate neurons that in normal conditions migrate only to the olfactory bulb. Nonetheless, NSCs in the two neurogenic regions share several key characteristics (Urban and Guillemot, 2014).

The NSC niche in neurogenic regions is comprised of varied types of cells and structures, which include astrocytes, neurons, axon projections and blood vessels. The primary function of this niche is to offer an apt milieu that maintains the bulk of NSCs in a quiescent and undifferentiated state (Morrison and Spradling, 2008; Urban and Guillemot, 2014). Furthermore, the niche presents a diversity of signals that regulate the behavior of NSCs and/or their progenitors to adjust the production of new cells according to the needs of the tissue (Faigle and Song, 2013; Urban and Guillemot, 2014). Activity of NSCs is determined by multiple signals arising from the milieu. A variety of cellular components existing in and around NSC niches such as astrocytes, oligodendrocyte progenitors, endothelial cells, pericytes, microglia, mature granule cells and GABA-ergic interneurons can influence NSC activity (Palmer *et al.*, 2000; Goldman and Chen, 2011). In addition, non-cellular components such as secreted molecules and the extracellular matrix proteins play roles (Palmer *et al.*, 2000; Hsieh, 2012). Studies have also shown that both neurons and astrocytes in NSC niches can influence self-renewal or differentiation of NSCs (Song *et al.*, 2002; Hsieh, 2012). Thus, adult neurogenesis is created through a multicellular niche, where NSCs react to instructive signals from other cell types, resulting in their proliferation, self-renewal and/or differentiation of their progeny into mature neurons or glia.

Putative NSCs in Non-Neurogenic Regions of the Adult Brain

Several reports reinforce the thought that some restricted extent of neurogenesis also occurs in so-called "non-neurogenic" regions of the brain under particular conditions (Gould, 2007). The regions include the hippocampus CA1 subfield (Rietze *et al.*, 2000), substantia nigra of the mesencephalon (Zhao *et al.*, 2003), neocortex (Cameron and Dayer, 2008), striatum (Bedard *et al.*, 2006), amygdala (Fowler *et al.*, 2008), piriform cortex (Shapiro *et al.*, 2007), and the hypothalamus (Yuan and Arias-Carrión *et al.*, 2011). However, in most of these regions, the progenitor cells do not differentiate into neurons under physiological conditions. Rather, they either maintain the properties of precursor cells or differentiate into glia (Gage and Temple, 2013). Remarkably, progenitors isolated from multiple adult brain regions maintain the ability for proliferation as well as differentiation into neurons *in vitro*, when expanded in FGF-2 and treated with differentiation factors, indicating that extrinsic factors play a key role in invigorating neural progenitors to differentiate into neurons (Palmer *et al.*, 1999). The presence of multipotent NSC-like cells in non-neurogenic adult brain regions demonstrating proficiency for proliferation and neuronal differentiation in the presence of apt neurotrophic factors is an exciting discovery. With the arrival of novel neurogenic compounds and drugs (Pieper *et al.*, 2010; Walker *et al.*, 2015), these cells may be amenable for extensive proliferation to produce large numbers of site-specific new neurons in neurodegenerative disease conditions.

Intrinsic Regulators of NSC Activity and Hippocampus Neurogenesis

Preservation of NSCs and cell fate specification of NSC-derived cells in the SGZ are facilitated through several transcription factors and signaling pathways. Several studies have shown that preservation of type 1 cells (primary NSCs) occurs via Notch signaling (Lugert *et al.*, 2010, 2012; Hsieh, 2012). The role of several other transcription factors in the maintenance of NSCs has also been observed, which comprise Pax-6 (paired domain and homeodomain-containing transcription factor), Ascl1 (another bHLH transcription factor), Fox03 (forkhead domain transcription factor), REST (repressor element1 silencing transcription factor), and TLX (nuclear hormone transcription factor) (Jessberger *et al.*, 2008; Renault *et al.*, 2009; Gao *et al.*, 2011). The development of type 2 cells (transient amplifying progenitors) and type 3 cells (neuroblasts) from types 1 and 2 cells involves a sequential up-regulation of transcription factors Neurogenin 2 (a bHLH transcription factor involved in neural fate-choice decision) and Tbr2 (T-brain gene 2). Differentiation of neuroblasts into mature neurons requires the expression of NeuroD1 (Neuronal differentiation 1; Gao *et al.*, 2009), controlled through Wnt/ß-catenin signaling (Kuwabara *et al.*, 2009; Seib *et al.*, 2013), and expression of Sox-3, Sox-11 and FoxG1 (Forkhead box G1, a Winged Helix transcriptional repressor) (Shen *et al.*, 2006; Wang *et al.*, 2006; Haslinger *et al.*, 2009). In contrast, the survival and maturation of newly generated neurons is thought to be influenced by Prox-1 (*prospero*-related homeobox gene) (Jessberger *et al.*, 2008) and CREB (cyclic AMP response element-binding protein) (Jagasia *et al.*, 2009).

Neurogenesis in the Adult Human Brain

The first evidence for the likely presence of NSCs in the adult human hippocampus came through demonstration of newly born neurons in the autopsied hippocampus of cancer patients who received 5′-bromodeoxyuridine (BrdU) injections for diagnostic purposes (Eriksson *et al.*, 1998). However, a recent study offered convincing proof for the occurrence of NSCs and neurogenesis in the DG of humans (Spalding *et al.*, 2013). This study employed a distinctive birth dating approach based on the peak of carbon isotope 14 (^{14}C) discharged into the atmosphere during the above ground nuclear bomb tests between 1945 and 1963 (Kempermann, 2013). This method depends on the principle that ^{14}C in the atmosphere gets integrated into the DNA of dividing human cells through consumption of plants that have absorbed ^{14}C from the atmosphere or eating animals that have consumed these plants (Welberg, 2013). As ^{14}C is amalgamated into the DNA during cell division, the ^{14}C content of a cell is thought to reflect ^{14}C levels in the atmosphere at the time of the birth of the cell. As atomic bomb testing in 1950s and 1960s produced an upsurge in atmospheric ^{14}C levels and quantities decayed after 1963 (due to the limited test ban treaty), the concentration of ^{14}C in cellular DNA enabled assessment of a cell's birth date (Welberg, 2013).

Spalding and colleagues, using hippocampi from post-mortem brains of persons who were born in various years in the 20th century, sorted neurons from glial cells, purified neuronal DNA and calculated ^{14}C levels (Spalding *et al.*, 2013). This study demonstrated that adult neurogenesis in the human brain is conspicuous mainly in the DG of hippocampus. As per the estimate, ~80% of DG granule cells undergo renewal in adulthood with ~700 new neurons added per day for an annual turnover rate of 1.75%, and the turnover rate of neurons is similar between men and women (Spalding *et al.*, 2013; Kempermann, 2013). Furthermore, the study showed that only a modest decrease in hippocampus neurogenesis occurs with aging, which is in sharp contrast to the major age-related decline observed in rodents (Kuhn *et al.*, 1996; Rao *et al.*, 2005, 2006; Hattiangady and Shetty, 2008). Thus, the occurrence of NSCs and neurogenesis in the adult human hippocampus has no doubt been verified.

NSC Activity and Hippocampus Function

Newly born neurons (granule cells) created by NSCs in the DG integrate into the prevailing hippocampus circuitry and become functional. Until about a month after their birth, they display an augmented receptiveness for long-term potentiation, a substrate underlying learning and memory formation (Schmidt-Heber *et al.*, 2004; Ming and Song, 2011). It has also been suggested that continuous turnover of DG granule cells is highly effective for meeting some of the unique computational needs of the hippocampus (Appleby *et al.*, 2011). Furthermore, behavioral studies implied that adult DG neurogenesis is important for hippocampus-dependent learning and memory (Braun and Jessberger, 2014). A multitude of correlative studies initially suggested a link between spatial memory function and the amount of newly generated neurons (Kempermann *et al.*, 1997; Van Praag *et al.*, 1999; Gould *et al.*, 1999; Drapeau *et al.*,

2003). Neurogenesis ablation via approaches such as whole brain radiation or administration of drugs targeting dividing NSCs and their progeny also supported a role for DG neurogenesis in hippocampus-dependent memory (Shors *et al.*, 2001; Snyder *et al.*, 2005). Yet, disputing results in some other studies have raised a few doubts on the purported role of DG neurogenesis in spatial learning and memory function.

Multiple follow-up studies nonetheless furnished sounder evidence that spatial learning cleverly introduces or eliminates newly born granule cells to the hippocampus circuitry depending on their stage of development and functional importance (Tronel *et al.*, 2010, Deng *et al.*, 2010). Likewise, computational models proposed a role for newly born granule cells in the encoding of temporal information as well as in the preservation of old memories during the encoding of new data (Aimone *et al.*, 2010, 2011). Investigations employing genetic ablation procedures also illustrated spatial learning deficits with the loss of hippocampal neurogenesis (Dupret *et al.*, 2008; Zhang *et al.*, 2008; Jessberger *et al.*, 2009). Another study, which exploits a combination of retroviral and optogenetic approaches to birth date and reversibly control a group of adult-born neurons in adult mice, showed that silencing a cohort of ~4-week-old newly born granule cells after water maze learning considerably disrupts retrieval of spatial memory (Gu *et al.*, 2012). Also, a number of studies through careful testing of DG circuitry, point to a decisive role for newly generated neurons in pattern separation function (Sahay *et al.*, 2011a,b; Kheirbek *et al.*, 2012; Nakashiba *et al.*, 2012; Ikrar *et al.*, 2013). Capability for pattern separation allows discernment of analogous experiences through storage of similar representations in a non-overlapping manner (Yassa and Stark, 2011). Constant addition of new granule cells seem to be necessary for maintaining normal hippocampal function, as it provides a pool of highly plastic immature cells to facilitate complex computational needs (Kempermann, 2012).

Diminished DG neurogenesis has also been associated with psychiatric illnesses (Bergmann and Frisen, 2013). It has been proposed that reduced neurogensis weakens pattern separation function and thereby impairs the ability for discerning threats from similar but safe situations. This alteration contributes to a generalized awareness of fear and anxiety in posttraumatic stress disorder (Kheirbek *et al.*, 2012; Bergmann and Frisen, 2013). Additionally, most antidepressant treatments increase DG neurogenesis and some of the effects of antidepressants in animal models are contingent on increased neurogenesis (Santarelli *et al.*, 2003). Thus, DG neurogenesis in the adult hippocampus appears vital for maintaining homeostasis in the hippocampus, particularly its ability for maintaining normal memory and mood function.

NSCs in Health and Disease

Since NSC activity and neurogenesis in the adult brain is now confirmed in virtually all mammalian species including humans, a series of chapters in this book (Chapters 1–12) focus on discussing current knowledge of: (i) mechanisms of NSC activity; (ii) the extent and functional significance of neurogenesis in the adult brain under normal, aged and disease environments; (iii) the susceptibility of NSCs and plasticity of neurogenesis to alcohol, drugs of abuse and anesthetic agents; and (iv) advanced techniques that trigger neurogenesis in non-neurogenic regions. A second series of chapters in this book (Chapters 13–18) are focused on discussing the promise and efficacy of grafting of NSCs and/or other stem cells for treating neurological disorders such as Parkinson's disease, stroke, temporal lobe epilepsy, Alzheimer's disease and spinal cord injury. The final chapter confers on advances that are made in manufacturing a variety of neural cell types from human PSCs that can be used as donor cells for cell transplantation.

NSC Activity and Neurogenesis in Normal, Aged and Disease Environments

The first chapter deliberates on how NSC activity and adult hippocampus neurogenesis are tied closely to activity of the hippocampus circuit, and how the plasticity of hippocampus circuitry depends upon the behavioral state of the organism as it interacts with its environment (Wojtowicz and Tan, 2015). The next chapter draws attention to important differences that exist in the SVZ-NSC niche organization and neurogenic capacity between rodents and humans. Authors suggest that any advancement in the ability to exploit the adult human SVZ-NSC niche for therapeutic ends must take into consideration its reduced capacity for neurogenesis as well as a likely diminished reparative potential (Eastman *et al.*, 2015). The third chapter considers the ability of NSCs to significantly enhance endogenous regenerative, reparative, and protective capacities in the adult as well as the aging brain after intracerebral transplantation (Madhavan, 2015). In Chapter 4, the consequences of radiation therapy and chemotherapeutic agents on NSC activity and neurogenesis, in the context of radiation-induced cognitive decline and chemotherapy-induced cognitive dysfunction, are conferred (Wood and Monje, 2015).

The next few chapters elucidate NSC behavior and/or plasticity of neurogenesis as well as their consequences on function in neurological conditions such as stroke, epilepsy, traumatic brain injury (TBI) and Alzheimer's disease. Shetty and Jin discuss the contribution of SVZ neurogenesis in replacing neurons that are lost due to ischemia or stroke in the adult brain, the link between stroke-induced SVZ neurogenesis and functional recovery after stroke, stroke-induced SVZ neurogenesis in the human brain and the promise of SVZ neurogenesis enhancing strategies for improved functional recovery after stroke (Shetty and Jin, 2015). Hosford and Danzer debate how altered NSC activity and neurogenesis in the hippocampus play roles in promoting temporal lobe epileptogenesis after brain injury or insults (Hosford and Danzer, 2015). They suggest that abnormal migration and integration of new granule cells generated from NSCs after brain injury or other insults establish recurrent excitatory connections, which in turn impairs the ability of DG to limit the flow of excitatory information through the hippocampus. Ahmed and Gray discuss the potential mechanisms that contribute to increased NSC activity and neurogenesis following traumatic brain injury (TBI), and the promise and challenges concerning harnessing of endogenous NSCs for repair after TBI (Ahmed and Gray, 2015). Lazarov confers the possible role of neurogenesis in the development of cognitive deficits in Alzheimer's disease and other neurodegenerative diseases characterized by loss of memory (Lazarov, 2015). This chapter highlights preclinical models of familial Alzheimer's disease where altered neurogenesis is one of the conspicuous features of the disease. The author however infers that advanced experimental tools for the detection of neurogenesis *in vivo* in humans will be essential for comprehending the role of neurogenesis in Alzheimer's disease progression or pathophysiology.

Wagner and colleagues review the role of NSCs in the alcoholic brain. It is intriguing that, while moderate to high-dose binge-like and chronic exposures reduce the proliferation of NSCs and the survival of newly born neurons, abstinence, on the other hand, induces reactive neurogenesis. The authors suggest that such reactive neurogenesis is likely beneficial for repopulating lost dentate granule cells in the DG (Wagner *et al.*, 2015). They emphasize that a better understanding of how alcohol affects NSCs could lead to the identification of novel pharmacological targets for the prevention or treatment of alcoholic neuropathology. Mandyam examines the link between hippocampus NSC activity and neurogenesis with the relapse of methamphetamine-seeking behavior in preclinical models of methamphetamine-addiction (Mandyam, 2015). The author suggests that strategies which reverse the maladaptive neuroplasticity (such as enhanced NSC proliferation and increased survival of newly born neurons) occurring during abstinence may normalize the methamphetamine-impaired hippocampus function as well as reduce the vulnerability to relapse in methamphetamine addicts. Liu and colleagues discuss NSC plasticity *in vitro* following exposure to anesthetic agents (Liu *et al.*, 2015). They point out that pediatric sedative or anesthesia-induced neurotoxicity depends on dosage, durations of exposure, routes of administration, receptor sub-type activated, and the stages of neural development at the time of exposure. Smith and colleagues discuss recent advances pertaining to *in vivo* reprogramming of resident glial cells in models of injury and neurodegenerative diseases (Smith *et al.*, 2015). They suggest that, while the current *in vivo* reprogramming approaches have several practical limitations that challenge its clinical utility, further refinement and innovation in the coming years would pave the way for patient-specific regenerative medicine through reprogramming of cells in the CNS.

Promise of NSC and/or Other Stem Cell Transplantation for Treating Neurological Disorders

In Chapter 13, Daadi deliberates on recent advances in NSC derivation from various sources, differentiation methods for obtaining specific dopaminergic lineage, and the current challenges to overcome prior to the clinical use of NSC-derived cells for treating Parkinson's disease (Daadi, 2015). The author suggests that the ideal stem cell-based cellular products will strike an optimal balance between the safety of the cells and the purity and scalability of derivation method of the midbrain dopaminergic neurons with a proven therapeutic innervation capacity. Pena and colleagues review the advantages and limitations of grafting of a variety of stem cells including NSCs for neuroprotection in stroke (dela Pena *et al.*, 2015). Authors emphasize that, while the successful entry of stem cell-based therapies in clinical studies is exciting, several factors need to be considered prior to the utilization of stem cell transplantation for stroke therapy. These include issues such as immunogenicity, tumorigenicity, survival, proliferation capacity and differentiation of the chosen stem cells as well as harvesting techniques.

Shetty and Hattiangady provide insights on NSC-based therapies for status epilepticus induced injury and chronic temporal lobe epilepsy (Shetty and Hattiangady, 2015). The authors point out that grafting of NSCs into the hippocampus early after an initial precipitating injury such as status epilepticus is beneficial for easing injury-induced epileptogenesis, spontaneous seizure development and cognitive and mood impairments. Additionally, they suggest that transplantation of NSCs into the hippocampus shortly or at prolonged periods after the onset of chronic epilepsy is efficacious for reducing the frequency and intensity of spontaneous seizures. However, the authors caution that prior to the clinical application of NSC grafts for treating SE or chronic epilepsy, additional critical studies on several aspects (e.g. long-term survival and behavior of grafted NSCs, long-lasting beneficial effects on seizures and co-morbidities such as memory and mood dysfunction, efficacy of possible combination therapies) are needed. Marsh and Blurton-Jones, in the following chapter, provide a critical overview of mechanisms by which NSC grafts mediate beneficial effects in preclinical models of Alzheimer's disease. They emphasize that, while NSC-based treatments for Alzheimer's disease offer an innovative therapeutic approach for an otherwise untreatable disease, there are several hurdles to overcome before the translation of NSC transplantation for treating Alzheimer's disease patients can be realized (Marsh and Blurton-Jones, 2015). They note that for a widespread disease such as AD, neuronal replacement represents an extremely daunting challenge that will likely take many decades of intense research to develop.

Haas and colleagues review the promise of transplantation of NSCs, neural progenitors, olfactory ensheathing cells and Schwann cells isolated from a variety of sources for treating spinal cord injury (Haas *et al.*, 2015). The authors note that a variety of these cells have demonstrated safety and some evidence of neurological recovery in clinical trials and the results obtained so far are encouraging for the design of future clinical trials. In the final chapter, Vemuri and Rao describe the landscape of scientific progress that is driving successful differentiation of human pluripotent stem cells (PSCs) towards multiple neural lineages. Specifically, they examine advances that are made in manufacturing a variety of human neural cell types from PSCs that can be used as donor cells for cell transplantation (Vemuri and Rao, 2015). They note that progress in the field has been rapid but hampered by several critical roadblocks, which include the stable maintenance of human PSCs, the long process of differentiation and the relative immaturity of the finally differentiated cells. They emphasize that further progress will require developing highly reproducible processes that are scalable and economical enough to justify the transition of using human PSC-derived cells for treating neurological disorders.

Acknowledgements

The author thanks the support from the National Institutes of Health (R01 awards), the Department of Veterans Affairs (VA Merit Review Awards), the State of Texas (Emerging Technology Funds) and the Department of Defense (Peer Reviewed Medical Research Program Grants) for his research on neural stem cells, adult neurogenesis and stem cell transplantation.

References

Ahmed AI, Gray WP (2015) Endogenous neural stem cell response to traumatic brain injury. In: *Neural Stem Cells in Health and Disease* (A.K. Shetty, Ed), World Scientific Press, in press, 2015.

Aimone JB, Deng W, Gage FG (2010) Adult neurogenesis: integrating theories and separating functions. *Trends Cogn Sci* 14:325–337.

Aimone JB, Deng W, Gage FH (2011) Resolving new memories: a critical look at the dentate gyrus, adult neurogenesis, and pattern separation. *Neuron* 70:589–596.

Altman J, Das GD (1965) Autoradiographic and histological evidence of postnatal hippocampal neurogenesis in rats. *J Comp Neurol* 124: 319–335.

Altman J (1969) Autoradiographic and histological studies of postnatal neurogenesis. IV. Cell proliferation and migration in the anterior forebrain, with special reference to persisting neurogenesis in the olfactory bulb. *J Comp Neurol* 137:433–457.

Appleby PA, Kempermann G, Wiskott L (2011) The role of additive neurogenesis and synaptic plasticity in a hippocampal memory model with grid-cell like input. *PLoS Comput Biol* 7:e1001063.

Bedard A, Gravel C, Parent A (2006) Chemical characterization of newly generated neurons in the striatum of adult primates. *Exp Brain Res* 170:501–512.

Bergmann O, Frisen J (2013) Neuroscience. Why adults need new brain cells. *Science* 340:695–696.

Braun SM, Jessberger S (2014) Review: Adult neurogenesis and its role in neuropsychiatric disease, brain repair and normal brain function. *Neuropathol Appl Neurobiol* 40:3–12.

Cameron HA, Dayer AG (2008) New interneurons in the adult neocortex: small, sparse, but significant? *Biol Psychiatry* 63:650–655.

Daadi MM (2015) Neural stem cell therapy for Parkinson's disease. In: *Neural Stem Cells in Health and Disease* (A.K. Shetty, Ed), World Scientific Press, in press, 2015.

Davis AA, Temple S (1994) A self-renewing multipotential stem cell in embryonic rat cerebral cortex. *Nature* 372:263–266.

dela Peña I, Antoine A, Reyes S, Hernandez D, Acosta S, Pabon M, Tajiri N, Kaneko Y, Borlongan CV (2015) Stem cell-based neuroprotective strategies in stroke. In: *Neural Stem Cells in Health and Disease* (A.K. Shetty, Ed), World Scientific Press, in press, 2015.

Deng W, Aimone JB, Gage FH (2010) New neurons and new memories: how does adult hippocampal neurogenesis affect learning and memory? *Nat Rev Neurosci* 11:339–350.

Drapeau E, Mayo W, Aurousseau C, Le Moal M, Piazza PV, and Abrous, DN (2003) Spatial memory performances of aged rats in the water maze predict levels of hippocampal neurogenesis. *Proc Natl Acad Sci USA* 100:14385–14390.

Dupret D, Revest JM, Koehl M, Ichas F, De Giorgi F, Costet P, Abrous DN, Piazza, PV (2008) Spatial relational memory requires hippocampal adult neurogenesis. *PLoS One* 3: e1959.

Eastman MB, Acabchuk RL, Conover JC (2015) Age-related changes to the subventricular zone stem cell niche. In: *Neural Stem Cells in Health and Disease* (A.K. Shetty, Ed), World Scientific Press, in press, 2015.

Englund C, Fink A, Lau C, Pham D, Daza RA, Bulfone A, Kowalczyk T, Hevner RF (2005) Pax6, Tbr2, and Tbr1 are expressed sequentially by radial glia, intermediate progenitor cells, and postmitotic neurons in developing neocortex. *J Neurosci* 25:247–251.

Eriksson PS, Perfilieva E, Bjork-Eriksson T, Alborn AM, Nordborg C, Peterson DA, Gage FH (1998) Neurogenesis in the adult human hippocampus. *Nat Med* 4:1313–1317.

Ernst A, Alkass K, Bernard S, Salehpour M, Perl S, Tisdale J, Possnert G, Druid H, Frisén J (2014) Neurogenesis in the striatum of the adult human brain. *Cell* 156:1072–1083.

Faigle R, Song H (2013) Signaling mechanisms regulating adult neural stem cells and neurogenesis. *Biochim Biophys Acta* 1830:2435–2448.

Fowler CD, Liu Y, Wang Z (2008) Estrogen and adult neurogenesis in the amygdala and hypothalamus. *Brain Res Rev* 57:342–351.

Gage FH, Temple S (2013) Neural stem cells: generating and regenerating the brain. *Neuron* 80:588–601.

Gao Z, Ure K, Ables JL, Lagace DC, Nave KA, Goebbels S, Eisch AJ, Hsieh J (2009) Neurod1 is essential for the survival and maturation of adult-born neurons. *Nat Neurosci* 12:1090–1092.

Gao Z, Ure K, Ding P, Nashaat M, Yuan L, Ma J, Hammer RE, Hsieh J (2011) The master negative regulator REST/NRSF controls adult neurogenesis by restraining the neurogenic program in quiescent stem cells. *J Neurosci* 31:9772–9786.

Goldman SA, Chen Z (2011) Perivascular instruction of cell genesis and fate in the adult brain. *Nat Neurosci* 14:1382–1389.

Goldman SA, Nottebohm F (1983) Neuronal production, migration, and differentiation in a vocal control nucleus of the adult female canary brain. *Proc Natl Acad Sci USA* 80:2390–2394.

Gould E (2007) How widespread is adult neurogenesis in mammals? *Nat Rev Neurosci* 8:481–488.

Gould E, Tanapat P, Hastings NB, Shors TJ (1999) Neurogenesis in adulthood: a possible role in learning. *Trends Cogn Sci* 3:186–192.

Gu Y, Arruda-Carvalho M, Wang J, Janoschka SR, Josselyn SA, Frankland PW, Ge S (2012) Optical controlling reveals time-dependent roles for adult-born dentate granule cells. *Nat Neurosci* 15:1700–1706.

Haslinger A, Schwarz TJ, Covic M, Lie DC (2009) Expression of Sox11 in adult neurogenic niches suggests a stage-specific role in adult neurogenesis. *Eur J Neurosci* 29:2103–2114.

Haas CJ, Bonner JF, Ghobrial G, Fischer I (2015) Neural stem cell therapy for spinal cord injury. In: *Neural Stem Cells in Health and Disease* (A.K. Shetty, Ed), World Scientific Press, in press, 2015.

Hattiangady B, Shetty AK (2008) Aging does not alter the number or phenotype of putative stem/progenitor cells in the neurogenic region of the hippocampus. *Neurobiol Aging* 29:129–147.

Hosford BE, Danzer SC (2015) Neurogenesis and dentate granule cell development in epilepsy. In: *Neural Stem Cells in Health and Disease* (A.K. Shetty, Ed), World Scientific Press, in press, 2015.

Hsieh J (2012) Orchestrating transcriptional control of adult neurogenesis. *Genes Dev* 26:1010–1021.

Ihrie RA, Alvarez-Buylla A (2011) Lake-front property: a unique germinal niche by the lateral ventricles of the adult brain. *Neuron* 70:674–686.

Ikrar T, Guo N, He K, Besnard A, Levinson S, Hill A, Lee HK, Hen R, Xu X, Sahay A (2013) Adult neurogenesis modifies excitability of the dentate gyrus. *Front Neural Circuits* 7:204.

Jagasia R, Steib K, Englberger E, Herold S, Faus-Kessler T, Saxe M, Gage FH, Song H, Lie DC (2009) GABA-cAMP response element-binding protein signaling regulates maturation and survival of newly generated neurons in the adult hippocampus. *J Neurosci* 29:7966–7977.

Jessberger S, Toni N, Clemenson GD Jr, Ray J, Gage FH (2008) Directed differentiation of hippocampal stem/progenitor cells in the adult brain. *Nat Neurosci* 11:888–893.

Jessberger S, Clark RE, Broadbent NJ, Clemenson GD Jr, Consiglio A, Lie DC, Squire LR, Gage FH (2009) Dentate gyrus-specific knockdown of adult neurogenesis impairs spatial and object recognition memory in adult rats. *Learn Mem* 16:147–154.

Kaplan MS, Hinds JW (1977) Neurogenesis in the adult rat: electron microscopic analysis of light radioautographs. *Science* 197:1092–1094.

Kempermann G, Kuhn HG, Gage FH (1997) More hippocampal neurons in adult mice living in an enriched environment. *Nature* 386:493–495.

Kempermann, G (2012) Youth culture in the adult brain. *Science* 335: 1175–1176.

Kempermann G (2013) Neuroscience — What the bomb said about the brain. *Science* 340:1180–1181.

Kheirbek MA, Klemenhagen KC, Sahay A, Hen R (2012) Neurogenesis and generalization: a new approach to stratify and treat anxiety disorders. *Nat Neurosci* 15:1613–1620.

Kuhn HG, Dickinson-Anson H, Gage FH (1996) Neurogenesis in the dentate gyrus of the adult rat: age-related decrease of neuronal progenitor proliferation. *J Neurosci* 16:2027–2033.

Kuwabara T, Hsieh J, Muotri A, Yeo G, Warashina M, Lie DC, Moore L, Nakashima K, Asashima M, Gage FH (2009) Wnt-mediated activation of NeuroD1 and retro-elements during adult neurogenesis. *Nat Neurosci* 12:1097–1105.

Lazarov O (2015) Neural stem cells in Alzheimer's disease. In: *Neural Stem Cells in Health and Disease* (A.K. Shetty, Ed), World Scientific Press, in press, 2015.

Liu F, Paule MG, Patterson TA, Wang C, Slikker W (2015) Studies on developmental exposures to anesthetic agents and stem cell derived models. In: *Neural Stem Cells in Health and Disease* (A.K. Shetty, Ed), World Scientific Press, in press, 2015.

Lugert S, Basak O, Knuckles P, Haussler U, Fabel K, Götz M, Haas CA, Kempermann G, Taylor V, Giachino C (2010) Quiescent and active hippocampal neural stem cells with distinct morphologies respond selectively to physiological and pathological stimuli and aging. *Cell Stem Cell* 6:445–456.

Lugert S, Vogt M, Tchorz JS, Müller M, Giachino C, Taylor V (2012) Homeostatic neurogenesis in the adult hippocampus does not involve amplification of Ascl1 (high) intermediate progenitors. *Nat Commun* 3:670.

Madhavan L (2015) Neural Stem Cells for Intrinsic Brain Repair in Aging and Neural Degeneration. In: *Neural Stem Cells in Health and Disease* (A.K. Shetty, Ed), World Scientific Press, in press, 2015.

Mandyam CD (2015) Neural stem cells in methamphetamine addiction In: *Neural Stem Cells in Health and Disease* (A.K. Shetty, Ed), World Scientific Press, in press, 2015.

Marsh SE, Blurton-Jones M (2015) Prospects of neural stem cell therapy for Alzheimer's disease. In: *Neural Stem Cells in Health and Disease* (A.K. Shetty, Ed), World Scientific Press, in press, 2015.

Ming GL, Song H (2011) Adult neurogenesis in the mammalian brain: significant answers and significant questions. *Neuron* 70:687–702.

Morrison SJ, Spradling AC (2008) Stem cells and niches: mechanisms that promote stem cell maintenance throughout life. *Cell* 132:598–611.

Nakashiba T, Cushman JD, Pelkey KA, Renaudineau S, Buhl DL, McHugh TJ, Rodriguez Barrera V, Chittajallu R, Iwamoto KS, McBain CJ, Fanselow MS, Tonegawa S (2012) Young dentate granule cells mediate pattern separation, whereas old granule cells facilitate pattern completion. *Cell* 149:188–201.

Noctor SC, Flint AC, Weissman TA, Dammerman RS, Kriegstein AR (2001) Neurons derived from radial glial cells establish radial units in neocortex. *Nature* 409:714–720.

Palmer TD, Markakis EA, Willhoite AR, Safar F, Gage FH (1999) Fibroblast growth factor-2 activates a latent neurogenic program in neural stem cells from diverse regions of the adult CNS. *J Neurosci* 19:8487–8497.

Palmer TD, Willhoite AR, Gage FH (2000) Vascular niche for adult hippocampal neurogenesis. *J Comp Neurol* 425:479–494.

Pieper AA, Xie S, Capota E, Estill SJ, Zhong J, Long JM, Becker GL, Huntington P, Goldman SE, Shen CH, Capota M, Britt JK, Kotti T, Ure K, Brat DJ, Williams NS, MacMillan KS, Naidoo J, Melito L, Hsieh J, De Brabander J, Ready JM, McKnight SL (2010) Discovery of proneurogenic, neuroprotective chemical. *Cell* 142:39–51.

Rao MS, Hattiangady B, Abdel-Rahman A, Stanley DP, Shetty AK (2005) Newly born cells in the ageing dentate gyrus display normal migration, survival and neuronal fate choice but endure retarded early maturation. *Eur J Neurosci* 21:464–476.

Rao MS, Hattiangady B, Shetty AK (2006) The window and mechanisms of major age-related decline in the production of new neurons within the dentate gyrus of the hippocampus. *Aging Cell* 5:545–558.

Renault VM, Rafalski VA, Morgan AA, Salih DA, Brett JO, Webb AE, Villeda SA, Thekkat PU, Guillerey C, Denko NC, Palmer TD, Butte AJ, Brunet A (2009) FoxO3 regulates neural stem cell homeostasis. *Cell Stem Cell* 5:527–539.

Reynolds BA, Weiss S (1992) Generation of neurons and astrocytes from isolated cells of the adult mammalian central nervous system. *Science* 255:1707–1710.

Rietze R, Poulin P, Weiss S (2000) Mitotically active cells that generate neurons and astrocytes are present in multiple regions of the adult mouse hippocampus. *J Comp Neurol* 424:397–408.

Sahay A, Scobie KN, Hill AS, O'Carroll CM, Kheirbek MA, Burghardt NS, Fenton AA, Dranovsky A, Hen R (2011a) Increasing adult hippocampal neurogenesis is sufficient to improve pattern separation. *Nature* 472:466–470.

Sahay A, Wilson DA, Hen R (2011b) Pattern separation: a common function for new neurons in hippocampus and olfactory bulb. *Neuron* 70:582–588.

Santarelli L, Saxe M, Gross C, Surget A, Battaglia F, Dulawa S, Weisstaub N, Lee J, Duman R, Arancio O, Belzung C, Hen R (2003) Requirement of hippocampal neurogenesis for the behavioral effects of antidepressants. *Science* 301:805–809.

Schmidt-Hieber C, Jonas P, Bischofberger J (2004) Enhanced synaptic plasticity in newly generated granule cells of the adult hippocampus. *Nature* 429:184–187.

Seib DR, Corsini NS, Ellwanger K, Plaas C, Mateos A, Pitzer C, Niehrs C, Celikel T, Martin-Villalba A (2013) Loss of Dickkopf-1 restores neurogenesis in old age and counteracts cognitive decline. *Cell Stem Cell* 12:204–214.

Shapiro LA, Ng KL, Kinyamu R, Whitaker-Azmitia P, Geisert EE, Blurton-Jones M, Zhou QY, Ribak CE (2007) Origin, migration and fate of newly generated neurons in the adult rodent piriform cortex. *Brain Struct Funct* 212:133–148.

Shen L, Nam HS, Song P, Moore H, Anderson SA (2006) FoxG1 haploinsufficiency results in impaired neurogenesis in the postnatal hippocampus and contextual memory deficits. *Hippocampus* 16:875–890.

Shetty AK, Hattiangady B (2015) Neural stem cell therapy for easing status epilepticus induced hippocampus dysfunction and chronic temporal lobe epilepsy. In: *Neural Stem Cells in Health and Disease* (A.K. Shetty, Ed), World Scientific Press, in press, 2015.

Shetty AK, Jin K. Neural stem cell activity and neurogenesis after stroke. In: *Neural Stem Cells in Health and Disease* (A.K. Shetty, Ed), World Scientific Press, in press, 2015.

Shors TJ, Miesegaes G, Beylin A, Zhao M, Rydel T, Gould E (2001) Neurogenesis in the adult is involved in the formation of trace memories. *Nature* 410:372–376.

Smith DK, Niu W, Zhang C-L (2015) Induced neurogenesis as a mechanism for adult central nervous system regeneration. In: *Neural Stem Cells in Health and Disease* (A.K. Shetty, Ed), World Scientific Press, in press, 2015.

Snyder JS, Hong NS, McDonald RJ, Wojtowicz JM (2005) A role for adult neurogenesis in spatial long-term memory. *Neuroscience* 130:843–852.

Spalding KL, Bergmann O, Alkass K, Bernard S, Salehpour M, Huttner HB, Boström E, Westerlund I, Vial C, Buchholz BA, Possnert G, Mash DC, Druid H, Frisén J (2013) Dynamics of hippocampal neurogenesis in adult humans. *Cell* 153:1219–1227.

Song H, Stevens CF, Gage FH (2002) Astroglia induce neurogenesis from adult neural stem cells. *Nature* 417:39–44.

Tronel S, Fabre A, Charrier V, Oliet SH, Gage FH, Abrous DN (2010) Spatial learning sculpts the dendritic arbor of adult-born hippocampal neurons. *Proc Natl Acad Sci USA* 107:7963–7968.

Urbán N, Guillemot F (2014) Neurogenesis in the embryonic and adult brain: same regulators, different roles. *Front Cell Neurosci* 8:396 eCollection 2014.

van Praag H, Christie BR, Sejnowski TJ, and Gage FH (1999) Running enhances neurogenesis, learning, and long-term potentiation in mice. *Proc Natl Acad Sci USA* 96:13427–13431.

Vemuri M, Rao MS (2015) Generating different neural cell types from IPSCs for screening and cell therapy for CNS disorders. In: *Neural Stem Cells in Health and Disease* (A.K. Shetty, Ed), World Scientific Press, in press, 2015.

Wagner JL, Barton EA, Geil CR, Leasure JL, Nixon K (2015) roles of neural stem cells in alcohol use disorders. In: *Neural Stem Cells in Health and Disease* (A.K. Shetty, Ed), World Scientific Press, in press, 2015.

Walker AK, Rivera PD, Wang Q, Chuang JC, Tran S, Osborne-Lawrence S, Estill SJ, Starwalt R, Huntington P, Morlock L, Naidoo J, Williams NS, Ready JM, Eisch AJ, Pieper AA, Zigman JM (2015) The P7C3 class of neuroprotective compounds exerts antidepressant efficacy in mice by increasing hippocampal neurogenesis. *Mol Psychiatry* 20:500–508.

Wang Y, Ristevski S, Harley VR (2006) SOX13 exhibits a distinct spatial and temporal expression pattern during chondrogenesis, neurogenesis, and limb development. *J Histochem Cytochem* 54:1327–1333.

Welberg L (2013) Neurogenesis: a bombshell of a finding. *Nat Rev Neurosci* 14:522.

Wood LS, Monje M (2015) Neural stem cells and the effects of cancer therapy. In: *Neural Stem Cells in Health and Disease* (A.K. Shetty, Ed), World Scientific Press, in press, 2015.

Wojtowicz JM, Tan YF (2015) Physiology of stem cells in the hippocampal dentate gyrus. In: *Neural Stem Cells in Health and Disease* (A.K. Shetty, Ed), World Scientific Press, in press, 2015.

Yao J, Mu Y, Gage FH (2012) Neural stem cells: mechanisms and modeling. *Protein Cell* 3:251–261.

Yassa MA, Stark CE (2011) Pattern separation in the hippocampus. *Trends Neurosci* 34:515–525.

Yuan TF, Arias-Carrion O (2011) Adult neurogenesis in the hypothalamus: evidence, functions, and implications. *CNS Neurol Disord Drug Targets* 10:433–439.

Zhang CL, Zou Y, He W, Gage FH, Evans RM (2008) A role for adult TLX-positive neural stem cells in learning and behaviour. *Nature* 451:1004–1007.

Zhao M, Momma S, Delfani K, Carlen M, Cassidy RM, Johansson CB, Brismar H, Shupliakov O, Frisen J, Janson AM (2003) Evidence for neurogenesis in the adult mammalian substantia nigra. *Proc Natl Acad Sci USA* 100:7925–7930.

Chapter 1

Physiology of Stem Cells in the Hippocampal Dentate Gyrus

J. Martin Wojtowicz and Yao Fang Tan

Introduction

Physiology of stem cells does not exist. This was our first thought when asked to write an introduction to this volume. A prevalent dogma is that stem cells are quiescent, "mysterious" cells endowed with the phenomenal powers of multipotentiality and self-renewal. These cells give rise to progeny when commanded by neurotrophins and growth factors, but are otherwise unique, independent, and not really a part of traditional hippocampal system. However, gradually, as the writing progressed we began to realize that indeed there is a physiology of stem cells and it amounts to the same physiology that is described in neuroscience textbooks dealing with brain in general, and hippocampus in particular. Although stem cells do not produce action potentials and do not express neuronal proteins, they are very much a part of the brain circuit. This participation is somewhat analogous to glial cells that were once thought to be passive and separate, but are now recognized as full-fledged partners in the brain circuitry working in tandem with neurons. In fact, stem cells express glial fibrillary acidic protein (GFAP) previously thought to be a sole characteristic of astroglia. Moreover, despite a lack of synapses, stem cells express typically neuronal receptors for the major central inhibitory transmitter gamma aminobutyric acid (GABA), and react to activation of these receptors by opening chloride channels and subsequent depolarization. This latter characteristic is similar to that of young neurons which are in large measure controlled by GABA as they progress through developmental stages of proliferation, migration and differentiation (Kilb *et al.*, 2013).

The evidence summarized in this chapter will show that stem cell physiology is inseparable from the physiology of the rest of the dentate gyrus (DG) and consequently the rest of the hippocampus. In addition to being the source of new neurons, stem cells are far more responsive to the activity of the surrounding neuronal circuitry than previously thought. At the membrane level, downstream responses to membrane depolarization and hyperpolarization lead to fundamental changes in the cell's behavior. Membrane depolarization from the resting state stimulates asymmetric division of stem cells to effectively produce neuronal precursors in the form of neuroblasts, which can divide further and ultimately develop into mature neurons. Membrane hyperpolarization results in an increased rate of symmetric divisions by mitosis and consequently increased replication of stem cells. Such responses of stem cells to changes in membrane potential represent a form of brain plasticity because the production of neuroblasts can have profound physiological consequences and elicit behavioural outcomes. Further, the physiological significance of stem cells is emphasized by their presence in the hippocampal DG, which is a gateway to the hippocampus, the key brain structure involved in learning and memory.

Essential Steps in Neuronal Development

Stem cells possess two basic properties, self-renewal and multipotentiality. Within the adult brain, there are two main regions where stem cells take residence during late embryonic development and persist postnatally for as long as the animal lives. The region that produces most progeny is the subventricular zone (SVZ) of the lateral ventricles. It has been estimated that as many as 50,000 cells are produced daily in the SVZ of adult laboratory rodents. Many of these cells die shortly after the first division but the remaining tens of thousands are carried via the rostral migratory stream (RMS) to the olfactory bulbs where they develop into functional interneurons (Lledo, 2011; Platel and Bordey, 2011) An analogous process occurs on a smaller scale in the hippocampus, a brain region that controls many forms of learning and memory. The migration of neuronal progenitors from the subgranular zone (SGZ) within the DG is limited to the granule cell layer, which measures only 100 μm in width so the migration path is relatively short. Nevertheless, the control mechanisms affect progenitor migration, proliferation, differentiation, maturation and survival. Collectively, these steps are known as adult neurogenesis (ANG). The name would suggest the process is very different from embryonic neurogenesis, but this is far from certain. In fact, many factors are known to control both embryonic and adult neurogenesis in a similar way. It is not even certain when one developmental process really ends and the other begins because in many species, including laboratory rodents such as mice and rats, the embryonic development of DG carries into a postnatal phase lasting prominently for 1–2 weeks after birth.

This period may be different in other species where the brain develops primarily in embryo, but it usually carries into the postnatal period to some extent (Kempermann, 2012). There is a phase in the animal's development when embryonic, postnatal and adult neurogenesis (ANG) appear to overlap. However, ANG proper presumably takes over when the animal reaches sexual maturity. This initial overlap may cause confusion when studying factors controlling cell development and those primarily controlling the animal's development. It would appear that ANG can serve different functions in animals of different ages, as would be expected, but superimposed on this age-dependence is the flexibility of the ANG process itself. The four crucial steps in each cell's development, which include proliferation, differentiation, maturation and survival, occur at different rates and are controlled uniquely according to the animal's age. Hence, it is crucial to always present and discuss ANG in terms of these steps and also as it relates to the animal's age. To emphasize this distinction, cell development should be viewed on a sliding scale of animal's development and its inevitable aging (see Figure 1).

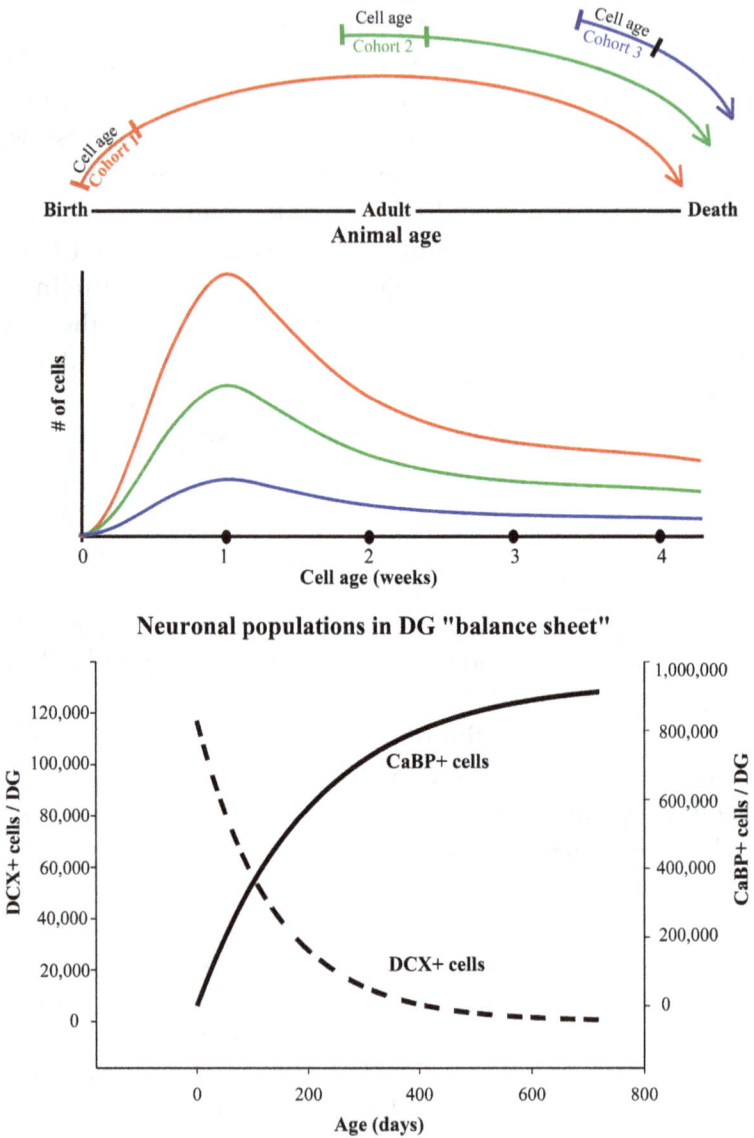

Figure 1. Sliding scale for adult neurogenesis (ANG). **Top:** Physiology and regulation of ANG is related to both the animal's age, and the cell age of each successive cohort. The early postnatal cohort is developing among numerous surrounding neurons of approximately the same age and in the context of high demand for hippocampal learning as the animal experiences the environment for the first time. The adult and aging cohorts experience a different environment, where the

Figure 1. (*Continued*) neuronal circuitry is mostly fully developed with very little free space so the new neurons have to displace the pre-existing cells. Because new neurons are a small minority among the mature ones, the microenvironment, essentially a support system in the sub-granular zone, may not be the same as in the young animal. The surrounding neuronal circuitry within the dentate gyrus (DG) also changes with age. The amount of GABA-ergic inhibition, and the synaptic density of excitatory inputs are reduced as the animal ages. Physiological/behavioural demands for new neurons in the mature animal may also be very different. Thus, the amount of new learning in the adult may be less than in a young animal, but recall of the pre-existing memories may be in high demand. Hence, the involvement of adult-born neurons in learning and memory processes may be animal and age specific. **Middle:** Survival curve for new neurons. For each new cohort of neurons shown in the top panel, the cell number is maximal during the first week, due to proliferation of neuroblasts. During the second week, cell numbers decline due to apoptosis. Cells that survive this decline persist for the rest of animal's life. The shape of the survival curve is similar for cohorts born in young (red), middle aged (green) and old (blue) animals but the overall number of produced cells is much smaller for the latter. **Bottom:** Balance sheet for ANG. The graph shows declining number of young neurons expressing doublecortin (DCX+) based on cell counts in rats of different ages. The rising curve represents the calculated number of neurons at 4 weeks of cell development. These neurons express calbindin (CaBP+), a mature neuronal marker Data is based on quantitative measurements of cells numbers in (McDonald and Wojtowicz, 2005). Note that in spite of reduced number of immature neurons, the addition of new neurons is still significant in adult animals due to a delay between cell birth and cell maturation.

Activity-dependent Regulation of ANG

Physiological/environmental regulation of ANG begins with stem cells (Figure 2). This is potentially the most powerful mode of regulation since in addition to changes in the rate of cell division, the cell fate can also be altered. Social isolation has been shown to increase the proportion of stem cells to neurons within adult hippocampus (Dranovsky *et al.*, 2011) whereas enriched environment had an opposite effect (Song *et al.*, 2013). The neurotransmitter GABA is a powerful regulatory factor at this early stage of cell development, and is in plentiful supply since it is a major inhibitory neurotransmitter utilized by hippocampal interneurons. Conveniently, there is a wide range of interneuron types with different soma locations, axonal arborizations and membrane properties (Freund and Buzsaki, 1996). It is well known that these interneurons can affect

Control of adult neurogenesis by neurotransmitters

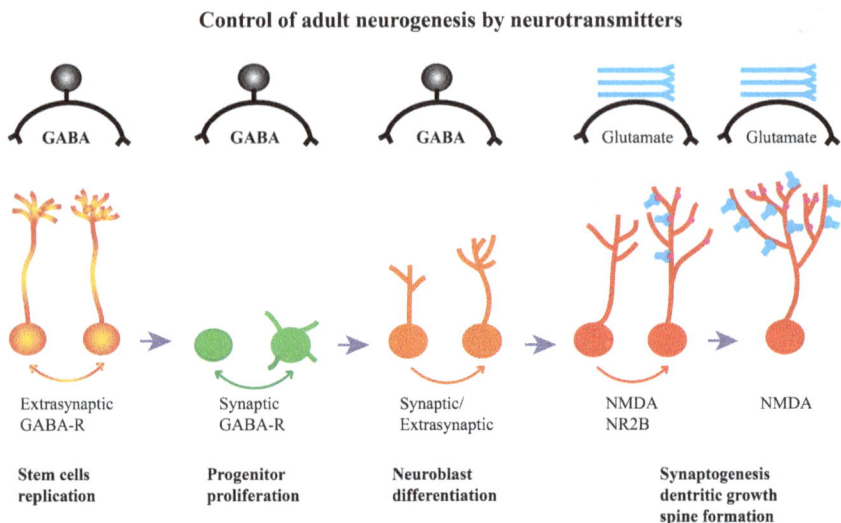

Figure 2. Regulation of ANG by GABA and Glutamate. Progression from stem cells to fully functional neurons is regulated by neurotransmitter GABA during early stages of cell development. This regulation is stage-specific and mediated by either synaptic or extrasynaptic GABA receptors. In some cases, a particular type of participating interneurons and subtype of GABA receptors has been identified (see text). At later stages of development glutamate, acting on glutamate (NMDA) receptors, regulates the rate of synaptogenesis, synaptic strength, dendritic growth and spine formation.

the activity of mature granule neurons but it is also becoming apparent that at least some of these interneurons affect the stem cells as well as adult-born, immature granule neurons (Armstrong *et al.*, 2011; Markwardt *et al.*, 2011). A subtype of these interneurons, basket cells, expressing a co-transmitter parvalbumin (PVA), are known to make synaptic contacts with proliferating cells in the SGZ (Song *et al.*, 2013). Stimulation or inhibition of these PVA interneurons can alter the rates of neuroblast proliferation and their differentiation into young neurons. Independently, stem cell division is altered by GABA release from PVA interneurons, but in this case the effect is mediated by extrasynaptic GABA receptors containing gamma-2 subunits (Song *et al.*, 2012). Activation of these receptors by ambient GABA promotes asymmetric division of stem cells. The resulting increase in the number of neuronal precursors can in turn lead to a subsequent increase in the number of new neurons. In contrast, inhibition of gamma-2 subunit-containing receptors or reduced concentration of GABA in their vicinity can promote symmetric stem cell replication at the expense of neuroblast production, but this only occurs in a specific neurogenic niche within the lower blade of the dentate gyrus (Dranovsky *et al.*, 2011).

The influence of GABA on ANG continues at later stages of cell development. A synthetic GABA agonist 4,5,6,7-Tetrahydroisoxazol [5,4,-c] pyridine-3-ol hydrochloride (THIP), also known as Gaboxadol, with its preferential affinity for delta GABA receptors stimulates neuronal production when given to the animal during the second week of cell development. At this stage, neuroblasts have stopped proliferating, express young neuronal marker doublecortin (DCX) and undergo a critical period for cell survival and differentiation (Whissell *et al.*, 2013). In support of this mechanism, the delta GABA receptor knockout mice show reduced neuronal maturation, and behavioral phenotype consistent with deficient ANG.

Glutamate takes over control of cell survival and growth when GABA influence ends. During the period between 3–6 weeks of cell development, new neurons are under control of NR2B-subtype of N-methyl-D-aspartate (NMDA) glutamate receptors. At later stages (two months and more) of cell development, glutamate-dependent neuronal plasticity persists, but at that time the main forms of plasticity being controlled by glutamate are synaptogenesis and dendritic growth (Tronel *et al.*, 2010).

Behavioral experiments provide supporting evidence for these regulatory mechanisms by GABA and glutamate. As noted above, social isolation and environmental enrichment have opposite effects on the stem cell population (Dranovsky *et al.*, 2011), consistent with the regulatory mechanism proposed by Song *et al.* 2012. At this stage, GABA is thought to be released into the extracellular space and act on extrasynaptic gamma-2 receptors. In addition, enriched environment has an effect on neuroblast expansion and ultimately on neurogenesis, presumably by activation of synaptic GABA receptors via PVA interneurons (Song *et al.*, 2013). Similarly, exposure to an enriched environment stimulates the formation of excitatory synapses onto the developing neurons. This process involves, at least partly, recruitment of previously silent NMDA synapses to more active status and consequent endowment of synapses with functional α-amino-3-hydroxy-5-methyl-4-isoxazolepropionic acid (AMPA) receptors (Chancey *et al.*, 2013). At later stages of neuronal development, adult-born neurons are primarily under the influence of excitatory, glutamatergic synapses and this regulation can involve rather specific environmental stimuli. In case of spatial learning for example, learning stimulates survival of relatively well-developed new neurons while inhibiting a less mature cohort (Dupret *et al.*, 2007). In addition, proliferation of neuroblasts at an even earlier stage of development is stimulated (Dupret *et al.*, 2007). Thus, control of neurogenesis by brain activity can have a complex pattern and is stage-sensitive.

Not surprisingly, in view of a tight relationship between newly born neurons and the existing circuitry of the DG, learning and memory can be influenced by changes in ANG. Upregulation of ANG by THIP, acting via GABA-delta receptors, facilitates the learning of contextual discrimination (Whissell *et al.*, 2013). In contrast, reduced ANG during aging or in pathological cases (i.e. Alzheimer's disease) results in impairment of memory (Drapeau and Abrous, 2008; Winocur *et al.*, 2014).

Specificity of regulatory mechanisms is partly dictated by the topography of the circuitry within the DG. Considering that GABA mediates regulation of the early stages of neurogenesis, it becomes apparent that such regulation may be relatively widespread along the longitudinal and transverse axes of the hippocampus due to wide topographical ramifications of the axonal arbour of the inhibitory interneurons (Figure 3). These arbours are often limited to certain regions of the DG as viewed in transverse hippocampal sections, but nevertheless cover large proportions of the DG and presumably make contacts with thousands of granule cells (Freund and Buzsaki, 1996). In contrast, the glutamatergic afferents in the perforant path make topographically limited, sparse connections with a relatively small number of granule neurons and are strictly delineated by specific strata within the molecular layer (Figure 3).

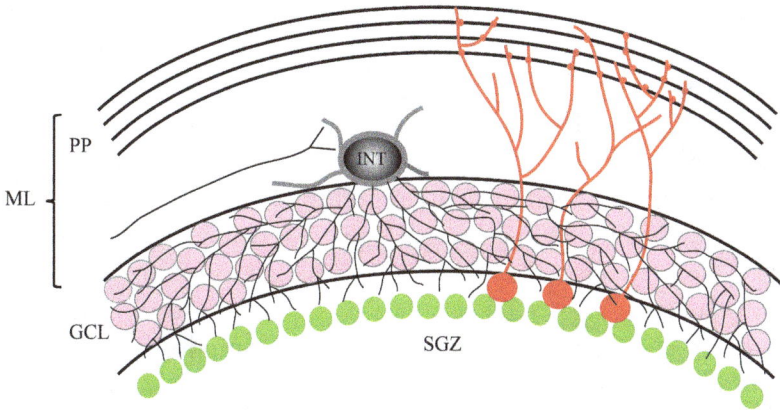

Figure 3. Topography of regulatory mechanisms in ANG. Profuse axonal arborisations by GABA-ergic interneurons suggest widespread control of ANG in DG. Example of an interneuron (INT) excited by an afferent axon and innervating numerous mature cells (purple) within granule cell layer (GCL) and immature neurons (green) within subgranular zone (SGZ). In contrast, the pinpoint projections of the perforant path (PP) onto the dendrites of granule cells (red) within the molecular layer (ML) suggest targeting of a limited number of neurons. Such differences in the topography of projections may explain some of the behavioural effects of ANG (see text).

The latter arrangement may be necessary for mediation of regulation during specific learning behaviors while the former is more suitable for regulation during behavioral "states" such as running, enriched sensory experience or sensory deprivation. In principle, this differentiation between generalized and localized regulation by GABA and glutamate respectively, may help to explain discrepancies among various studies involving regulation of ANG at different stages and involving behavioral tasks mediated by only some hippocampal regions.

Age-dependent Regulation of ANG

Rate of ANG declines with an animal's age and is often associated with cognitive decline. However, this decline should be seen in the context of all other age-associated changes in the neuronal circuitry of the DG. In fact, the DG has been identified as one of the most age-sensitive regions of the hippocampus in terms of afferent inputs, synaptic strength, cell activity, blood flow and synaptic plasticity (Barnes, 1994; Small *et al.*, 2004; Burke and Barnes, 2010). Since ANG is closely regulated by activity within the hippocampal neuronal circuit, it is not surprising that the rate of proliferation is dramatically lower as the animal ages (McDonald and Wojtowicz, 2005). Nevertheless, it has been shown that proliferation can be sharply increased in older animals by external stimuli, suggesting that some regulatory mechanisms are still functional and can be potentially recruited by behavioral or experimental manipulations. However, the conditions for complete restoration of ANG may no longer be present, presumably due to unfavorable tissue micro-environment (Kempermann and Gage, 2002; Rai *et al.*, 2007; Tan *et al.*, 2010). It is also unclear whether the retained capacity for upregulation of ANG is sufficient to make a functional difference. Thus, although the regulatory mechanisms are still present in older animals, they may not be as efficient as those taking place in younger animals.

Summary

Remarkable diversity of GABA interneurons within the DG in terms of their connectivity, responsiveness to afferent stimuli and release of peptide co-transmitters is utilized as an ANG-controlling system. This system is particularly important at earlier stages of development when glutamatergic afferents are not yet developed. Neuronal development is further shaped by the development of glutamatergic synaptic inputs, increasing strength of the synapses on dendritic spines, and growth of the dendritic tree. Superimposed on these influences are the additional effects of other transmitters and neuromodulators such as acetylcholine and serotonin (Cooper-Kuhn *et al.*, 2004; Klempin *et al.*, 2013). Thus, ANG is tied closely to activity of the hippocampal circuit, which in turn reflects the behavioral state of the animals as they interact with their environment. Importantly, regulation of ANG begins and ends with stem cells. They provide the source of proliferating progenitors that are produced in excess in young animals, but become scarce or inactive in old age. The adaptive decline of ANG with age could be at times pathological and may precede other pathological changes, such as in Alzheimer's disease, in the neuronal circuitry within the DG (Krezymon *et al.*, 2013). Early detection of such changes and their remedy may well be dependent on early interventions to ANG.

Acknowledgments

This work was supported by an operating grant from CIHR (MOP:119271) and NSERC (RGPIN 194616-11) discovery grant to JMW. We also thank Dr. Christina Merkley for helpful comments on the manuscript.

References

Armstrong C, Szabadics J, Tamas G, Soltesz I (2011) Neurogliaform cells in the molecular layer of the dentate gyrus as feed-forward GABA-ergic modulators of entorhino-hippocampal interplay. *J Comp Neurol* 519:1476–1491.

Barnes CA (1994) Normal aging: regionally specific changes in hippocampal synaptic transmission. *Trends Neurosci* 17:13–18.

Burke SN, Barnes CA (2010) Senescent synapsys and hippocampal circuit dynamics. *Trends Neurosci* 33:153–161.

Chancey JH, Adlaf EW, Sapp MC, Pugh PC, Wadiche JI, Overstreet-Wadiche LS (2013) GABA depolarization is required for experience-dependent synapse unsilencing in adult-born neurons. *J Neurosci* 33:6614–6622.

Cooper-Kuhn CM, Winkler J, Kuhn HG (2004) Decreased neurogenesis after cholinergic forebrain lesion in the adult rat. *J Neurosci Res* 77:155–165.

Dranovsky A, Picchini AM, Moadel T, Sisti AC, Yamada A, Kimura S, Leanardo ED, Hen R (2011) Experience dictates stem cell fate in the adult hippocampus. *Neuron* 70:908–923.

Drapeau E, Abrous DN (2008) Stem cell review series: role of neurogenesis in age-related memory disorders. *Aging Cell* 7:569–589.

Dupret D, Fabre A, Dobrossy MD, Pantier A, Rodriguez JJ, Lamarque S, Lemaire V, Oliet SHR, Piazza PV, Abrous DN (2007) Spatial learning depends on both the addition and removal of new hippocampal neurons. *PLoS Biology* 5:1683–1694.

Freund TF, Buzsaki G (1996) Interneurons of the hippocampus. *Hippocampus* 6:347–470.

Kempermann G (2012) New neurons for survival of the fittest. *Nat Rev Neurosci* 13:727–736.

Kempermann G, Gage FG (2002) Genetic influence on phenotypic differentiation in adult hippocampal neurogenesis. *Dev Brain Res* 134:13–21.

Kilb W, Kirischuk S, Luhman H (2013) Role of tonic GABAergic currents during pre- and early postnatal rodent development. *Front Neural Circuits* 7:139.

Klempin F, Beis D, Mosienko V, Kempermann G, Bader M, Alenina N (2013) Serotonin is required for exercise-induced adult hippocampal neurogenesis. *J Neurosci* 33:8270–8275.

Krezymon A, Richetin K, Halley H, Roybon L, Lassalle JM, Frances B, Verret L, Rampon C (2013) Modifications of hippocampam circuits and early disruption of adult neurogenesis in the Tg2576 mouse model of Alzheimer's disease. *PLoS One* 8:e76497.

Lledo PM (2011) Wiring new neurons with old circuits. In: *Neurogenesis in the Adult Brain I* (Seki T, Sawamoto K, Parent JM, Alvarez-Buylla A, ed.), pp. 371–393. Tokyo: Springer.

Markwardt SJ, Dieni CV, Wadiche JI, Overstreet-Wadiche LS (2011) Ivy/ neurogliaform interneurons coordinate activity in the neurogenic niche. *Nat Neurosci* 14:1407–1409.

McDonald HY, Wojtowicz JM (2005) Dynamics of neurogenesis in the dentate gyrus of adult rats. *Neurosci Lett* 385:70–75.

Platel JC, Bordey A (2011) Control of adult-born neuron production by converging GABA and glutamate signals. In: *Neurogenesis in the Adult Brain I* (Seki T, Sawamoto K, Parent JM, Alvarez-Buylla A, ed.), pp. 395–406. Tokyo: Springer.

Rai KS, Hattiangady B, Shetty AK (2007) Enhanced production and dendritic growth of new dentate granule cells in the middle-aged hippocampus folowing intracerebroventricular FGF-2 infusions. *Eur J Neurosci* 26:1765–1779.

Small SA, Chawla MK, Buonocore M, Rapp PR, Barnes CA (2004) Imaging correlates of brain function in monkeys and rats isolates a hippocampal subregion differentially. *Proc Natl Acad Sci USA* 101:7181–7186.

Song J, Sun J, Moss J, Wen Z, Sun GJ, Hsu D, Zhong C, Davoudi H, Christian KM, Toni N, Ming G-L, Song H (2013) Parvalbumin interneurons mediate neuronal circuitry-neurogenesis coupling in the adult hippocampus. *Nat Neurosci* 16:1728–1732.

Song J, Zhong C, Bonaguidi MA, Sun GJ, Hsu D, Gu Y, Meletis K, Huang ZJ, Ge S, Enikolopov G, Deisseroth K, Luscher B, Christian M, Ming GI (2012) Neuronal circuitry mechanism regulating adult quiescent neural stem-cell fate decision. *Nature* 489:150–154.

Tan YF, Preston E, Wojtowicz JM (2010) Enhanced postischemic neurogenesis in aging rats. *Front Neurosci* 4:pii, 163.

Tronel S, Fabre A, Charrier V, Oliet SHR, Gage FH, Abrous DN (2010) Spatial learning sculpts the dendritic arbor of adult hippocampal neurons. *Proc Natl Acad Sci USA* 107:7963–7968.

Whissell PD, Rosenzweig S, Lecker I, Wang DS, Wojtowicz JM, Orser BA (2013) γ-aminobutyric acid type A receptors that contain the δ subunit promote memory and neurogenesis in the dentate gyrus. *Ann Neurol* 74:611–621.

Winocur G, Wojtowicz JM, Huang J, Tannock IF (2014) Physical exercise prevents suppression of hippocampal neurogenesis and reduces cognitive impairment in chemotherapy-treated rats. *Psychopharmacology* 231:2311–2320.

Chapter 2

Age-Related Changes to the Subventricular Zone Stem Cell Niche

Matthew B. Eastman, Rebecca L. Acabchuk, and Joanne C. Conover

Along the lateral walls of the lateral ventricles of the adult rodent brain lies a stem cell niche capable of an array of regenerative and reparative functions that persist throughout adulthood. In humans, this same region shows robust neurogenesis in neonatal development; however, in contrast to rodents, little to no neurogenesis is detected in adulthood and it is unclear whether stem cells persist and can be prompted to support regenerative repair following injury or disease. Here, we compare and contrast the molecular and cellular characteristics of the rodent and human subventricular stem cell niche with a particular focus on changes that occur during the process of aging. We also address the potential to exploit the adult human stem cell niche for therapeutic ends, while acknowledging the obstacles and limitations that currently exist.

Introduction

The subventricular zone (SVZ) stem cell niche is generally defined as the assembly of cells that lies subjacent to the ependymal cell monolayer that lines the lateral wall of the lateral ventricles (also frequently referred to as the subependymal zone) (Doetsch, 2003; Mirzadeh *et al.*, 2008; Shen *et al.*, 2008; Tavazoie *et al.*, 2008). It is one of two major stem cell niches associated with the adult brain, the other being the dentate gyrus of the hippocampus (see Chapter 1). The cellular composition and organization of the rodent SVZ stem cell niche has been described in detail, and the stem cells associated with the SVZ niche are characterized as neural stem cells due to their ability to support adult neurogenesis (Luskin, 1993; Doetsch and Alvarez-Buylla, 1996; Doetsch *et al.*, 1997; Wichterle *et al.*, 1997; Doetsch *et al.*, 1999b). Specifically, the SVZ stem cell niche allows regenerative replacement of GABAergic interneuron populations of the granule and periglomerular layers of the olfactory bulb in rodents. While SVZ neurogenesis in the rodent brain was found to continue throughout adulthood, albeit at reduced levels in advanced age (Maslov *et al.*, 2004; Luo *et al.*, 2006; Bouab *et al.*, 2011; Capilla-Gonzalez *et al.*, 2014a; Capilla-Gonzalez *et al.*, 2014b), studies have revealed that following injury SVZ stem cells possess regenerative functions that include generation of new oligodendrocytes, ependymal cells and new neurons capable of migrating to sites of injury (Wiltrout *et al.*, 2007; Conover and Notti, 2008; Luo *et al.*, 2008; Conover and Shook, 2011; Shook *et al.*, 2012; Maki *et al.*, 2013). In contrast, studies of the human SVZ revealed that little if any neurogenesis continues in the adult brain (Quinones-Hinojosa *et al.*, 2006; Sanai *et al.*, 2007; Sanai *et al.*, 2011; Wang *et al.*, 2011). However, activation of stem cells in the SVZ region following injury has been suggested (Macas *et al.*, 2006; Curtis *et al.*, 2007), opening the possibility for stem cell function in multiple injury situations. Ultimately, questions remain: to what extent do quiescent stem cells persist in the human SVZ, how and when are quiescent stem cells activated, and what is their regenerative capacity? In this chapter we will discuss how the SVZ stem cell niche changes with age in mice and in humans, the effect aging has on stem cell behavior, the molecular mechanisms required for stem cell niche maintenance through aging and how SVZ functions are implicated in diseases often associated with aging. While much of the analysis of the SVZ in aging will be based on mouse studies, analysis of the human SVZ, its reduced neurogenic capacity, and the consequence this imposes on the aging brain will also be discussed.

SVZ Niche Changes in Development, Adulthood and Aging

Rodents

In the developing brain, the neural tube gives rise to the three primary brain vesicles that make up the nascent ventricular system. The three-vesicle stage expands further to give five-vesicles, the most anterior being the lateral ventricles of the telencephalon from which the cerebral cortex is derived. Stem cells line the ventricle surface as a neuroepithelium and early in development, their symmetric division enlarges the ventricle surface. Later stem cells, which at this stage are referred to as radial glia, undergo asymmetric division to generate neurons and then glial cells that populate the developing brain structures. Toward the end of embryonic development, the radial glia of the ventricular zone (VZ) generate an epithelial layer of ependymal cells to line the ventricles (Spassky *et al.*, 2005). These ciliated cells form a barrier between the cerebrospinal and the brain parenchyma, but also act to maintain CSF-interstitial fluid homeostasis and support interstitial solute clearance (Cserr and VanDyke, 1971; Spassky *et al.*, 2005; Del Bigio, 2010; Johanson *et al.*, 2011). Along the lateral wall of the lateral ventricles, stem cells are retained just subjacent to the ependymal cell layer and each stem cell maintains an apical process with a single cilium at the ventricle surface allowing contact with the CSF. This region under the ependyma of the lateral ventricles is referred to as the subependymal layer (or subventricular zone, SVZ, as we will refer to it here) and consists of the stem cells, transit amplifying progenitor cells (Type C cells) and neuroblasts — the stem cell niche (Doetsch *et al.*, 1997; Garcia-Verdugo *et al.*, 1998; Doetsch *et al.*, 1999b; Doetsch *et al.*, 1999a). It should be noted that a stem cell niche with associated robust neurogenesis is found only along the lateral wall of the lateral ventricle; neither the medial walls of the lateral ventricle, the third ventricle, nor the fourth ventricle support robust neurogenesis in the adult mouse (Luo *et al.*, 2006). However, it has recently been reported that hypothalamic neurogenesis via tanycytes of the third ventricle are involved in feeding/metabolic disorders and obesity in rodents (Kokoeva *et al.*, 2005; Xu *et al.*, 2005; Pierce and Xu, 2010; Lee *et al.*, 2012).

The SVZ stem cells resemble their predecessors, the radial glia, based on their apical, ventricle-contacting process and basal process that extends to underlying blood vessels. With this organization, the stem cells span the extent of the stem cell niche from ventricle surface to the blood vessels at the basal boundary of the niche (Shen *et al.*, 2008; Tavazoie *et al.*, 2008) (Figure 1A). Examination of whole mount preparations of the lateral ventricle surface reveals a unique organization of ependymal cell rosettes that have a core of stem cell processes, descriptively referred to as pinwheel structures (Mirzadeh *et al.*, 2008; Nam and Benezra, 2009). The SVZ stem cells cycle through stages of quiescence and active proliferation, generating a daughter transient amplifying Type C progenitor cell that can go through several divisions before generating neuroblasts (Doetsch *et al.*, 1997; Doetsch *et al.*, 1999b; Temple, 2001; Tramontin *et al.*, 2003; Alvarez-Buylla and Lim, 2004; Mirzadeh *et al.*, 2008; Tavazoie *et al.*, 2008). These newly generated neuroblasts (approximately 30,000/day) migrate along a very discrete pathway, the rostral migratory stream (RMS), to the olfactory bulb, directed in large part

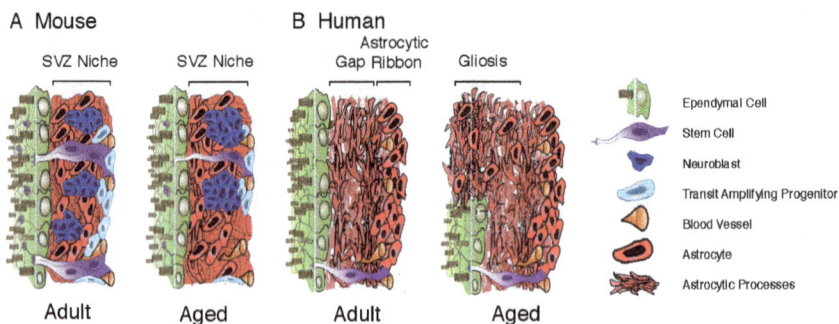

Figure 1. Schematic representations show the cytoarchitectural organization of the mouse (A) and human (B) SVZ stem cell niche in young adult and aged adult tissue.

by astrocytes that form glial tubes through which the neuroblasts migrate. These glial tubes are thought to maintain the strict boundaries required en route to the olfactory bulb. In rodents, SVZ stem cells are retained throughout adulthood and neurogenesis is supported throughout the course of aging (Tropepe *et al.*, 1997; Doetsch *et al.*, 1999b; Jin *et al.*, 2003; Enwere *et al.*, 2004; Maslov *et al.*, 2004; Luo *et al.*, 2006; Luo *et al.*, 2008; Ahlenius *et al.*, 2009; Conover and Shook, 2011; Shook *et al.*, 2012). However, with increasing age, the SVZ stem cell niche becomes attenuated and SVZ neurogenesis declines, as does the number of new neuroblasts that reach the olfactory bulb (see below, **Aging's Effect on SVZ Stem Cell Numbers and Neurogenesis**). However, the capacity for neuroblasts to migrate along the RMS does not appear to be affected by age (Mobley *et al.*, 2013) and while fewer neuroblasts are generated, all the different subtypes of GABAergic interneurons are still produced in old age in the same relative proportions as in young mice.

Humans

The human fetal forebrain VZ is similar in organization to the rodent, with one important exception, the developing human forebrain has an additional proliferative stem cell layer subjacent to the VZ that lacks ventricle and CSF contact and resides as a separate, internal zone, termed the outer SVZ (oSVZ) (Hansen *et al.*, 2010; Betizeau *et al.*, 2013). Together, both the VZ and oSVZ stem cells contribute to the development of the cerebral cortex with the oSVZ providing an additional population of neuronal progenitors that give rise to the substantially increased numbers of neurons that make up the folds (gyri and sulci) associated with the human cerebral cortex, a key characteristic of the human and non-human primate brain. Since the oSVZ layer is important for producing large numbers of new neurons found in the human (and non-human primate) cortex, it is not surprising that rodents lacking an oSVZ have a smooth cerebral cortex surface that lacks sulci and gyri.

In early fetal development, the VZ has direct contact with the CSF; however, during the first and second trimester, ependymal cell differentiation begins and a layer of ependymal cells is generated to cover the ventricle surface (McAllister, 2012), replacing the VZ cells and ultimately signaling the winding down of cortical neurogenesis. While some stem cells maintain ventricle contact through an apical process that projects through the ependymal cells, leaving the cell body just below the ependymal cell monolayer, by 2 years of age SVZ and VZ stem cell contributions to neurogenesis declines and newly generated neuroblasts are rarely detected along the lateral ventricles (Quinones-Hinojosa *et al.*, 2006; Sanai *et al.*, 2011; Wang *et al.*, 2011). Neuroblasts that are generated in early postnatal development migrate either along the RMS to the olfactory bulb or along an additional migratory pathway (medial migratory stream, MMS) to the prefrontal cortex. The MMS appears to be depleted of cells expressing markers of immature neurons by 8 months (Sanai *et al.*, 2011). By 18 months, the SVZ and RMS are both greatly depleted of neuroblasts (Sanai *et al.*, 2004; Sanai *et al.*, 2011; Wang *et al.*, 2011). While there seems to be consensus that SVZ neurogenesis does not continue into adulthood in humans, at least at the robust level found in rodents; it is unclear to what extent stem cells are retained along the ventricles and contribute to neurogenesis and other regenerative or reparative functions following injury.

The absence of neurogenesis along the lateral ventricles in humans is visibly revealed in the organization of the adult human SVZ compared to the rodent (compare Figure 1A and B). In humans, the ependymal cell lining is bordered by an acellular zone of astrocytic processes that project from a band of astrocytes, referred to as the 'astrocyte ribbon' (Sanai *et al.*, 2004; Zecevic, 2004; Guerrero-Cazares *et al.*, 2011). This organization is thought to be the result of the loss of neuroblasts that would typically migrate through a dense array of astrocytes that form the glial tubes. The glial tubes or at least the processes of astrocytes that made up the tubes remain, but the areas where the neuroblasts had once migrated are devoid of cell bodies leaving an acellular zone. Why astrocytes remain clustered as an 'astrocyte ribbon' is not clear, especially since astrocytes in the brain parenchyma tend to 'tile' and do not typically cluster together, except in the cases of injury or lesion where a glial scar forms (Sofroniew, 2009). Ultimately, the lack of neurogenesis along the lateral ventricles in adult humans and the contrasting robust neurogenesis that exists in rodents highlights the need for a better understanding of the key characteristics required to maintain an adult neurogenic stem cell niche in the brain. In the next section, we will focus on how the rodent (mouse) lateral ventricle stem cell numbers and neurogenesis change with aging.

Aging's Effect on SVZ Stem Cell Numbers and Neurogenesis

In rodents, neurogenesis serves the primary function of supplying the olfactory bulb with newly generated GABAergic interneurons that populate either the granule cell or periglomerular layers of the olfactory bulb. Interneurons of the granule layer are subdivided into deep, superficial or calretinin-expressing interneurons, whereas interneurons of the periglomerular layer are subdivided into calretinin-, calbindin- or tyrosine hydroxylase-expressing interneurons (Price and Powell, 1970; Kosaka *et al.*, 1995; Lledo *et al.*, 2008). Several groups have reported a diminution of the SVZ in aged mice (20–24 months old) with the total number of proliferating cells in the niche reduced by 50–75% (Tropepe *et al.*, 1997; Doetsch *et al.*, 1999; Jin *et al.*, 2003; Enwere *et al.*, 2004; Maslov *et al.*, 2004; Luo *et al.*, 2006; Ahlenius *et al.*, 2009; Shook *et al.*, 2012). Similarly, a 75% reduction in the number of thymidine analog label-retaining neuroblasts that reach the olfactory bulb has been reported. This reduction in new neurons for the olfactory bulb was suggested to result from a functional decline in fine odor discrimination (Tropepe *et al.*, 1997; Enwere *et al.*, 2004; Lledo and Saghatelyan, 2005). However, Moreno *et al.* (Moreno *et al.*, 2014) provided data that suggests that a specific impairment of perceptual learning and not basic discrimination ability occurs in aging. This is supported by the perseveration of the olfactory network (number of cells and synapses) (Richard *et al.*, 2010) despite the drastic reduction in the level of neurogenesis (Mandairon and Didier, 2010; Richard *et al.*, 2010; Rey *et al.*, 2012). In other words, it was found that odor enrichment did not increase neurogenesis in old mice as it does in young adult mice, and this might contribute to an inability to perform olfactory perceptual learning. Interestingly, increasing noradrenergic release can restore this deficit in old mice.

Examination of cell proliferation solely in the SVZ is not an adequate means to measure stem cell numbers, as stem cells are typically quiescent with only approximately 2.5% dividing at any one particular time (Shook *et al.*, 2012). Accurate assessment of changes in stem cell numbers has been difficult due to the lack of stem cell-specific markers. One technique to address stem cell changes over the course of aging is to take advantage of morphological characteristics of SVZ stem cells in combination with cell-specific markers. SVZ stem cells are positive for GFAP (Doetsch *et al.*, 1999b; Maslov *et al.*, 2004) and they possess an apical process that contacts the ventricle surface. Using whole mount preparations of the lateral ventricle walls, the stem cell populations can be identified based on the presence of a GFAP-positive apical process extending through the ependymal cell layer and the presence of a basal body that anchors the single primary cilium. Thus, by using both the cytoarchitectural organization of stem cells at the ventricle lining, as well as their cellular identity as GFAP-positive astrocytes that are still in the cell cycle, it was found that a steady decline in stem cell number occurs with age, with an 86% decline in total stem cells/mm² of ependyma in 2-year-old versus 3-month-old mice (Shook *et al.*, 2012). The largest declines are seen between 6 months and 1 year (Luo *et al.*, 2006), indicating a relatively early start for stem cell loss (Luo *et al.*, 2006; Shook *et al.*, 2012) (Figure 1A). Fewer stem cell processes were found within each pinwheel structure with an associated reduction of 78% in total pinwheel units/mm². Regional analysis revealed that loss of stem cells and pinwheels was spatially uniform with no one particular region being either adversely or beneficially affected, and the ratio of olfactory bulb interneuron subtypes was conserved in aged animals (Shook *et al.*, 2012). This is of particular interest since different regions of the SVZ differentially pattern resident stem cells for generation of each of the six unique interneuron subtypes (Hack *et al.*, 2005; Kohwi *et al.*, 2005; Merkle *et al.*, 2007; Ihrie and Alvarez-Buylla, 2011; Ihrie *et al.*, 2011).

Surprisingly, while overall neurogenic output of the aged SVZ is reduced, no significant change in the number of actively proliferating stem cells/mm^2 of ventricle surface is detected. Instead, actively mitotic stem cells found within the SVZ increased from 2.5% to 17% of the total stem cell population over the course of aging (3 months to 2 years) (Stoll *et al.*, 2011; Shook *et al.*, 2012). Because aged mice maintain a proliferative SVZ stem cell population, the decline in SVZ neurogenesis must then be attributed to factors acting downstream of stem cell activation (Shook *et al.*, 2012). Jin *et al.* (Jin *et al.*, 2003) demonstrated that after infusion of FGF or EGF, the level of total proliferation (neurogenesis) in the aged SVZ was comparable to young adults, and aged stem cells isolated using a nestin-GFP mouse can generate the same number of neurospheres as young stem cells (Ahlenius *et al.*, 2009). These data suggest that the aged stem cell niche maintains the same proliferative potential as the young niche, but a decline in available growth factors or other niche-associated factors likely contribute to the diminished neurogenic potential. Thus, the loss of neurogenic capacity appears to result from events downstream of stem cell activation, perhaps at the level of the transit amplifying progenitor population, Type C cells. Alternatively, neuroblasts may not go through as many rounds of division in the aged versus the young adult SVZ.

It remains to be determined by which mechanism the aged SVZ increases the number of stem cells that are activated versus those that remain quiescent. One possibility may depend on the unique fractone network within the SVZ (Mercier *et al.*, 2002; Kerever *et al.*, 2007; Shen *et al.*, 2008; Kerever *et al.*, 2014) (see below, **Extracellular Matrix and Signaling Mechanisms Affecting SVZ Functions**). In addition, a negative feedback loop between stem cells and their immediate progeny, Type C cells, has been shown to inhibit stem cell proliferation (Aguirre *et al.*, 2010). This feedback loop, functioning through the interaction of Notch and EGF receptor pathways, has been shown to maintain the balance between stem cells and progeny numbers in the young adult mouse. Based on the reduced number of Type C cells in aged mice (Luo *et al.*, 2006), increased stem cell activation may result. Additional investigations are required to determine the mechanisms controlling increased stem cell activation in the aged SVZ.

In summary, with increased age, total stem cell numbers decline in a spatially uniform manner across the entire ventricle surface in mice. This results in regional subpopulations of stem cells being equally affected and as a consequence the aged SVZ generates the same ratio of OB interneurons, albeit in reduced numbers. However, the aged SVZ maintains the same number of mitotically active stem cells as the young adult when dividing stem cells are normalized to the total number of stem cells; this results in an age-related increase in the percentage of proliferative stem cells to quiescent cells. Therefore, declines in neurogenesis appear to be the result of factors acting downstream of stem cell activation.

Extracellular Matrix and Signaling Mechanisms Affecting SVZ Functions

Signaling between adult stem cells and their surrounding environment is an important component for the regulation of proliferation, cell fate choice and appropriate migration [reviewed in (Scadden, 2006)]. Because of the importance of the stem cell niche to stem cell activity, the origin of observed age-related differences in stem cell behavior may be broadly categorized as cell-intrinsic (cell-autonomous) or cell-extrinsic (i.e., brought about by changes in the surrounding environment). Intrinsic changes due to aging are those that occur at the level of an individual stem cell and are thought to contribute to stem cell senescence, depletion of the progenitor pool and a decline in neurogenesis (Ferron *et al.*, 2009). Cell-intrinsic changes such as the 'Hayflick limit,' which puts a cap on the number of cell divisions (Hayflick and Moorhead, 1961), are usually considered independent of the external environment and are a property of the biology of an individual cell.

External factors, such as changes in environmental factors or signaling between cells via secreted soluble or cell surface factors can influence cell behaviors, such as proliferation, quiescence, and migration. However, extracellular factors rely on intracellular signaling for their effects on proliferation, and these simplified categories are not mutually exclusive and observed changes in adult stem cell behavior are likely the result of a combination of both intrinsic and extrinsic factors (Figure 2). In this section, we will focus on recently described age-related changes that affect neural stem cell proliferation within the rodent SVZ stem cell niche from a cell-signaling perspective.

Fractones and growth factors

The extracellular matrix (ECM) provides the three-dimensional scaffold in which the adult stem cells interact with both their supporting structures and their regulatory factors [reviewed in (Scadden, 2006)]. ECM components can have a direct effect on multiple adult stem cell functions; for example, laminin-integrin adhesions can regulate proliferation and promote migration (Emsley and Hagg, 2003). To achieve these types of direct interactions (e.g., proliferation, symmetric/asymmetric division choices, migration) the ECM proteins are known to bind and sequester soluble regulatory factors, such as those from the systemic circulation, thereby creating local concentrations of signaling molecules specific to the stem cell niche (Kerever *et al.*, 2007; Douet *et al.*, 2013).

An intimate association of stem cells within the SVZ with underlying blood vessels and perivascular structures also exists (Mercier *et al.*, 2002; Shen *et al.*, 2008) and allows for regulation of adult neurogenesis by the vasculature, which has been shown to impact neural stem cell function through factors that increase self-renewal and proliferation (Shen *et al.*, 2008). Adult stem cells in the SVZ lie adjacent to a unique vascular niche that is largely devoid of both the pericyte coverage and astrocytic end-feet that make up the blood-brain barrier found throughout the rest of the brain (Tavazoie *et al.*, 2008). Specialized structures called fractones are projections of the blood vessel basal lamina. They consist of laminins, collagens, and proteoglycans that contact every cell type in the region due to an intricate branching morphology that is much different from the flat, sheet-like basal lamina of other epithelial tissues (Mercier *et al.*, 2002). Named for their branching structure resembling fractals, fractones

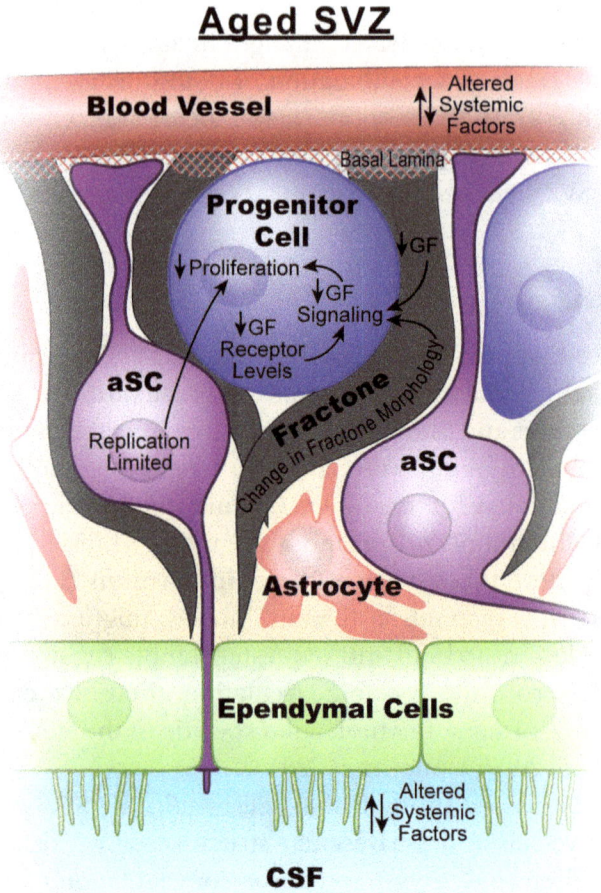

Figure 2. Age-related changes in intrinsic and extrinsic factors on progenitor cell proliferation in the SVZ. Decreased levels of proliferation in the aged SVZ can be brought about by a combination of intrinsic and extrinsic factors. Adult stem cells may undergo only a limited number of divisions throughout their lifetime. Changes in the extracellular environment, such as an increase in neurogenesis-inhibiting systemic factors and decreased levels of growth factors and their receptors, may lead to decreased progenitor cell proliferation. Fractones, extensions of the blood vessel basal lamina unique to the SVZ and reported to sequester and activate growth factors, undergo morphological changes with age that may contribute to reductions in growth factor signaling.

have been implicated in binding regulatory factors, thereby creating local microenvironments of growth factor concentrations in proximity to the stem cells of the SVZ (Mercier *et al.*, 2002; Kerever *et al.*, 2007; Douet *et al.*, 2013; Kerever *et al.*, 2014). Morphological changes to fractones have been observed with aging, with fractones in aged tissue described as larger and more penetrative within the SVZ when examined by electron microscopy (Capilla-Gonzalez *et al.*, 2014). Fractone morphology within the aged mouse SVZ, visualized as laminin-immunoreactive puncta in lateral ventricle whole mount preparations, shifts to less well defined, more diffusely immunoreactive, larger puncta through aging (Figure 2). It is unknown whether these changes in ECM fractones precede age-associated declines in neurogenesis, but experimental disruption of fractones with infused heparatinase has been shown to impair neurogenesis by reducing growth factor signaling in young mice (Mercier *et al.*, 2002; Kerever *et al.*, 2007; Douet *et al.*, 2013; Kerever *et al.*, 2014). Additionally, changes in fractone morphology similar to those observed in aging have been reported in experiments which reduce SVZ proliferation via irradiation or DNA mutagens (Achanta *et al.*, 2012; Capilla-Gonzalez *et al.*, 2012; Capilla-Gonzalez *et al.*, 2014a), and these studies postulate that observed changes in fractone morphology may be in response to decreased proliferation within the region. Therefore, structural changes to the specialized ECM can have a severe impact on cell proliferation by disrupting growth factor signaling important for neurogenesis within the region.

Declines in growth factor signaling within the aged SVZ have been linked to decreased proliferation of neural progenitor cells. Specifically, diminished levels of epidermal growth factor receptor (EGFR) signaling within the aged SVZ have been linked to declines in fine olfactory discrimination tasks, and declines in EGFR ligand, transforming growth factor alpha (TGFα), together with decreased EGFR have been described to contribute to impaired SVZ neurogenesis in the aged mouse brain (Enwere *et al.*, 2004), which can decrease by as much as 75% (Enwere *et al.*, 2004; Luo *et al.*, 2006). Infusion of EGF into the lateral ventricles of aged mice resulted in only a modest increase in proliferating cells, compared to infusion in a young adult mouse, indicating a compromised ability of the aged adult neural progenitor cell population (including neural stem cells and transient amplifying progenitors) to respond to EGF signaling (Enwere *et al.*, 2004). However, reduced EGFR signaling did not diminish the overall regenerative capacity of the aged SVZ in response to experimental stem cell depletion, indicating that the aged SVZ retains the ability to replenish the stem cell niche to age-typical functional levels after insult, even though EGFR signaling is reduced (Enwere *et al.*, 2004). The effect of EGFR signaling on neurogenesis in the SVZ is at least partially mediated by the mammalian target of rapamycin (mTOR) pathway. mTORC1 activity is reduced in the aged SVZ and thought to contribute to the decline of the transitory amplifying cell pool, and interference of mTOR signaling by infusion of rapamycin causes a dramatic decline in proliferating cells (Paliouras *et al.*, 2012). While infusion of EGF into the lateral ventricles of aged mice can increase proliferation, this increase is blocked by co-infusion with rapamycin, suggesting that EGF promotes neurogenesis in an mTORC1-dependent manner (Paliouras *et al.*, 2012). Declining levels of EGF and mTOR signaling in the aged brain can therefore be implicated in the decline in SVZ neurogenesis.

Expression of fibroblast growth factor receptor 2 (FGFR-2) has been associated with GFAP-positive cells in the adult neurogenic regions, which includes the adult stem cells, and has been shown to decline in the SVZ of aged mice (Chadashvili and Peterson, 2006). Additionally, fibroblast growth factor 2 (FGF-2) has been shown to co-localize with fractones, extensions of the blood vessel basal lamina that associate intimately with the SVZ stem cell niche and may be required for growth factor activation of stem cells (Douet *et al.*, 2013). If fractone density is diminished or morphology disrupted in aging, the reduced activation by FGF-2 may be partially responsible for diminished neurogenesis in aging. Even though the number of neural progenitor cells is diminished in aged mice, infusion of FGF-2 into the aged SVZ can restore neurogenesis to youthful levels, as measured by BrdU label retention, while infusion of FGF-2 in young adult mice results in only a modest increase in proliferation (Jin *et al.*, 2003). Taken together, these results indicate that the response of the aged SVZ to FGF-2-mediated signaling is enhanced compared to young animals. Such increased sensitivity to FGF-2 could partially mediate the increased level of proliferation reported specifically in the adult stem cell population in aging (Shook *et al.*, 2012), even when the proliferation of the overall neural progenitor cell population in the aged SVZ is decreased.

Vascular endothelial growth factor (VEGF) family signaling is also implicated in the regulation of neurogenesis in the SVZ. Specifically, VEGF receptor 3 (VEGFR-3) has been detected on stem cells and is activated by ligand VEGF-C to promote neurogenesis, independent of angiogenesis (Calvo *et al.*, 2011). Overexpression of VEGF in the SVZ increased the number of BrdU+ neuroblasts in young animals, but the effect was severely diminished in aged mice, indicating that the ability to respond to neurogenic VEGF signaling is compromised in the aged SVZ (Gao *et al.*, 2009).

Taken together, examination of growth factor signaling indicates that there is a dramatic decrease in the ability of the stem cell population to respond to neurogenesis-promoting signals from growth factors such as EGFs, FGFs, and VEGFs, possibly due to declining receptor numbers and changes in ECM fractones that can concentrate and activate these factors. There is some ability of the remaining neural progenitors to respond to proliferative signals, and, in the case of FGF-2, the population of adult neural progenitor cells can respond with a proportionally greater increase in proliferation than young adult neural progenitors, and can even attain the level of BrdU+ cells seen in untreated young-adult animals (Jin *et al.*, 2003). Such changes in signaling responses may help to explain the relative increase in activation seen in the adult stem cell population that occurs with increased age (Shook *et al.*, 2012).

Systemic factors

Declines in the neurogenic output of the SVZ parallel the loss of regenerative potential seen in other adult stem cell niches, specifically epithelial tissues such as skin [reviewed in (Mimeault and Batra, 2010)] and intestine [reviewed in (Liu and Rando, 2011)], indicating that there is some degree of global regenerative impairment with aging. Such a global decline in overall progenitor cell proliferation may be mediated in part by changes in systemic factors in aging, as has been described for the muscle satellite stem cell niche (Carlson *et al.*, 2009). Similar investigations into systemic contribution to neurogenic decline with age have utilized heterochronic transplantation paradigms to demonstrate the effect of aged sera on postnatal neurogenesis. These studies show impairment of neurogenesis in the presence of aged sera, but have largely concentrated on the neurogenic subgranular zone of the hippocampal dentate gyrus (Villeda *et al.*, 2011). However, because of the SVZ's close association with blood vessels and unique perivascular cytoarchitecture, changes in systemic circulation most likely contribute to the impairment of neurogenesis seen in the SVZ as well. The combination of reduced growth factors from the systemic circulation, combined with the changed fractone morphology observed in the aged SVZ, could severely compromise the neurogenesis-promoting effects of growth factors in the region. Systemic perturbations due to aging brought about by global declines in endocrine function, such as decreased gonadotropin releasing hormone (GnRH) signaling, can bring about deleterious changes within an organism, including impairment of neurogenesis through changes in global immunity and neuroendocrine function regulated by hypothalamic GnRH signaling (Zhang *et al.*, 2013).

Systemic factors are only a part of extrinsic regulation of adult neurogenesis, and it is important to note that systemic changes may not be completely decoupled from local changes in growth factor levels within the stem cell niche, and are divided here simply for ease of presentation. Altered levels of growth factors and growth factor receptors in the aged SVZ alone do not tell the entire story of the decline adult neurogenesis in the aged brain, and structural changes to the ECM such as altered fractone structure and signal activation mechanisms need further investigation. Diminished levels of growth factor receptors may simply be a consequence of declining stem cell and progenitor cell numbers, and the inability of exogenous growth factor infusion to restore neurogenesis to youthful levels may be a consequence of these lower numbers or changes in the ability of these cells to respond to growth factors. It is surprising that the aged SVZ is able to maintain a similar number of actively proliferating adult neural stem cells as a young animal, and there is an increase in the relative proportion of proliferating adult stem cells in the aging brain (Shook *et al.*, 2012). Growth factor signaling may have differential effects with age on different types of adult neural progenitor cells, including stem cells, transient amplifying progenitor cells, and neuroblasts. Still, reports have demonstrated that the aged SVZ is at least partially responsive to infusion of many growth factors, indicating that age-related observations in neurogenesis are at least in part due to changes in the aged extracellular signaling environment SVZ.

SVZ Reparative Functions in Injury and Disease

The discovery of neurogenesis in the adult brain has generated excitement that the innate capacity of the SVZ may be used to treat neurologic disorders. However, the extent of the regenerative and reparative capacity of the human SVZ is still under investigation and while many studies, using both human tissue analysis and mouse models of disease, link alterations in SVZ functions to specific diseases, the significance of these findings remain mainly unresolved and often controversial. Below we review current studies that examine SVZ alterations in injury and disease, comparing results from both rodents and humans. We pay special attention to the role of the SVZ in age-related, idiopathic expansion of the lateral ventricle volume (ventriculomegaly), which would impact the integrity of the SVZ niche.

Stroke

Ischemic stroke causes hypoxic conditions and is known to result in increased neurogenesis in the SVZ of mice. Experimental rodent models of global and focal ischemia demonstrate increased levels of neural progenitor cell proliferation in the SVZ and migration of neuroblasts to the site of injury (Arvidsson *et al.*, 2002; Wiltrout *et al.*,

2007). This migration occurs in tandem with angiogenesis and vascular remodeling, suggesting that blood vessels provide a scaffold for neuroblast migration (Ohab *et al.*, 2006). However, it is not only neuroblasts that migrate out of the SVZ in response to injury, but also GFAP-positive astrocytes. It has been reported that the predominant SVZ response to focal cerebral ischemia is this glial response, with neuroblasts making up only a small percentage of the responding cells (Li *et al.*, 2010). The presence of SVZ cells at the site of injury combined with the lack of evidence for newly integrated neurons suggests that the role of SVZ cell migration is to provide a supportive rather than a regenerative role in injury conditions. Indeed, SVZ-derived neuroblasts appear to assist in the survival of neurons adjacent to the lesion by exerting neurotrophic effects (Sabelstrom *et al.*, 2013). For instance, SVZ neural progenitors have been found to protect nearby striatal neurons from glutamatergic excitotoxicity by releasing endogenous endocannabinoids (Butti *et al.*, 2012) and additional non-neuronal functions might also include phagocytosis (Jin *et al.*, 2010; Sun *et al.*, 2013). Experimentally induced ischemic stroke also appears to affect the cells of the SVZ niche, as ciliary dysfunction in ependymal cells and reactive astrocytosis have been observed (Young *et al.*, 2013).

While animal models of stroke clearly indicate activation of SVZ-derived 'repair' mechanisms, it is more difficult to assess the effect of stroke on the human SVZ. Doublecortin-positive cells have been identified in surgically resected tissue following primary intracerebral hemorrhage (Jin *et al.*, 2006) and while the morphology of these cells resembles migrating neuroblasts, the site of origin of these cells, their capacity for long-term survival, and their functional integration within the disrupted circuits have yet to be validated.

Multiple sclerosis

Demyelinating lesions associated with multiple sclerosis (MS) are caused by loss of oligodendrocytes, the axon myelinating cells of the CNS. Newly generated cells from the SVZ are thought to contribute to the regeneration of oligodendrocytes in nearby demyelinated lesions. Several studies using rodent models of MS support this claim, demonstrating increased proliferation in the SVZ and newly generated cells migrating to the site of the lesion to replace lost oligodendrocytes (Picard-Riera *et al.*, 2002; Maki *et al.*, 2013). Green fluorescent protein (GFP) retrovirus labeling has shown that SVZ-derived oligodendrocyte progenitor cells (OPCs) re-directed migration to the site of the lesion and established synaptic contacts with axons (Etxeberria *et al.*, 2010). However, another investigation using longitudinal bioluminescence imaging found that while SVZ proliferation did increase in response to the demyelinating insult, no SVZ neuroblasts or OPCs migrated to the site of the lesion (Guglielmetti *et al.*, 2014). The reason for conflicting reports is unclear, but consensus may be complicated by the types of model used, variations in inflammatory responses, or other reasons yet to be identified. In particular, inflammation, which plays a central role in MS, may interfere with repair mechanisms. Inhibition of microglia activation in a mouse model of MS increased the number of OPCs originating from the SVZ and their differentiation into mature oligodendrocytes (Rasmussen *et al.*, 2011). While additional studies are required to confirm the potential of SVZ stem cells to contribute to oligodendrogenesis in MS mouse models, therapeutic strategies such as erythropoietin (EPO) treatment are currently being evaluated as potential methods to increase SVZ-derived oligodendrogenesis (Kaneko *et al.*, 2013).

Studies using human post-mortem tissue have investigated changes in the cellular composition of the SVZ in MS patients. An increased width of the SVZ hypocelluar gap region has been attributed to reactivation of SVZ stem cells and increased numbers of proliferating progenitor cells in response to demyelination (Nait-Oumesmar *et al.*, 2008). However, SVZ stem cells can also differentiate into astrocytes (Benner, 2013). Therefore, increased proliferation in this region could be due to reactive gliosis rather than oligodendrogenesis. Reactive gliosis can be found throughout demyelinating lesions in MS as astrocytes play a critical role in forming glial scars and regulating inflammation, oxidative stress, blood brain barrier repair and controlling vasogenic edema. Distinguishing between reactive gliosis, neurogenesis and oligodendrogenesis in proliferation studies will contribute to a better understanding of the contribution of endogenous SVZ-mediated repair in MS.

Other neurodegenerative diseases

It is still unclear if the SVZ stem cell niche responds to or contributes to neurodegenerative pathologies in diseases often associated with aging, such as Parkinson disease, Huntington's disease, amyotrophic lateral sclerosis, and Alzheimer's disease. Several animal models of Parkinson disease have shown reduced precursor proliferation in the SVZ due to loss of dopaminergic input (Lennington *et al.*, 2011; Freundlieb *et al.*, 2006; Baker *et al.*, 2004; Winner *et al.*, 2004, 2008b). However, while previous research found a reduction in SVZ proliferation in humans with Parkinson disease (Hoglinger *et al.*, 2004), more recent findings conclude that dopamine depletion likely has no effect in the human SVZ (van den Berge *et al.*, 2011). Several rodent studies are aimed at utilizing the SVZ for regenerative repair by stimulating SVZ stem cells to produce dopaminergic neurons for the striatum [reviewed in (Geraerts *et al.*, 2007)]. A recent study was able to generate SVZ-derived striatal neurogenesis in a Parkinsonian rodent model by reducing intrinsic inhibitory signals in the SVZ microenvironment (Jing *et al.*, 2012). While these studies provide inspiration for future therapeutic treatment, much work is still needed prior to transitioning to application in humans.

The role of the SVZ in amyotrophic lateral sclerosis and Alzheimer's disease is inconclusive in both mouse and human, with some studies finding increased activation of neuroblast production (Shan *et al.*, 2006; Galan *et al.*, 2011; Rodriguez and Verkhratsky, 2011), and others finding reduced levels (Liu and Martin, 2006). Similarly, while SVZ proliferation and differentiation was not found to be altered a mouse model of Huntington's disease (Phillips *et al.*, 2005; Simpson *et al.*, 2011), studies on human tissue with Huntington's disease have found both increased (Curtis *et al.*, 2003) and decreased neurogenesis (Ernst *et al.*, 2014). Similar to findings in stroke models, mouse models of traumatic brain injury show limited numbers of neuroblasts migrating from the ipsilateral SVZ to the site of injury using a cortical impact model (Ramaswamy *et al.*, 2005). While a solid link has not yet been made between SVZ functions and neuropathological decline, new studies aim to stimulate SVZ and hippocampus neurogenesis in rodent models of Alzheimer's disease and Parkinson disease with the hope of recruiting the brain's endogenous mechanisms of self-repair (Geraerts *et al.*, 2007; Tiwari *et al.*, 2014).

Involvement of SVZ in glioblastoma

Glioblastoma, the most commonly diagnosed malignant brain tumor in adults, has garnered significant attention based on the possible relationship between glioblastoma-initiating cells and stem cells of the SVZ. Imaging studies have linked the proximity of a glioblastoma tumor to the SVZ with increased morbidity, although the exact reason for this correlation remains to be determined. In mouse models of genetically induced glioma, tumorigenic cells arise from the SVZ stem cell niche (Alcantara Llaguno *et al.*, 2009) and transplanting human glioblastoma cells into the cortex of nude mice causes SVZ cells to migrate and integrate into the resultant tumor (Najbauer *et al.*, 2012). Outcome assessments of patients with glioblastoma multiforme (GBM) found that those who received higher irradiation doses to the ipsilateral SVZ had greater overall survival rates (Gupta *et al.*, 2012; Chen *et al.*, 2013), supporting the notion that the SVZ may be the source of tumorigenic cells in GBM. However, rodent studies indicate that SVZ progenitor cells may also have potential anti-tumorigenic properties. In a mouse model of GBM using implanted tumor cells, SVZ cells migrate to the site of tumor implantation, accumulate around the tumor, and contribute to the apoptosis of the tumor cells (Glass *et al.*, 2005). The authors also noted that this anti-tumorigenic capacity of neural progenitor cells observed in rodents was diminished with age. While it is still unclear whether the SVZ contributes to tumor growth, new adjunct therapies to treat glioblastoma are being aimed at the SVZ (Kast *et al.*, 2014). Further research is critical in clarifying whether SVZ-derived progenitor cells that migrate to the site of the tumor contribute to tumor growth, or conversely, function to help contain the tumor.

Ventriculomegaly

Due to the location of the SVZ along the lateral walls of the lateral ventricles, ventricle enlargement (ventriculomegaly) as seen in normal human aging would impact the neurogenic or reparative capacity of the SVZ niche. In aged mice, regenerative stem cell-mediated repair appears to be sufficient to maintain a healthy intact ependyma throughout aging (Shook *et al.*, 2013) and aged mice do not succumb to ventriculomegaly. In humans, while the ability to utilize regenerative repair in response to ventricular enlargement and/or injury may be available in infancy, it may not be a sufficient option in aged humans (Sanai *et al.*, 2011; Wang *et al.*, 2011; Bergmann *et al.*, 2012; Shook *et al.*, 2013). Rather, inspection of aged human tissue most often reveals large expanses of ependymal cell loss replaced by astrocytic gliosis, or 'scarring' (Shook *et al.*, 2013) (Figure 1B). While ependymal cell stretching appears somewhat variable across regions, there is no evidence of cell stretching sufficient to accommodate the amount of ventricle volume expansion seen in normal human aging (Shook *et al.*, 2013). Therefore, disruption in the ependymal monolayer with replacement by glial scars appears to be the mechanism by which the ventricle lining responds to surface area expansion in ventriculomegaly. The repercussions of periventricular gliosis instead of regenerative ependymal cell repair would be significant and ultimately compromise the organization and function of the SVZ stem cell niche. In addition, there would be loss of the bidirectional transport system provided by the ependymal cells lining the ventricles (Roales-Bujan *et al.*, 2012). The ependyma provides both a barrier and transport system for cerebral spinal fluid (CSF) and interstitial fluid exchange (Del Bigio, 2010; Johanson *et al.*, 2011; Roales-Bujan *et al.*, 2012), helping to clear toxins and maintain physiologic balance (Johanson *et al.*, 2011; Roales-Bujan *et al.*, 2012). Fluid-attenuated inversion recovery MRI (FLAIR-MRI) scans of aged humans typically show ventriculomegaly with associated periventricular hyperintensities, indicative of edema (Fazekas *et al.*, 1993; Sener, 2002). Furthermore, large expanses of ependymal cell loss imply loss of motile cilia, which would reduce CSF microcurrents and ventricle surface laminar flow. While the impact of SVZ alterations that occur due to age or disease-related ventriculomegaly requires additional research, it is likely that the associated loss of ependymal cells contributes to detrimental alterations in barrier and molecular exchange mechanisms shared by the CSF and parenchyma, with potential repercussions beyond the SVZ niche.

Conclusion

Significant advances have been made in our understanding of the rodent and human SVZ stem cell niche and how it changes through aging. However, important species-specific differences exist in stem cell niche organization and neurogenic capacity between rodents and humans. Therefore, any advancement in the ability to exploit the adult human stem cell niche for therapeutic ends must take into consideration its reduced capacity for neurogenesis and also likely diminished reparative potential. While efforts to enhance the neurogenic and reparative capacity of the SVZ may provide the best way forward, current work on the human SVZ is limited by tissue availability, inherent variability among the human population based on genetics, health history, medication usage, co-morbidity, and limitations presented by the inability to adequately label and track stem cells of the human SVZ stem cell niche. Ultimately, comparative analysis using different species, as well as analysis of different organ system adult stem cell niches will provide the best understanding of the potential of this brain stem cell niche, while also acknowledging its limitations.

References

Achanta P, Capilla-Gonzalez V, Purger D, Reyes J, Sailor K, Song H, Garcia-Verdugo JM, Gonzalez-Perez O, Ford E, Quinones-Hinojosa A (2012)

Subventricular zone localized irradiation affects the generation of proliferating neural precursor cells and the migration of neuroblasts. *Stem Cells* 30:2548–2560.

Aguirre A, Rubio ME, Gallo V (2010) Notch and EGFR pathway interaction regulates neural stem cell number and self-renewal. *Nature* 467:323–327.

Ahlenius H, Visan V, Kokaia M, Lindvall O, Kokaia Z (2009) Neural stem and progenitor cells retain their potential for proliferation and differentiation into functional neurons despite lower number in aged brain. *J Neurosci* 29:4408–4419.

Alcantara Llaguno S, Chen J, Kwon CH, Jackson EL, Li Y, Burns DK, Alvarez-Buylla A, Parada LF (2009) Malignant astrocytomas originate from neural stem/progenitor cells in a somatic tumor suppressor mouse model. *Cancer Cell* 15:45–56.

Alvarez-Buylla A, Lim DA (2004) For the long run: maintaining germinal niches in the adult brain. *Neuron* 41:683–686.

Arvidsson A, Collin T, Kirik D, Kokaia Z, Lindvall O (2002) Neuronal replacement from endogenous precursors in the adult brain after stroke. *Nat Med* 8:963–970.

Bergmann O, Liebl J, Bernard S, Alkass K, Yeung MS, Steier P, Kutschera W, Johnson L, Landen M, Druid H, Spalding KL, Frisen J (2012) The age of olfactory bulb neurons in humans. *Neuron* 74:634–639.

Betizeau M, Cortay V, Patti D, Pfister S, Gautier E, Bellemin-Menard A, Afanassieff M, Huissoud C, Douglas RJ, Kennedy H, Dehay C (2013) Precursor diversity and complexity of lineage relationships in the outer subventricular zone of the primate. *Neuron* 80:442–457.

Bouab M, Paliouras GN, Aumont A, Forest-Berard K, Fernandes KJ (2011) Aging of the subventricular zone neural stem cell niche: evidence for quiescence-associated changes between early and mid-adulthood. *Neuroscience* 173:135–149.

Butti E, Bacigaluppi M, Rossi S, Cambiaghi M, Bari M, Cebrian Silla A, Brambilla E, Musella A, De Ceglia R, Teneud L, De Chiara V, D'Adamo P, Garcia-Verdugo JM, Comi G, Muzio L, Quattrini A, Leocani L, Maccarrone M, Centonze D, Martino G (2012) Subventricular zone neural progenitors protect striatal neurons from glutamatergic excitotoxicity. *Brain* 135:3320–3335.

Calvo CF *et al.* (2011) Vascular endothelial growth factor receptor 3 directly regulates murine neurogenesis. *Genes Dev* 25:831–844.

Capilla-Gonzalez V, Cebrian-Silla A, Guerrero-Cazares H, Garcia-Verdugo JM, Quinones-Hinojosa A (2014a) Age-related changes in astrocytic and ependymal cells of the subventricular zone. *Glia.*

Capilla-Gonzalez V, Gil-Perotin S, Ferragud A, Bonet-Ponce L, Canales JJ, Garcia-Verdugo JM (2012) Exposure to N-ethyl-N-nitrosourea in adult mice alters structural and functional integrity of neurogenic sites. *PLoS One* 7:e29891.

Capilla-Gonzalez V, Guerrero-Cazares H, Bonsu JM, Gonzalez-Perez O, Achanta P, Wong J, Garcia-Verdugo JM, Quinones-Hinojosa A (2014b) The subventricular zone is able to respond to a demyelinating lesion after localized radiation. *Stem Cells* 32:59–69.

Carlson ME, Conboy MJ, Hsu M, Barchas L, Jeong J, Agrawal A, Mikels AJ, Agrawal S, Schaffer DV, Conboy IM (2009) Relative roles of TGF-beta1 and Wnt in the systemic regulation and aging of satellite cell responses. *Aging Cell* 8:676–689.

Chadashvili T, Peterson DA (2006) Cytoarchitecture of fibroblast growth factor receptor 2 (FGFR-2) immunoreactivity in astrocytes of neurogenic and non-neurogenic regions of the young adult and aged rat brain. *J Comp Neurol* 498:1–15.

Chen L, Guerrero-Cazares H, Ye X, Ford E, McNutt T, Kleinberg L, Lim M, Chaichana K, Quinones-Hinojosa A, Redmond K (2013) Increased subventricular zone radiation dose correlates with survival in glioblastoma patients after gross total resection. *Int J Radiat Oncol Biol Phys* 86:616–622.

Conover JC, Notti RQ (2008) The neural stem cell niche. *Cell Tissue Res* 331:211–224.

Conover JC, Shook BA (2011) Aging of the subventricular zone neural stem cell niche. *Aging Dis* 2:49–63.

Cserr HF, VanDyke DH (1971) 5-hydroxyindoleacetic acid accumulation by isolated choroid plexus. *Am J Physiol* 220:718–723.

Curtis MA, Faull RL, Eriksson PS (2007) The effect of neurodegenerative diseases on the subventricular zone. *Nat Rev Neurosci* 8:712–723.

Curtis MA, Penney EB, Pearson AG, van Roon-Mom WM, Butterworth NJ, Dragunow M, Connor B, Faull RL (2003) Increased cell proliferation and neurogenesis in the adult human Huntington's disease brain. *Proc Nat Acad Sci USA* 100:9023–9027.

Del Bigio MR (2010) Ependymal cells: biology and pathology. *Acta Neuropathol* 119:55–73.

Doetsch F (2003) A niche for adult neural stem cells. *Curr Opin Genet Dev* 13:543–550.

Doetsch F, Alvarez-Buylla A (1996) Network of tangential pathways for neuronal migration in adult mammalian brain. *Proc Nat Acad Sci USA* 93:14895–14900.

Doetsch F, Garcia-Verdugo JM, Alvarez-Buylla A (1997) Cellular composition and three-dimensional organization of the subventricular germinal zone in the adult mammalian brain. *J Neurosci* 17:5046–5061.

Doetsch F, Garcia-Verdugo JM, Alvarez-Buylla A (1999a) Regeneration of a germinal layer in the adult mammalian brain. *Proc Natl Acad Sci USA* 96:11619–11624.

Doetsch F, Caille I, Lim DA, Garcia-Verdugo JM, Alvarez-Buylla A (1999b) Subventricular zone astrocytes are neural stem cells in the adult mammalian brain. *Cell* 97:703–716.

Douet V, Kerever A, Arikawa-Hirasawa E, Mercier F (2013) Fractone-heparan sulphates mediate FGF-2 stimulation of cell proliferation in the adult subventricular zone. *Cell Prolif* 46:137–145.

Emsley JG, Hagg T (2003) alpha6beta1 integrin directs migration of neuronal precursors in adult mouse forebrain. *Exp Neurol* 183:273–285.

Enwere E, Shingo T, Gregg C, Fujikawa H, Ohta S, Weiss S (2004) Aging results in reduced epidermal growth factor receptor signaling, diminished olfactory neurogenesis, and deficits in fine olfactory discrimination. *J Neurosci* 24:8354–8365.

Ernst A, Alkass K, Bernard S, Salehpour M, Perl S, Tisdale J, Possnert G, Druid H, Frisen J (2014) Neurogenesis in the striatum of the adult human brain. *Cell* 156:1072–1083.

Etxeberria A, Mangin JM, Aguirre A, Gallo V (2010) Adult-born SVZ progenitors receive transient synapses during remyelination in corpus callosum. *Nat Neurosci* 13:287–289.

Fazekas F, Kleinert R, Offenbacher H, Schmidt R, Kleinert G, Payer F, Radner H, Lechner H (1993) Pathologic correlates of incidental MRI white matter signal hyperintensities. *Neurology* 43:1683–1689.

Ferron SR, Marques-Torrejon MA, Mira H, Flores I, Taylor K, Blasco MA, Farinas I (2009) Telomere shortening in neural stem cells disrupts neuronal differentiation and neuritogenesis. *J Neurosci* 29:14394–14407.

Galan L, Gomez-Pinedo U, Vela-Souto A, Guerrero-Sola A, Barcia JA, Gutierrez AR, Martinez-Martinez A, Jimenez MS, Garcia-Verdugo JM, Matias-Guiu J (2011) Subventricular zone in motor neuron disease with frontotemporal dementia. *Neurosci Lett* 499:9–13.

Gao P, Shen F, Gabriel RA, Law D, Yang E, Yang GY, Young WL, Su H (2009) Attenuation of brain response to vascular endothelial growth factor-mediated angiogenesis and neurogenesis in aged mice. *Stroke* 40:3596–3600.

Garcia-Verdugo JM, Doetsch F, Wichterle H, Lim DA, Alvarez-Buylla A (1998) Architecture and cell types of the adult subventricular zone: in search of the stem cells. *J Neurobiol* 36:234–248.

Geraerts M, Krylyshkina O, Debyser Z, Baekelandt V (2007) Concise review: therapeutic strategies for Parkinson disease based on the modulation of adult neurogenesis. *Stem Cells* 25:263–270.

Guerrero-Cazares H, Gonzalez-Perez O, Soriano-Navarro M, Zamora-Berridi G, Garcia-Verdugo JM, Quinones-Hinojosa A (2011) Cytoarchitecture of the lateral ganglionic eminence and rostral extension of the lateral ventricle in the human fetal brain. *J Comp Neurol* 519:1165–1180.

Guglielmetti C, Praet J, Rangarajan JR, Vreys R, De Vocht N, Maes F, Verhoye M, Ponsaerts P, Van der Linden A (2014) Multimodal imaging of subventricular zone neural stem/progenitor cells in the cuprizone mouse model reveals increased neurogenic potential for the olfactory bulb pathway, but no contribution to remyelination of the corpus callosum. *Neuroimage* 86:99–110.

Gupta T, Nair V, Paul SN, Kannan S, Moiyadi A, Epari S, Jalali R (2012) Can irradiation of potential cancer stem-cell niche in the subventricular zone influence survival in patients with newly diagnosed glioblastoma? *J Neurooncol* 109:195–203.

Hack MA, Saghatelyan A, de Chevigny A, Pfeifer A, Ashery-Padan R, Lledo PM, Gotz M (2005) Neuronal fate determinants of adult olfactory bulb neurogenesis. *Nat Neurosci* 8:865–872.

Hansen DV, Lui JH, Parker PR, Kriegstein AR (2010) Neurogenic radial glia in the outer subventricular zone of human neocortex. *Nature* 464:554–561.

Hayflick L, Moorhead PS (1961) The serial cultivation of human diploid cell strains. *Exp Cell Res* 25:585–621.

Hoglinger GU, Rizk P, Muriel MP, Duyckaerts C, Oertel WH, Caille I, Hirsch EC (2004) Dopamine depletion impairs precursor cell proliferation in Parkinson disease. *Nat Neurosci* 7:726–735.

Ihrie RA, Alvarez-Buylla A (2011) Lake-front property: a unique germinal niche by the lateral ventricles of the adult brain. *Neuron* 70:674–686.

Ihrie RA, Shah JK, Harwell CC, Levine JH, Guinto CD, Lezameta M, Kriegstein AR, Alvarez-Buylla A (2011) Persistent sonic hedgehog signaling in adult brain determines neural stem cell positional identity. *Neuron* 71:250–262.

Jin K, Wang X, Xie L, Mao XO, Greenberg DA (2010) Transgenic ablation of doublecortin-expressing cells suppresses adult neurogenesis and worsens stroke outcome in mice. *Proc Nat Acad Sci USA* 107:7993–7998.

Jin K, Sun Y, Xie L, Batteur S, Mao XO, Smelick C, Logvinova A, Greenberg DA (2003) Neurogenesis and aging: FGF-2 and HB-EGF restore neurogenesis in hippocampus and subventricular zone of aged mice. *Aging Cell* 2:175–183.

Jin K, Wang X, Xie L, Mao XO, Zhu W, Wang Y, Shen J, Mao Y, Banwait S, Greenberg DA (2006) Evidence for stroke-induced neurogenesis in the human brain. *Proc Natl Acad Sci USA* 103:13198–13202.

Jing X, Miwa H, Sawada T, Nakanishi I, Kondo T, Miyajima M, Sakaguchi K (2012) Ephrin-A1-mediated dopaminergic neurogenesis and angiogenesis in a rat model of Parkinson's disease. *PLoS One* 7:e32019.

Johanson C, Stopa E, McMillan P, Roth D, Funk J, Krinke G (2011) The distributional nexus of choroid plexus to cerebrospinal fluid, ependyma and brain: toxicologic/pathologic phenomena, periventricular destabilization, and lesion spread. *Toxicol Pathol* 39:186–212.

Kaneko N, Kako E, Sawamoto K (2013) Enhancement of ventricular-subventricular zone-derived neurogenesis and oligodendrogenesis by erythropoietin and its derivatives. *Front Cell Neurosci* 7:235.

Kast RE, Ellingson BM, Marosi C, Halatsch ME (2014) Glioblastoma treatment using perphenazine to block the subventricular zone's tumor trophic functions. *J Neurooncol* 116:207–212.

Kerever A, Schnack J, Vellinga D, Ichikawa N, Moon C, Arikawa-Hirasawa E, Efird JT, Mercier F (2007) Novel extracellular matrix structures in the neural stem cell niche capture the neurogenic factor fibroblast growth factor 2 from the extracellular milieu. *Stem Cells* 25:2146–2157.

Kerever A, Mercier F, Nonaka R, de Vega S, Oda Y, Zalc B, Okada Y, Hattori N, Yamada Y, Arikawa-Hirasawa E (2014) Perlecan is required for FGF-2 signaling in the neural stem cell niche. *Stem Cell Res* 12:492–505.

Kohwi M, Osumi N, Rubenstein JL, Alvarez-Buylla A (2005) Pax6 is required for making specific subpopulations of granule and periglomerular neurons in the olfactory bulb. *J Neurosci* 25:6997–7003.

Kokoeva MV, Yin H, Flier JS (2005) Neurogenesis in the hypothalamus of adult mice: potential role in energy balance. *Science* 310:679–683.

Lee DA, Bedont JL, Pak T, Wang H, Song J, Miranda-Angulo A, Takiar V, Charubhumi V, Balordi F, Takebayashi H, Aja S, Ford E, Fishell G,

Blackshaw S (2012) Tanycytes of the hypothalamic median eminence form a diet-responsive neurogenic niche. *Nat Neurosci* 15:700–702.

Lennington JB, Pope S, Goodheart AE, Drozdowicz L, Daniels SB, Salamone JD, Conover JC (2011) Midbrain dopamine neurons associated with reward processing innervate the neurogenic subventricular zone. *J Neurosci* 31:13078–13087.

Li L, Harms KM, Ventura PB, Lagace DC, Eisch AJ, Cunningham LA (2010) Focal cerebral ischemia induces a multilineage cytogenic response from adult subventricular zone that is predominantly gliogenic. *Glia* 58:1610–1619.

Liu L, Rando TA (2011) Manifestations and mechanisms of stem cell aging. *J Cell Biol* 193:257–266.

Liu Z, Martin LJ (2006) The adult neural stem and progenitor cell niche is altered in amyotrophic lateral sclerosis mouse brain. *J Comp Neurol* 497:468–488.

Lledo PM, Saghatelyan A (2005) Integrating new neurons into the adult olfactory bulb: joining the network, life-death decisions, and the effects of sensory experience. *Trends Neurosci* 28:248–254.

Luo J, Shook BA, Daniels SB, Conover JC (2008) Subventricular zone-mediated ependyma repair in the adult mammalian brain. *J Neurosci* 28:3804–3813.

Luo J, Daniels SB, Lennington JB, Notti RQ, Conover JC (2006) The aging neurogenic subventricular zone. *Aging Cell* 5:139–152.

Luskin MB (1993) Restricted proliferation and migration of postnatally generated neurons derived from the forebrain subventricular zone. *Neuron* 11:173–189.

Macas J, Nern C, Plate KH, Momma S (2006) Increased generation of neuronal progenitors after ischemic injury in the aged adult human forebrain. *J Neurosci* 26:13114–13119.

Maki T, Liang AC, Miyamoto N, Lo EH, Arai K (2013) Mechanisms of oligodendrocyte regeneration from ventricular-subventricular zone-derived progenitor cells in white matter diseases. *Front Cell Neurosci* 7:275.

Mandairon N, Didier A (2010) The brain's fight against aging. *Proc Nat Acad Sci USA* 107:15316–15317.

Maslov AY, Barone TA, Plunkett RJ, Pruitt SC (2004) Neural stem cell detection, characterization, and age-related changes in the subventricular zone of mice. *J Neurosci* 24:1726–1733.

McAllister JP, 2nd (2012) Pathophysiology of congenital and neonatal hydrocephalus. *Semin Fetal Neonatal Med* 17:285–294.

Mercier F, Kitasako JT, Hatton GI (2002) Anatomy of the brain neurogenic zones revisited: fractones and the fibroblast/macrophage network. *J Comp Neurol* 451:170–188.

Merkle FT, Mirzadeh Z, Alvarez-Buylla A (2007) Mosaic organization of neural stem cells in the adult brain. *Science* 317:381–384.

Mimeault M, Batra SK (2010) Recent advances on skin-resident stem/progenitor cell functions in skin regeneration, aging and cancers and novel anti-aging and cancer therapies. *J Cell Mol Med* 14:116–134.

Mirzadeh Z, Merkle FT, Soriano-Navarro M, Garcia-Verdugo JM, Alvarez-Buylla A (2008) Neural stem cells confer unique pinwheel architecture to the ventricular surface in neurogenic regions of the adult brain. *Cell Stem Cell* 3:265–278.

Moreno M, Richard M, Landrein B, Sacquet J, Didier A, Mandairon N (2014) Alteration of olfactory perceptual learning and its cellular basis in aged mice. *Neurobiol Aging* 35:680–691.

Nait-Oumesmar B, Picard-Riera N, Kerninon C, Baron-Van Evercooren A (2008) The role of SVZ-derived neural precursors in demyelinating diseases: from animal models to multiple sclerosis. *J Neurological Sci* 265:26–31.

Najbauer J, Huszthy PC, Barish ME, Garcia E, Metz MZ, Myers SM, Gutova M, Frank RT, Miletic H, Kendall SE, Glackin CA, Bjerkvig R, Aboody KS (2012) Cellular host responses to gliomas. *PLoS One* 7:e35150.

Nam HS, Benezra R (2009) High levels of Id1 expression define B1 type adult neural stem cells. *Cell Stem Cell* 5:515–526.

Ohab JJ, Fleming S, Blesch A, Carmichael ST (2006) A neurovascular niche for neurogenesis after stroke. *J Neurosci* 26:13007–13016.

Paliouras GN, Hamilton LK, Aumont A, Joppe SE, Barnabe-Heider F, Fernandes KJ (2012) Mammalian target of rapamycin signaling is a key regulator of the transit-amplifying progenitor pool in the adult and aging forebrain. *J Neurosci* 32:15012–15026.

Phillips W, Morton AJ, Barker RA (2005) Abnormalities of neurogenesis in the R6/2 mouse model of Huntington's disease are attributable to the in vivo microenvironment. *J Neurosci* 25:11564–11576.

Picard-Riera N, Decker L, Delarasse C, Goude K, Nait-Oumesmar B, Liblau R, Pham-Dinh D, Evercooren AB (2002) Experimental autoimmune encephalomyelitis mobilizes neural progenitors from the subventricular zone to undergo oligodendrogenesis in adult mice. *Proc Natl Acad Sci USA* 99:13211–13216.

Pierce AA, Xu AW (2010) *De novo* neurogenesis in adult hypothalamus as a compensatory mechanism to regulate energy balance. *J Neurosci* 30:723–730.

Quinones-Hinojosa A, Sanai N, Soriano-Navarro M, Gonzalez-Perez O, Mirzadeh Z, Gil-Perotin S, Romero-Rodriguez R, Berger MS, Garcia-Verdugo JM, Alvarez-Buylla A (2006) Cellular composition and cytoarchitecture of the adult human subventricular zone: a niche of neural stem cells. *J Comp Neurol* 494:415–434.

Ramaswamy S, Goings GE, Soderstrom KE, Szele FG, Kozlowski DA (2005) Cellular proliferation and migration following a controlled cortical impact in the mouse. *Brain Res* 1053:38–53.

Rasmussen S, Imitola J, Ayuso-Sacido A, Wang Y, Starossom SC, Kivisakk P, Zhu B, Meyer M, Bronson RT, Garcia-Verdugo JM, Khoury SJ (2011) Reversible neural stem cell niche dysfunction in a model of multiple sclerosis. *Ann Neurol* 69:878–891.

Rey NL, Sacquet J, Veyrac A, Jourdan F, Didier A (2012) Behavioral and cellular markers of olfactory aging and their response to enrichment. *Neurobiol Aging* 33:626 e629–626 e623.

Richard MB, Taylor SR, Greer CA (2010) Age-induced disruption of selective olfactory bulb synaptic circuits. *Proc Nat Acad Sci USA* 107:15613–15618.

Roales-Bujan R, Paez P, Guerra M, Rodriguez S, Vio K, Ho-Plagaro A, Garcia-Bonilla M, Rodriguez-Perez LM, Dominguez-Pinos MD, Rodriguez EM, Perez-Figares JM, Jimenez AJ (2012) Astrocytes acquire morphological and functional characteristics of ependymal cells following disruption of ependyma in hydrocephalus. *Acta Neuropathologica* 124:531–546.

Rodriguez JJ, Verkhratsky A (2011) Neurogenesis in Alzheimer's disease. *J Anat* 219:78–89.

Sabelstrom H, Stenudd M, Reu P, Dias DO, Elfineh M, Zdunek S, Damberg P, Goritz C, Frisen J (2013) Resident neural stem cells restrict tissue damage and neuronal loss after spinal cord injury in mice. *Science* 342:637–640.

Sanai N, Berger MS, Garcia-Verdugo JM, Alvarez-Buylla A (2007) Comment on "Human neuroblasts migrate to the olfactory bulb via a lateral ventricular extension". *Science* 318:393; author reply 393.

Sanai N, Tramontin AD, Quinones-Hinojosa A, Barbaro NM, Gupta N, Kunwar S, Lawton MT, McDermott MW, Parsa AT, Manuel-Garcia Verdugo J, Berger MS, Alvarez-Buylla A (2004) Unique astrocyte ribbon in adult human brain contains neural stem cells but lacks chain migration. *Nature* 427:740–744.

Sanai N, Nguyen T, Ihrie RA, Mirzadeh Z, Tsai HH, Wong M, Gupta N, Berger MS, Huang E, Garcia-Verdugo JM, Rowitch DH, Alvarez-Buylla A (2011) Corridors of migrating neurons in the human brain and their decline during infancy. *Nature* 478:382–386.

Scadden DT (2006) The stem-cell niche as an entity of action. *Nature* 441:1075–1079.

Sener RN (2002) Callosal changes in obstructive hydrocephalus: observations with FLAIR imaging, and diffusion MRI. *Comput Med Imaging Graph* 26:333–337.

Shan X, Chi L, Bishop M, Luo C, Lien L, Zhang Z, Liu R (2006) Enhanced de novo neurogenesis and dopaminergic neurogenesis in the substantia nigra of 1-methyl-4-phenyl-1,2,3,6-tetrahydropyridine-induced Parkinson's disease-like mice. *Stem Cells* 24:1280–1287.

Shen Q, Wang Y, Kokovay E, Lin G, Chuang SM, Goderie SK, Roysam B, Temple S (2008) Adult SVZ stem cells lie in a vascular niche: a quantitative analysis of niche cell-cell interactions. *Cell Stem Cell* 3:289–300.

Shook BA, Manz DH, Peters JJ, Kang S, Conover JC (2012) Spatiotemporal changes to the subventricular zone stem cell pool through aging. *J Neurosci* 32:6947–6956.

Shook BA, Lennington JB, Acabchuk RL, Halling M, Sun Y, Peters J, Wu Q, Mahajan A, Fellows DW, Conover JC (2013) Ventriculomegaly associated with ependymal gliosis and declines in barrier integrity in the aging human and mouse brain. *Aging Cell.*

Simpson JM, Gil-Mohapel J, Pouladi MA, Ghilan M, Xie Y, Hayden MR, Christie BR (2011) Altered adult hippocampal neurogenesis in the YAC128 transgenic mouse model of Huntington disease. *Neurobiol Dis* 41:249–260.

Sofroniew MV (2009) Molecular dissection of reactive astrogliosis and glial scar formation. *Trends Neurosci* 32:638–647.

Spassky N, Merkle FT, Flames N, Tramontin AD, Garcia-Verdugo JM, Alvarez-Buylla A (2005) Adult ependymal cells are postmitotic and are derived from radial glial cells during embryogenesis. *J Neurosci* 25:10–18.

Stoll EA, Habibi BA, Mikheev AM, Lasiene J, Massey SC, Swanson KR, Rostomily RC, Horner PJ (2011) Increased re-entry into cell cycle mitigates age-related neurogenic decline in the murine subventricular zone. *Stem Cells* 29:2005–2017.

Sun C, Sun H, Wu S, Lee CC, Akamatsu Y, Wang RK, Kernie SG, Liu J (2013) Conditional ablation of neuroprogenitor cells in adult mice impedes recovery of poststroke cognitive function and reduces synaptic connectivity in the perforant pathway. *J Neurosci* 33:17314–17325.

Tavazoie M, Van der Veken L, Silva-Vargas V, Louissaint M, Colonna L, Zaidi B, Garcia-Verdugo JM, Doetsch F (2008) A specialized vascular niche for adult neural stem cells. *Cell Stem Cell* 3:279–288.

Temple S (2001) The development of neural stem cells. *Nature* 414:112–117.

Tiwari SK, Agarwal S, Seth B, Yadav A, Nair S, Bhatnagar P, Karmakar M, Kumari M, Chauhan LK, Patel DK, Srivastava V, Singh D, Gupta SK, Tripathi A, Chaturvedi RK, Gupta KC (2014) Curcumin-loaded nanoparticles potently induce adult neurogenesis and reverse cognitive deficits in Alzheimer's disease model via canonical Wnt/beta-catenin pathway. *ACS Nano* 8:76–103.

Tramontin AD, Garcia-Verdugo JM, Lim DA, Alvarez-Buylla A (2003) Postnatal development of radial glia and the ventricular zone (VZ): a continuum of the neural stem cell compartment. *Cereb Cortex* 13:580–587.

Tropepe V, Craig CG, Morshead CM, van der Kooy D (1997) Transforming growth factor-alpha null and senescent mice show decreased neural progenitor cell proliferation in the forebrain subependyma. *J Neurosci* 17:7850–7859.

van den Berge SA, van Strien ME, Korecka JA, Dijkstra AA, Sluijs JA, Kooijman L, Eggers R, De Filippis L, Vescovi AL, Verhaagen J, van de Berg WD, Hol EM (2011) The proliferative capacity of the subventricular zone is maintained in the parkinsonian brain. *Brain* 134:3249–3263.

Villeda SA *et al.* (2011) The ageing systemic milieu negatively regulates neurogenesis and cognitive function. *Nature* 477:90–94.

Wang C, Liu F, Liu YY, Zhao CH, You Y, Wang L, Zhang J, Wei B, Ma T, Zhang Q, Zhang Y, Chen R, Song H, Yang Z (2011) Identification and characterization of neuroblasts in the subventricular zone and rostral migratory stream of the adult human brain. *Cell Res* 21:1534–1550.

Wichterle H, Garcia-Verdugo JM, Alvarez-Buylla A (1997) Direct evidence for homotypic, glia-independent neuronal migration. *Neuron* 18:779–791.

Wiltrout C, Lang B, Yan Y, Dempsey RJ, Vemuganti R (2007) Repairing brain after stroke: a review on post-ischemic neurogenesis. *Neurochem Int* 50:1028–1041.

Xu Y, Tamamaki N, Noda T, Kimura K, Itokazu Y, Matsumoto N, Dezawa M, Ide C (2005) Neurogenesis in the ependymal layer of the adult rat 3rd ventricle. *Exp Neurol* 192:251–264.

Young CC, van der Harg JM, Lewis NJ, Brooks KJ, Buchan AM, Szele FG (2013) Ependymal ciliary dysfunction and reactive astrocytosis in a reorganized subventricular zone after stroke. *Cereb Cortex* 23:647–659.

Zecevic N (2004) Specific characteristic of radial glia in the human fetal telencephalon. *Glia* 48:27–35.

Zhang G, Li J, Purkayastha S, Tang Y, Zhang H, Yin Y, Li B, Liu G, Cai D (2013) Hypothalamic programming of systemic ageing involving IKK-beta, NF-kappaB and GnRH. *Nature* 497:211–216.

Zitnik G, Martin GM (2002) Age-related decline in neurogenesis: old cells or old environment? *J Neurosci Res* 70:258–263.

Chapter 3

Neural Stem Cells for Intrinsic Brain Repair in Aging and Neural Degeneration

Lalitha Madhavan

Neural stem cells (NSCs) offer a promising avenue to develop rational therapeutic strategies to treat age-related neurological diseases. On one hand, NSCs represent a renewable source for generating an array of neuronal and glial cell types, which can be used for cellular replacement in neurodegenerative disease scenarios. On the other hand, NSCs have the natural ability to interact with other cells in the surrounding neural environment through direct physical interactions, and indirectly through diffusible factors, to stimulate endogenous plasticity and tissue repair which can result in functional improvements. Such NSC interactions with host cells become quite relevant in the context of the complexity and the challenges posed by the chronically deteriorating brain environment present during aging and neural degeneration. In particular, the capacity of immature NSCs to prevail in such pathological situations, and in fact activate cell survival and regeneration mechanisms in the host brain, allows for the possibility of actually countering degenerative processes and impeding disease progression. Here, we discuss such NSC potential to modify the brain environment and its prospects with respect to aging and neural degeneration.

Introduction

Once NSCs are transplanted into the brain, they start to dynamically interact with cellular and molecular components in their local microenvironment or 'niche.' Niche is a terminology originating from the field of ecology, and is a description of the habitat of an organism and the entirety of environmental interactions that allow the organism to survive in this habitat. It has become clear that, in addition to intrinsic factors, cell extrinsic interactions between NSCs and their niche are critical in determining the behavior and fate of both grafted (donor) and host (recipient) cells after neural transplantation (Alvarez-Buylla and Lim, 2004; Ourednik and Ourednik, 2005, 2007; Garzon-Muvdi and Quinones-Hinojosa, 2009; Madhavan and Collier, 2010).

As alluded to in other chapters, endogenous NSCs exist throughout life in the mammalian brain largely in specialized niches localized in the subventricular zone (SVZ) and the dentate gyrus (DG) of the hippocampus (Alvarez-Buylla and Lim, 2004; Riquelme *et al.*, 2008). The microenvironment of these regions have evolved to be able to maintain the population of stem cells in a state that represents a fine balance between cell proliferation, differentiation and/or cell death. In fact it is known that these niches comprise of cellular structures, and a variety of extracellular matrix (ECM) and soluble (diffusible) factors, all of which aid NSC survival, proliferation/self-renewal, and multipotentiality (Figure 1). Also, multiple studies demonstrate that NSCs in these niches can respond to a variety of insults, including those occurring in degenerative disorders such as Parkinson's disease, ischemic stroke, and multiple sclerosis, pointing to a remarkable plasticity and regenerative potential in the mammalian brain (Arvidsson *et al.*, 2002; Rocha *et al.*, 2005; Thored *et al.*, 2006; Madhavan *et al.*, 2009; Madhavan *et al.*, 2012; Mecha *et al.*, 2013).

Recent studies indicate that exogenously grown NSCs are in fact able to 'recreate' such tightly regulated, regenerative, and injury responsive niches, upon transplantation (Ourednik and Ourednik, 2007; Madhavan and Collier, 2010). Akin to NSCs in endogenous niches, the grafted NSCs establish lines of communication with host

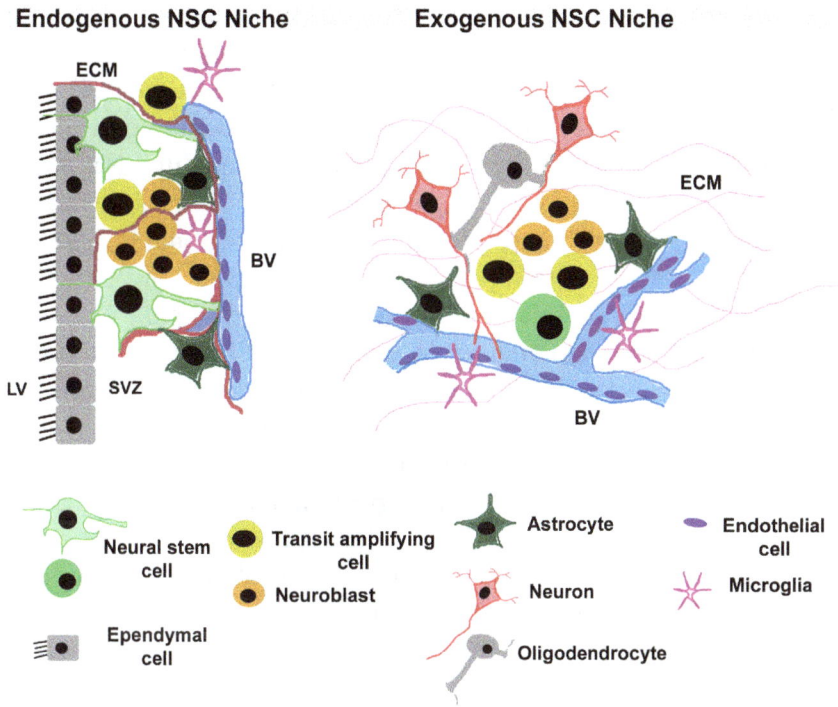

Figure 1. Endogenous and Exogenous (transplanted) NSC niches share similar attributes. The endogenous subventricular zone (SVZ) niche (shown to the left) is located adjacent to the lateral ventricle (LV) in the forebrain. Bonafide neural stem cells (a type of glial cell), also called type B cells, reside adjacent to the ependymal cell layer which separates the stem cells from the ventricular cavity. These Type B neural stem cells give rise to transit amplifying type C cells, which then generate type A neuroblasts that migrate away towards the olfactory bulb. In addition to ependymal cells, the B cells also contact multiple other cell types and the SVZ vasculature. In particular astrocytes, endothelial cells, neighboring microglia, and the extracellular matrix which pervades the SVZ, are all in close apposition to type B NSCs, allowing direct as well as indirect diffusible factor based interactions. Such specific and tightly regulated communication between the cellular and extracellular SVZ components is known to be crucial for the maintenance of the regenerative function of this niche. Similar to endogenous niches, NSCs upon transplantation are known to strategically settle adjacent to the parenchymal vasculature to create exogenous niches (shown to the right). As in the endogenous niches, close interplay with endothelial cells, astrocytes, oligodendrocytes, microglia, and ECM components are pivotal in determining the behavior and fate of NSCs, as well as host cells, in these exogenous or supplementary niches.

cells in their extracellular niche, through diffusible factors, cell to cell, and cell to ECM interactions among others (Figure 1). Through such interactions, not only are the NSCs able to affect the activity of surrounding host cells, but are also influenced and altered in return during this process. Such networking between implanted NSCs and host brain cells can significantly control the behavior and fate of both interacting donor and host elements. The regional location of donor cells, age of the host, presence of pathology or injury, and the timing of donor cell implantation with respect to the pathology, can all influence the specific nature of emerging NSC-host interactions to determine when and which molecular pathways become activated or suppressed. In essence, such finely tuned graft-host interactions can activate multiple mechanisms involved in cell survival, cell proliferation, cell differentiation, cell migration, neurite outgrowth, and synaptogenesis in a physiologically relevant manner. Further, these interactions can also result in the modulation of inflammation and injury. Ultimately, these effects can repair and protect neural tissues to restore physiological equilibrium. Therefore, understanding the tenets of such powerful graft and host signaling will be essential in realizing the therapeutic purpose of NSCs.

Indirect NSC Based Effects Through Diffusible Factors

It is well established that NSCs can spontaneously express, both *in vitro* and *in vivo*, a number of diffusible factors. These factors can act in autocrine and paracrine ways to support NSC survival, and self-renewal, as well as allow the NSCs to adapt to and influence their extracellular niche. Two predominant groups of NSC-derived diffusible factors have been identified from the literature so far: (1) Trophic; and (2) Immune modulatory. These factors can have persistent and broad-based effects on the host environment of the transplanted NSCs, including the stimulation of neurogenesis, axo-dendritic outgrowth, reduction of oxidative stress, and regulation of the immune response. Eventually, such trophic and immune factor-based phenomena can lead to protection and repair of cells and neural circuitries helping to reinstate tissue homeostasis.

Trophic factors

As mentioned, NSCs exhibit an innate ability to express a variety of trophic factors upon implantation into the adult, aged, and/or diseased nervous system. Basically, it has been found that these NSC-derived beneficial proteins, can help resist degenerative processes, and promote neural health and function ameliorating symptoms in the context of both primary and secondary neurodegenerative conditions such as Parkinson's disease (PD), spinal cord disorders, and stroke.

Parkinson's disease

In models of PD, NSC-derived trophic factors can stimulate plasticity in host tissues, and lead to protective and restorative effects. Our recent studies in a 6-hydroxydopamine (6-OHDA, toxin inducing degeneration of the nigrostriatal dopaminergic system) rodent model indicate that trophic molecules such as glial-derived neurotrophic factor (GDNF), sonic hedgehog (SHH), and stromal-derived factor 1 alpha (SDF1α), can be expressed by implanted NSCs (Madhavan *et al.*, 2009). It was observed that the trophic factor expression by the NSCs was associated with the stimulation of endogenous neurogenesis in the SVZ, the migration of newborn doublecortin (Dcx) expressing neuroblasts into the striatal parenchyma, protection of tyrosine hydroxylase (TH^+) dopamine neurons in the substantia nigra, and the amelioration of behavioral deficits (Madhavan *et al.*, 2009; Madhavan *et al.*, 2012). Using lentiviral RNA interference to silence trophic factor expression in the *ex vivo* grown NSCs, before implantation, it was subsequently confirmed that SHH was in fact a major mediator of the observed NSC-mediated plasticity and neuroprotection. Not only this, SHH silencing in the donor NSCs essentially ablated the endogenous neurogenesis response and inhibited the migration of new Dcx-expressing precursors into the striatum (Madhavan *et al.*, 2015).

Given the robust activation of endogenous NSCs, and the correlation of this response with neuroprotection in the abovementioned studies, the plausible contribution of endogenous neural precursors to the observed nigrostriatal system protection was also explored. In these experiments, the mitotic inhibitor cytosine arabinoside (Ara-C) was used to first deplete the pool of endogenous NSCs (and block their activation and influence), prior to donor NSC implantation. Under these conditions, it was observed that the neuroprotective efficacy of the grafted NSCs was significantly reduced. Not only this, although the survival of the grafted cells was not affected, their phenotypic fate was significantly altered. In particular, grafts in animals in which the endogenous NSC response had been suppressed via Ara-C, were determined to contain a notably reduced fraction of undifferentiated (nestin$^+$) cells, which also co-expressed SHH. Interestingly, in the RNA interference experiments mentioned previously, the silencing of SHH in the donor cells before implantation had also lead to a reduction in the nestin$^+$ population in the grafted cells *in vivo*. These results strongly indicated the immature nestin/SHH expressing donor population as a critical group of cells mediating host neuroprotection and neurogenesis (Madhavan *et al.*, 2012).

It has also become evident that the potential of immature NSCs to induce endogenous tissue repair is particularly effective when they are implanted during early stages of the disease. In our own studies, it has been determined that the efficacy of NSC-mediated nigrostriatal neuroprotection and neurogenesis is maximum when the cells are transplanted before, or soon after, the administration of 6-OHDA, which is a stage when degenerative mechanisms are just beginning and not well established (Madhavan *et al.*, 2009, 2012, 2015). In a study by Yasuhara *et al.*, (2006) a similar effect was observed wherein NSCs, when grafted in tandem with 6-OHDA administration, were able to elicit the protection of substantia nigra TH$^+$ dopamine neurons and the nigrostriatal circuit (Yasuhara *et al.*, 2006). As in our study, the NSC-mediated neuroprotection was accompanied by endogenous SVZ neurogenesis and behavioral recovery. When the mechanisms underlying the phenomenon were investigated *in vitro*, in this case, it was revealed that the trophic molecule stem cell factor (SCF) was a major contributor. Specifically, SCF was found to up-regulate the anti-apoptotic factor, Bcl2 (B-cell CLL/lymphoma 2), and related molecular pathways to result in neuroprotection.

In the context of PD, other studies attest to the multiple endogenous effects that can be induced by trophic factors expressed by transplanted NSCs. Ourednik *et al.* (2002) utilized NSCs in an aged mouse model of chronic PD, and observed that donor cell-derived GDNF could rescue dysfunctional substantia nigra dopamine neurons (Ourednik *et al.*, 2002). Although the restoration of dopaminergic function was graft-dependent, it was determined that the effects was not predominantly due to the differentiation of donor NSCs to TH$^+$ dopamine neurons. On the contrary, a vast majority of recovered midbrain dopamine neurons were actually protected host cells. Similar to the Ourednik study, a report by Redmond *et al.* (2007) showed neuroprotection in a parkinsonian primate model (Redmond *et al.*, 2007). Again, it was not the differentiation of the NSCs which was responsible, but the expression of GDNF by grafted NSCs which were found closely interacting with host substantia nigra TH$^+$ cells and their projections along the nigrostriatal pathway. This behavior of the NSCs was associated with a lower number of nigrostriatal cells (20%) containing aggregates of alpha synuclein, a protein implicated as a major contributor to the degeneration of the dopamine neurons, in NSC-grafted animals compared to controls where 80% of the cells showed aggregates.

Stroke and ischemia

In models of stroke and ischemia, the evidence for NSC-mediated endogenous host plasticity is strong. Andres *et al.* have reported, in an ischemic model of stroke, that transplanted human NSCs expressed trophic factors and stimulated the re-expression of axon guidance factors to result in dendritic sprouting and enhance axonal plasticity (Andres *et al.*, 2011). More specifically, given that a bilateral reorganization of neural circuits is crucial to behavioral recovery observed after stroke, the authors investigated the potential of human NSC transplants to enhance such structural plasticity after unilateral middle cerebral artery occlusion. They observed that the human NSCs could significantly increase dendritic plasticity (enhanced dentritic extension and branching), in both the ipsi (same cerebral hemisphere)

parts and contralateral (opposite hemisphere) parts of affected cortical regions. The pattern of dendritic plasticity closely correlated with
stem cell-induced functional recovery in the animals. Importantly,
axonal transport, which is normally reduced in ischemic neural tissue,
was rescued by NSC implantation providing a cellular basis for the
improved axonal sprouting and function. In addition to the axonal
plasticity, NSC- grafted animals exhibited remarkable rewiring of cor-
ticocortical, corticothalamic and descending cortical tracts from the
contralateral side. Through further analysis, NSC expressed trophic
factors, vascular endothelial growth factor (VEGF) and thrombo-
spondins 1 and 2, and the axon guidance molecule, Slit, were determined as mediators of the observed dendritic and axonal plasticity,
and subsequent functional recovery of the ischemic cortical tissue.

It is also quite well established in stroke models that there is an
attempt by endogenous NSCs to promote neural plasticity and repair.
In particular, NSCs in the SVZ of adult rats subjected to an ischemic
insult continually produce new neuroblasts which travel into the
injured striatum, a phenomenon which occurs for several months
after stroke (Arvidsson *et al.*, 2002; Thored *et al.*, 2006). These
newborn neuroblasts have been shown to differentiate into mature
neurons which migrate to the stroke boundary with many integrating
into the local neural circuitry (Yamashita *et al.*, 2006). Similarly, there
is evidence for enhanced SVZ proliferation and neuroblast formation
after stroke in humans (Macas *et al.*, 2006; Minger *et al.*, 2007; Marti-
Fabregas *et al.*, 2010). However, in these studies, only a fraction of the
newborn neurons survive long-term, and it is unclear whether and to
what extent they contribute to the spontaneous functional recovery
observed after stroke (Arvidsson *et al.*, 2002). Mine *et al.* (2013)
addressed this issue by taking advantage of the ability of implanted
human NSCs to secrete soluble trophic factors in order to improve
the survival of endogenous SVZ neuroblasts and their progeny in the
striatum (Mine *et al.*, 2013). More specifically, upon implanting
human NSCs in a middle cerebral artery occlusion model of stroke,
they observed that the NSC implants could enhance endogenous SVZ
proliferation, the generation and survival of newborn neuroblasts,
and the maturation of the neuroblasts into neurons that could

project to correct target regions to cause behavioral improvements. In addition, the implanted NSCs also acted by altering the striatal microenvironment encountered by the new neurons, to a more supportive state, by modulating inflammation.

In other work, human NSCs transplanted into the rat cortex, during early stages of stroke, survived and migrated towards to the ischemic lesion, and induced functional recovery (Horie *et al.*, 2011). It was determined that the human NSCs were able to stimulate neovascularization, increase blood brain barrier (BBB) integrity, and mediate immune suppression (which are all postulated to significantly influence post-stroke recovery) via the expression of VEGF. In particular, VEGF was noted to increase blood vessel formation through the phosphorylation of the VEGF2 receptor resulting in increased VEGF signaling. Also, VEGF was found to support BBB integrity by enhancing tight junctions between endothelial cells, as well as B-dystroglycan protein expression which binds astrocytes to the endothelial cell extracellular matrix. Finally, VEGF also modulated the inflammatory response after stroke by reducing the number of microglia in the ischemic tissue.

Spinal cord and myelin disorders

Several studies support a role for NSC-derived diffusible factors in spinal cord disorders. In one investigation, NSCs grafted into cystic dorsal column lesions in the cervical spinal cord of adult rats expressed NT-3 (neurotrophin-3) and supported the growth of host axons (Lu *et al.*, 2003; Tuszynski *et al.*, 2003). In addition, when the NSCs were genetically modified to produce increased amounts of NT-3, this lead to significantly improved NSC effects on host axons. Interestingly, NT-3 specifically stimulated the extension of dorsal sensory axons while inhibiting the expression of GDNF and brain derived neurotrophic factor (BDNF), to cause the reduction of local motor axon growth. This phenomenon indicated that the trophic effects were quite tightly and strategically regulated.

With respect to Amytrophic Lateral Sclerosis (ALS), Corti *et al.* (2007) have shown that NSC implantation into a superoxide dismutase-1 (SOD1) mouse model led to neuroprotection through increased spinal cord levels of VEGF and insulin-like growth factor-1 (IGF-1) (Corti *et al.*, 2007). More specifically, the transplanted transgenic mice exhibited a delayed onset and progression of disease, and survived significantly longer than non-treated animals. Additionally, upon examination of the spinal cord, a significant protection of host motor neurons was revealed. Both VEGF- and IGF1-dependent pathways were significantly activated in transplanted animals compared to controls, suggesting a role of these neurotrophins in motor neuron protection.

In addition to inducing axonal extension and neuroprotection, NSC-based trophic effects have also been shown to improve endogenous remyelination in the central nervous system. This has been demonstrated in elegant studies conducted in mice with experimental chronic autoimmune encephalomyelitis (EAE) (Pluchino *et al.*, 2003). In this model, NSC administration resulted in significant numbers of donor cells populating demyelinating areas of the brain. It was observed that especially oligodendrocyte progenitors were markedly increased in these demyelinating regions, with large proportion of them being of donor origin. These donor oligodendrocyte precursors had in fact remyelinated axons, and additionally reduced astrogliosis and the extent of demyelination and axonal loss. These changes culminated in a suppression of the functional impairment caused by EAE. More recent EAE studies have built on this information and indicated that platelet-derived growth factor AA (PDGF-AA) and fibroblast growth factor II (FGF-II) secreted by NSCs are responsible for the activation of host oligodendrocyte progenitor cells, and their further maturation into remyelinating oligodendrocytes (Einstein *et al.*, 2009).

In summary, there is significant evidence that exogenous NSCs, via the secretion of physiologically relevant trophic factors, can stimulate multiple host-based adaptive phenomena such as the activation of endogenous NSCs, stimulation of axonal outgrowth and transport, suppression of pathological protein aggregates, stimulation of myelination, control of oxidative stress, and the inhibition of apoptosis. These phenomena are most effective when the NSCs are

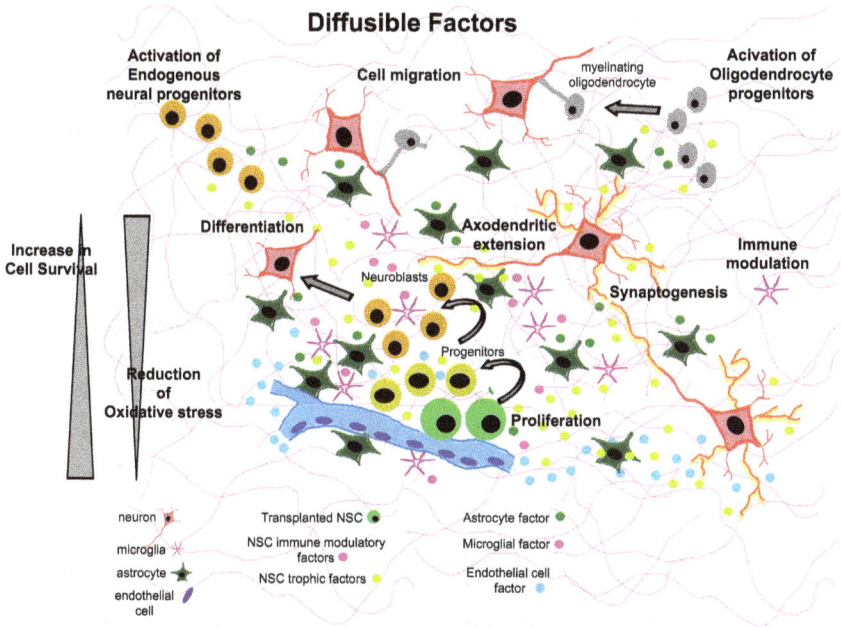

Figure 2. Grafted NSCs can spontaneously express a variety of diffusible factors known to have trophic, immune-modulatory, and cell survival effects. Through cell surface receptors, these soluble factors can directly influence neuronal, glial and vascular cells in their environment, which can in return (and also independently) express similar or additional diffusible molecules. The totality of diffusible factors emanating from these NSC-host interactions can spread over considerable distances in the parenchyma to stimulate neurogenesis, gliogenesis, axodendritic outgrowth, synaptogenesis, modulation of host immune (microglial) activity, and the reduction of oxidative stress.

grafted during early stages of the disease process, and can lead to the substantially improved survival and functioning of host cells (Figure 2).

Immune modulatory factors

A second group of diffusible molecules, mediating the communication between grafted NSCs and their environmental niche, are immune modulators. Many acute as well as chronic neural disorders are characterized by a heightened activation of the immune system and inflammation, events which likely contribute to disease progression. Inflammation could be the primary trigger leading to secondary degeneration in pathologies such as multiple sclerosis (MS), spinal cord injury, brain trauma, stroke, and EAE. Alternatively, inflammation could also occur secondarily after the onset of neurodegeneration in conditions such as PD and Huntington's disease. There is accumulating evidence in some of these disorders that the brain attempts to initiate self-repair through the stimulation of endogenous neurogenesis and gliogenesis. However, it has also been proposed that the presence of inflammation may impede the potency of such regenerative attempts by possibly disturbing the homeostasis of resident stem cell niches (Martino and Pluchino, 2006). In this respect, supplementing the brain with NSCs, via transplantation, appears to modulate inflammation, to create more favorable environments which support host intrinsic regeneration and repair.

In our own studies in a parkinsonian model, implanted NSCs were able to modulate microglial activity and induce efficient neuroprotection through the trophic factor SHH (Madhavan *et al.*, 2012, 2015). Results indicated that SHH, which was expressed by both the grafted NSCs as well as endogenous NSCs (which had been stimulated) directly influenced the immune response. More specifically, it was observed that the inhibition of the endogenous NSC activation via the administration of mitotic inhibitor Ara-C, or diminishing SHH expression in the grafted NSCs using RNA silencing, significantly increased the number of activated cd68$^+$ microglia adjacent to grafted NSCs. Both endogenous NSC depletion, as well as SHH silencing, also drastically reduced the number of undifferentiated nestin-expressing NSCs within donor grafts suggesting a key role for this cell type in regulating the immune response. In particular, the presence of this nestin expressing immature NSC population resulted in a reduction in the glial scar, and the greater survival and function of the grafted NSCs.

In this context, there is supporting evidence that particularly undifferentiated NSCs can interact with immune cells through a variety of cytokines and chemokines to significantly modify inflammation ridden environments such as that in EAE. More specifically,

NSCs have been shown to induce the apoptosis of infiltrating T-lymphocytes (main cell type, along with B cells, in adaptive immune response) to reduce the progression of EAE (Pluchino *et al.*, 2003). Similarly in models of stroke, a lower infiltration of mononuclear cells at the borders of ischemic areas, where NSCs accumulate, has been reported (Kelly *et al.*, 2004).

The molecular dynamics underlying NSC interactions with immune cells have also been investigated. For example, in a report by Cao *et al.* (2011) NSC-expressed factors such as LIF (leukemia inhibitory factor) which can control the differentiation of encephalitogenic T helper 17 (Th17) cells to ameliorate EAE (Cao *et al.*, 2011). In this study, it was established that LIF counteracts IL-6 (interleukin-6)-induced Th17 cell differentiation through ERK (extracellular signal related kinase), and SOCS3 (suppressor of cytokine signaling) dependent inhibition of STAT3 (signal transducer and activator of transcription). T cell-NSC interactions have also been further analyzed in *in vitro* co-culture models where nitric oxide and prostaglandin E2 were found to be involved in the suppression of T cells. Further, NSC secreted HO-1 (hemoxygenase-1) has been implicated in T cell suppression since NSCs pretreated with the HO-1 inhibitor SnPP (protoporphyrin 1X) before co-culture with T cells showed a reduction in their immune suppressive activity (Bonnamain *et al.*, 2012).

In addition to T cells, NSCs have also been shown to affect the maturation of another immune cell type, dendritic cells (DCs). DCs are antigen-presenting cells (also known as *accessory cells*) of the immune system. Their main function is to process antigen material and present it on the cell surface to the T cells of the immune system. Thus, DCs basically act as messengers between the innate and the adaptive immune systems. In this respect, studies have shown a significant down-regulation of co-stimulatory molecules (CD80/B7.1, CD86/B7.2) on dendritic cells extracted from the lymph nodes of NSC injected EAE mice (Pluchino *et al.*, 2009). This finding was also confirmed in NSC-DC co-cultures, and further investigation revealed the involvement of a NSC specific BMP4 (bone morphogenic protein 4) dependent pathway that had hindered DC maturation.

While modulating inflammatory components in the neural environment, NSCs can reciprocally be influenced by immune cells via their own expression of immune-related receptors such as toll-like receptors (TLRs). Toll-like receptors (TLRs) are a class of proteins that play a key role in the innate immune system. They are single membrane-spanning receptors, usually expressed in sentinel cells such as macrophages and dendritic cells, that recognize structurally conserved molecules derived from microbes. In this regard, Rolls *et al.* (2007) showed that NSCs express TLR2 and 4 receptors, which can control their proliferative and differentiation potential (Rolls *et al.*, 2007). The *in vitro* pharmacological activation of TLR2 was able to promote neuronal differentiation with no effects on self-renewal. TLR4 on the other hand was able to inhibit neuronal differentiation and self-renewal. These observations were confirmed *in vivo*, in TLR-2 deficient mice which have impaired hippocampal neurogenesis. Also, the absence of TLR-4 resulted in enhanced NSC proliferation and differentiation. A more recent study indicates that TL-3 can regulate NSC proliferation by inhibiting SHH signaling (Yaddanapudi *et al.*, 2011). These results suggest that the activation of TLRs may regulate neurogenesis in response to injury and inflammation, and that NSCs within major germinal niches in the brain, through TLRs, may adapt their proliferation and differentiation in response to invading inflammatory agents. Because TLRs have evolved not only to recognize a wide array of invading agents (bacterial, viral and fungal), but also signals present during cellular injury and repair, it is plausible that these molecules may modulate proliferation, differentiation and other NSC functions in a number of neurological conditions (Zuany-Amorim *et al.*, 2002).

In a nutshell, NSC-immune system interactions, transpiring through diffusible factors, can temper and even reconfigure deleterious inflammatory environments. Such inflammatory modulation can strengthen endogenous regenerative and reparative processes to result in therapeutic consequences. Also, there is the emergence of the concept that immature undifferentiated NSCs are plausibly the main orchestrators of immune modulatory as well as trophic therapeutic effects. In essence, the undifferentiated NSCs seem to be able to call upon a number of essential intrinsic molecular programs, which had previously allowed them to survive and function in their native environments during early development, to now bear upon the host adult nervous system. The re-utilization of such innate programs would allow implanted NSCs to establish enriched environments in the adult brain, which would serve as hubs of tissue plasticity to support their own survival and function while also influencing the fate of neighboring cells in their microenvironment (Figure 2).

Direct NSC-based Effects

Although indirect effects mediated via diffusible factors have been typically implicated as underlying NSC ability to induce endogenous tissue repair and regeneration, more direct influences on host cells by NSCs have also been established. This section discusses such direct NSC effects mediated through cell-cell, cell-ECM (extra cellular matrix), and gap junction based communication.

Cell-Cell and Cell-ECM interactions

A broad spectrum of growth promoting, and guidance molecules, are active in the central nervous system during neural development and maturation. This includes ECM components such as laminin, and cell adhesion molecules or CAMs (Kamiguchi, 2007). It is known that CAMs associated with growth cones, present at the tips of developing axons of neuronal cells, as well as CAM receptors such as integrins, are crucial for axodendritic outgrowth and correct targeting of post-synaptic structures in the developing nervous system. In this context, it seems natural that transplanted NSCs, trying to integrate into host tissues, would utilize such well-versed interactions between various types of CAMs, as well as CAMs and ECM components, active during development, to influence host cell biology in the adult nervous system. A strong example of such NSC-host interactions has been demonstrated by Ourednik *et al.* (2009) who focused on L1, one of the well-known CAM molecules. L1, which is a glycoprotein, and member of the immunoglobulin superfamily, has been shown to mediate cell survival, neurite outgrowth, axonal extension, synaptic plasticity, and cell migration in the nervous system (Ourednik *et al.*, 2009). Ourednik *et al.* showed that L1 could have another important function, namely improving the neuroprotective efficacy of transplanted NSCs. This effect was shown in experiments where L1 overexpressing NSCs were implanted into aged mice treated chronically with low doses of 1-methyl-4-phenyl-1,2,3,6-tetrahydropyridine (MPTP), which is toxic to substantia nigra dopaminergic neurons. This MPTP regimen induced a dysfunction and protracted loss of nigral dopamine neurons in the model. Under these conditions, an improved survival and migration of grafted NSCs was found, resulting in faster and more robust recovery/protection of host TH neurons, compared to control animals transplanted with non-engineered NSCs. In addition, the efficacy of the L1 overexpressing NSCs was much improved when host astrocytes were also expressing L1. In previous experiments, the authors had shown, in transgenic animals overexpressing L1 in astrocytes, that a robust improvement in the development of major motor and sensory corticospinal tracts occurs. Together, these results indicate that CAMs such as L1 can be powerful regulators NSC biology. These molecules can mediate critical interactions between grafted NSCs and host brain cells, creating another avenue via which NSCs can be influenced and exert their plastic and reparative effects as well. Such CAM-based NSC approaches could be seen to be particularly useful in conditions such as spinal cord injury and ALS, where long distance regeneration of axons would need to occur for meaningful therapeutic improvement.

Gap junctions

Communication via gap junctions has also been recently shown as an important mechanism through which NSCs can exert direct influences on host brain cells. Gap junctions are specialized membrane channels that allow a cell into cell exchange of ions and small molecules (Belousov and Fontes, 2013). Jaderstad *et al.* (2010) investigated the role of these channels in mediating the function of transplanted NSCs (Jaderstad *et al.*, 2010). The authors found in organotypic slice cultures, using calcium imaging, electrophysiology, and dye-coupling techniques, that engrafted human NSCs can integrate functionally and affect host brain cells via gap junction coupling. These gap junctions were formed early after transplantation, and supported interactions between donor NSCs and host cells via synchronized calcium currents.

The role of gap junctions was also further analyzed *in vivo* in animal models of cerebellar Purkinje neuron degeneration (SCA1 and *nervous* mouse mutants). In both these models, grafted NSCs were again able to establish gap junction communication with at-risk host cells, and in fact rescue them (Jaderstad *et al.*, 2010). As a consequence, enhanced host cell survival and function, and behavioral improvements were observed in the NSC-implanted animals. It was inferred that the transfer of plasticity inducing molecules via the gap junctions was plausibly responsible for these neuroprotective effects.

There is also evidence that gap junctions, in addition to acting as conduits to pass molecular signals from one cell to another, can play a crucial role in neuronal migration (Elias *et al.*, 2007). It has been reported that the two fused gap junction hemi-channels can in fact serve as a form of adhesion between the migrating neurons and the neural stem cell fibers. To establish the role of gap junctions in neuronal migration, this study focused on the activity of specific Connexins (Cx), in a series of experiments in the developing rat brain. In particular, two of these proteins were investigated — Cx26 and Cx43 — because it was determined that they were expressed at high levels in migrating neurons and along radial fibers. Blocking the activity of either Connexin subunit significantly impaired neuronal migration to the neocortex, resulting in a notable change in the final distribution and location of the neurons.

These reports indicate that gap junctions between NSCs and neighboring cells in their environment can act as conduits for the transfer of plasticity inducing and protective molecules, and also

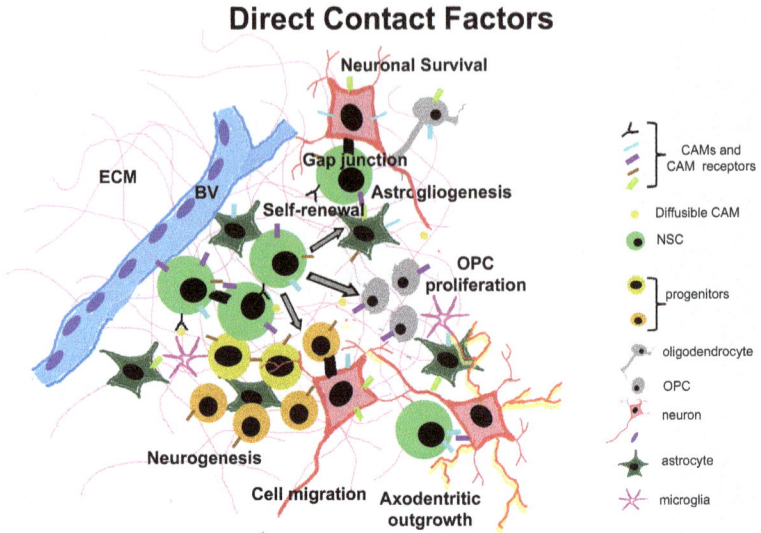

Figure 3. Transplanted NSCs can also exert endogenous plastic and reparative influences on the nervous system via direct cell-cell and cell-extracellular matrix (ECM) interactions. A number of cell adhesion molecules (CAMs) such as integrins, L1, N-Cadherin can mediate physical communications between NSCs and host cells. ECM molecules such as laminin and fibronectin can mediate the NSC-ECM communication. Additionally, other direct interactions can be mediated via gap junction channels forming in between NSCs and host neurons. Such CAM, ECM, and gap junction-based interactions with NSCs can result in improved survival, and a multitude of regenerative effects on host cells including neurogenesis, gliogenesis and remyelination, and neuritic extension.

directly influence cell migration. Such effects when articulated in pathological environments can be envisioned to help support the survival and function of otherwise endangered host populations, and result in therapeutic effects (Figure 3).

Innate Stress Resistance as a Core Feature Supporting NSC-based Therapeutic Effects

NSCs need to be able to survive and function optimally in unfavorable environments ridden with increasing oxidative stress, inflammation, and other cellular stresses, in order to exert their therapeutic effects during aging and neurodegeneration. Such age-associated environmental changes are recognized to negatively affect the function of endogenous NSCs residing in the brain's two major neurogenic niches, the SVZ and DG of the hippocampus, and have been discussed, in part, in other chapters in this book (Conover and Shook, 2011; Encinas *et al.*, 2011). Nevertheless, it is important to note that the endogenous NSCs still do persist in the aging brain, and are able to increase their regenerative activity under suitable conditions (Ourednik *et al.*, 2002; Hattiangady *et al.*, 2007; Park *et al.*, 2009). In this regard, there are indications that the high expression of molecules that help counteract various environmental stresses, such as antioxidants, DNA repair genes, and detoxification enzymes, maybe naturally enriched in NSCs (Ivanova *et al.*, 2002; Ramalho-Santos *et al.*, 2002). It is possible that NSC populations may have evolutionarily developed such intrinsic abilities to combat the build-up of reactive oxygen species (ROS, which lead to oxidative stress) that can threaten their very existence during aging and pathology.

In this context, it has been documented that SOD1 is expressed highly in postnatal NSCs in the SVZ and its continuation, the rostral migratory stream, as well as the SGZ of hippocampus (Faiz *et al.*, 2006). Some of our own work has also compared NSCs and mature neural cell types in terms of their sensitivity to oxidative stress (Madhavan *et al.*, 2006). More specifically NSCs, from the early postnatal brain, and their differentiated neuronal and glial counterparts, were exposed to 3-nitropropionic acid (3-NP) which induces the generation of ROS and oxidative stress. Firstly, it was observed that the undifferentiated NSCs, at a basal level, harbored lower ROS and higher antioxidants as compared to mature neural cells. This finding supports the aforementioned idea that a higher expression of antioxidant mechanisms may be a fundamental NSC feature. Secondly, when the cells were challenged with 3-NP, NSCs were quickly able to upregulate the expression of antioxidants such as glutathione peroxidase (GPx), superoxide dismutase 2 (SOD2) and uncoupling protein 2 (UCP2) to survive robustly. In contrast, the mature neural cells were marked by substantially increasing ROS levels and exhibited apoptosis and cell death. In support of these *in vitro* results, analysis of antioxidant expression in SVZ NSCs of adult mice *in vivo* revealed a high steady state expression of GPx and UCP2 compared to surrounding neural cells. Essentially, these findings indicate that adult NSCs are probably well equipped to manage oxidative stress and perhaps, other forms of pathological insults as well.

The abovementioned studies were followed up by further *in vivo* investigations, in which postnatal NSCs were implanted into a 3-NP mouse model of Huntington's disease (Madhavan *et al.*, 2005, 2007). Here the NSCs were able to protect striatal neurons and reduce behavioral symptoms. Examination of mechanisms underlying the neuroprotection using an *in vitro* co-culture system and also *in vivo* histology revealed that under 3-NP induced oxidative stress, the NSCs were able to express trophic factors such as BDNF, ciliary neurotrophic factor (CNTF), and VEGF. The implanted NSCs were also able to recruit host astrocytes which also contributed to the trophic factor pool via the expression of CNTF and VEGF. This led to the up-regulation of the expression of the antioxidant superoxide dismutase-2 (SOD2) in the endangered host striatal neurons while the NSCs themselves maintained high levels of SOD2. VEGF was the major factor determined to directly participate in signaling events leading to the increased expression of SOD2. In the end, this study indicated that NSCs can survive in oxidatively challenged environments, and induce protective effects in host cells through the direct activation of antioxidant defense mechanisms which were controlled by trophic factor signaling. Thus, high antioxidant expression may be one innate feature of NSCs which allows them to survive and wield their beneficial influence on host brain cells upon transplantation.

In support of these studies, there is evidence from oligodendrocyte progenitor cells (OPCs) that indicates that ROS can also act as an important regulator of the stem cell function with respect to determining the balance between self-renewal/proliferation and differentiation (Smith *et al.*, 2000; Noble *et al.*, 2003; Prozorovski *et al.*, 2008). More specifically, a reducing intracellular state promotes proliferation through a better response to mitogens and promotes survival. On the other hand, an oxidizing intracellular milieu encourages differentiation and apoptosis (Noble *et al.*, 2005). As in OPCs, there is evidence for similar redox regulation in NSCs. The growth factor fibroblast growth factor (FGF), used to culture NSCs, reduces oxidative stress indicating that pathways promoting NSC proliferation and self-renewal may in part function through the regulation of ROS (Limoli *et al.*, 2004). In addition, it has been reported that Forkhead Box O (FOXO) proteins, which are sensitive to oxidative stress, may promote NSC proliferation by controlling ROS through the expression of detoxification enzymes such as peroxiredoxin, glutathione peroxidase 1, and sestrin3 (Paik *et al.*, 2007). Thus, clearly, it is important for such intrinsic protective mechanisms to be maintained within NSCs to allow for their robust survival functioning in challenging microenvironments present during aging and neurodegeneration (Paik *et al.*, 2009; Renault *et al.*, 2009).

Conclusions

To conclude, NSCs can significantly enhance endogenous regenerative, reparative, and protective capacities in the adult as well as the aging brain after transplantation. These phenomena are a testament to powerful mechanisms by which NSCs may exert their therapeutic effects, in addition to their more traditional roles in cell replacement. The basis of these NSC effects lies not only in their intrinsic capabilities, but importantly in their interactions with the 'niche' or local environment of the brain. In particular, these graft-host interactions, which are critical in determining donor and host cell behavior and fate, can surface in the form of an intricate network between endogenous NSCs, transplanted NSCs, and other mature host cells, to lead to regeneration and repair. Such NSC networking particularly seems to be effective in early stages of neural degeneration when pathology has not completely taken root. Hence, by capitalizing upon this NSC capacity, it may after all be possible to tackle the significant challenge posed by age-related neural disorders. Indeed, slowing, impeding, or even preventing age-related neural degeneration may become a distinct future possibility.

References

Alvarez-Buylla A, Lim DA (2004) For the long run: maintaining germinal niches in the adult brain. *Neuron* 41:683–686.

Andres RH, Horie N, Slikker W, Keren-Gill H, Zhan K, Sun G, Manley NC, Pereira MP, Sheikh LA, McMillan EL, Schaar BT, Svendsen CN, Bliss TM, Steinberg GK (2011) Human neural stem cells enhance structural plasticity and axonal transport in the ischaemic brain. *Brain* 134:1777–1789.

Arvidsson A, Collin T, Kirik D, Kokaia Z, Lindvall O (2002) Neuronal replacement from endogenous precursors in the adult brain after stroke. *Nat Med* 8:963–970.

Belousov AB, Fontes JD (2013) Neuronal gap junctions: making and breaking connections during development and injury. *Trends Neurosci* 36:227–236.

Bonnamain V, Mathieux E, Thinard R, Thebault P, Nerriere-Daguin V, Leveque X, Anegon I, Vanhove B, Neveu I, Naveilhan P (2012) Expression of heme oxygenase-1 in neural stem/progenitor cells as a potential mechanism to evade host immune response. *Stem Cells* 30:2342–2353.

Cao W, Yang Y, Wang Z, Liu A, Fang L, Wu F, Hong J, Shi Y, Leung S, Dong C, Zhang JZ (2011) Leukemia inhibitory factor inhibits T helper 17 cell differentiation and confers treatment effects of neural progenitor cell therapy in autoimmune disease. *Immunity* 35:273–284.

Conover JC, Shook BA (2011) Aging of the subventricular zone neural stem cell niche. *Aging Dis* 2:49–63.

Corti S, Locatelli F, Papadimitriou D, Del Bo R, Nizzardo M, Nardini M, Donadoni C, Salani S, Fortunato F, Strazzer S, Bresolin N, Comi GP (2007) Neural stem cells LewisX+ CXCR4+ modify disease progression in an amyotrophic lateral sclerosis model. *Brain* 130:1289–1305.

Einstein O, Friedman-Levi Y, Grigoriadis N, Ben-Hur T (2009) Transplanted neural precursors enhance host brain-derived myelin regeneration. *J Neurosci* 29:15694–15702.

Elias LA, Wang DD, Kriegstein AR (2007) Gap junction adhesion is necessary for radial migration in the neocortex. *Nature* 448:901–907.

Encinas JM, Michurina TV, Peunova N, Park JH, Tordo J, Peterson DA, Fishell G, Koulakov A, Enikolopov G (2011) Division-coupled astrocytic differentiation and age-related depletion of neural stem cells in the adult hippocampus. *Cell Stem Cell* 8:566–579.

Faiz M, Acarin L, Peluffo H, Villapol S, Castellano B, Gonzalez B (2006) Antioxidant Cu/Zn SOD: expression in postnatal brain progenitor cells. *Neurosci Lett* 401:71–76.

Garzon-Muvdi T, Quinones-Hinojosa A (2009) Neural stem cell niches and homing: recruitment and integration into functional tissues. *ILAR J* 51:3–23.

Hattiangady B, Shuai B, Cai J, Coksaygan T, Rao MS, Shetty AK (2007) Increased dentate neurogenesis after grafting of glial restricted progenitors or neural stem cells in the aging hippocampus. *Stem Cells* 25:2104–2117.

Horie N, Pereira MP, Niizuma K, Sun G, Keren-Gill H, Encarnacion A, Shamloo M, Hamilton SA, Jiang K, Huhn S, Palmer TD, Bliss TM, Steinberg GK (2011) Transplanted stem cell-secreted vascular endothelial growth factor effects poststroke recovery, inflammation, and vascular repair. *Stem Cells* 29:274–285.

Ivanova NB, Dimos JT, Schaniel C, Hackney JA, Moore KA, Lemischka IR (2002) A stem cell molecular signature. *Science* 298:601–604.

Jaderstad J, Jaderstad LM, Li J, Chintawar S, Salto C, Pandolfo M, Ourednik V, Teng YD, Sidman RL, Arenas E, Snyder EY, Herlenius E (2010) Communication via gap junctions underlies early functional and beneficial interactions between grafted neural stem cells and the host. *Proc Nat Acad Sci USA* 107:5184–5189.

Kamiguchi H (2007) The role of cell adhesion molecules in axon growth and guidance. *Adv Exp Med Biol* 621:95–103.

Kelly S, Bliss TM, Shah AK, Sun GH, Ma M, Foo WC, Masel J, Yenari MA, Weissman IL, Uchida N, Palmer T, Steinberg GK (2004) Transplanted human fetal neural stem cells survive, migrate, and differentiate in ischemic rat cerebral cortex. *Proc Nat Acad Sci USA* 101:11839–11844.

Limoli CL, Giedzinski E, Rola R, Otsuka S, Palmer TD, Fike JR (2004) Radiation response of neural precursor cells: linking cellular sensitivity to cell cycle checkpoints, apoptosis and oxidative stress. *Rad Res* 161:17–27.

Lu P, Jones LL, Snyder EY, Tuszynski MH (2003) Neural stem cells constitutively secrete neurotrophic factors and promote extensive host axonal growth after spinal cord injury. *Exp Neurol* 181:115–129.

Macas J, Nern C, Plate KH, Momma S (2006) Increased generation of neuronal progenitors after ischemic injury in the aged adult human forebrain. *J Neurosci* 26:13114–13119.

Madhavan L, Collier TJ (2010) A synergistic approach for neural repair: cell transplantation and induction of endogenous precursor cell activity. *Neuropharmacology* 58:835–844.

Madhavan L, Ourednik V, Ourednik J (2005) Grafted neural stem cells shield the host environment from oxidative stress. *Ann NY Acad Sci* 1049:185–188.

Madhavan L, Ourednik V, Ourednik J (2006) Increased "vigilance" of antioxidant mechanisms in neural stem cells potentiates their capability to resist oxidative stress. *Stem Cells* 24:2110–2119.

Madhavan L, Ourednik V, Ourednik J (2007) Neural stem/progenitor cells initiate the formation of cellular networks that provide neuroprotection by growth factor–modulated antioxidant expression. *Stem Cells* 26:254–265.

Madhavan L, Daley BF, Paumier KL, Collier TJ (2009) Transplantation of subventricular zone neural precursors induces an endogenous precursor cell response in a rat model of Parkinson's disease. *J Comp Neurol* 515:102–115.

Madhavan L, Daley BF, Sortwell CE, Collier TJ (2012) Endogenous neural precursors influence grafted neural stem cells and contribute to neuroprotection in the parkinsonian rat. *Eur J Neurosci* 35:883–895.

Madhavan L, Daley BF, Davidson BL, Boudreau RL, Lipton JW, Cole-Strauss A, Steece-Collier K, and Collier TJ (2015) Sonic hedgehog controls the phenotypic fate and therapeutic efficacy of grafted neural precursor cells in a model of nigrostriatal degeneration.

Marti-Fabregas J, Romaguera-Ros M, Gomez-Pinedo U, Martinez-Ramirez S, Jimenez-Xarrie E, Marin R, Marti-Vilalta JL, Garcia-Verdugo JM (2010) Proliferation in the human ipsilateral subventricular zone after ischemic stroke. *Neurology* 74:357–365.

Martino G, Pluchino S (2006) The therapeutic potential of neural stem cells. *Nat Rev Neuroscience* 7:395–406.

Mecha M, Feliu A, Carrillo-Salinas FJ, Mestre L, Guaza C (2013) Mobilization of progenitors in the subventricular zone to undergo oligodendrogenesis in the Theiler's virus model of multiple sclerosis: implications for remyelination at lesions sites. *Exp Neurol* 250:348–352.

Mine Y, Tatarishvili J, Oki K, Monni E, Kokaia Z, Lindvall O (2013) Grafted human neural stem cells enhance several steps of endogenous neurogenesis and improve behavioral recovery after middle cerebral artery occlusion in rats. *Neurobiol Dis* 52:191–203.

Minger SL, Ekonomou A, Carta EM, Chinoy A, Perry RH, Ballard CG (2007) Endogenous neurogenesis in the human brain following cerebral infarction. *Regen Med* 2:69–74.

Noble M, Mayer-Proschel M, Proschel C (2005) Redox regulation of precursor cell function: insights and paradoxes. *Antioxid Redox Signa* 7:1456–1467.

Noble M, Smith J, Power J, Mayer-Proschel M (2003) Redox state as a central modulator of precursor cell function. *Annals NY Acad Sci* 991:251–271.

Ourednik J, Ourednik V, Lynch WP, Schachner M, Snyder EY (2002) Neural stem cells display an inherent mechanism for rescuing dysfunctional neurons. *Nat Biotechnol* 20:1103–1110.

Ourednik V, Ourednik J (2005) Graft/Host relationships in the developing and regenerating CNS of mammals. *Ann N Y Acad Sci* 1049:172–184.

Ourednik V, Ourednik J (2007) Plasticity of the central nervous system and formation of "auxiliary niches" after stem cell grafting: an essay. *Cell Transplant* 16:263–271.

Ourednik V, Ourednik J, Xu Y, Zhang Y, Lynch WP, Snyder EY, Schachner M (2009) Cross-talk between stem cells and the dysfunctional brain is facilitated by manipulating the niche: evidence from an adhesion molecule. *Stem Cells* 27:2846–2856.

Paik JH, Kollipara R, Chu G, Ji H, Xiao Y, Ding Z, Miao L, Tothova Z, Horner JW, Carrasco DR, Jiang S, Gilliland DG, Chin L, Wong WH, Castrillon DH, DePinho RA (2007) FoxOs are lineage-restricted redundant tumor suppressors and regulate endothelial cell homeostasis. *Cell* 128:309–323.

Paik JH, Ding Z, Narurkar R, Ramkissoon S, Muller F, Kamoun WS, Chae SS, Zheng H, Ying H, Mahoney J, Hiller D, Jiang S, Protopopov A, Wong WH, Chin L, Ligon KL, DePinho RA (2009) FoxOs cooperatively regulate diverse pathways governing neural stem cell homeostasis. *Cell Stem Cell* 5:540–553.

Park DH, Eve DJ, Sanberg PR, Musso Iii J, Bachstetter AD, Wolfson A, Schlunk A, Baradez MO, Sinden JD, Bickford PC, Gemma C (2009) Increased neuronal proliferation in the dentate gyrus of aged rats following neural stem cell implantation. *Stem Cells Dev* 19:175–180.

Pluchino S, Quattrini A, Brambilla E, Gritti A, Salani G, Dina G, Galli R, Del Carro U, Amadio S, Bergami A, Furlan R, Comi G, Vescovi AL, Martino G (2003) Injection of adult neurospheres induces recovery in a chronic model of multiple sclerosis. *Nature* 422:688–694.

Pluchino S, Zanotti L, Brambilla E, Rovere-Querini P, Capobianco A, Alfaro-Cervello C, Salani G, Cossetti C, Borsellino G, Battistini L, Ponzoni M, Doglioni C, Garcia-Verdugo JM, Comi G, Manfredi AA,

Martino G (2009) Immune regulatory neural stem/precursor cells protect from central nervous system autoimmunity by restraining dendritic cell function. *PloS One* 4:e5959.

Prozorovski T, Schulze-Topphoff U, Glumm R, Baumgart J, Schroter F, Ninnemann O, Siegert E, Bendix I, Brustle O, Nitsch R, Zipp F, Aktas O (2008) Sirt1 contributes critically to the redox-dependent fate of neural progenitors. *Nat Cell Biol* 10:385–394.

Ramalho-Santos M, Yoon S, Matsuzaki Y, Mulligan RC, Melton DA (2002) "Stemness": transcriptional profiling of embryonic and adult stem cells. *Science* 298:597–600.

Redmond DE, Jr., Bjugstad KB, Teng YD, Ourednik V, Ourednik J, Wakeman DR, Parsons XH, Gonzalez R, Blanchard BC, Kim SU, Gu Z, Lipton SA, Markakis EA, Roth RH, Elsworth JD, Sladek JR, Jr., Sidman RL, Snyder EY (2007) Behavioral improvement in a primate Parkinson's model is associated with multiple homeostatic effects of human neural stem cells. *Proc Nat Acad Sci USA* 104:12175–12180.

Renault VM, Rafalski VA, Morgan AA, Salih DA, Brett JO, Webb AE, Villeda SA, Thekkat PU, Guillerey C, Denko NC, Palmer TD, Butte AJ, Brunet A (2009) FoxO3 regulates neural stem cell homeostasis. *Cell Stem Cell* 5:527–539.

Riquelme PA, Drapeau E, Doetsch F (2008) Brain micro-ecologies: neural stem cell niches in the adult mammalian brain. Philos Trans R Soc Lond B Biol Sci 363:123–137.

Rocha MJ, Chen Y, Oliveira GR, Morris M (2005) Physiological regulation of brain angiotensin receptor mRNA in AT1a deficient mice. *Exp Neurol* 195:229–235.

Rolls A, Shechter R, London A, Ziv Y, Ronen A, Levy R, Schwartz M (2007) Toll-like receptors modulate adult hippocampal neurogenesis. *Nat Cell biol* 9:1081–1088.

Smith J, Ladi E, Mayer-Proschel M, Noble M (2000) Redox state is a central modulator of the balance between self-renewal and differentiation in a dividing glial precursor cell. *Proc Nat Acad Sci USA* 97:10032–10037.

Thored P, Arvidsson A, Cacci E, Ahlenius H, Kallur T, Darsalia V, Ekdahl CT, Kokaia Z, Lindvall O (2006) Persistent production of neurons from adult brain stem cells during recovery after stroke. *Stem Cells* 24:739–747.

Tuszynski MH, Grill R, Jones LL, Brant A, Blesch A, Low K, Lacroix S, Lu P (2003) NT-3 gene delivery elicits growth of chronically injured corticospinal axons and modestly improves functional deficits after chronic scar resection. *Exp Neurol* 181:47–56.

Yaddanapudi K, De Miranda J, Hornig M, Lipkin WI (2011) Toll-like receptor 3 regulates neural stem cell proliferation by modulating the Sonic Hedgehog pathway. *PloS One* 6:e26766.

Yamashita T, Ninomiya M, Hernandez Acosta P, Garcia-Verdugo JM, Sunabori T, Sakaguchi M, Adachi K, Kojima T, Hirota Y, Kawase T, Araki N, Abe K, Okano H, Sawamoto K (2006) Subventricular zone-derived neuroblasts migrate and differentiate into mature neurons in the post-stroke adult striatum. *J Neurosci* 26:6627–6636.

Yasuhara T, Matsukawa N, Hara K, Yu G, Xu L, Maki M, Kim SU, Borlongan CV (2006) Transplantation of human neural stem cells exerts neuroprotection in a rat model of Parkinson's disease. *J Neurosci* 26:12497–12511.

Zuany-Amorim C, Hastewell J, Walker C (2002) Toll-like receptors as potential therapeutic targets for multiple diseases. *Nat Rev Drug Discov* 1:797–807.

Chapter 4

Neural Stem Cells and the Effects of Cancer Therapy

Lauren S.Y. Wood and Michelle Monje

Radiotherapy and chemotherapy extend and improve the lives of cancer patients. However, use of these therapies frequently results in a debilitating neuropsychiatric syndrome characterized by impaired memory function, attention, speed of information processing and multitasking; these deficits are particularly severe and memory dysfunction prominent when cancer therapy is directed at the central nervous system (CNS). The cellular mechanism underlying these neurocognitive deficits involves damage to neural stem and precursor cell populations. This chapter highlights what is known about the consequences of radiation therapy and chemotherapeutic agents upon these cell populations in the context of radiation-induced cognitive decline and chemotherapy-induced cognitive dysfunction.

Introduction

Cancer therapy has a long history of extending, improving and saving lives. Over a period of forty years from 1969 to 2009, the mortality rate of childhood cancer decreased by 68% largely due to advances made in how cancer is treated. In 2013, there were an estimated 14 million survivors of cancer in the United States

(American Cancer Society, 2013). The two major mainstays of treatment for cancer — radiotherapy and chemotherapy — however, are not without their devastating side effects.

Soon after the discovery of X-rays by Wilhelm Roentgen in 1895, the application of this new technology as radiation therapy to the human body and the field of medicine quickly followed, with consequences ranging from the less severe (e.g. hair loss) to traumatic inflammatory injury in the regions of exposure, such as skin, gastrointestinal tract, and even brain (Daniel, 1896; Stevens, 1896; Walsh, 1897). X-rays were demonstrated to damage DNA and predispose individuals to cancer; Roentgen himself died of intestinal carcinoma in 1923 (Bauer *et al.*, 1938; Howel and Roberts, 1928; The Nobel Foundation, 1967).

Chemotherapeutic agents were first described as potential agents of chemical warfare — with nitrogen mustards as a chief example — during World War II, and were subsequently applied to blood cancers once it was appreciated that a mechanism of action was to suppress cells of the bone marrow (Gilman and Philips, 1946; Goodman *et al.*, 1946). However, notable toxicity has been recognized from the beginning of chemotherapeutics use, including short-term effects such as nausea, vomiting, loss of appetite, and longer-term yet typically impermanent effects such as leukopenia, thrombocytopenia, and anemia (Gilman and Philips, 1946).

It is not surprising then that an increased survival rate in cancer patients — patients treated with chemotherapy and/or radiation — is associated with chronic health issues related to cancer therapy. Childhood cancer survivors utilize healthcare more frequently as adults compared to healthy counterparts (Rebholz *et al.*, 2011). Some of the major problems that patients struggle with after cancer therapy are deficits in memory, attention and concentration in pediatric and adult populations alike, representing an important neuropsychiatric component to the side effects associated with chemotherapy and radiation therapy (Siegel *et al.*, 2011; Oeffinger *et al.*, 2010; Langer *et al.*, 2002; Armstrong *et al.*, 2009; Kesler *et al.*, 2011).

Neural stem cells in the postnatal brain

As chemotherapy and radiotherapy exert their effects on dividing cells, leading them to halt the progression of and even eliminate cancers, cognitive impairment seen in patients suggests a dysfunction induced by cancer treatments in mitotically active neural stem and precursor cells. Neural stem and precursor cell populations serve an important role in the postnatal development and plasticity of the nervous system. The ability to generate new cells in the postnatal brain is vital for processes such as learning and memory, and maintenance and repair (Snyder *et al.*, 2005; Clelland *et al.*, 2009). The subgranular zone (SGZ) of the dentate gyrus in the hippocampus and the subventricular zone (SVZ) contain two major populations of neural stem cells. Hippocampal neural stem cells primarily contribute to new neuron production — neurogenesis — in the SGZ, which is important for some types of memory function. The SVZ contains stem cells that contribute neuroblasts which migrate to the olfactory bulb for olfactory bulb neurogenesis, and oligodendrocyte precursor cells that travel throughout the brain for myelin remodeling or repair (Doetsch *et al.*, 1999; for review see Zhao, Deng and Gage, 2008). However, the existence of neurogenesis within the adult human olfactory bulb remains controversial, as this phenomenon has predominantly been studied in rodents (Bergmann *et al.*, 2012).

Neural precursor cell function depends not only on the integrity of the cell, but also on the integrity of the neurogenic or gliogenic microenvironment (Monje *et al.*, 2002). Figure 1 delineates the major neural stem and precursor populations in the postnatal brain and the differentiation lineages of a neural stem cell. This figure highlights neural stem and precursor cell populations thought to contribute to cognitive functioning, in addition to the niches (microenvironments) frequently affected by cancer therapy.

While cancer therapies involve treatment modalities outside of chemo- and radiotherapy including steroids, hormones, and targeted therapeutic agents, this chapter will highlight the effects of traditional cancer therapy on cognition — specifically the neurocognitive sequelae seen after radio- and chemotherapies — and what is known about the underlying cellular etiology.

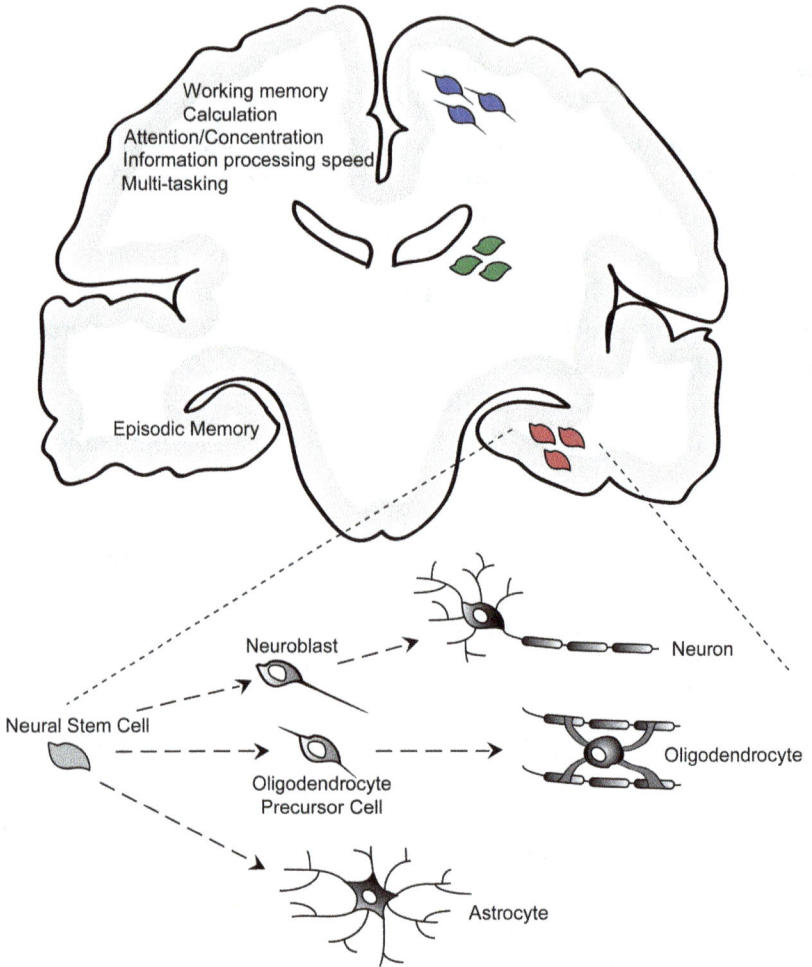

Figure 1. Neural precursor populations in the postnatal human brain. Coronal section view of the human brain with neural stem cell and progenitor cell populations in their native locations, and neural stem cell differentiation lineages. Oligodendrocyte precursor cells (blue) exist throughout the brain, whereas there are two known neural stem cell niches: subventricular zone (green cells) and subgranular zone of the dentate gyrus of the hippocampus (red cells). The cognitive functions associated with particular areas of the brain and mediated by maturation of precursor cell populations of those areas are listed on the corresponding left half of the brain. Adapted from Gibson and Monje, 2012.

Neurocognitive Sequelae of Radiotherapy

Stages of radiation encephalopathy can be classified according to time elapsed after radiation therapy: acute (during irradiation); early-delayed (or sub-acute, up to 6 months after irradiation); late-delayed (or chronic, 6 months and after) (Sheline *et al.*, 1980). The acute stage can include anxiety, confusion, nausea and vomiting due to radiation-induced cerebral edema, from which recovery can be expected; in rare cases, severe cerebral edema and death can occur (Centers for Disease Control and Prevention [CDC], 2005). Early-delayed toxicity can manifest itself as encephalopathy, cognitive dysfunction, somnolence syndrome (excessive drowsiness, headache, fever, nausea, vomiting), and/or worsening of pre-existing neuro-logical symptoms; these subacute symptoms are thought to result from transient radiation-induced demyelination. Late-delayed toxicity can be comprised of cognitive dysfunction (called radiation-induced cognitive decline), hydrocephalus *ex vacuo*, cerebral atrophy, dementia, and necrosis (Keime-Guibert *et al.*, 1998; Malamud *et al.*, 1954; Pennybacker and Russell, 1948; Crompton and Layton, 1961).

With a focus on the neurocognitive sequelae, adults and children undergoing radiation therapy that involves the central nervous system (CNS) exhibit a constellation of chronic neurocognitive deficits including issues with episodic memory (encoding new information), speed of information processing, concentration and attention (Armstrong *et al.*, 2009; Langer *et al.*, 2002; Anderson *et al.*, 2000; Crossen *et al.*, 1994). Episodic memory is localized to the hippocampus, whereas attention, concentration and speed of information processing are associated with subcortical white matter, particularly of the frontal lobes.

The severity of symptoms can range from mild cognitive impairment to frank dementia, and appear to be dependent upon the dose of radiation delivered, fractionation schedule, volume of the brain irradiated, and concurrent administration of chemotherapy (Imperato *et al.*, 1990; Lawrence *et al.*, 2010). Patient demographics that are associated with increased severity of neurocognitive seque-lae include extremes of age of the patient (especially less than age 7 or older than age 65) and female sex (Sheline *et al.*, 1980; Christie *et al.*, 1995; Edelstein *et al.*, 2011; Cousens *et al.*, 1988; Campbell *et al.*, 2007). While efforts have been made to refine cancer therapies involving radiotherapy by limiting the maximum dosage at a given time and limiting exposure to unaffected areas when possible, chronic neurocognitive deficits continue to persist; severity of symptoms appear to worsen over time since exposure to radiation (Crompton and Layton, 1961; Crossen *et al.*, 1994). Leukoencephalopathy, or white matter pathology, present on neuroimaging is common after radiation therapy and is associated with neurocognitive sequelae; however, the lack of leukoencephalopathy is not necessarily predictive of a positive neurocognitive outcome (Keime-Guibert *et al.*, 1998; Armstrong *et al.*, 1995; Ebi *et al.*, 2013).

Cellular and Molecular Mechanisms Underlying Neurocognitive Sequelae of Radiotherapy

An early study of the pathological effects of whole-brain radiation in macaques by Clemente and Holst in 1954 focused on three major components of the brain affected by radiation therapy: (1) neurons; (2) glia and myelin; (3) vasculature. The literature describing the pathogenesis of radiation encephalopathy continues to build, and as such, hypotheses regarding the mechanisms underlying neurocognitive deficits tend to fall into these categories, and the interdependence of these components must be emphasized. As the focus of this chapter is upon neural stem cells, the direct effect of cancer therapy upon the vasculature of the brain will not be discussed.

Neurons and neurogenesis

Sensitivity of neural stem cells and neurogenesis to irradiation has been extensively studied. Apoptosis — or programmed cell death — in the brain after radiation exposure in juvenile rat brains occurs acutely within the SVZ, one of two recognized neural stem cell niches (Bellinzona *et al.*, 1996; Tada *et al.*, 1999). Similarly, fractionated radiotherapy in rodents induces apoptosis in the neural stem cells of the dentate gyrus of the hippocampus, a brain structure vital to learning and memory, and one that serves as the other major site of adult neurogenesis aside from the SVZ (Peissner *et al.*, 1999; Tada *et al.*, 2000). Following this early apoptosis, the population of neural stem cells in the hippocampus recovers, but a near complete ablation of hippocampal neurogenesis has also been described after exposure to radiation in both rodent models (Monje *et al.*, 2002; Mizumatsu *et al.*, 2003) and in humans (Monje *et al.*, 2007). Neuronal precursor proliferation and differentiation were found to be vulnerable to low and clinically-relevant doses of radiation within the subgranular zone (SGZ) of the hippocampus, where neural stem cells reside (Parent *et al.*, 1999; Snyder *et al.*, 2001).

Furthermore, researchers have also been able to demonstrate deficits in hippocampal learning and memory in young and adult rodents exposed to radiation therapy; these models exhibit increased apoptosis and hindered neurogenesis within the dentate gyrus, further supporting a link between neurocognitive deficits and radiation therapy through damage to neural stem cells (Madsen *et al.*, 2003; Rola *et al.*, 2004).

While the neural stem cell populations do recover in number by one month following a single fraction of clinically-relevant irradiation in the rat, the growth potential of these cells was found to be limited in a dose-dependent fashion (Monje *et al.*, 2002). Furthermore, the neurogenic microenvironment is chronically altered. Experimental manipulation demonstrated that irradiated neural precursor cells are able to differentiate *in vitro*, but transplanted non-irradiated neural precursor cells are unable to differentiate in an irradiated hippocampus, suggesting that the neurogenic microenvironment plays a large role in radiation-induced damage to hippocampal neurogenesis (Monje *et al.*, 2002).

Cognitive dysfunction following irradiation is not due only to impairment of neurogenesis. While mature neurons exposed to radiation doses in the clinical range generally survive the exposure, this does not mean that neuronal function following radiation is entirely normal. Electrophysiological recordings conducted in the irradiated hippocampi of guinea pigs demonstrated that excitatory post-synaptic potentials of afferent neurons were less able to generate an action potential within the hippocampus, suggesting that radiation exposure alters the ability of mature neurons to transmit signals and perhaps their ability to encode memories (Pellmar *et al.*, 1990). The receptor implicated in radiation-induced neuronal dysfunction is vital to synaptic plasticity: the N-methyl-D-aspartate (NMDA) receptor. Coupled with impaired performance in memory tests, adult rats exhibited an up-regulation of NMDA receptor subunits after whole-brain irradiation within the hippocampus, which may lead to or reflect altered signal transmission at the synapse (Shi *et al.*, 2006). Researchers have also investigated neuronal dysfunction following irradiation by looking at the expression levels of immediate early genes (IEG), or genes that are expressed immediately after cellular activation and in the brain can serve as a proxy for neuronal activation. Mice exposed to radiation and allowed to explore a novel environment to induce IEG expression showed significantly fewer neurons expressing the IEG and an overall lower expression level within the hippocampus chronically (Rosi *et al.*, 2008). Overall, these results suggest that neuronal dysfunction secondary to irradiation may also contribute to cognitive impairment.

Glia and gliogenesis: oligodendrocytes and myelin

One type of glial cell affected by radiation is the oligodendrocyte, the myelinating cell of the central nervous system. Irradiation of the CNS has been noted histologically and on neuroimaging to specifically damage white matter and cause demyelination in humans particularly in the late-delayed phase after high-dose irradiation (Keime-Guibert *et al.*, 1998; Martins *et al.*, 1977; Dooms *et al.*, 1986; Asai *et al.*, 1989; Valk and Dillon, 1991); animal models have been generated to reproduce this (Chiang *et al.*, 1993a; Sano *et al.*, 2000; Panagiotakos *et al.*, 2007). Given this consequence, researchers investigated the oligodendrocyte as a target cell of high dose radiation in the CNS. Studies showed that the identity of the cells undergoing apoptosis in the white matter of the irradiated rodent CNS were oligodendrocytes (Li *et al.*, 1996; Shinohara *et al.*, 1997; Kurita *et al.*, 2001). A model of mouse designed to lack expression of p53, a tumor suppressor gene, demonstrated that oligodendrocytes without this gene did not undergo apoptosis after exposure to high-dose radiation compared to wild-type mice with p53 intact. The expressed protein of the gene p53 normally functions as a regulator of the cell cycle; it induces cell death if cellular DNA is irreparably damaged. This knockout mouse study suggests that p53 is the mechanism by which normal oligodendrocytes undergo apoptosis after DNA damage from irradiation (Chow *et al.*, 2000).

Histopathological analysis of specimens from humans who underwent radiotherapy showed a long-lasting consequence on the oligodendrocyte and its precursors. In the early-delayed period after radiation, there was a loss of oligodendrocyte precursor cells and a loss in the late-delayed period of mature oligodendrocytes; this latter finding was accompanied by a disorganization of the myelin sheaths, which was confirmed in a rodent model (Panagiotakos *et al.*, 2007). These findings suggest the mechanism for the late-delayed leukoencephalopathy and for the deficits in executive function (such as attention, task-switching, and working memory) observed in patients undergoing radiotherapy, particularly with high-dose radiation exposure. They reflect a targeted depletion of oligodendrocyte precursor cells by radiation that are unable to proliferate and differentiate into mature oligodendrocytes needed for adequate myelination of axons. In contrast to neurogenesis in the hippocampus, however, oligodendrocyte precursor cells and gliogenesis are relatively preserved at clinically relevant doses of radiation (Monje *et al.*, 2002; Mizumatsu *et al.*, 2003). This is consistent with the observation that frank leukoencephalopathy is less common at the modern radiation doses used clinically.

Glia and gliogenesis: astrocytes

Astrocytes function as support cells in the CNS and react to injury, including irradiation of the CNS; in doing so, they are capable of both protecting and harming the CNS. Reactive astrocytosis — activation and migration of astrocytes to a site of injury — occurs secondary to radiotherapy in humans, which has been replicated in rodents after high-dose and fractionated radiotherapy (Asai *et al.*, 1989; Chiang *et al.*, 1993b; Yuan *et al.*, 2006). The accumulation of astrocytes ultimately results in a glial scar, which impedes regeneration and healing within the brain, thereby potentially impairing cognition by impeding hippocampal or frontal subcortical white matter function. Activation of astrocytes appears to be facilitated by microglia, as demonstrated *in vitro* (Hwang *et al.*, 2006).

Despite the harmful end result secondary to astrocyte involvement, astrocytes may also play a helpful role after radiation exposure. A review by Tofilon and Fike suggests that astrocytes may determine the CNS's radioresponsiveness given their protective effects upon the cells targeted by radiation exposure (Tofilon and Fike, 2000). Astrocytes co-cultured with cortical neurons were able to protect the neurons from free radical damage induced by irradiation, especially at lower dosages in the clinical range (Noel and Tofilon, 1998).

Aside from a possible neuroprotective role, astrocytes induce and maintain the blood brain barrier (BBB), which tightly regulates the brain homeostasis by strictly limiting the passive and active transport of ions, molecules, and proteins into the brain (Janzer and Raff, 1987). The BBB is compromised secondary to CNS irradiation, and astrocytes play an important role in this phenomenon. Astrocyte proliferation appeared to precede BBB permeability after fractionated irradiation, in which the dosing strategy more closely resembles the delivery in the clinical setting (Yuan *et al.*, 2006; Zhou *et al.*, 2011). While the cytokine tumor necrosis factor (TNF)-α has been shown to be both protective and damaging to the CNS [for review see (Shohami *et al.*, 1999)], its secretion by astrocytes and microglia increases the expression of the intracellular adhesion molecule ICAM-1 on the endothelial cells of the BBB, facilitating the entry of immune cells (e.g. lymphocytes) from the systemic circulation and fluid, thus leading to brain edema and enhancing inflammation within the brain (Kyrkanides *et al.*, 1999; Olschowka *et al.*, 1997). Peaks in expression of TNF-α correlate to the acute and late-delayed phases of irradiation (Daigle *et al.*, 2001), and TNF-α itself inhibits neurogenesis (Mizumatsu *et al.*, 2003). Breakdown of the BBB causing edema and a disruption of brain homeostasis can contribute to many of the acute symptoms observed in patients undergoing cranial irradiation, such as nausea, vomiting, and headache. It may also cause the late-delayed necrosis and neurocognitive deficits observed.

Neuroinflammation after radiation: microglia

A microglial inflammatory response accompanies neural stem cell and neuronal sensitivity to CNS radiation exposure. While microglia do not originate from neural stem cells, activated microglia and an upregulation of inflammatory cytokines are believed to negatively regulate neurogenesis following irradiation (Mizumatsu *et al.*, 2003). Microglia act as the resident macrophage of the CNS, having differentiated through the monocyte lineage of the hematopoietic stem cell. These cells are activated in response to a variety of signals, from infectious material such as pathogen-associated molecules or self-generated responses to infection or injury such as complement and cytokines. Many microglial phenotypes exist, and each one is capable of switching rapidly between these subtypes depending on the type of immune response needed.

An increase in the number of microglia present in the brain is correlated with increased irradiation dosages (Chiang *et al.*, 1993b). A study analyzing the effects of whole brain irradiation on mice at different ages confirms previous reports of increased proliferation of microglia in the brain. There also appear to be regional- and age-differences, where younger mice appeared to mount more robust proliferative microglial responses in the corpus callosum compared to older mice, and areas of the hippocampus reflected less of an inflammatory response. The authors suggest that microglia may become less capable of responding to whole brain irradiation damage with age, as there was a decreased proliferative response (Hua *et al.*, 2012).

Early research honed in on interleukin-6 (IL-6), a mediator of the inflammatory response produced by inflammatory microglia, as a cytokine with the potential to affect neurogenesis or even promote neurodegeneration. A related molecule acting through the same JAK/STAT signaling pathway, ciliary neurotrophic factor, was first demonstrated to direct differentiation of neural precursors to a glial fate (Bonni *et al.*, 1997). *In vivo*, IL-6 expressed in the brains of transgenic mice yielded deficits in an avoidance learning task; this is paralleled by another study that demonstrated reduction in hippocampal neurons in adult mice whose astrocytes chronically produced IL-6 (Heyser *et al.*, 1997; Vallières *et al.*, 2002). In fact, microglial IL-6 was found to specifically block neuronal differentiation of hippocampal neural stem cells, and administering an anti-inflammatory drug to an irradiated rodent restored neurogenesis, suggesting that inflammation is a modulator of neurocognitive deficits via its effects on neurogenesis and is therefore a potential therapeutic target to ameliorate radiation-induced memory dysfunction (Monje *et al.*, 2003).

Neurocognitive Sequelae of Chemotherapy

Unlike radiotherapy which can be used to target regions of interest while protecting others, chemotherapy is generally systemic, in that treatments are introduced intravenously, enterally, and intrathecally or intraventricularly. This affects a wider range of non-cancerous tissues than does radiotherapy and increases the chance of side effects, including chemotherapy-induced cognitive dysfunction (CICD), also known as chemotherapy-related cognitive impairment or, as it is known colloquially, 'chemo-brain.' While the health burden after treatment with chemotherapy is acknowledged to be high, reports of chronic cognitive impairment vary, from limited to severe (Oeffinger *et al.*, 2010; Langer *et al.*, 2002; Moleski, 2000). Current methods of studying CICD may not be sensitive enough to pick up mild cognitive impairment which can have significant effects on quality of life; furthermore, the cognitive tests used are not implemented in a uniform fashion, as definitions of cognitive impairment, control groups used (if one is used at all), and study design (e.g. cross-sectional versus longitudinal) can vary from study to study (Shilling *et al.*, 2006; Vardy *et al.*, 2007). Another major difficulty associated with studying CICD is the variability in cancer treatment regimens from patient to patient.

Many different classes of chemotherapeutics exist, as seen in Table 1, and are used in combination with one another at different dosages in patients with the same type of cancer, and frequently alongside radiation therapy. While there is some debate that 'chemobrain' may not be due to the chemotherapy itself but perhaps to

Table 1. Types of chemotherapeutics by class, with descriptions of mechanism of action, example drug names, and ways in which each drug can be used.

Category	Mechanism of action	Drug names	Major examples of clinical use in cancers
Anti-metabolites	Inhibits DNA synthesis thereby halting cell cycle progression	Methotrexate (MTX)	Osteosarcoma, leukemia
		5-fluorouracil (5-FU)	Colorectal
		Cytarabine	Leukemia
Alkylating agents	Damages DNA by attaching an alkyl group to DNA	Cyclophosphamide	Brain, breast, retinoblastoma, leukemia
		Carmustine (BCNU)	Lymphoma, glioblastoma
		ThioTEPA	Breast, bladder
Microtubule inhibitors	Stabilize or block microtubule formation to halt mitosis	Vincristine	Leukemia, lymphoma
		Paclitaxel	Breast, ovarian
Platinum-based	Cross-link DNA to prevent mitosis	Cisplatin	Testicular, ovarian, brain
		Oxaliplatin	Colorectal
Topoisomerase inhibitors	Prevent the topoisomerase enzymes from uncoiling DNA during translation and replication	Topotecan	Lung, ovarian

the biology of the cancer or to endocrine dysfunction (Ahles and Saykin, 2007; Ahles *et al.*, 2012), the remainder of this chapter will focus on what is known about the effects of chemotherapeutics on neural stem cells, and how this may contribute to the cognitive deficits observed in patients after chemotherapy.

Great strides are being made in targeting agents directly to tumors in attempts to limit toxicity and enhance specificity, yet traditional agents are still the mainstay in cancer therapy. It was widely believed that very few chemotherapeutics could cross the BBB when administered systemically; this population includes methotrexate (MTX) and 5-fluorouracil (5-FU). However, positive emission tomography studies have demonstrated that radiolabelled chemotherapeutics administered systemically or intravenously to animals or humans are capable of crossing the BBB in small but detectable amounts, and that these levels are capable of causing neurological harm while being too low to kill tumor cells (Gangloff *et al.*, 2005; Ginos *et al.*, 1987; Mitsuki *et al.*, 1991; Dietrich *et al.*, 2006). These findings are confirmed in the patient populations frequently examined for the neurocognitive effects of chemotherapy, such as in breast cancer and lymphoma patients who receive systemic/intravenous treatments (i.e. there is no direct introduction of chemotherapy to the CNS through intrathecal or intraventricular routes) (Ahles *et al.*, 2002; Ahles *et al.*, 2003).

The stages of the neurological sequelae as a result of chemotherapy exposure are divided clinically into the acute and delayed phases. The acute stage can include seizures, somnolence, and focal neurological deficits (e.g. motor, visual) (Walker *et al.*, 1986; Copeland *et al.*, 1988; Osterlundh *et al.*, 1997). The delayed or late stage can include more irreversible changes, such as dementia and cerebral atrophy. CICD is seen both acutely and chronically, with some patients experiencing resolution of symptoms over time (Filley and Kleinschmidt-DeMasters, 2001; Reid-Arndt *et al.*, 2010; Koppelmans *et al.*, 2012). Similarly to cognitive deficits secondary to radiotherapy, female sex and younger age of exposure to chemotherapy predicts poorer neurocognitive outcome, and radiotherapy and chemotherapy combined appear to have a negative synergistic effect (Von der Weid *et al.*, 2003; Bleyer *et al.*, 1990). Chemotherapeutic agents tend to affect a similar constellation of neurocognitive domains as compared to radiotherapy, but as a more subtle syndrome. CICD can include deficits in aspects of memory, attention, processing speed, and executive function; the neural structures underlying these processes include the hippocampus, frontal lobes, and subcortical white matter (Jansen *et al.*, 2005; Duffner, 2006; Komotar *et al.*, 2009; Shilling *et al.*, 2005). Animal studies have been able to replicate chronic cognitive dysfunction that result from administration of commonly used cancer drugs, such as MTX and 5-FU — memory functions which can be localized to the hippocampus and the frontal cortex, such as the spatial Morris water maze task and non-matching to sample learning, respectively (Winocur *et al.*, 2006; Winocur *et al.*, 2012; Fardell *et al.*, 2010).

Coupled with these symptoms are often structural and functional changes to areas vital to cognition that are appreciated on gross inspection, histology, and imaging. Areas such as white matter tracts, prefrontal cortex and parahippocampal gyrus — involved in attention tasks — and hippocampus — involved in learning, memory, and recall — appear to be smaller than normal in human patients exposed to chemotherapy. This suggests cell death, loss of white matter integrity, and diminished cell proliferation after chemotherapy (Inagaki *et al.*, 2007; Zeller *et al.*, 2013; Carey *et al.*, 2008).

Leukoencephalopathy has been appreciated upon gross examination of the brain of many patients treated with intraventricular MTX, who suffered from debilitating consequences of their cancer treatment chronically (Shapiro *et al.*, 1973; Norrell *et al.*, 1974). Furthermore, magnetic resonance imaging (MRI) and diffusion tensor imaging (DTI) demonstrate leukoencephalopathy typically affecting white matter of the frontal lobes in patients treated with systemic or intrathecal MTX. Severity can range from mild and possibly reversible leukoencephalopathy to a disseminated necrotizing leukoencephalopathy that usually results in death (Haykin *et al.*, 2006; Ziereisen *et al.*, 2006; Oka *et al.*, 2003).

Similar findings apply to other commonly used chemotherapeutics, such as carmustine (BCNU), cisplatin, cytarabine, and 5-FU (Filley and Kleinschmidt-DeMasters, 2001; Kleinschmidt-DeMasters, 1986; Cossaart *et al.*, 2003; Moore-Maxwell *et al.*, 2004; Fassas *et al.*, 1994). Application of dynamic imaging, such as functional MRI (fMRI), and electrophysiology demonstrated altered activity within brain regions of chemotherapy-treated patients who reported symptoms of CICD; regions that were hypoactive on fMRI imaging suggesting less active involvement during tasks compared to controls included the dorsolateral prefrontal cortex (working memory, planning), posterior parietal cortex (spatial attention), and inferior frontal gyrus (inhibition) (Silverman *et al.*, 2007; De Ruiter *et al.*, 2011). These observed changes suggest alterations in the cellular makeup of these structures and in the connection amongst the structures vital to learning and memory, which may stem from defects involving the neural precursor cell from which neurons in the hippocampus originate, and the oligodendrocyte precursor cell, from which myelinating oligodendrocytes originate.

Cellular and Molecular Mechanisms Underlying Neurocognitive Sequelae of Chemotherapy

Neurons and neurogenesis

Neurons were previously seen as immune to the effects of chemotherapy, as chemotherapeutics were known to target dividing cells, and neurons were understood to be incapable of dividing (Gregorios *et al.*, 1989). In light of evidence for hippocampal neurogenesis throughout life, chemotherapy may target sensitive neural precursor cell populations. The effects of chemotherapeutic agents on neuronal function (electrophysiological properties, synaptic plasticity, etc.) remain to be studied in detail.

Neuronal stem cells exhibit sensitivity to a variety of chemotherapeutic agents, and frequently at doses less than what are required to be toxic to cancer cells. However, there can be variability amongst the chemotherapeutic agents in their time course of action, as well as differential sensitivities of neural precursor cell populations to specific agents. A seminal study by Dietrich *et al.* analyzed the effects of BCNU, cisplatin, and cytarabine on various neural stem cells *in vitro* and *in vivo*. BCNU and cisplatin both negatively affect the viability of restricted progenitors and neural stem cells (both human and rat) *in vitro*; *in vivo*, apoptosis was observed within neural stem cell niches. Cells of the SVZ and dentate gyrus both appeared sensitive to BCNU, with SVZ cells exhibiting perhaps the most sensitivity to BCNU. The majority of acutely apoptotic cells included neuronal progenitor cells (neuroblasts) (Dietrich *et al.*, 2006). Neuroblasts were identified by expression of the neuroblast-specific marker doublecortin (DCX), a surrogate for hippocampal neurogenesis (Brown *et al.*, 2003; Rao and Shetty, 2004). Apoptotic cells in these regions were observed in BCNU-treated animals up to 6 weeks, suggesting a chronic effect of the chemotherapy. Cells of the dentate gyrus appeared most sensitive to cisplatin, followed by the SVZ. In animals treated with cytarabine, the SVZ demonstrated more sensitivity in the chronic period compared to the other areas, and with overall lower percentages of apoptotic cells compared to the other two drugs analyzed in this study: BCNU and cisplatin. Neuronal progenitor cells of the SVZ were affected most acutely by cytarabine with recovery over time, whereas the neuronal progenitor cell population of the dentate gyrus remained diminished chronically (Dietrich *et al.*, 2006).

Other commonly used chemotherapeutics such as 5-FU, MTX, doxorubicin and cyclophosphamide demonstrated similar findings in killing neural stem cells and neuronal progenitors. 5-FU revealed a similar picture to BCNU, in that the majority of apoptotic cells in the SVZ and dentate gyrus *in vivo* co-stained with DCX, suggesting sensitivity of neuronal progenitors (Han *et al.*, 2008). MTX also appears to target neural stem cells, as evidenced by an acute increase in apoptosis within the dentate gyrus after MTX exposure, and a decrease in the total number of DCX-positive cells reaching an overall lower level than normal over a two-week period (Yang *et al.*, 2011; Yang *et al.*, 2012). In a model of breast cancer therapy, rats treated with either doxorubicin or cyclophosphamide showed a decrease in the number of neuronal progenitors within the hippocampus compared to controls (Christie *et al.*, 2012).

In addition to studies on cell survival, researchers have extended their analysis to include the effects of individual agents on cell proliferation and animal behavior. While 5-FU caused cellular apoptosis of neuronal precursors within the dentate gyrus in one animal model as discussed earlier (Han *et al.*, 2008), another study demonstrated that three consecutive days of systemic 5-FU had no effect on neuronal precursor proliferation (Mignone and Weber, 2006). In contrast, MTX, thioTEPA, and cyclophosphamide all appear to cause a decrease in hippocampal cell proliferation within the dentate gyrus. A dose-dependent decrease in proliferation was observed in MTX-treated animals coupled with impaired hippocampal-dependent learning, demonstrated by deficits in the passive avoidance task, Morris water maze task and novel object recognition test (Yang *et al.*, 2011; Yang *et al.*, 2012; Seigers *et al.*, 2008; Seigers *et al.*, 2009). ThioTEPA-treated animals also exhibited a dose-dependent decrease in hippocampal cell proliferation *in vivo* in the acute and chronic time periods tested; there was also a deficit observed in performance on the object recognition test (Mignone and Weber, 2006; Mondie *et al.*, 2010). Cyclophosphamide exposure in animals demonstrated an acutely transient decrease in proliferating cells and number of DCX positive cells; an acute deficit in object recognition paralleled the cellular finding (Yang *et al.*, 2010). This finding was confirmed as previously discussed, and both cyclophosphamide and doxorubicin independently yielded cognitive deficits in novel place recognition and contextual fear conditioning tasks (Christie *et al.*, 2012).

Combinations of chemotherapeutics also have negative effects on neuroblast proliferation. A study analyzing those commonly used together in breast cancer regimens — cyclophosphamide, MTX, 5-FU — demonstrated in rats deficits in object-in-place test and temporal order memory, both associated with frontal memory processes (Briones and Woods, 2014; Barker *et al.*, 2007).

In addition to promoting apoptosis and hindering cellular proliferation, chemotherapy negatively affects the ability of neuroblasts to mature. Rats exposed to doxorubicin or cyclophosphamide demonstrated a defect in neuronal maturation within the hippocampus (Christie *et al.*, 2012).

Mature neurons are also damaged by chemotherapy, potentially further contributing to cognitive deficits. *In vitro*, chemotherapeutic agents cause neuronal cell death, including taxol, camptothecin (a topoisomerase inhibitor), and cisplatin, although supporting glial cells may protect mature neurons *in vivo*, as wide-spread neuronal apoptosis is not observed with chemotherapy exposure *in vivo* (Figueroa-Masot *et al.*, 2001; Morris *et al.*, 1996; Gozdz *et al.*, 2003). Young rats exposed to systemic cisplatin, cyclophosphamide, thioTEPA, or ifosfamide all demonstrated significant neurotoxicity, perhaps mediated by excitotoxicity and caspase-mediated apoptosis (Rzeski *et al.*, 2004).

The function of neurons may also be affected by chemotherapy, specifically long-term potentiation (LTP) and synaptic plasticity. Briefly, LTP is a process vital to learning and memory particularly in the hippocampus, which strengthens the connection between two neurons that are able to communicate effectively with one another. Electrophysiological studies performed on mice exposed to 5-FU and MTX exhibited a chronic defect in their ability to filter extraneous auditory stimuli as demonstrated in abnormal auditory event-related potentials, which suggests a neuronal dysfunction underlying attention deficits. These mice also demonstrated increased freezing times during contextual fear conditioning, a task involving the hippocampus and amygdala, suggesting an increased vulnerability to a noxious stimulus in the environment (Gandal *et al.*, 2008).

With the evidence that chemotherapy has the capacity to kill neurons and neuronal stem cells, diminish proliferative capacity, and affect animal cognition, the phenomenon of CICD may be able to be explained, at least partly, by research focusing on neural stem cells. Exposure of the brain on such a large scale to neuronotoxic drugs may be causing the changes in patient cognition after chemotherapy.

Glia and gliogenesis: oligodendrocytes and myelin

Dysfunction of oligodendrocyte lineage cells and defects in myelin may underlie a large part of the neurocognitive deficits seen after chemotherapy treatment. It is likely that defects in these myelinating cells cause the cognitive defects that localize to white matter tracts, and the leukoencephalopathy seen on imaging in humans and animals after treatment with chemotherapy.

Oligodendrocyte precursor cells within stem cell niches, such as in the SVZ, appear to be targeted by chemotherapy, as observed with neuronal progenitors. After exposure to MTX, glial precursors appeared to apoptose based upon morphological features, and this population decreased in number over time (Morris *et al.*, 1995). When MTX is applied at high doses used in breast cancer treatment alongside cyclophosphamide and 5-FU, a decrease in pre-myelinating oligodendrocyte precursors was observed; this was partially rescued by the administration of an anti-inflammatory agent, suggesting that high-dose chemotherapy can cause inflammation within the brain, thereby negatively affecting the oligodendrocyte precursor cell population (Briones and Woods, 2014). Mature oligodendrocytes and oligodendrocyte precursor cells demonstrate an *in vitro* sensitivity to 5-FU, at levels lower than those required to kill tumor cells; *in vivo*, cells of the oligodendrocyte lineage (precursor and mature) underwent apoptosis after exposure. Acutely, there was an increase in oligodendrocyte lineage cells, perhaps reflecting a response to cell death; however, chronically, mature oligodendrocytes demonstrated a loss of the oligodendrocyte lineage marker Olig2, suggesting a change in the expression profile of chemotherapy-exposed cells (Han *et al.*, 2008). BCNU and cisplatin each reveal the marked sensitivity of oligodendrocyte precursor cells and mature oligodendrocytes to treatment *in vitro* and *in vivo*, also at levels lower than what is required to kill tumor cells, like 5-FU. Cytarabine also elicited a reduction in the oligodendrocyte precursor cell population acutely *in vivo*, but recovery was seen over time (Dietrich *et al.*, 2006).

If chemotherapy indeed hinders the function of oligodendrocyte lineage cells or decreases their number, white matter pathology is likely to follow. Existing myelin sheaths may not be able to be maintained, and new myelin may not be laid down along axons properly or in adequate quantity. Indeed, much of the research previously discussed also delved into the effects of chemotherapy on myelin. After exposure to intraventricular MTX, the thickness of the corpus callosum decreased in treated animals, suggested a decrement in the density of white matter (Seigers *et al.*, 2009). After infusion of intraventricular high-dose MTX, rats exhibited extensive leukoencephalopathy acutely, which could be grossly appreciated (Shapiro *et al.*, 1973). 5-FU also exhibited a decrease in the intensity of staining for myelin basic protein, a component of myelin sheaths making up white matter (Han *et al.*, 2008).

Despite research that correlates marker staining and corpus callosum thickness with effects of chemotherapy on myelin, electron microscopy remains the gold standard for the study of myelination, as it allows for direct analysis of the myelin sheaths themselves (Gregorios *et al.*, 1989). Myelin sheath pathology was confirmed in the 5-FU study, in that demyelinated axons and splitting of myelin sheaths were observed; although, processing of tissue for electron microscopy can cause damage to the myelin sheaths in such a manner (Han *et al.*, 2008). A combination of 5-FU, cyclophosphamide and MTX resulted in a decrease in the thickness of myelin sheaths, suggesting a loss in myelin or less myelination taking place (Briones and Woods, 2014). Considering the human leukoencephalopathy observed after chemotherapy exposure, such pathology elicited in an animal model helps to define the mechanism underlying white-matter tract-related aspects of CICD.

Glia and gliogenesis: astrocytes

Reactive astrocytosis is observed in human patients exposed to chemotherapy throughout the brain and particularly in deep white matter (Shapiro *et al.*, 1973; Cossaart *et al.*, 2003). MTX injected intraperitoneally and intraventricularly in rats demonstrated reactive astrocytosis within 24 hours after exposure, which is also confirmed *in vitro* (Gregorios *et al.*, 1989; Gregorios and Soucy, 1990). Astrocytes, in general, appear to be less susceptible than other types of CNS cells to undergo cell death at high concentrations of drug (Dietrich *et al.*, 2006; Han *et al.*, 2008; Wick *et al.*, 2004).

With any activation or dysfunction of astrocytes, a number of mechanisms may facilitate injury to other cells of the CNS, and contribute to CICD as a result. One suggested mechanism is the decreased uptake of the excitatory neurotransmitter glutamate by astrocytes, which can cause excitotoxicity in neurons and oligodendrocytes, or cell death caused by increased ion influx via glutamate activation of cell receptor ion channels (Rothman and Olney, 1986; McDonald *et al.*, 1998; Rothstein *et al.*, 1996). Another possible mechanism is the formation of glial scars by reactive astrocytosis to wall off a site of injury to protect the CNS, as discussed in the context of radiotherapy; here in response to chemotherapy exposure, this process may contribute to neurodegeneration and possibly the neurocognitive sequelae secondary to chemotherapy exposure (Sofroniew, 2009).

Neuroinflammation after chemotherapy: microglia

As previously discussed, while microglia are not descendents of neural stem cells, they may play an important role in modifying the effects of chemotherapy on neural stem cells and the pathogenesis of CICD. There appeared to be transient, and minimal to no activation of microglia, after exposing rats to 5-FU or doxorubicin respectively (Han *et al.*, 2008; Christie *et al.*, 2012). However, after MTX or cyclophosphamide exposure, activated microglia appeared in the brain in significant numbers (Christie *et al.*, 2012; Seigers *et al.*, 2010). The limited studies performed on the role of microglia in the brain when exposed to chemotherapy suggest that, like the other cell types of the CNS, the type of chemotherapy administered can preferentially target certain cell types. Microglial activation could play a role in various forms of chemotherapy-induced neurotoxicity, from inhibition of neurogenesis (Monje *et al.*, 2003) to alterations in myelin integrity (Miron *et al.*, 2013). Future studies will elucidate this likely critical issue.

Conclusion

Cancer therapy in the form of radiation and traditional chemotherapy can have a profound effect on neural stem and precursor cells, contributing to long-term cognitive dysfunction and decrement in quality of life. While much progress has been made in understanding the side effects of cancer therapy on the CNS, much work remains in understanding how to protect neural stem cells and potentially prevent radiation-induced cognitive decline and CICD. Deepening our understanding of the effects of cancer therapy on neural stem and precursor cells will elucidate strategies to protect these vulnerable and important populations of cells.

References

Ahles T, Root JC, Ryan EL (2012) Cancer- and cancer treatment-associated cognitive change: an update on the state of the science. *J Clin Oncol* 30:3675–3686.

Ahles TA, Saykin AJ (2007) Candidate mechanisms for chemotherapy-induced cognitive changes. *Nat Rev Cancer* 7:192–201.

Ahles T, Saykin AJ, Furstenberg CT, Cole B, Mott L, Skalla K, Whedon MB, Bivens S, Mitchell T, Greenberg ER, Silberfarb PM (2002) Neuropsychologic impact of standard-dose systemic chemotherapy in long-term survivors of breast cancer and lymphoma. *J Clin Oncol* 20:485–493.

Ahles TA, Saykin AJ, Noll WW, Furstenberg CT, Guerin S, Cole B, Mott LA (2003) The relationship of APOE genotype to neuropsychological performance in long-term cancer survivors treated with standard dose chemotherapy. *Psychooncology* 12:612–619.

American Cancer Society (2013). Cancer Facts & Figures 2013. American Cancer Society, 1–62.

Anderson VA, Godber T, Smibert E, Weiskop S, Ekert H (2000) Cognitive and academic outcome following cranial irradiation and chemotherapy in children: a longitudinal study. *Br J Cancer* 82:255–262.

Armstrong GT, Liu Q, Yasui Y, Huang S, Ness KK, Leisenring W, Hudson MM, Donaldson SS, King AA, Stovall M, Krull KR, Robison LL, Packer RJ (2009) Long-term outcomes among adult survivors of childhood central nervous system malignancies in the Childhood Cancer Survivor Study. *J Natl Cancer Inst* 101:946–958.

Armstrong C, Ruffer J, Corn B, DeVries K, Mollman J (1995) Biphasic patterns of memory deficits following neuropsychologic outcome and proposed mechanisms. *J Clin Oncol* 13:2263–2271.

Asai A, Matsutani M, Kohno T, Nakamura O, Tanaka H, Fujimaki T, Funada N, Matsuda T, Nagata K, Takakura K (1989) Subacute brain atrophy after radiation therapy for malignant brain tumor. *Cancer* 63:1962–1974.

Barker GRI, Bird F, Alexander V, Warburton EC (2007) Recognition memory for objects, place, and temporal order: a disconnection analysis of the role of the medial prefrontal cortex and perirhinal cortex. *J Neurosci* 27:2948–2957.

Bauer H, Demerec M, Kaufmann BP (1938) X-Ray induced chromosomal alterations in drosophila melanogaster. *Genetics* 610:610–630.

Bellinzona M, Gobbel G, Shinohara C, Fike J (1996) Apoptosis is induced in the subependyma of young adult rats by ionizing irradiation. *Neurosci Lett* 208:163–166.

Bergmann O, Liebl J, Bernard S, Alkass K, Yeung MSY, Steier P, Kutschera W, Johnson L, Landén M, Druid H, Spalding KL, Frisén J (2012) The age of olfactory bulb neurons in humans. *Neuron* 74:634–639.

Bleyer WA, Fallavollita J, Robison L, Balsom W, Meadows A, Heyn R, Sitarz A, Ortega J, Miller D, Constine L, Nesbit M, Sather H, Hammond D (1990) Influence of age, sex, and concurrent intrathecal methotrexate therapy on intellectual function after cranial irradiation during childhood: a report from the children's cancer study group. *Pediatr Hematol* 7:329–338.

Bonni A, Sun Y, Nadal-Vicens M, Bhatt A, Frank D, Rozovsky I, Stahl N, Yancopoulos G, Greenberg M (1997) Regulation of Gliogenesis in the Central Nervous System by the JAK-STAT Signaling Pathway. *Science* 278:477–483.

Briones TL, Woods J (2014) Dysregulation in myelination mediated by persistent neuroinflammation: Possible mechanisms in chemotherapy-related cognitive impairment. *Brain Behav Immun* 35:23–32.

Brown JP, Couillard-Després S, Cooper-Kuhn CM, Winkler J, Aigner L, Kuhn HG (2003) Transient expression of doublecortin during adult neurogenesis. *J Comp Neurol* 467:1–10.

Campbell L, Scaduto M, Sharp W, Dufton L, Van Slyke D, Whitlock J, Compas B (2007) A meta-analysis of the neurocognitive sequelae of treatment for childhood acute lymphocytic leukemia. *Pediatr Blood Cancer* 49:65–73.

Carey ME, Haut MW, Reminger SL, Hutter JJ, Theilmann R, Kaemingk KL (2008) Reduced frontal white matter volume in long-term childhood leukemia survivors: a voxel-based morphometry study. *Am J Neuroradiol* 29:792–797.

Centers for Disease Control and Prevention (2005) Acute Radiation Syndrome: A Fact Sheet for Clinicians.

Chiang CS, McBride WH, Withers HR (1993a) Myelin-associated changes in mouse brain following irradiation. *Radiother Oncol* 27:229–236.

Chiang C, McBride W, Withers H (1993b) Radiation-induced astrocytic and microglial responses in mouse brain. *Radiother Oncol* 29:60–68.

Chow BM, Li YQ, Wong CS (2000) Radiation-induced apoptosis in the adult central nervous system is p53-dependent. *Cell Death Differ* 7: 712–720.

Christie D, Leiper AD, Chessells JM, Vargha-Khadem F (1995) Intellectual performance after presymptomatic cranial radiotherapy for leukaemia: effects of age and sex. *Arch Dis Child* 73:136–140.

Christie L-A, Acharya MM, Parihar VK, Nguyen A, Martirosian V, Limoli CL (2012) Impaired cognitive function and hippocampal neurogenesis following cancer chemotherapy. *Clin Cancer Res* 18:1954–1965.

Clelland CD, Choi M, Romberg C, Clemenson GD, Fragniere A, Tyers P, Jessberger S, Saksida LM, Barker RA, Gage FH, Bussey TJ (2009) A functional role for adult hippocampal neurogenesis in spatial pattern separation. *Science* 325:210–213.

Clemente C, Holst E (1954) Pathological changes in neurons, neuroglia, and blood-brain barrier induced by x-irradiation of heads of monkeys. *AMA Arch Neurol Psychiatry* 71:66–79.

Copeland D, Dowell R, Fletcher J, Bordeaux J, Sullivan M, Jaffe N, Frankel L, Ried H, Cangir A (1988) Neuropsychological effects of childhood cancer treatment. *J Child Neurol* 3:S68–S72.

Cossaart N, SantaCruz KS, Preston D, Johnson P, Skikne BS (2003) Fatal chemotherapy-induced encephalopathy following high-dose therapy for metastatic breast cancer: a case report and review of the literature. *Bone Marrow Transplant* 31:57–60.

Cousens P, Waters B, Said J, Stevens M (1988) Cognitive effects of cranial irradiation in leukaemia: a survey and meta-analysis. *J Child Psychol Psychiatry* 29:839–852.

Crompton M, Layton D (1961) Delayed radionecrosis of the brain following therapeutic x-radiation of the pituitary. *Brain* 84:85–101.

Crossen JR, Garwood D, Glatstein E, Neuwelt E (1994) Neurobehavioral sequelae of cranial irradiation in adults: a review of radiation-induced encephalopathy. *J Clin Oncol* 12:627–642.

Daigle J, Hong J, Chiang C, McBride W (2001) The role of tumor necrosis factor signaling pathways in the response of murine brain to irradiation. *Cancer Res* 61:8859–8865.

Daniel J (1896) The X-rays. *Science* III: 562–563.

De Ruiter MB, Reneman L, Boogerd W, Veltman DJ, van Dam FSAM, Nederveen AJ, Boven E, Schagen SB (2011) Cerebral hyporesponsiveness and cognitive impairment 10 years after chemotherapy for breast cancer. *Hum Brain Mapp* 32:1206–1219.

Dietrich J, Han R, Yang Y, Mayer-Pröschel M, Noble M (2006) CNS progenitor cells and oligodendrocytes are targets of chemotherapeutic agents *in vitro* and *in vivo*. *J Biol* 5.

Doetsch F, Caillé I, Lim D, García-Verdugo JM, Alvarez-Buylla A (1999) Subventricular zone astrocytes are neural stem cells in the adult mammalian brain. *Cell* 97:703–716.

Dooms GC, Hecht S, Brant-Zawadzki M, Berthiaume Y, Norman D, Newton TH (1986) Brain radiation lesions: MR imaging. *Radiology* 158:149–155.

Duffner P (2006) The long term effects of chemotherapy on the central nervous system. *J Biol* 5:21.1–21.4.

Ebi J, Sato H, Nakajima M, Shishido F (2013) Incidence of leukoencephalopathy after whole-brain radiation therapy for brain metastases. *Int J Radiat Oncol Biol Phys* 85:1212–1217.

Edelstein K, D'agostino N, Bernstein LJ, Nathan PC, Greenberg ML, Hodgson DC, Millar BA, Laperriere N, Spiegler BJ (2011) Long-term neurocognitive outcomes in young adult survivors of childhood acute lymphoblastic leukemia. *J Pediatr Hematol Oncol* 33:450–458.

Fardell JE, Vardy J, Logge W, Johnston I (2010) Single high dose treatment with methotrexate causes long-lasting cognitive dysfunction in laboratory rodents. *Pharmacol Biochem Behav* 97:333–339.

Fassas A, Gattani A, Morgello S (1994) Cerebral demyelination with 5-fluorouracil and levamisole. *Cancer Invest* 12:379–383.

Figueroa-Masot X, Hetman M, Higgins M, Kokot N, Xia Z (2001) Taxol induces apoptosis in cortical neurons by a mechanism independent of Bcl-2 phosphorylation. *J Neurosci* 21:4657–4667.

Filley C, Kleinschmidt-DeMasters BK (2001) Toxic leukoencephalopathy. *N Engl J Med* 345:425–432.

Gandal M, Ehrlichman R, Rudnick N, Siegel S (2008) A novel electrophysiological model of chemotherapy-induced cognitive impairments in mice. *Neuroscience* 157:95–104.

Gangloff A, Hsueh W, Kesner A, Kiesewetter D, Pio B, Pegram M, Beryt M, Townsend A, Czernin J, Phelps M, Silverman D (2005) Estimation of paclitaxel biodistribution and uptake in human-derived xenografts in vivo with 18F-fluoropaclitaxel. *J Nucl Med* 46:1866–1871.

Gibson E, Monje M (2012) Effect of cancer therapy on neural stem cells: implications for cognitive function. *Curr Opin Oncol* 24:672–678.

Gilman A, Philips FS (1946) The biological actions and therapeutic applications of the B-chloroethyl amines and sulfides. *Science* 103: 409–415.

Ginos JZ, Cooper AJ, Dhawan V, Lai JC, Strother SC, Alcock N, Rottenberg DA (1987) [13N]cisplatin PET to assess pharmacokinetics of intra-arterial versus intravenous chemotherapy for malignant brain tumors. *J Nucl Med* 28:1844–1852.

Goodman L, Wintrobe MM, Dameshek W, Goodman M, Gilman A, McLennan M (1946) Nitrogen Mustard Therapy: Use of methyl-bis(beta-chloroethyl)amine hydrochloride and tris(beta-chloroethyl) amine hydrochloride for Hodgkin's Disease, Lymphosarcoma, Leukemia and Certain Allied and Miscellaneous Disorders. *JAMA*:126–132.

Gozdz A, Habas A, Jaworski J, Zielinska M, Albrecht J, Chlystun M, Jalili A, Hetman M (2003) Role of n-methyl-d-aspartate receptors in the neuroprotective activation of extracellular signal-regulated kinase 1/2 by Cisplatin. *J Biol Chem* 278:43663–43671.

Gregorios JB, Soucy D (1990) Effects of methotrexate on astrocytes in primary culture: light and electron microscopic studies. *Brain Res* 516:20–30.

Gregorios J, Gregorios A, Mora J, Marcillo A, Fojaco R, Green B (1989) Morphologic alterations in rat brain following systemic and intraventricular methotrexate injection: light and electron microscopic studies. *J Neuropathol Exp Neurol* 48:33–47.

Han R, Yang YM, Dietrich J, Luebke A, Mayer-Pröschel M, Noble M (2008) Systemic 5-fluorouracil treatment causes a syndrome of delayed myelin destruction in the central nervous system. *J Biol* 7:12.

Haykin M, Gorman M, van Hoff J, Fulbright R, Baehring J (2006) Diffusion-weighted MRI correlates of subacute methotrexate-related neurotoxicity. *J Neurooncol* 76:153–157.

Heyser CJ, Masliah E, Samimi A, Campbell IL, Gold LH (1997) Progressive decline in avoidance learning paralleled by inflammatory neurodegeneration in transgenic mice expressing interleukin 6 in the brain. *Proc Natl Acad Sci USA* 94:1500–1505.

Howel W, Roberts R (1928) Splenomedullary leukaemia in an X-ray worker. *Lancet* 748–751.

Hua K, Schindler MK, McQuail JA, Forbes ME, Riddle DR (2012) Regionally distinct responses of microglia and glial progenitor cells to whole brain irradiation in adult and aging rats. *PLoS One* 7:e52728.

Hwang S-Y, Jung J-S, Kim T-H, Lim S-J, Oh E-S, Kim J-Y, Ji K-A, Joe E-H, Cho K-H, Han I-O (2006) Ionizing radiation induces astrocyte gliosis through microglia activation. *Neurobiol Dis* 21:457–467.

Imperato JP, Paleologos NA, Vick NA (1990) Effects of treatment on long-term survivors with malignant astrocytomas. *Ann Neurol* 28:818–822.

Inagaki M, Yoshikawa E, Matsuoka Y, Sugawara Y, Nakano T, Akechi T, Wada N, Imoto S, Murakami K, Uchitomi Y (2007) Smaller regional volumes of brain gray and white matter demonstrated in breast cancer survivors exposed to adjuvant chemotherapy. *Cancer* 109:146–156.

Jansen CE, Miaskowski C, Dodd M, Dowling G, Kramer J (2005) A meta-analysis of studies of the effects of cancer chemotherapy on various domains of cognitive function. *Cancer* 104:2222–2233.

Janzer R, Raff M (1987) Astrocytes induce blood-brain barrier properties in endothelial cells. *Nature* 325:253–257.

Keime-Guibert F, Napolitano M, Delattre J-Y (1998) Neurological complications of radiotherapy and chemotherapy. *J Neurol* 245:695–708.

Kesler S, Kent J, O'Hara R (2011) Prefrontal Cortex and Executive Function Impairments in Primary Breast Cancer. *Arch Neurol* 68:1447–1453.

Kleinschmidt-DeMasters BK (1986) Intracarotid BCNU leukoencephalopathy. *Cancer* 57:1276–1280.

Komotar RJ, Otten ML, Garrett MC, Anderson RCE (2009) Treatment of early childhood medulloblastoma by postoperative chemotherapy alone-a critical review. *Clin Med Oncol* 3:13–14.

Koppelmans V, Breteler MMB, Boogerd W, Seynaeve C, Gundy C, Schagen SB (2012) Neuropsychological performance in survivors of breast cancer more than 20 years after adjuvant chemotherapy. *J Clin Oncol* 30:1080–1086.

Kurita H, Kawahara N, Asai A, Ueki K, Shin M, Kirino T (2001) Radiation-induced apoptosis of oligodendrocytes in the adult rat brain. *Neurol Res* 23:869–874.

Kyrkanides S, Olschowka JA, Williams JP, Hansen JT, Banion MKO (1999) TNFa and IL-1b mediate intercellular adhesion molecule-1 induction via microglia-astrocyte interaction in CNS radiation injury. *J Neuroimmunol* 95:95–106.

Langer T, Martus P, Ottensmeier H, Hertzberg H, Beck JD, Meier W (2002) CNS late-effects after ALL therapy in childhood. Part III: neuropsychological performance in long-term survivors of childhood ALL: impairments of concentration, attention, and memory. *Med Pediatr Oncol* 38:320–328.

Lawrence YR, Li XA, el Naqa I, Hahn CA, Marks LB, Merchant TE, Dicker AP (2010) Radiation dose-volume effects in the brain. *Int J Radiat Oncol Biol Phys* 76:S20–S27.

Li YQ, Guo YP, Jay V, Stewart PA, Wong CS (1996) Time course of radiation-induced apoptosis in the adult rat spinal cord. *Radiother Oncol* 39:35–42.

Madsen T, Kristjansen PE, Bolwig T, Wörtwein G (2003) Arrested neuronal proliferation and impaired hippocampal function following fractionated brain irradiation in the adult rat. *Neuroscience* 119:635–642.

Malamud N, Boldrey EB, Welch WK, Fadell EJ (1954) Necrosis of brain and spinal cord following x-ray therapy. *J Neurosurg* 11:353–362.

Martins AN, Johnston JS, Col LT, Henry JM, Stoffel TJ, Chino GDI, Min M (1977) Delayed radiation necrosis of the brain. *J Neurosurg* 47:336–345.

McDonald J, Althomsons S, Hyrc K, Choi D, Goldberg M (1998) Oligodendrocytes from forebrain are highly vulnerable to AMPA/kainate receptor-mediated excitotoxicity. *Nat Med* 4:291–297.

Mignone RG, Weber ET (2006) Potent inhibition of cell proliferation in the hippocampal dentate gyrus of mice by the chemotherapeutic drug thioTEPA. *Brain Res* 1111:26–29.

Miron VE, Boyd A, Zhao J-W, Yuen TJ, Ruckh JM, Shadrach JL, van Wijngaarden P, Wagers AJ, Williams A, Franklin RJM, ffrench-Constant C (2013) M2 microglia and macrophages drive oligodendrocyte differentiation during CNS remyelination. *Nat Neurosci* 16:1211–1218.

Mitsuki S, Diksic M, Conway T, Yamamoto YL, Villemure JG, Feindel W (1991) Pharmacokinetics of 11C-labelled BCNU and SarCNU in gliomas studied by PET. *J Neurooncol* 10:47–55.

Mizumatsu S, Monje M, Morhardt D (2003) Extreme Sensitivity of Adult Neurogenesis to Low Doses of X-Irradiation. *Cancer Res* 63:4021–4027.

Moleski M (2000) Neuropsychological, Neuroanatomical, and Neurophysiological Consequences of CNS Chemotherapy for Acute Lymphoblastic Leukemia. *Arch Clin Neuropsychol* 15:603–630.

Mondie CM, Vandergrift KA, Wilson CL, Gulinello ME, Weber ET (2010) The chemotherapy agent, thioTEPA, yields long-term impairment of hippocampal cell proliferation and memory deficits but not depression-related behaviors in mice. *Behav Brain Res* 209:66–72.

Monje ML, Mizumatsu S, Fike JR, Palmer TD (2002) Irradiation induces neural precursor-cell dysfunction. *Nat Med* 8:955–962.

Monje ML, Toda H, Palmer TD (2003) Inflammatory blockade restores adult hippocampal neurogenesis. *Science* 302:1760–1765.

Monje ML, Vogel H, Masek M, Ligon KL, Fisher PG, Palmer TD (2007) Impaired human hippocampal neurogenesis after treatment for central nervous system malignancies. *Ann Neurol* 62:515–520.

Moore-Maxwell CA, Datto MB, Hulette CM (2004) Chemotherapy-induced toxic leukoencephalopathy causes a wide range of symptoms: a series of four autopsies. *Mod Pathol* 17:241–247.

Morris E, Geller H (1996) Induction of neuronal apoptosis by camptothecin, an inhibitor of Topoisomerase-I: Evidence for Cell Cycle-independent Toxicity. *J Cell Biol* 134:757–770.

Morris GM, Hopewell JW, Morris AD (1995) A comparison of the effects of methotrexate and misonidazole on the germinal cells of the subependymal plate of the rat. *Br J Radiol* 68:406–412.

The Nobel Foundation (1967) Nobel Lectures, Physics 1901–1921. Elsevier Publishing Company.

Noel F, Tofilon PJ (1998) Astrocytes protect against X-ray-induced neuronal toxicity *in vitro. Neuroreport* 9:1133–1137.

Norrell H, Wilson C, Slagel D, Clark D (1974) Leukoencephalopathy following the administration of methotrexate into the cerebrospinal fluid in the treatment of primary brain tumors. *Cancer* 33:923–932.

Oeffinger KC, Nathan PC, Kremer LCM (2010) Challenges after curative treatment for childhood cancer and long-term follow up of survivors. *Hematol Oncol Clin North Am* 24:129–149.

Oka M, Terae S, Kobayashi R, Sawamura Y, Kudoh K, Tha KK, Yoshida M, Kaneda M, Suzuki Y, Miyasaka K (2003) MRI in methotrexate-related leukoencephalopathy: Disseminated necrotising leukoencephalopathy in comparison with mild leukoencephalopathy. *Neuroradiology* 45:493–497.

Olschowka JA, Kyrkanides S, Harvey BK, O'Banion MK, Williams JP, Rubin P, Hansen JT (1997) ICAM-1 induction in the mouse CNS following irradiation. *Brain Behav Immun* 11:273–285.

Osterlundh G, Bjure J, Lannering B, Kjellmer I, Uvebrant P, Márky I (1997) Studies of cerebral blood flow in children with acute lymphoblastic leukemia: case reports of six children treated with methotrexate examined by single photon emission computed tomography. *J Pediatr Hematol Oncol* 19:28–34.

Panagiotakos G, Alshamy G, Chan B, Abrams R, Greenberg E, Saxena A, Bradbury M, Edgar M, Gutin P, Tabar V (2007) Long-term impact of radiation on the stem cell and oligodendrocyte precursors in the brain. *PLoS One* 2:e588.

Parent JM, Tada E, Fike JR, Lowenstein DH (1999) Inhibition of dentate granule cell neurogenesis with brain irradiation does not prevent seizure-induced mossy fiber synaptic reorganization in the rat. *J Neurosci* 19:4508–4519.

Peissner W, Kocher M, Treuer H, Gillardon F (1999) Ionizing radiation-induced apoptosis of proliferating stem cells in the dentate gyrus of the adult rat hippocampus. *Brain Res Mol Brain Res* 71:61–68.

Pellmar TC, Schauer D, Zeman GH (1990) Time- and dose-dependent changes in neuronal activity produced by X radiation in brain slices. *Radiat Res* 122:209–214.

Pennybacker J, Russell DS (1948) Necrosis of the Brain Due To Radiation Therapy: Clinical and Pathological Observations. *J Neurol Neurosurg Psychiatry* 11:183–198.

Rao M, Shetty A (2004) Efficacy of doublecortin as a marker to analyse the absolute number and dendritic growth of newly generated neurons in the adult dentate gyrus. *Eur J Neurosci* 19:234–246.

Rebholz CE, Reulen RC, Toogood AA, Frobisher C, Lancashire ER, Winter DL, Kuehni CE, Hawkins MM (2011) Health care use of long-term survivors of childhood cancer: the British Childhood Cancer Survivor Study. *J Clin Oncol* 29:4181–4188.

Reid-Arndt SA, Hsieh C, Perry MC (2010) Neuropsychological functioning and quality of life during the first year after completing chemotherapy for breast cancer. Psychooncology 19:535–544.

Rola R, Raber J, Rizk A, Otsuka S, VandenBerg SR, Morhardt DR, Fike JR (2004) Radiation-induced impairment of hippocampal neurogenesis is associated with cognitive deficits in young mice. *Exp Neurol* 188: 316–330.

Rosi S, Andres-Mach M, Fishman KM, Levy W, Ferguson RA, Fike JR (2008) Cranial irradiation alters the behaviorally induced immediate-early gene arc (activity-regulated cytoskeleton-associated protein). *Cancer Res* 68:9763–9770.

Rothman SM, Olney JW (1986) Glutamate and the pathophysiology of hypoxic–ischemic brain damage. *Ann Neurol* 19:105–111.

Rothstein JD, Dykes-Hoberg M, Pardo CA, Bristol LA, Jin L, Kuncl RW, Kanai Y, Hediger MA, Wang Y, Schielke JP, Welty DF (1996) Knockout of glutamate transporters reveals a major role for astroglial transport in excitotoxicity and clearance of glutamate. *Neuron* 16:675–686.

Rzeski W, Pruskil S, Macke A, Felderhoff-Mueser U, Reiher AK, Hoerster F, Jansma C, Jarosz B, Stefovska V, Bittigau P, Ikonomidou C (2004) Anticancer agents are potent neurotoxins *in vitro* and *in vivo*. *Ann Neurol* 56:351–360.

Sano K, Morii K, Sato M, Mori H, Tanaka R (2000) Radiation-induced diffuse brain injury in the neonatal rat model. *Neurol Med Chir (Tokyo)* 40:495–500.

Seigers R, Schagen SB, Beerling W, Boogerd W, van Tellingen O, van Dam FSAM, Koolhaas JM, Buwalda B (2008) Long-lasting suppression of hippocampal cell proliferation and impaired cognitive performance by methotrexate in the rat. *Behav Brain Res* 186:168–175.

Seigers R, Schagen SB, Coppens CM, van der Most PJ, van Dam FSAM, Koolhaas JM, Buwalda B (2009) Methotrexate decreases hippocampal cell proliferation and induces memory deficits in rats. *Behav Brain Res* 201:279–284.

Seigers R, Timmermans J, van der Horn HJ, de Vries EFJ, Dierckx RA, Visser L, Schagen SB, van Dam FSAM, Koolhaas JM, Buwalda B (2010) Methotrexate reduces hippocampal blood vessel density and activates microglia in rats but does not elevate central cytokine release. *Behav Brain Res* 207:265–272.

Shapiro W, Chernik N, Posner J (1973) Necrotizing encephalopathy following intraventricular instillation of methotrexate. *Arch Neurol* 28:96–102.

Sheline G, Wara W, Smith V (1980) Therapeutic irradiation and brain injury. *Int J Radiat Oncol Biol Phys* 6:1215–1228.

Shi L, Adams M, Long A, Carter C, Bennett C, Sonntag W, Nicolle M, Robbins M, D'Agostino Jr. R, Brunso-Bechtold J (2006) Spatial learning and memory deficits after whole-brain irradiation are associated with changes in NMDA receptor subunits in the hippocampus. *Radiat Res* 166:892–899.

Shilling V, Jenkins V, Morris R, Deutsch G, Bloomfield D (2005) The effects of adjuvant chemotherapy on cognition in women with breast cancer-preliminary results of an observational longitudinal study. *Breast* 14:142–150.

Shilling V, Jenkins V, Trapala IS (2006) The (mis)classification of chemofog -methodological inconsistencies in the investigation of cognitive impairment after chemotherapy. *Breast Cancer Res Treat* 95:125–129.

Shinohara C, Gobbel G, Lamborn K (1997) Apoptosis in the subependyma of young adult rats after single and fractionated doses of X-rays. *Cancer Res* 57:2694–2702.

Shohami E, Ginis I, Hallenbeck JM (1999) Dual role of tumor necrosis factor alpha in brain injury. *Cytokine Growth Factor Rev* 10:119–130.

Siegel R, Ward E, Brawley O, Jemal A (2011) Cancer statistics, 2011. *CA Cancer J Clin* 61:212–236.

Silverman DHS, Dy CJ, Castellon SA, Lai J, Pio BS, Abraham L, Waddell K, Petersen L, Phelps ME, Ganz PA (2007) Altered frontocortical, cerebellar, and basal ganglia activity in adjuvant-treated breast cancer survivors 5–10 years after chemotherapy. *Breast Cancer Res Treat* 103:303–311.

Snyder JS, Hong NS, McDonald RJ, Wojtowicz JM (2005) A role for adult neurogenesis in spatial long-term memory. *Neuroscience* 130:843–852.

Snyder JS, Kee N, Wojtowicz JM (2001) Effects of adult neurogenesis on synaptic plasticity in the rat dentate gyrus. *J Neurophysiol* 85: 2423–2431.

Sofroniew MV (2009) Molecular dissection of reactive astrogliosis and glial scar formation. *Trends Neurosci* 32:638–647.

Stevens LG (1896) Injurious effects on the skin. *Br Med J* 1:998.

Tada E, Parent JM, Lowenstein DH, Fike JR (2000) X-irradiation causes a prolonged reduction in cell proliferation in the dentate gyrus of adult rats. *Neuroscience* 99:33–41.

Tada E, Yang C, Gobbel GT, Lamborn KR, Fike JR (1999) Long-term impairment of subependymal repopulation following damage by ionizing irradiation. *Exp Neurol* 160:66–77.

Tofilon P, Fike J (2000) The radioresponse of the central nervous system: a dynamic process. *Radiat Res* 153:357–370.

Valk P, Dillon W (1991) Radiation injury of the brain. *Am J Neuroradiol* 12:45–62.

Vallières L, Campbell IL, Gage FH, Sawchenko PE (2002) Reduced hippocampal neurogenesis in adult transgenic mice with chronic astrocytic production of interleukin-6. *J Neurosci* 22:486–492.

Vardy J, Rourke S, Tannock IF (2007) Evaluation of cognitive function associated with chemotherapy: a review of published studies and recommendations for future research. *J Clin Oncol* 25:2455–2463.

Von der Weid N, Mosimann I, Hirt A, Wacker P, Nenadov Beck M, Imbach P, Caflisch U, Niggli F, Feldges A, Wagner HP (2003) Intellectual outcome in children and adolescents with acute lymphoblastic leukaemia treated with chemotherapy alone: age- and sex-related differences. *Eur J Cancer* 39:359–365.

Walker RW, Allen JC, Rosen G, Caparros B (1986) Transient cerebral dysfunction secondary to high-dose methotrexate. *J Clin Oncol* 4: 1845–1850.

Walsh D (1897) Deep tissue traumatism from roentgen ray exposure. *Br Med J*:272–273.

Wick A, Wick W, Hirrlinger J, Gerhardt E, Dringen R, Dichgans J, Weller M, Schulz JB (2004) Chemotherapy-induced cell death in primary cerebellar granule neurons but not in astrocytes: in vitro paradigm of differential neurotoxicity. *J Neurochem* 91:1067–1074.

Winocur G, Vardy J, Binns MA, Kerr L, Tannock I (2006) The effects of the anti-cancer drugs, methotrexate and 5-fluorouracil, on cognitive function in mice. *Pharmacol Biochem Behav* 85:66–75.

Winocur G, Henkelman M, Wojtowicz JM, Zhang H, Binns M, Tannock IF (2012) The effects of chemotherapy on cognitive function in a mouse model: a prospective study. *Clin Cancer Res* 18:3112–3121.

Yang M, Kim J-S, Kim J, Jang S, Kim S-H, Kim J-C, Shin T, Wang H, Moon C (2012) Acute treatment with methotrexate induces hippocampal dysfunction in a mouse model of breast cancer. *Brain Res Bull* 89:50–56.

Yang M, Kim J-S, Kim J, Kim S-H, Kim J-C, Kim J, Wang H, Shin T, Moon C (2011) Neurotoxicity of methotrexate to hippocampal cells *in vivo* and *in vitro*. *Biochem Pharmacol* 82:72–80.

Yang M, Kim J-S, Song M-S, Kim S-H, Kang SS, Bae C-S, Kim J-C, Wang H, Shin T, Moon C (2010) Cyclophosphamide impairs hippocampus-dependent learning and memory in adult mice: Possible involvement of hippocampal neurogenesis in chemotherapy-induced memory deficits. *Neurobiol Learn Mem* 93:487–494.

Yuan H, Gaber MW, Boyd K, Wilson CM, Kiani MF, Merchant TE (2006) Effects of fractionated radiation on the brain vasculature in a murine model: blood-brain barrier permeability, astrocyte proliferation, and ultrastructural changes. *Int J Radiat Oncol Biol Phys* 66:860–866.

Zeller B, Tamnes CK, Kanellopoulos A, Amlien IK, Andersson S, Due-Tønnessen P, Fjell AM, Walhovd KB, Westlye LT, Ruud E (2013) Reduced neuroanatomic volumes in long-term survivors of childhood acute lymphoblastic leukemia. *J Clin Oncol* 31:2078–2085.

Zhao C, Deng W, Gage FH (2008) Mechanisms and functional implications of adult neurogenesis. *Cell* 132:645–660.

Zhou H, Liu Z, Liu J (2011) Fractionated radiation-induced acute enceph-alopathy in a young rat model: cognitive dysfunction and histologic findings. *Am J Neuroradiol* 32:1795–1800.

Ziereisen F, Dan B, Azzi N, Ferster A, Damry N, Christophe C (2006) Reversible acute methotrexate leukoencephalopathy: atypical brain MR imaging features. *Pediatr Radiol* 36:205–212.

Chapter 5

Neural Stem Cell Activity and Neurogenesis After Stroke

Ashok K. Shetty and Kunlin Jin

Stroke is one of the foremost causes of mortality and morbidity in the world today. Systemic thrombolysis with tissue plasminogen activator remains the only established therapy available for ischemic stroke but can be employed in only a minority of patients because of its adverse effects when administered at delayed time points after stroke. For most stroke survivors, a lengthy program of rehabilitation with a life-long process of clinical support is the sole option for treatment. Hence, findings in animal models that neural stem cells in the brain react to ischemic brain injuries with enhanced proliferation, newly born immature neurons generated from neural stem cells migrate to the injured brain regions, and proliferating cells with the ability to give rise to neurons are found in ischemic regions of the brain, have raised hopes of rebuilding damaged brain regions through endogenous neuronal cell replacement. The purpose of this chapter is to confer current knowledge pertaining to the contribution of neurogenesis in replacing neurons that are lost due to ischemia or stroke in the adult brain, and possible relationship between stroke-induced neurogenesis and functional recovery after stroke. Additionally, the extent of stroke-induced neurogenesis in the human brain and the efficacy of neurogenesis enhancing strategies for improved functional recovery after stroke are also discussed.

Introduction

Maintenance of neural stem cells (NSCs) and manifestation of neurogenesis throughout life have been proven convincingly in two distinct zones of the adult brain of mammals. These comprise the subventricular zone (SVZ) covering the lateral ventricles of the forebrain and the subgranular zone (SGZ) of the dentate gyrus (DG) in the hippocampus (Ihrie and Alvarez-Buylla, 2011; Ming and Song, 2011; Yao *et al.*, 2012). In the SVZ, NSCs proliferate and produce a large pool of neuroblasts. These immature neurons then migrate along a pathway called the rostral migratory stream (RMS) and enter the olfactory bulb (OB) where they differentiate into mature olfactory interneurons (Ihrie and Alvarez-Buylla, 2011). On the other hand, NSCs in the SGZ proliferate and produce immature dentate granule cells and glia. Newly born dentate granule cells migrate into the granule cell layer (GCL) of the DG, mature and establish afferent connectivity with perforant path axons coming from the entorhinal cortex and efferent connectivity with the CA3 pyramidal neuron dendrites. (Ming and Song, 2011; Yao *et al.*, 2012).

Neurogenesis also occurs in the adult human brain. Eriksson and colleagues (1998) provided the first glimpse of neurogenesis occurring in the hippocampus of the adult human brain. A recent study demonstrated even stronger evidence for widespread neurogenesis in the DG of humans all through adulthood (Spalding *et al.*, 2013). An interesting finding is that neurogenesis does not decline significantly with aging in the human hippocampus, in contrast to substantial reductions typically seen in rodents (Kuhn *et al.*, 1996; Rao *et al.*, 2005, 2006; Hattiangady and Shetty, 2008). A clear validation of neurogenesis in the adult human brain has been instrumental in triggering a great deal of interest for examining the behavior of NSCs and the magnitude of neurogenesis in different regions of the adult brain in neurological disease conditions. One such disease is stroke, which can be classified into two major categories: ischemic and hemorrhagic. Ischemic strokes are caused by interruption of the blood supply, while hemorrhagic strokes result from the rupture of a blood vessel or an abnormal vascular structure. About 87% of strokes are ischemic, the rest are hemorrhagic. Currently, stroke is the fourth leading cause of death in the United States and the prominent cause for disability world-wide. Systemic thrombolysis with tissue plasminogen activator (tPA) remains the only proven treatment available for patients afflicted with ischemic stroke (Brott and Bogousslavsky, 2000; Adams *et al.*, 2007). However, because of an increased risk of hem-orrhage beyond 4.5 hours post stroke, only certain stroke patients (1–2%) can benefit from tPA. About one-third of these people failed to survive the event, and even among those who survived stroke, 90% of them suffered permanent deficits (Jorgensen *et al.*, 1997; Wang *et al.*, 2012). A lengthy program of rehabilitation fol-lowed by a life-long process of clinical support remains the best available treatment for many stroke survivors today. Even with rehabilitation therapy, 50–95% of stroke survivors remain impaired (Mayo *et al.*, 1999). From this perspective, the finding in animal prototypes that NSCs in the SVZ of forebrain and SGZ of the hip-pocampus react swiftly to stroke or ischemic brain injuries with enhanced proliferation of NSCs and increased generation of new neurons has offered hope for facilitating self-repair of the injured brain. Because of this, a new track of stroke-related research aimed towards amelioration of brain dysfunction via mobilization of NSCs in the forebrain has emerged (Wang *et al.*, 2012).

Subventricular Zone Neurogenesis following Focal Ischemia in Animal Models

The focal ischemia model used most often in rodents involves occlu-sion of the middle cerebral artery (MCAO), which causes localized brain infarction (Ginsberg *et al.*, 1989) and recapitulates many of the pathophysiological features of stroke. Ischemic brain injury trig-gers endogenous molecular and cellular repair mechanisms that contribute to recovery and may include ischemic activation of neu-rogenesis in the young adult brain (Cramer and Chopp, 2000). Studies in many animal prototypes have shown that focal cerebral ischemia triggers an enhanced proliferation of NSCs in the SVZ, resulting in increased production of neuroblasts (Jin *et al.*, 2001).

It has been shown that bilateral proliferation begins as early as 48 hours after transient focal ischemia in the SVZ, which then peaks at 1–2 weeks and returns to sham levels at 3–4 weeks post-ischemia (Jin *et al.*, 2001). Interestingly, these rapidly produced neuroblasts take a detour from their normal migratory behavior of entering the RMS and reaching the olfactory bulb. Instead, they migrate into peripheral areas of stroke-induced damage in the cerebral cortex and the striatum (Parent *et al.*, 2002; Jin *et al.*, 2003; Ohab *et al.*, 2006). A study by Thored and colleagues reported that, neuroblasts in the SVZ could migrate to injured areas like the striatum for up to a year after ischemia (Thored *et al.*, 2009), which suggested the existence of an extensive window of opportunity for therapeutic action. This finding also led to the notion that the SVZ can serve as a steady reservoir of newborn neurons for replenishing neurons that are lost due to ischemia or other injury.

Newly born neurons that migrate to ischemic regions can undergo maturation and acquire markers of mature neurons such as the microtubule associated protein-2 and neuron-specific nuclear antigen (NeuN). An elegant investigation by Arvidsson and colleagues (2002) has demonstrated that stroke-generated new neurons can differentiate into mature, medium-sized spiny neurons in the stroke-affected striatum region. This finding revealed that stroke-induced factors could promote the differentiation of NSC-derived new neuroblasts into specific neuronal types that are demolished by the ischemic injury. Several mechanisms likely underlie such specific differentiation. Some studies have suggested that increased erythropoitin (EPO) expression after stroke is instrumental in promoting NSC proliferation in the SVZ, the migration of newly born neuroblasts into the peripheral zones of the infarct region and angiogenesis in the damaged brain areas (Wang *et al.*, 2004; Tsai *et al.*, 2006). Another study points out that post-stroke neuroblast migration is linked to the vascular production of stromal-derived factor-1 and angiopoietin-1 (Ohab *et al.*, 2006). Additional investigations have documented the establishment of synapses between stroke-generated newly differentiated neurons and the existing striatal neurons (Yamashita *et al.*, 2006). Electrophysiological studies also demonstrate appropriate synaptic integration of newly added neurons (Lai *et al.*, 2008). However, the number of adult-born striatal neurons that survive long-term is equivalent to only 0.2% of striatal neurons that die in response to the ischemic injury (Arvidsson *et al.*, 2002). This may suggest that the microenvironment in peripheral regions of the infarct is not particularly conducive for maturation and/or integration of large numbers of newly born neurons. A study using a global cerebral ischemia model has also demonstrated the capability of NSCs for functional neuronal replacement after injury in the hippocampal CA1 subfield of young adult rats (Nakatomi *et al.*, 2002). Specifically, NSCs exhibited considerable activation in the SVZ bordering the CA1 region of the hippocampus after ischemic injury, which resulted in generation of new neuroblasts, migration towards the injured CA1 pyramidal cell layer and extensive repopulation of lost neurons with new pyramidal neurons. Additionally, infusion of growth factors into the lateral ventricle boosted the restoration of the damaged CA1 pyramidal cell layer and facilitated the integration of newly added neurons into the hippocampus circuitry and improved function (Nakatomi *et al.*, 2002). Thus, strategies that make the microenvironment in peripheral regions of the infarct suitable for maturation of a larger population of newly born neurons may further improve functional recovery after stroke.

Does Stroke-induced Neurogenesis in the SVZ Contribute to Functional Recovery?

The presence of NSCs in the adult mammalian brain has awakened new interest and optimism in potential treatments for a variety of acquired cerebral disorders including stroke. It is, however, unclear what role, if any, adult NSCs play in contributing to post-injury recovery or in neurodegenerative diseases because of the limitations of currently available techniques for tracking newly born cells. Typically, neural precursor cells in the adult brain are identified through 5′-bromodeoxyuridine (BrdU) labeling and their fate is then followed with specific differentiation markers. However, this procedure suffers several limitations including issues of sensitivity and permanence. Furthermore, while a mouse model expressing green fluorescent protein (GFP) gene under the control of the nestin promoter has been generated to genetically label NSCs *in vivo* (Yamaguchi *et al.*, 2000; Fukuda *et al.*, 2003), tracking the fate of NSCs in normal and diseased brains is not possible. This is because, the nestin promoter is inactivated once newborn cells undergo maturation resulting in the loss of GFP expression (Yu *et al.*, 2005). Injections of retroviruses or lentiviruses encoding GFP also have limited use, as this procedure labels only a few neural precursor cells and injections themselves can cause some brain damage (Mozdziak and Schultz, 2000; Kay *et al.*, 2001).

To understand the functional implications of post-stroke neurogenesis, several studies have employed NSC and neurogenesis ablation approaches after ischemia. These studies have uncovered that blocking of post-stroke neurogenesis is detrimental, as it leads to exacerbation of ischemia-induced neurological deficits. For example, whole-brain ionizing radiation ablating NSCs in the SGZ impaired performance on a water-maze task after global cerebral ischemia in guinea pig and mouse (Raber *et al.*, 2004; Zhu *et al.*, 2009). However, as ablation of NSCs by ionizing radiation may also affect astrocytic, microglial, and endothelial cell lineages, the observed impairment could not be attributed to loss of NSCs alone. To circumvent this, another study specifically targeted NSCs by using transgenic mice that expressed the herpes simplex virus-1 thymidine kinase (HSV-TK) under the ontrol of DCX promoter (DCX-TK mice).

Administration of ganciclovir (GCV, a synthetic analogue of 2′-deoxy-guanosine) to these animals resulted in phosphorylation of GCV into GCV-monophosphate in cells containing HSV-TK (i.e. in DCX+ newly born neurons). The GCV-monophosphate was then sequentially converted into GCV-diphosphate and GCV-triphosphate by host kinases. Becuse GCV-triphosphate causes premature DNA chain termination and apoptosis, immature DCX+ and recently divided neurons in the SVZ and the SGZ of DCX-TK mice were specifically depleted with 14 days of GCV treatment. Induction of stroke via MCAO in these mice resulted in larger infarcts and more severe sensorimotor behavioral deficits than control mice when examined a day after the induction of MCAO (Jin *et al.*, 2010; Figure 1), implying that neurogenesis contributes to recovery after acute stroke (Sun *et al.*, 2012; Wang *et al.*, 2012). Collectively, these results have supported the concept that targeted addition of new neurons by NSCs following stroke plays an important role in post-stroke functional recovery (Zhang *et al.*, 2004; Zhu *et al.*, 2009; Wang *et al.*, 2012). This prompted a great interest in developing therapies that are efficacious for increasing the activity of NSCs and neurogenesis after stroke.

Global Ischemia-induced Hippocampus Neurogenesis in Animal Models

Global cerebral ischemia is induced by permanent occlusion of the vertebral arteries and transient occlusion of the common carotid arteries (in rats) or through transient occlusion of the common carotid arteries (in gerbils and mice), followed by reperfusion. Several studies have demonstrated that global cerebral ischemia induces NSC proliferation and neurogenesis in the SGZ of the hippocampus, but not the SVZ (Liu *et al.*, 1998; Jin *et al.*, 2001). Some studies also reveal that post-stroke generated neurons are recruited into the hippocampal networks (Geibig *et al*, 2012). Other studies have examined potential mechanisms underlying such phenomenon. It has been suggested that stroke stimulates DG neurogenesis through multiple mechanisms. These comprise: (1) activation of cAMP response element binding protein (Zhu *et al.*, 2004); (2) Ca^{2+} influx through L-type voltage-gated Ca^{2+} channels (Luo *et al.*, 2005); and (3) reduced neuronal nitric oxide synthase (nNOS) and up-regulation of inducible NOS (iNOS) expression (Luo *et al.*, 2007).

Does Stroke-induced Neurogenesis in the SGZ Contribute to Functional Recovery?

The functional implications of increased hippocampus neurogenesis following stroke are yet to be ascertained. Some studies suggest

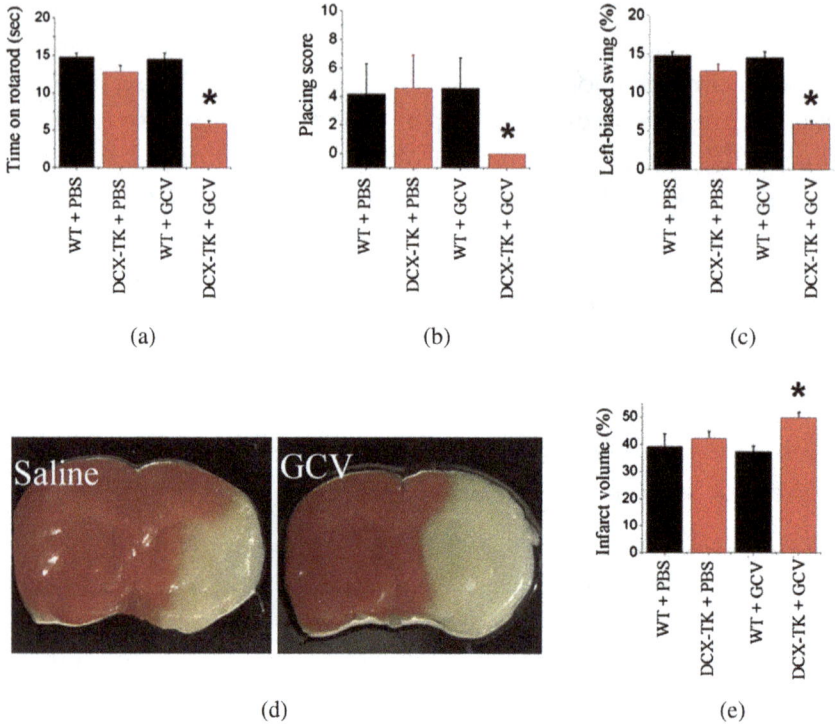

Figure 1. Focal cerebral ischemia in DCX-TK mice. WT (black bars) and DCX-TK transgenic (DCX-TK, red bars) mice were treated for 14 days with saline vehicle (PBS) or GCV, then underwent MCAO to induce focal cerebral ischemia. Twenty-four hours later, behavioral testing was performed and mice were killed for measurement of infarct size. (a) Rotarod scores, expressed as time (s) mice remained on the rod; lower scores represent more severe deficits. (b) Limb-placing test scores — lower scores represent more severe deficits. (c) Elevated body swing test scores, expressed as percentage turns away from the ischemic hemisphere — lower scores represent more severe deficits. (d) Infarct areas (white) in TTC — (red) stained coronal brain sections from PBS- and GCV-treated DCX-TK mice. (e) Infarct volumes (expressed as percentage hemispheric volume) in PBS- and GCV-treated WT (black) and DCX-TK (red) mice. *$P < 0.05$. *Reproduced from: Jin et al. (2010) Transgenic ablation of doublecortin-expressing cells suppresses adult neurogenesis and worsens stroke outcome in mice. Proc Natl Acad Sci USA 107:7993–7998.*

that it helps in the recovery from hippocampus-dependent learning and/or memory deficits (Raber *et al.*, 2004; Luo *et al.*, 2007) but direct evidence in support of that possibility is not available. For example, whole-brain ionizing radiation ablating dividing neuronal precursors in the SGZ, two weeks prior to 5 min of global cerebral ischemia of guinea pigs, greatly inhibited neurogenesis as well as impaired performance on a water-maze task (Raber *et al.*, 2004). Another study points out that enhancement of DG neurogenesis after stroke increases aberrant integration of newly born neurons into the hippocampus circuitry. Although it remains to be seen whether this anomalous circuitry underlies cognitive deficits and/or epilepsy after stroke (Niv *et al.*, 2012), it appears prudent to develop targeted approaches that specifically enhance SVZ neurogenesis, in order to prevent the formation of abnormal hippocampus circuitry from newly born dentate granule cells.

Stroke-Induced Neurogenesis in the Human Brain

There have been only a few studies on post-stroke neurogenesis in the human brain. Jin and colleagues (Jin *et al.*, 2006) were the first to provide a proof for stroke-induced neurogenesis in the human brain. They investigated the status of neurogenesis in brain sections taken from human brain biopsies performed for the diagnosis of cerebral lesions that proved to be ischemic strokes. Only negligible or no proliferating cells were found in control specimens obtained from the cerebral cortex of autopsied patients who died without the history of brain injury/pathology. In contrast, the cortical region adjacent to the infarct core (ischemic penumbra) in specimens taken from stroke patients demonstrated significant numbers of proliferating Ki-67+ cells, a fraction of which co-expressed the immature neuronal marker doublecortin (DCX; Figure. 2). Examination of NSC markers such as mini-chromosome maintenance protein-2 (MCM2) and proliferating cell nuclear antigen (PCNA) in Ki-67+ cells established that Ki-67 labeling reflected recent proliferation of NSC-like cells.

Furthermore, the ischemic penumbra displayed sizable numbers of cells positive for neuron-specific markers such as DCX and beta-III tubulin (Tuj-1). Some of the DCX+ or TuJ-1+ cells were also positive for Ki-67, implying that these are newly born neurons. While characterization of biopsy specimens in this study did not allow

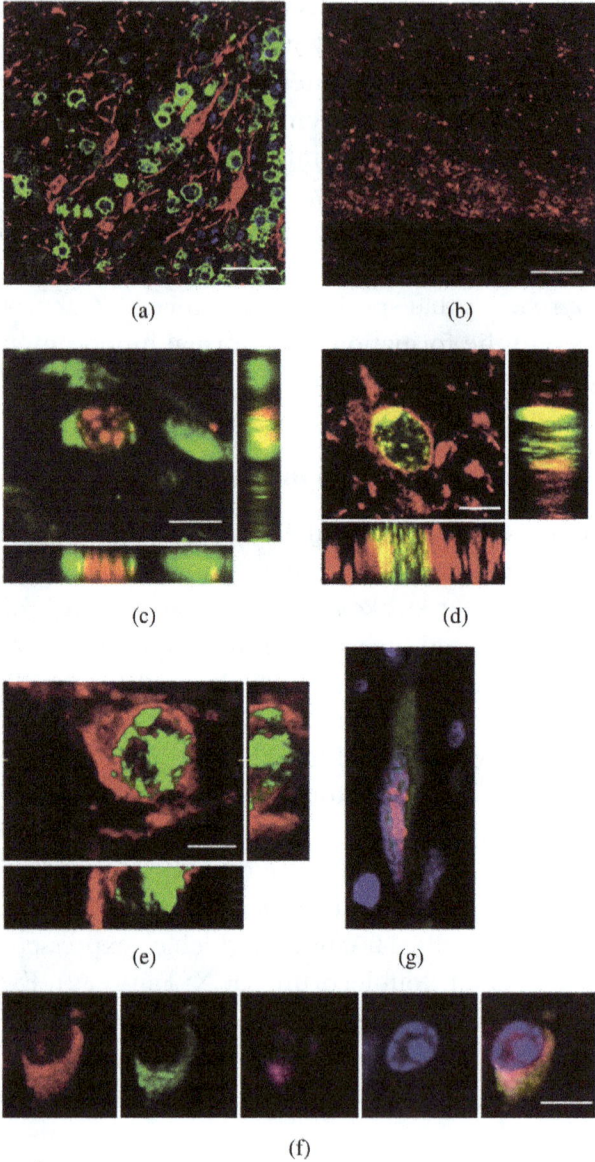

Figure 2. Neuronal characteristics of cells in the ischemic penumbra of the human cerebral cortex after stroke. (a) The early neuronal marker doublecortin (DCX, green) is expressed in the cytoplasm of numerous cells in the ischemic penumbra, where its expression does not overlap with that of the astroglial marker glial fibrillary acidic protein (GFAP, red). Scale bar, 150 μm. (b) The neuronal

←

Figure 2. (*Continued*) marker βIII-tubulin (red) is highly expressed in the ischemic penumbra (center of panel), less highly expressed in adjacent normal cortex (top of panel), and is absent in the ischemic core (bottom of panel). Scale bar, 200 μm. (c) DCX (green) is expressed in the cytoplasm of a cell with Ki-67-positive (red) nucleus. Scale bar, 5 μm. (d) βIII-tubulin (red) is expressed in the cytoplasm of a cell with Ki-67-positive (green) nucleus. Scale bar, 7 μm. (e) TUC-4 (red) is expressed in the cytoplasm of a cell with Ki-67-positive (green) nucleus. Scale bar, 5 μm. (f) ENCAM (red), DCX (green), and TUC-4 (purple) are co-localized; the nucleus is counterstained with DAPI (blue). Scale bar, 10 μm. (g) A cell with a Ki-67-stained nucleus (red) and DCX-positive cytoplasm (green) exhibits characteristic migratory morphology, with a leading process and trailing nucleus; nuclei are counterstained with DAPI (blue). *Reproduced from: Jin et al. (2006) Evidence for stroke-induced neurogenesis in the human brain. Proc Natl Acad Sci USA 103:13198–13202.*

detection of the origin of newly born neurons, their perivascular location insinuated that newly born neurons have likely derived from the SVZ and migrated alongside blood vessels into the ischemic region or areas around the ischemic region. However, it is currently unknown whether newly migrated neurons into these regions endure or contribute to brain repair after stroke in humans.

Neurogenesis Regulation and Manipulation

If endogenous neurogenesis indeed contributes to a more favorable outcome from stroke as suggested in several studies (Zhu *et al.*, 2009; Zhang *et al.*, 2004; Jin *et al.*, 2010), it has vital therapeutic implications. Specifically, non-invasive strategies that enhance endogenous neurogenesis (e.g. antidepressant treatment, physical exercise or exposure to enriched environment) may be used in the clinical management of stroke. Indeed, investigations in animal prototypes have revealed the potential of multiple strategies for enhancing forebrain neurogenesis and improving functional recovery via stimulation of NSCs following stroke. Kobayashi and colleagues (2006) showed that several steps of striatal neurogenesis after stroke can be enhanced through intrastriatal infusion of glial cell line-derived neurotrophic factor (GDNF), which is a neurotrophic factor belonging to the transforming growth factor beta superfamily and well known to promote the survival of various neuronal populations.

Wang and collaborators (2007), on the other hand, demonstrated that stroke-induced striatal neurogenesis can also be enhanced through administration of the vascular endothelial growth factor (VEGF), which is another neurotrophic factor well known to stimulate vasculogenesis and angiogenesis and have neuroprotective properties. Furthermore, Bambakidis *et al.* (2012) showed that improved NSC proliferation and neurological recovery following stroke could be obtained via intrathecal administration of sonic hedgehog (Shh), which is a soluble signaling protein known to promote the proliferation of adult NSCs. A study by Shruster and colleagues (2012) has suggested that enhanced neurogenesis and improved neurological function after focal ischemic injury in mice can also be achieved through overexpression of Wnt signaling, which is a pathway linked to stem cell expansion in several systems. Moreover, a recent study suggests that grafting of NSCs is effective for augmenting endogenous neurogenesis and improving functional recovery after stroke in rats (Mine *et al.*, 2013). Several other strategies have also been found to boost neurogenesis and improve functional recovery following stroke. These include strategies such as physical exercise (Zhang *et al.*, 2013), intravenous administration of bone marrow derived mesenchymal stem cells (MSCs) or umbilical cord derived MSCs (Yang *et al.*, 2013; Iskander *et al.*, 2013; Tsai *et al.*, 2014; Tsuji *et al.*, 2014), improved social environment provided through housing of a mouse that underwent stroke with a healthy cage mate (Venna *et al.*, 2014).

Conclusions

The recent demonstration of neurogenesis in several regions of the adult brain of humans, the ability of newly born immature neurons in the SVZ to migrate to the injured brain regions, the competence of the hippocampus to enhance neurogenesis in response to even remote brain injury, and the presence of proliferating cells with the ability to give rise to neurons in regions of the brain afflicted with ischemia have reinvigorated our hopes of rebuilding damaged tissues through endogenous neuronal cell replacement. However, molecular mechanisms regulating NSC function at different stages of life and after injury remain to be comprehended. Moreover, though many studies in animal prototypes point out the usefulness of increased neurogenesis by NSCs in the SVZ and SGZ for recovery of function after stroke or ischemia, it is currently unclear whether NSCs contribute to the recovery of function of the injured adult human brain. Answers to these questions will be important for understanding the role of neurogenesis in brain repair such as after stroke, for which effective treatment remains elusive.

References

Adams HP Jr, del Zoppo G, Alberts MJ, Bhatt DL, Brass L, Furlan A, Grubb RL, Higashida, RT, Jauch EC, Kidwell C *et al.* (2007) Guidelines for the early management of adults with ischemic stroke: a guideline from the American Heart Association/American Stroke Association Stroke Council, Clinical Cardiology Council, Cardiovascular Radiology and Intervention Council, and the Atherosclerotic Peripheral Vascular Disease and Quality of Care Outcomes in Research Interdisciplinary Working Groups: the American Academy of Neurology affirms the value of this guideline as an educational tool for neurologists. *Stroke* 38:1655–1711.

Arvidsson A, Collin T, Kirik D, Kokaia Z, Lindvall O (2002) Neuronal replacement from endogenous precursors in the adult brain after stroke. *Nat Med* 8:963–970.

Bambakidis NC, Petrullis M, Kui X, Rothstein B, Karampelas I, Kuang Y, Selman WR, LaManna JC, Miller RH (2012) Improvement of neurological recovery and stimulation of neural progenitor cell proliferation by intrathecal administration of Sonic hedgehog. *J Neurosurg* 116:1114–1120.

Brott, T, Bogousslavsky, J 2000 Treatment of acute ischemic stroke. *N Engl J Med* 343:710–722.

Cramer SC, Chopp M 2000 Recovery recapitulates ontogeny. *Trends Neurosci* 23:265–271.

Fukuda S, Kato F, Tozuka Y, Yamaguchi M Miyamoto Y, and Hisatsune T (2003) Two distinct subpopulations of nestin-positive cells in adult mouse dentate gyrus. *J Neurosci* 23:9357–9366.

Geibig CS, Keiner S, Redecker C (2012) Functional recruitment of newborn hippocampal neurons after experimental stroke. *Neurobiol Dis* 46:431–439.

Ginsberg MD, Busto R 1989 Rodent models of cerebral ischemia. *Stroke* 20:1627–1642.

Hattiangady B, Shetty AK (2008) Aging does not alter the number or phenotype of putative stem/progenitor cells in the neurogenic region of the hippocampus. *Neurobiol Aging* 29, 129–147.

Ihrie, RA, Alvarez-Buylla A (2011) Lake-front property: a unique germinal niche by the lateral ventricles of the adult brain. *Neuron* 70: 674–686.

Iskander A, Knight RA, Zhang ZG, Ewing JR, Shankar A, Varma NR, Bagher-Ebadian H, Ali MM Arbab AS, Janic B (2013) Intravenous administration of human umbilical cord blood-derived AC133+ endothelial progenitor cells in rat stroke model reduces infarct volume: magnetic resonance imaging and histological findings. *Stem Cells Transl Med* 2:703–714.

Jin K, Minami M, Lan JQ, Mao XO, Batteur S, Simon RP, Greenberg DA (2001) Neurogenesis in dentate subgranular zone and rostral subventricular zone after focal cerebral ischemia in the rat. *Proc Natl Acad Sci U S A* 98:4710–4715.

Jin K, Sun Y, Xie L, Peel A, Mao XO, Batteur S, Greenberg DA (2003) Directed migration of neuronal precursors into the ischemic cerebral cortex and striatum. *Mol Cell Neurosci* 2003 Sep;24(1):171–89.

Jin K, Wang X, Xie L, Mao XO, Greenberg DA (2010) Transgenic ablation of doublecortin-expressing cells suppresses adult neurogenesis and worsens stroke outcome in mice. *Proc Natl Acad Sci U S A* 107:7993–7998.

Jin, K Wang X, Xie L, Mao XO, Zhu W, Wang Y, Shen J, Mao Y, Banwait S, Greenberg DA (2006) Evidence for stroke-induced neurogenesis in the human brain. *Proc Natl Acad Sci U S A* 103:13198–13202.

Jorgensen HS, Nakayama H, Raaschou HO, Olsen TS (1997) Acute stroke care and rehabilitation: an analysis of the direct cost and its clinical and social determinants. The Copenhagen Stroke Study. *Stroke* 28:1138–1141.

Kay MA, Glorioso JC, Naldini L (2001) Viral vectors for gene therapy: the art of turning infectious agents into vehicles of therapeutics. *Nat Med* 7:33–40.

Kobayashi T, Ahlenius H, Thored P, Kobayashi R, Kokaia Z, Lindvall O (2006) Intracerebral infusion of glial cell line-derived neurotrophic factor promotes striatal neurogenesis after stroke in adult rats. *Stroke* 37:2361–2367.

Kuhn HG, Dickinson-Anson H, Gage FH (1996) Neurogenesis in the dentate gyrus of the adult rat: age-related decrease of neuronal progenitor proliferation. *J Neurosci* 16:2027–2033.

Lai B, Mao XO, Xie L, Jin K, Greenberg, DA (2008) Electrophysiological neurodifferentiation of subventricular zone-derived precursor cells following stroke. *Neurosci Lett* 442:305–308.

Liu J, Solway K, Messing RO, Sharp, FR (1998) Increased neurogenesis in the dentate gyrus after transient global ischemia in gerbils. *J Neurosci* 18:7768–7778.

Luo CX, Zhu XJ, Zhang AX, Wang W, Yang XM, Liu SH, Han X, Sun J, Zhang SG, Lu Y, Zhu DY (2005) Blockade of L-type voltage-gated calcium channel inhibits ischemia-induced neurogenesis by down-regulating iNOS expression in adult mouse. *J Neurochem* 94: 1077–1086.

Luo CX, Zhu XJ, Zhou QG, Wang B, Wang W, Cai HH Sun YJ, Hu M, Jiang J, Hua Y, Han X, Zhu DY (2007) Reduced neuronal nitric oxide synthase is involved in ischemia-induced hippocampal neurogenesis by up-regulating inducible nitric oxide synthase expression. *J Neurochem* 103:1872–1882.

Mayo NE, Wood-Dauphinee S, Ahmed S, Gordon C, Higgins J, McEwen S, Salbach N (1999) Disablement following stroke. *Disabil Rehabil* 21: 258–268.

Mine Y, Tatarishvili J, Oki K, Monni E, Kokaia Z, Lindvall O (2013) Grafted human neural stem cells enhance several steps of endogenous neurogenesis and improve behavioral recovery after middle cerebral artery occlusion in rats. *Neurobiol Dis* 52:191–203.

Ming GL, Song H (2011) Adult neurogenesis in the mammalian brain: significant answers and significant questions. *Neuron* 70:687–702.

Mozdziak P, Schultz E (2000) Retroviral labeling is an appropriate marker for dividing cells. *Biotech Histochem* 75:141–146.

Nakatomi H, Kuriu T, Okabe S, Yamamoto S, Hatano O, Kawahara N, Tamura A, Kirino T, Nakafuku M (2002) Regeneration of hippocampal pyramidal neurons after ischemic brain injury by recruitment of endogenous neural progenitors. *Cell* 110:429–441.

Niv F, Keiner S, Krishna, Witte OW, Lie DC, Redecker C (2012) Aberrant neurogenesis after stroke: a retroviral cell labeling study. *Stroke* 43: 2468–2475.

Ohab JJ, Fleming S, Blesch A, Carmichael ST (2006) A neurovascular niche for neurogenesis after stroke. *J Neurosci* 26:13007–13016.

Parent JM, Vexler ZS, Gong C, Derugin N, Ferriero DM (2002) Rat forebrain neurogenesis and striatal neuron replacement after focal stroke. *Ann Neurol* 52:802–813.

Raber J, Fan Y, Matsumori Y, Liu Z, Weinstein PR, Fike JR, Liu J (2004) Irradiation attenuates neurogenesis and exacerbates ischemia-induced deficits. *Ann Neurol* 55:381–389.

Rao MS, Hattiangady B, Abdel-Rahman A, Stanley DP, Shetty AK (2005) Newly born cells in the ageing dentate gyrus display normal migration, survival and neuronal fate choice but endure retarded early maturation. *Eur J Neurosci* 21:464–476.

Rao MS, Hattiangady B, Shetty AK (2006) The window and mechanisms of major age-related decline in the production of new neurons within the dentate gyrus of the hippocampus. *Aging Cell* 5:545–558.

Shruster A, Ben-Zur T, Melamed E, Offen D (2012) Wnt signaling enhances neurogenesis and improves neurological function after focal ischemic injury. *PLoS One* 7:e40843.

Spalding KL, Bergmann O, Alkass K, Bernard S, Salehpour M, Huttner HB, Bostrom E, Westerlund I, Vial C, Buchholz BA *et al.* (2013) Dynamics of hippocampal neurogenesis in adult humans. *Cell* 153:1219–1227.

Sun F, Wang X, Mao X, Xie L, Jin K (2012) Ablation of neurogenesis attenuates recovery of motor function after focal cerebral ischemia in middle-aged mice. *PLoS One* 7:e46326.

Thored P, Arvidsson A, Cacci E, Ahlenius H, Kallur T, Darsalia V, Ekdahl CT, Kokaia Z, Lindvall O (2006) Persistent production of neurons from adult brain stem cells during recovery after stroke. *Stem Cells* 24:739–747.

Tsai MJ, Tsai SK, Hu BR, Liou DY, Huang SL, Huang MC, Huang WC, Cheng H, Huang SS (2014) Recovery of neurological function of ischemic stroke by application of conditioned medium of bone marrow mesenchymal stem cells derived from normal and cerebral ischemia rats. *J Biomed Sci* 21:5.

Tsai PT, Ohab JJ, Kertesz N, Groszer M, Matter C, Gao J, Liu X, Wu H, Carmichael ST (2006) A critical role of erythropoietin receptor in neurogenesis and post-stroke recovery. *J Neurosci* 26:1269–1274.

Tsuji M, Taguchi A, Ohshima M, Kasahara Y, Sato, Y Tsuda H, Otani K, Yamahara K, Ihara M, Harada-Shiba M, Ikeda T, Matsuyama T (2014) Effects of intravenous administration of umbilical cord blood CD34 cells in a mouse model of neonatal stroke. *Neuroscience* [Epub ahead of print].

Venna V.R, Xu Y, Doran SJ, Patrizz A, McCullough LD (2014) Social interaction plays a critical role in neurogenesis and recovery after stroke. *Transl Psychiatry* 4:e351.

Wang X, Mao X, Xie L, Sun F, Greenberg DA, Jin K (2012) Conditional depletion of neurogenesis inhibits long-term recovery after experimental stroke in mice. *PLoS One* 7:e38932.

Wang L, Zhang Z, Wang Y, Zhang R, Chopp M (2004b) Treatment of stroke with erythropoietin enhances neurogenesis and angiogenesis and improves neurological function in rats. *Stroke* 35:1732–1737.

Wang YQ, Guo X, Qiu MH, Feng XY, Sun FY (2007) VEGF overexpression enhances striatal neurogenesis in brain of adult rat after a transient middle cerebral artery occlusion. *J Neurosci Res* 85:73–82.

Yamaguchi M, Saito H, Suzuki M, Mori K (2000) Visualization of neurogenesis in the central nervous system using nestin promoter-GFP transgenic mice. *Neuroreport* 11:1991–1996.

Yamashita T, Ninomiya M, Hernandez Acosta P, Garcia-Verdugo JM, Sunabori T, Sakaguchi M, Adachi K, Kojima T, Hirota Y, Kawase T *et al.* (2006) Subventricular zone-derived neuroblasts migrate and differentiate into mature neurons in the post-stroke adult striatum. *J Neurosci* 26:6627–6636.

Yang B, Migliati E, Parsha K, Schaar K, Xi X, Aronowski J, Savitz, SI (2013) Intra-arterial delivery is not superior to intravenous delivery of autologous bone marrow mononuclear cells in acute ischemic stroke. *Stroke* 44:3463–3472.

Yao J, Mu Y, Gage FH (2012) Neural stem cells: mechanisms and modeling. *Protein Cell* 3:251–261.

Yu TS, Dandekar M, Monteggia LM, Parada LF, Kernie SG (2005) Temporally regulated expression of Cre recombinase in neural stem cells. *Genesis* 41:147–153.

Zhang L, Hu X, Luo J, Li L, Chen X, Huang R, Pei Z (2013) Physical exercise improves functional recovery through mitigation of autophagy, attenuation of apoptosis and enhancement of neurogenesis after MCAO in rats. *BMC Neurosci* 14:46-2202-14-46.

Zhang R, Zhang Z, Wang L, Wang Y, Gousev A, Zhang L, Ho KL, Morshead C, Chopp M (2004) Activated neural stem cells contribute to stroke-induced neurogenesis and neuroblast migration toward the infarct boundary in adult rats. *J Cereb Blood Flow Metab* 24:441–448.

Zhu DY, Lau L, Liu SH, Wei JS, Lu YM (2004) Activation of cAMP-response-element-binding protein (CREB) after focal cerebral ischemia stimulates neurogenesis in the adult dentate gyrus. *Proc Natl Acad Sci USA* 101:9453–9457.

Zhu C, Huang Z, Gao J, Zhang Y, Wang X, Karlsson N, Li Q, Lannering B, Bjork-Eriksson T, Georg Kuhn H *et al.* (2009) Irradiation to the immature brain attenuates neurogenesis and exacerbates subsequent hypoxic-ischemic brain injury in the adult. *J Neurochem* 111:1447–1456.

Chapter 6

Neurogenesis and Dentate Granule Cell Development in Epilepsy

Bethany E. Hosford and Steve C. Danzer

Temporal lobe epilepsy is associated with dramatic changes in hippocampal granule cell neurogenesis, affecting cell proliferation, survival, and integration. In adult animals, epileptogenic brain injuries typically lead to an acute increase in granule cell neurogenesis, which is sometimes followed by a decrease in cell production in chronic stages of the disease. Seizure-induced changes in neural progenitor cell proliferation are age-dependent, with distinct effects on the neonatal and aged brain. Many of the new neurons produced in the burst of neurogenesis following an epileptogenic injury develop aberrantly. Abnormalities include the formation of recurrent excitatory connections among granule cells, which can be mediated by aberrant sprouting of granule cell mossy fiber axons, formation of basal dendrites, or ectopic cell migration. These abnormal connections are hypothesized to contribute to epileptogenesis. Notably, however, not all new granule cells integrate abnormally, and some may act to maintain homeostasis, making the net effect of granule cell neurogenesis in epilepsy uncertain. Here, we discuss different lines of evidence favoring both pro-epileptogenic and protective roles these cells may have on hippocampal circuitry.

Introduction

Epilepsy is a neurological condition defined by the occurrence of two or more unprovoked seizures. Epilepsy can develop as a consequence of a wide variety of brain insults including genetic mutations, birth defects, traumatic brain injury, cerebral infections, *status epilepticus*, tumors, and stroke. There are many different types of epilepsy syndromes which can vary widely in severity, prognosis, and etiology. For the present review we will focus on temporal lobe epilepsy, which as the name suggests, affects cerebral structures within the temporal lobes of the brain including the entorhinal cortex, amygdala, and hippocampus [for review see (Bertram, 2009)]. Involvement of the hippocampus is most pertinent to the present review, as seizures often exert dramatic effects on the production, development, integration, and physiology of hippocampal dentate granule cells.

Dentate granule cells are an intriguing neuronal population exhibiting several unique developmental features that potentially make them vulnerable to seizures and epileptogenic brain injury. Granule cells are produced very late in development; much later than almost all other neurons. Approximately 70% of the granule cell population is generated after birth in rodents (Schlessinger *et al.*, 1975; Bayer, 1980; Altman and Bayer, 1990a; 1990b), while more than 30% of the granule cell population is generated within the first three months after birth in non-human primates (Lavenex *et al.*, 2007; Jabès *et al.*, 2010). Studies in humans are more limited for obvious ethical reasons; however, both histological and imaging data support a late development of the hippocampal formation (Giedd *et al.*, 1996; Seress *et al.*, 2001). Even more intriguing, production of dentate granule cells, unlike most other neuronal populations, continues throughout life and into old age. After this latter discovery in mammals decades ago (Altman and Das, 1965; Kaplan and Hinds, 1977; Bayer *et al.*, 1982), and with the first demonstration of postnatal granule cell neurogenesis in humans in the late 90s (Eriksson *et al.*, 1998), epilepsy researchers began to examine the impact of seizures on this unusual cell population. Recent studies support the general concept that the protracted generation of dentate granule cells renders the dentate gyrus uniquely vulnerable to epileptogenic brain injury. In this chapter, we review changes in granule cell proliferation and development that occur in the epileptic brain. The functional consequences of granule cell disruption remain controversial; therefore, we will review several hypotheses on whether these abnormalities are pro-epileptogenic or protective.

Changes in Granule Cell Proliferation and Survival Following Seizures

Adult-generated dentate granule cells are produced from hippocampal neural progenitor cells located in the subgranular zone of the dentate gyrus. Granule cell neurogenesis is a very dynamic process and progenitor cell proliferation can be regulated by a variety of agents including growth factors, neurotransmitters, steroid hormones, and activity. Importantly, the net number of granule cells added to the dentate gyrus can be regulated by controlling the number of new cells produced and the percentage of these new cells that survive and integrate stably. Different factors can regulate different aspects of granule cell neurogenesis; therefore, changes in cell proliferation and cell survival can be controlled independently (e.g. increased proliferation and decreased survival may occur simultaneously). This complex biology can produce paradoxical and seemingly conflicting findings which should be kept in mind when reviewing the literature. Epilepsy, the focus of the present chapter, adds an additional level of complexity to the story. The initial injuries that produce epilepsy, as well as the resulting seizures, can substantially alter many cues that regulate granule cell neurogenesis, and correspondingly, impact the proliferation and integration of granule cells. In this section, we discuss the effects epileptogenic insults and seizures can have on neural progenitor cell behavior in the neonatal, mature, and aged brain. Moreover, because epilepsy is a progressive disorder, we discuss changes in progenitor cell behavior that can occur as the disease evolves from an acute phase to a more chronic phase.

Acute seizures increase granule cell neurogenesis in the mature brain

In the late 90s, Parent and colleagues (1997) described increased proliferative behavior of hippocampal neural progenitor cells following seizure activity in rodents. Using bromodeoxyuridine (BrdU), a synthetic nucleoside that incorporates into the DNA of mitotically active cells, they were able to assess neurogenesis at different time points following seizures. Subsequent analysis of BrdU immunoreactivity revealed significant increases in neurogenesis during the first two weeks following *status epilepticus* induced by the cholinergic agonist pilocarpine (Figure 1). Similar increases in neurogenesis have now been described in many adult animal models of epilepsy including hippocampal kindling (Bengzon *et al.*, 1997), amygdala kindling (Parent *et al.*, 1998), systemic kainic acid (Covolan *et al.*, 2000), intracerebroventricular kainic acid (Gray and Sundstrom, 1998) electroconvulsive shock seizures (Scott *et al.*, 2000, Madsen *et al.*, 2000), and tetanus toxin (Jiruska *et al.*, 2013). The increase in neurogenesis in epilepsy models is not universal, with intrahippocampal infusion of kainic acid being a notable exception (Kralic *et al.*, 2005).

Dentate granule cells generated after an epileptogenic insult functionally integrate into the brain and can persist for long periods of time. Granule cells born after self-sustaining *status epilepticus*, for example, were still present when the animals were examined six months later (Bonde *et al.*, 2006). Similarly, viral fate-mapping techniques have demonstrated that granule cells produced following kainic acid-induced *status epilepticus* can persist for up to a year in rodents (Jessberger *et al.*, 2007). Not all newborn granule cells survive, however. In the normal brain, many adult-generated granule cells are eliminated via naturally occurring cell death (also known as apoptosis). This natural pruning mechanism is hypothesized to eliminate neurons that are not effectively utilized by the brain (Buss *et al.*, 2009). In support of this hypothesis, processes that increase the activity of dentate granule cells, such as hippocampal-dependent learning tasks, can improve the survival of newborn cells in rodents (Gould *et al.*, 1999; Leuner *et al.*, 2004; Hairston

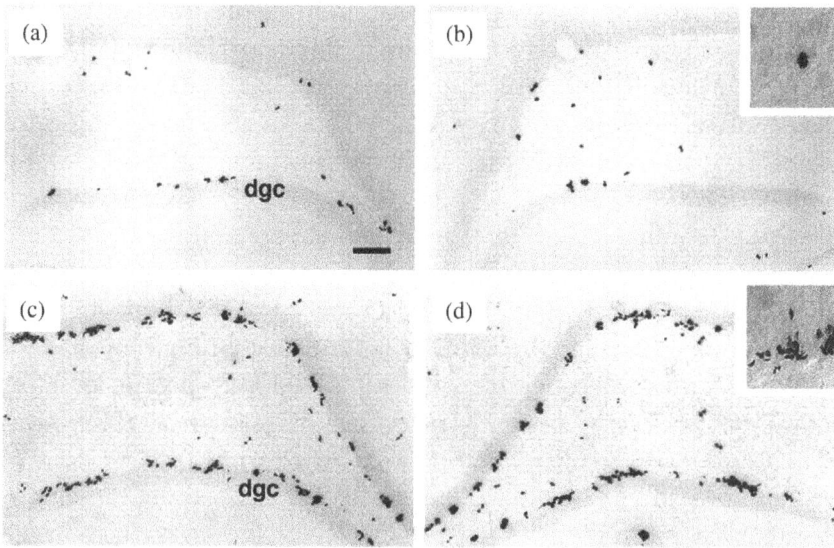

Figure 1. Acute seizures can increase dentate granule cell neurogenesis in the mature rodent brain. BrdU immunoreactivity within dentate gyri of control rat (a and b) and pilocarpine treated rat (c and d) 13 hours post treatment. Insets show magnification of granular layer. Neural proliferation rates are dramatically increased following pilocarpine treatment compared to saline treated controls. Scale bar is 100 μm. Figure reprinted with permission from Parent *et al.*, 1997. Copyright © 1997 by the Society for Neuroscience.

et al., 2005; Dalla *et al.*, 2007). Seizures induced through hippocampal kindling have also been shown to improve the survival of granule cells generated one week prior to seizure induction (Scott and Burnham, 2006), leading to the hypothesis that seizures — which can dramatically increase neuronal activity levels — promote newborn granule cell survival. On the other hand, evidence suggests that this effect may depend on the severity of the insult, with more modest injuries promoting survival, while more severe insults decrease survival (Mohapel *et al.*, 2004).

Effects of acute seizures in the neonatal and aged brain

Developing animals and children exhibit a high incidence of seizures (Hauser, 1994; Silverstein and Jensen, 2007). This is likely due in part to a reduced seizure threshold in the immature brain relative to the mature brain, making children particularly suscepti- ble to febrile seizures (Sanchez and Jensen, 2001). The high inci- dence of seizures in children has led to an extensive literature aimed at determining whether and how they impact the developing brain [for review see (Ben-Ari and Holmes, 2006)]. Somewhat para- doxically, studies of animal models of neonatal seizures have revealed that although the immature brain is more prone to exhibit- ing seizures, the seizures themselves appear to be less damaging. For example, in contrast to the adult brain, the developing brain is rela- tively resistant to cell death in the hilus and CA3 pyramidal layer following *status epilepticus* (Sankar *et al.*, 1998; Liu *et al.*, 1999, Haas *et al.*, 2001) and insults which usually cause the development of recurrent seizures later in life are not necessarily epileptogenic to the neonatal brain (Sankar *et al.*, 1998). Nevertheless, seizures in the developing brain do appear to be harmful. Seizures in developing rodents lead to impairments in hippocampal-dependent learning tasks later in adulthood. Furthermore, while seizures in the imma- ture brain tend not to lead to the development of epilepsy, neonatal seizures can lead to reduced seizure thresholds and increased sus- ceptibility to seizures in adulthood [for reviews see (Holmes, 2005; Sankar and Rho, 2007)].

Neonatal seizures affect postnatal neurogenesis. The affect appears to be highly variable and dependent on the age of the ani- mal and the amount of time passed following seizures. In contrast to the seizure-induced rapid increase in neurogenesis observed in adult rodents, McCabe and colleagues (2001) found a reduction in neurogenesis during the first week following flurothyl-induced sei- zures in one day old rats. Similar results have been obtained from rodents subjected to intracerebroventricular kainic acid- (Dong *et al.*, 2003) and pilocarpine- (Xiu-Yu *et al.*, 2007; Shi *et al.*, 2007) induced seizures during the first week of life. Interestingly, when neurogenesis was analyzed in these animals several weeks later, granule cell production was increased relative to controls, suggest- ing a bimodal response to seizures during the earliest stages of postnatal development. When animals were subjected to seizures during their second and third weeks of life, however, neural proliferation increased, similar to the mature brain (Sankar *et al.*, 2000; Bender *et al.*, 2003). These data support the idea that a critical developmental stage must be reached before seizures begin to increase neurogenic activity.

Acute effects of seizures on neural progenitor cell behavior in the aged brain (equivalent to 20–30 months old rodent) differ from younger adults as well. During normal aging, postnatal hippocampal neurogenesis continues, but at a decreasing rate (Kuhn *et al.*, 1996). It has been reported that *status epilepticus* in the aged brain, in contrast to the adult brain, does not increase neurogenesis (Rao *et al.*, 2008). A separate study, however, found a dramatic increase in the production of immature neurons following *status epilepticus* (Shapiro *et al.*, 2011). Differences in methodology — including rat strain, model of *status epilepticus*, and timing of tissue analysis following the brain injury — may account for some of these differences. Additional studies are needed to assess the potential of the aged brain for seizure-induced neurogenesis.

Chronic seizures and disruption of the dentate gyrus lead to decreased neurogenesis

In contrast to increased neural progenitor cell behavior observed following acute seizures in the mature brain, Hattiangady and colleagues (2004) demonstrated that hippocampal neurogenesis can be dramatically decreased in the chronic phases of epilepsy. Rather than merely assessing progenitor cell behavior days to weeks following the epileptic injury, researchers measured doublecortin expression, a marker for immature neurons, two weeks and five months following *status epilepticus* induced by systemic administration of kainic acid. Two weeks after the injury the investigators observed the expected increase in neurogenesis, consistent with prior studies. Five months after the injury, however, they found a significant reduction in the number of immature neurons compared to age-matched control animals (Figure 2). A follow-up study by the same group indicated that in the chronic phases of epilepsy, basal

Temporal Hippocampus

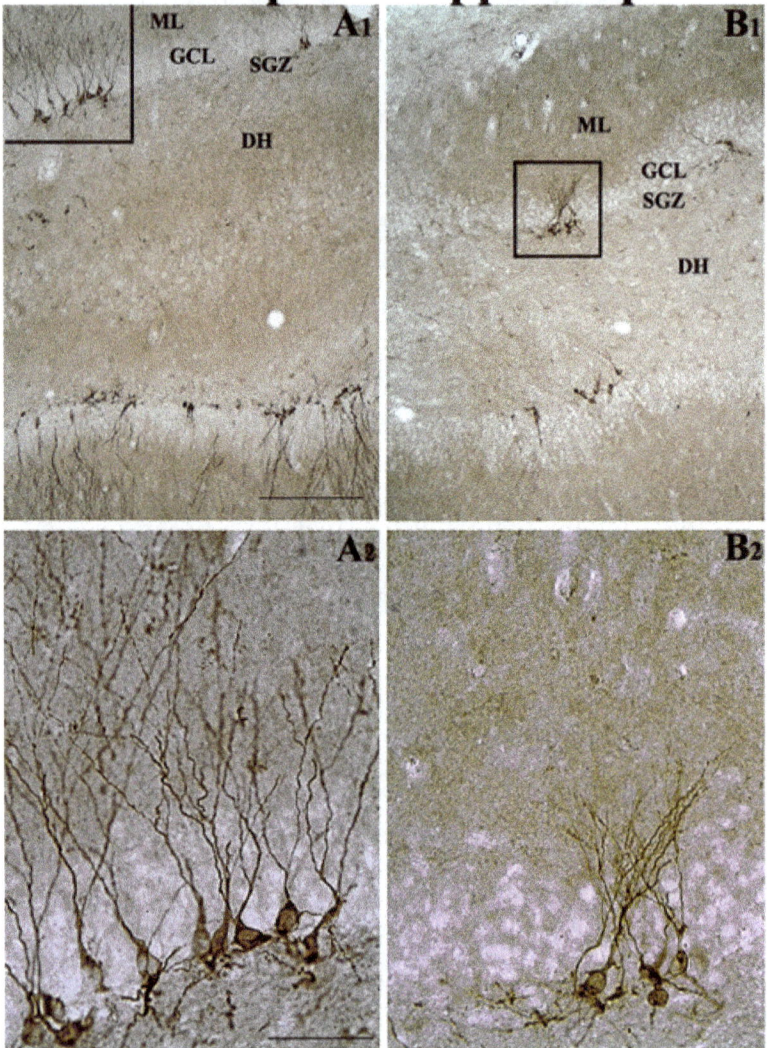

Figure 2.   Chronic seizures can decrease dentate granule cell neurogenesis in the mature rodent brain. Doublecortin immunoreactivity within dentate gyrus of control rat (A_1) and kainic acid treated rat (B_1) five months post treatment. Image (A_2) and image (B_2) show magnified area in boxes indicated in (A_1) and (B_1), respectfully. Neural proliferation rates are dramatically decreased several months following kainic acid treatment compared to saline treated controls. Scale bar for (A_1 and B_1) is 200 µm and scale bar for (A_2 and B_2) is 50 µm. Figure reprinted with permission from (Hattiangady *et al.*, 2004). Copyright © 2004 by the Elsevier Inc.

proliferation was unchanged; however the majority of these cells differentiated into glial cells (Hattiangady and Shetty, 2010). In this model of chronic epilepsy, the dramatic shift in the ratio of neurons to glia generated from neural progenitor cells underlies decreased neurogenesis [for review see (Kuruba *et al.*, 2009)].

Reduced neurogenesis in chronic epilepsy may be model specific or exhibit temporal dynamics, which vary among animals. Bonde and colleagues (2006), for example, did not observe a reduction in doublecortin positive immature neurons in mice examined six months after self-sustained *status epilepticus*, and Avanzi and colleagues (2010) found a slight increase in doublecortin immunoreactivity 20 months following pilocarpine-induced *status epilepticus*. Alternatively, Danzer (2012) observed reduced neurogenesis months after pilocarpine-induced *status epilepticus*; but only in a subset of animals that also exhibited pronounced hippocampal cell loss. Hippocampal cell loss in this model is reminiscent of hippocampal sclerosis in human temporal lobe epilepsy, characterized by pronounced loss of principle cells and gliosis. It is conceivable that cell loss could lead to the disruption of the neurogenic niche, and since cell loss can develop progressively over time, patterns of neurogenesis may exhibit complex temporal and model-specific dynamics.

Consistent with the idea that progressive hippocampal damage may disrupt the neurogenic niche in chronic epilepsy, the intrahippocampal kainic acid model of epilepsy, which produces rapid disruption of the dentate architecture, is associated with an acute reduction in neurogenesis (Kralic *et al.*, 2005). In this model, kainic acid is infused into the hippocampus unilaterally, resulting in focal *status epilepticus*. Cell proliferation is briefly increased days after the insult, but rapidly drops to levels below those seen in control animals. Moreover, the brief increase in proliferation does not lead to more neurons; rather, the new cells assume a glial fate, similar to the findings of Hattiangady and Shetty in chronic epilepsy (2010). Impaired neurogenesis in the injected hemisphere is associated with profound dispersion of the granular layer and neuronal hypertrophy. The contralateral hippocampus, on the other hand, does not exhibit reduced neurogenesis, and exhibits only modest structural changes (Murphy *et al.*, 2012). These observations suggest that severe disruption of the dentate gyrus may also disrupt the neurogenic subgranular zone, impairing cell proliferation and cell fate decisions.

If reduced neurogenesis is a common feature of at least some chronic epilepsy conditions, it is likely to have significant consequences on other cerebral functions. Granule cells are critical for hippocampal dependent learning and memory [for review see (Kitabatake *et al.*, 2007; Deng *et al.*, 2010)] and reductions in neurogenesis may underlie the cognitive impairments associated with temporal lobe epilepsy [for review see (Hattiangady and Shetty, 2008)]. Likewise, depression, which is often a comorbidity associated with epilepsy, can be accompanied by decreases in neurogenesis; perhaps contributing to the increased susceptibility of epileptic individuals to the disorder [for reviews see (Kanner, 2008; Danzer *et al.*, 2012)].

Neurogenesis in the epileptic human brain

Evidence for increased neurogenesis during the acute phase of epileptogenesis is well accepted in animal models; however, the extent to which this occurs in humans is unclear. While the majority of animal studies focus on the time period shortly after an epileptogenic brain injury, human tissue studies examine much later disease stages, as patients typically undergo years of treatment with anticonvulsants before surgery is considered. Tissue from these patients may be more reflective of chronic stages of the disease, even in very young patients. Other confounding variables in human tissue studies, including the history of anticonvulsant treatment and the availability of appropriate human tissue controls, likely affect findings. Despite these caveats, human studies are essential for testing hypotheses and providing critical information about the condition in patients.

Evidence for both increased and decreased granule cell proliferation in human epilepsy has been obtained using resected hippocampi from patients with temporal lobe epilepsy. Increased immunoreactivity for the neural progenitor marker nestin has been found within the dentate gyri of patients, suggesting an increased proliferative capacity of the hippocampus in temporal lobe epilepsy (Blümcke *et al.*, 2001; Crespel *et al.*, 2005; Wang *et al.*, 2009). Likewise, the expression of the immature neuronal marker doublecortin was found to be increased in one study examining adult patients with temporal lobe epilepsy (Liu *et al.*, 2008); however, expression was found to be decreased in a separate study (D'Alessio *et al.*, 2010). The latter study specifically analyzed tissue sections from adults with hippocampal sclerosis; therefore, these conflicting findings may reflect differing neurogenic potentials of the epileptic hippocampus and the severely damaged sclerotic hippocampus. In support of this hypothesis, Mathern and colleagues (2002) found decreased immunoreactivity for the immature neuronal marker polysialic acid neural cell adhesion molecule (PSA-NCAM) in children with epilepsy who exhibited reduced cell density within the dentate gyrus, indicative of cell loss. More information concerning changes in granule cell neurogenesis in response to seizures in human cases of temporal lobe epilepsy can be reviewed elsewhere (Siebzehnrubl and Blümcke, 2008).

To compliment these immunohistochemical studies, Coras and colleagues (2010) generated *in vitro* cell cultures of neural progenitor cells excised from patients with temporal lobe epilepsy. The results of this study indicated that while some patients with temporal lobe epilepsy have neural progenitor cells capable of rapid cell division, other patients have neural progenitor cells with a reduced capacity for cell division. These findings suggest that progenitor cells in some temporal lobe epilepsy patients exhibit increased proliferation while others exhibit decreased proliferation. In a related study, Paradisi and colleagues (2010), using a similar methodology, found that cell proliferation negatively correlated with disease duration. Neural progenitor cells extracted from patients who had experienced temporal lobe epilepsy for only a few years exhibited high proliferation rates, whereas progenitor cells from patients with over a 20-year history of epilepsy exhibited significantly decreased proliferation rates. In addition, progenitor cells extracted from patients with hippocampal sclerosis showed decreased potential for proliferation. Whether these *in vitro* findings are representative of neurogenesis within the intact human brain has yet to be determined, however the results are consistent with the idea that disease duration may have a negative impact on neurogenesis rates.

Role of the Dentate Gyrus in Temporal Lobe Epileptogenesis

Under normal conditions, dentate granule cells mature and integrate in a highly organized fashion within the dentate gyrus. The apical dendrites of these cells project to the hippocampal fissure and their axons arborize in the dentate hilus and CA3 stratum lucidum. Granule cells make up one part of the classic 'trisynaptic circuit,' with layer II neurons from the entorhinal cortex synapsing on granule cells via the perforant path, granule cells synapsing on CA3 pyramidal cells via their mossy fiber axons, and CA3 pyramidal cells synapsing on CA1 pyramidal cells via their Schaffer collaterals. Hippocampal circuits are now understood to be much more complicated, with additional connections between hippocampal subregions and robust innervation of local circuit neurons. A unique feature of dentate granule cells is the strength of feedforward and feedback inhibitory control maintained over the dentate gyrus. While CA3 pyramidal cells were historically considered to be the primary target of granule cells, it is now recognized that granule cells contact 10 times as many inhibitory interneurons (Acsády *et al.*, 1998; Acsády and Káli, 2007). These interneurons provide feedforward inhibition to CA3 pyramidal cells, while CA3 pyramidal cells can provide feedback inhibition to the dentate gyrus by exciting other inhibitory networks (Scharfman, 2007). In addition, granule cells excite glutamatergic mossy cells that excite GABAergic basket cells which innervate granule cells; providing another channel for robust feedback inhibition (Scharfman and Myers, 2013). This elaborate connectivity, particularly the high 10:1 ratio of inhibitory to excitatory neuron innervation by granule cells, is unusual and may allow the dentate gyrus to play a uniquely important role in temporal lobe epilepsy.

Subsequent analysis of this unusual circuit has led to the proposal that dentate granule cells act collectively as a 'synaptic gate' (Hsu, 2007). Specifically, while a large amount of activity enters the dentate via the perforant path, physiological studies demonstrate that very little of this activity actually makes it through to CA3 pyramidal cells (Ang *et al.*, 2006). Conceptually, this gating function of the dentate may be extremely important for maintaining excitatory/inhibitory balance in the brain. Failure of this gating function is hypothesized to promote epileptogenesis, and physiological studies support the conclusion that the dentate gate is compromised in tissue from epileptic animals (Heinemann *et al.*, 1992; Behr *et al.*, 1998; Gloveli *et al.*, 1998; Pathak *et al.*, 2007; Shao and Dudek, 2011). While the need for such an unusually robust gate remains speculative, two features of hippocampal circuitry are likely contributory factors. Firstly, the hippocampal circuit is organized as a loop, with hippocampal outputs feeding back to entorhinal cortex inputs. Unchecked excitatory transmission through this circuit could create reverberatory waves of excitation that might provoke seizures. Secondly, the granule cell to CA3 pyramidal cell synapse is one of the strongest synapses in the brain. Granule cell synaptic terminals, called giant mossy fiber boutons, can exceed 5 μm in diameter (approximately 10 times larger than a typical cortical synapse) and are loaded with synaptic vesicles. Moreover, a single granule cell synapse can sufficiently depolarize its target CA3 pyramidal cell to cause it to fire an action potential, earning this structure the title 'detonator synapse' (Urban *et al.*, 2001; Henze *et al.*, 2002). It seems reasonable, therefore, that robust inhibitory control is needed to keep this synapse in check, and correspondingly, failure of this system could be epileptogenic (Lawrence and McBain, 2003).

The hypothesis that temporal lobe epileptogenesis results in part from failure of the dentate gate originates from a long history of studies demonstrating remarkable anatomical and physiological changes within the dentate gyrus during epileptogenesis. In most temporal lobe epilepsy models, a subset of cells within the dentate gyrus develop new axon pathways, develop new patterns of dendritic projections, and exhibit changes in somatic organization and structure. Over the last decade, a series of studies has demonstrated that many of these changes are unique to recently-generated dentate granule cells. More specifically, granule cells born shortly before an epileptogenic brain injury and cells born after the injury develop the abnormal morphologies observed in epilepsy (Figure 3). Therefore, while most epileptogenic insults increase the production of granule cells, many of these cells do not integrate correctly into hippocampal circuitry. Improper integration of recently-generated granule cells in the epileptic brain may compromise the ability of the dentate gate to adequately regulate synaptic transmission throughout the hippocampus, leading to the hypothesis that recently-generated granule cells may contribute to epileptogenesis. In the following sections we review anatomical studies, which largely support a pro-epileptogenic role for recently-generated granule cells, and physiological studies which provide more mixed support for the hypothesis.

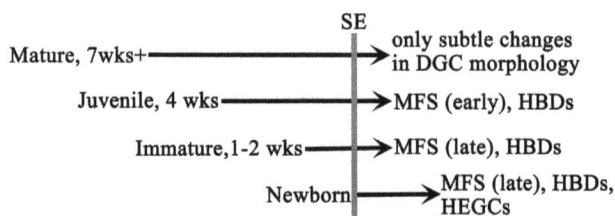

Figure 3. Timeline depicting plasticity of dentate granule cells in regards to their stage of maturation. At the time of an epileptogenic insult, such as *status epilepticus*, cells that are mature exhibit only subtle changes in cell morphology. However, younger cells may develop gross abnormalities. Juvenile cells may form hilar basal dendrites and contribute to early mossy fiber sprouting soon after the epileptogenic insult. Immature cells may form hilar basal dendrites, exhibit changes within their apical dendritic trees, and contribute to late mossy fiber sprouting. Newborn cells, born after the epileptogenic insult, may form hilar basal dendrites, contribute to late mossy fiber sprouting, and migrate to ectopic locations in the hippocampus. SE = *status epilepticus*, DGC = dentate granule cell, MFS = mossy fiber sprouting, HBDs = hilar basal dendrites, HEGCs = hilar ectopic granule cells. Figure modified with permission from (Danzer, 2012).

Mossy fiber sprouting

The most well-studied, and arguably the most controversial, granule cell pathology is mossy fiber axon sprouting. Mossy fiber sprouting was described by Nadler and colleagues (1980) following administration of epileptogenic drugs in rodents. The phenomenon occurs when mossy fiber axons, which are normally restricted to the dentate hilus and CA3 stratum lucidum, project additional collaterals into the inner molecular layer of the dentate gyrus (Figure 4).

This region contains the proximal dendrites of granule cells, and sprouted mossy fiber axons form functional granule cell to granule cell synapses with these dendrites (Frotscher and Zimmer, 1983; Tauck and Nadler, 1985). In addition to rodent models of epilepsy, mossy fiber sprouting has become a pathological hallmark of temporal lobe epilepsy in humans, having been confirmed in numerous studies using postmortem and resected tissue (Scheibel *et al.*, 1974; Sutula *et al.*, 1989; de Lanerolle *et al.*, 1989; Houser *et al.*, 1990; Babb *et al.*, 1991).

Mossy fiber sprouting has long been hypothesized to contribute to epileptogenesis (Tauck and Nadler, 1985; Nadler, 2003; Sutula and Dudek, 2007). Anatomical and physiological studies largely support the conclusion that mossy fiber sprouting creates *de novo* recurrent excitatory circuits, but investigators have also proposed that sprouting may reestablish inhibitory control over the dentate gyrus (Sloviter, 1992; Sloviter *et al.*, 2006). The complexity of the circuit, the frequent need to study the phenomenon in reduced preparations (thus transecting many pathways), and the expression of both inhibitory (Gutiérrez and Heinemann, 2006; Sperk *et al.*, 2012) and excitatory neurotransmitters by granule cells in epileptic tissue samples have made attempts to determine the physiological effect of mossy fiber sprouting extremely difficult. Furthermore, efforts to establish a positive correlation between mossy fiber sprouting and seizure frequency have produced mixed results, with some studies finding positive relationships and others suggesting that the degree of sprouting has little impact on seizure frequency (Buckmaster, 2012). The most definitive approach would be to selectively eliminate mossy fiber sprouting

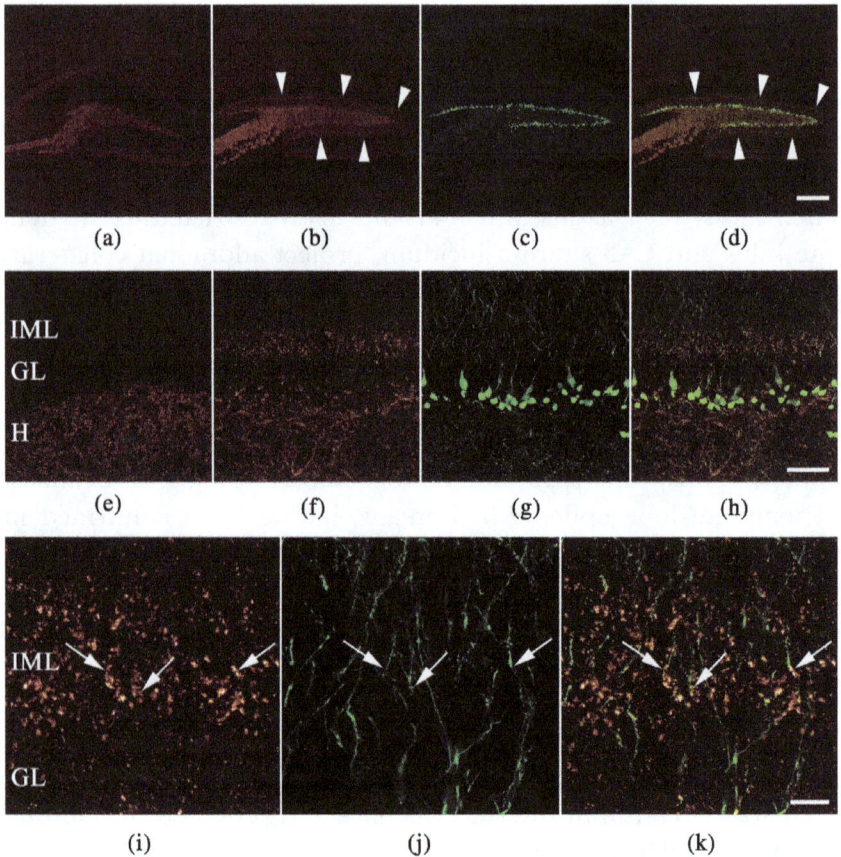

Figure 4. Recently-generated dentate granule cells can contribute to mossy fiber sprouting. Zinc transporter 3 (ZnT3), a protein found within mossy fiber axon terminals, is shown in red. Green fluorescent protein (GFP), which in this image is labeling dentate granule cells born as early as 5 weeks prior to pilocarpine-induced status epilepticus, is shown in green. Dentate gyrus (a) and magnification of hilus, granular layer, and inner molecular layer (e) of a pilocarpine treated mouse that did not develop spontaneous seizures. Dentate gyrus (b, c, and d) and magnification of hilus, granular layer, and inner molecular layer (f, g, and h) of a pilocarpine treated mouse that developed robust, frequent spontaneous seizures. Arrowheads indicate the band of aberrant mossy fiber sprouting visible in the inner molecular layer. Magnification of inner molecular layer (i, j, and k) showing ZnT3 positive mossy fiber axon terminals apposed to GFP positive dendrites, suggestive of granule cell to granule cell synapses (arrows). Scale bar for (a–d) is 250 μm, scale bar for (e–h) is 50 μm and scale bar for (i–k) is 10 μm. IML = inner molecular layer, GL = granular layer, H = hilus.

from epileptic animals. While optimal methodologies for achieving this have yet to be developed, some intriguing results have been found using an inhibitor of the AKT-mTOR (protein kinase B-mammalian target of rapamycin) pathway. The mTOR pathway is involved in many cellular processes including axon growth, and administration of rapamycin, an inhibitor of the AKT-mTOR pathway, has consistently been found to suppress mossy fiber sprouting in animal models of epilepsy (Buckmaster *et al.*, 2009; Zeng *et al.*, 2009; Huang *et al.*, 2010; Buckmaster and Lew, 2011; Tang *et al.*, 2012; Heng *et al.*, 2013). While several investigators found that this treatment also reduced or eliminated seizures in these animals, other investigators did not (Buckmaster and Lew, 2011; Buckmaster, 2012; Heng *et al.*, 2013). Furthermore, mossy fiber sprouting is not required for epilepsy, as animal models of the disease that lack the pathology have been described (Pun *et al.*, 2012). Nonetheless, this should not be taken as evidence that sprouting does not contribute in any way to the epilepsy syndrome, but it does raise questions about its relative importance.

It is now apparent that granule cells, born shortly before and after an epileptogenic brain injury, are responsible for mossy fiber sprouting. The first clue that this was the case came from data generated by Parent and colleagues (1997), who observed sprouted mossy fiber axons projecting from granule cells born after pilocarpine-induced *status epilepticus.* A subsequent study by the same group found that blocking neurogenesis with radiation treatment following *status epilepticus* did not prevent mossy fiber sprouting, leading to the preliminary conclusion that adult neurogenesis did not play a major role in the process (Parent *et al.*, 1999). In an elegant follow-up study (Kron *et al.*, 2010), the story was found to be more complicated. Radiation was used to transiently suppress neurogenesis at different time points relative to pilocarpine-induced *status epilepticus.* Specifically, one cohort of animals received radiation five weeks prior to *status epilepticus* and another received radiation four days following *status epilepticus.* The extent of mossy fiber sprouting was then assessed four and ten weeks after the insult. Unlike their previous study, suppression of neurogenesis did reduce mossy fiber sprouting at four weeks, but only when radiation was applied five weeks prior to the epileptogenic injury. Intriguingly, animals that received radiation four days following *status epilepticus* did not show reduced sprouting at four weeks, but did show reduced sprouting at ten weeks. Together these findings indicate that 'juvenile' granule cells, born up to five weeks before *status epilepticus*, quickly develop mossy fiber axon sprouts, while newborn granule cells, born shortly after the insult, do not contribute to mossy fiber sprouting until a couple of months after the injury (Figure 3).

Hilar basal dendrites

Within the rodent brain, mature dentate granule cells possess a single axon which typically originates from the hilar (basal) side of the cell and subsequently projects into the hilus. Apical dendrites, on the other hand, typically originate from the opposite side of the cell from the axon (the molecular layer or apical side) and project into the molecular layer. During the first week of development, immature granule cells transiently grow basal dendrites that project into the hilus (Seress and Pokorny, 1981; Jones *et al.*, 2003); however, these structures eventually retract and are absent once the cells have fully matured. In contrast to this normal anatomy, Spigelman and colleagues (1998) observed the presence of hilar basal dendrites on some mature granule cells within hippocampi of rodents that developed epilepsy following *status epilepticus* induced by perforant path stimulation. Dentate granule cells in other rodent models of *status epilepticus*, including kainic acid (Buckmaster and Dudek, 1999), pilocarpine (Ribak *et al.*, 2000), and intrahippocampal kainic acid (Murphy *et al.*, 2012), were also found to exhibit abnormal basal dendrites (Figure 5). Hilar basal dendrites are innervated by granule cell mossy fiber axon terminals in the hilus, forming functional granule cell to granule cell synapses (Ribak *et al.*, 2000; Thind *et al.*, 2008; Murphy *et al.*, 2011).

It is hypothesized that recurrent connections mediated by hilar basal dendrites promote hyperexcitability within the hippocampus (Ribak *et al.*, 2012). In support of this hypothesis, physiological data

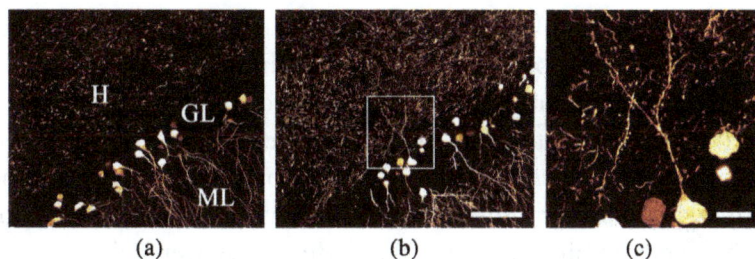

Figure 5. Recently-generated dentate granule cells can form hilar basal dendrites. Hilus, granular layer, and inner molecular layer from a control mouse (a) and a pilocarpine treated mouse (b). Note the absence of basal dendrites from the control animal and the presence of a basal dendrite on a granule cell from the epileptic animal. Area in box is shown magnified in (c). Scale bar for (a) and (b) is 50 μm and scale bar for (c) is 10 μm. H = hilus, GL = granular layer, ML = molecular layer.

on granule cells with and without basal dendrites in non-human primates suggests that cells with basal dendrites receive more excitatory current than cells without basal dendrites (Austin and Buckmaster, 2004); however, a separate study produced different results in rodent tissue (Becker *et al.*, 2012). In this latter study, the investigators recorded from cells with and without hilar basal dendrites in organotypic entorhino-hippocampal slice cultures. Granule cells in these cultures often develop hilar basal dendrites (Murphy and Danzer, 2011), perhaps reflecting a form of *in vitro* epileptogenesis (Dyhrfjeld-Johnsen *et al.*, 2010). Recordings from the two types of cells revealed similar intrinsic properties, and paired patch clamp recordings of adjacent granule cells revealed minimal granule cell to granule cell connectivity. Whether these findings are predictive of the *in vivo* condition in epileptic animals or reflect features unique to the culture system has not been determined. The significance of granule cell basal dendrites in human epilepsy presents an additional complexity. Unlike the rodent brain, hilar basal dendrites are normal features of some granule cells within the brains of humans and non-human primates (Seress and Mrzljak, 1987). Hilar basal dendrites have been found on dentate granule cells within human temporal lobe epilepsy samples (von Campe *et al.*, 1997; da Silva *et al.*, 2006), but the extent to which they are present in greater numbers relative to the normal brain remain unclear. The limited availability of control tissue has precluded making definitive conclusions.

Hilar basal dendrites selectively form on dentate granule cells located on the inner third of the granule cell body layer, nearest the hilar border (Ribak *et al.*, 2000). This region also contains the most recently-generated granule cells. This observation led to the hypothesis that cells exhibiting hilar basal dendrites were also recently-generated granule cells. Several studies, using a combination of neuronal birthdating and transgenic fate-mapping techniques, have now confirmed that granule cells with hilar basal dendrites arise from neural progenitor cells active a couple weeks before, or after, an epileptogenic insult (Figure 3) (Jessberger *et al.*, 2007; Walter *et al.*, 2007; Murphy *et al.*, 2011; Kron *et al.*, 2010). Whether the basal dendrites arise *de novo* from the affected cells, or reflect a failure to retract the normally transient basal dendrites exhibited by immature cells remains uncertain. Several lines of evidence favor the latter possibility. Firstly, basal dendrites arise from immature granule cell populations that would still possess these transient basal dendrites at the time of the insult; but not from more mature cells that would have already lost these processes. Secondly, in animals exposed to epileptogenic insults, these transient basal dendrites develop immature synapses, which are lacking in normal animals (Shapiro and Ribak, 2006). Finally, in culture conditions, increasing neuronal activity appears to stabilize transient basal dendrites, causing them to persist as the granule cells mature (Nakahara *et al.*, 2009). Taken together, these findings suggest a scenario in which normally transient basal dendrites are stabilized in the epileptic environment by the abnormally high levels of activity (Shapiro and Ribak, 2005).

Hilar ectopic granule cells

As dentate granule cells mature, they migrate short distances away from the subgranular zone to their appropriate location in the inner third of the granular layer. Normal granule cell localization within the dentate gyrus allows this structure to maintain a highly

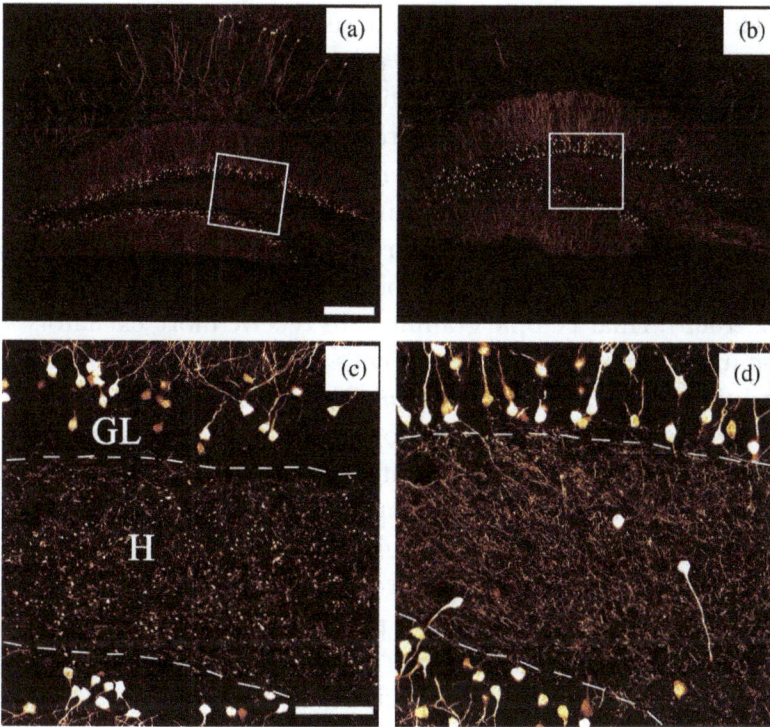

Figure 6. Newborn dentate granule cells can migrate to ectopic locations. Dentate gyrus from a control mouse (a) and a pilocarpine treated mouse (b). Image (c) and image (d) show magnified area in boxes indicated in (a) and (b), respectfully. All granule cells are localized within the granular layer of the dentate gyrus in the control animal, whereas some granule cells were found in ectopic locations in the hilus of the epileptic animal. Scale bar for (a) and (b) is 200 μm and scale bar for (c) and (d) is 50 μm. GL = granular layer, H = hilus.

organized cellular arrangement, with cell bodies contained within the dense granular layer, dendritic trees projecting throughout the molecular layer, and axons projecting into the hilus. In the epileptic brain of rodents and humans, however, the structure of the dentate gyrus can be disrupted by the aberrant migration of granule cells to ectopic locations in the dentate hilus (Figure 6) (Parent *et al.*, 1997; Parent *et al.*, 2006) or near the hilar/CA3 border (Scharfman *et al.*, 2000).

Hilar ectopic granule cells are postsynaptic to granule cell mossy fiber axon terminals (Dashtipour *et al.*, 2001; Pierce *et al.*, 2005). In addition to their abnormal migration into the hilus, ectopic granule cells exhibit several unique features giving them distinct properties compared to granule cells properly located in the cell body layer. Detailed anatomical analyses using electron microscopy demonstrate that excitatory mossy fiber terminals are the predominant source of input onto hilar ectopic granule cell dendrites (Pierce *et al.*, 2005). Hilar ectopic granule cells receive more excitatory synaptic input compared to granule cells located in the granular layer (Dashtipour *et al.*, 2001; Zhan *et al.*, 2010), which is likely a result of a greater ratio of asymmetric to symmetric synapses, suggesting more excitatory and less inhibitory input (Pierce *et al.*, 2005). Furthermore, these cells exhibit spontaneous and evoked bursting; features typically absent from granule cells in normal animals (Scharfman *et al.*, 2003; Cameron *et al.*, 2011; Myers *et al.*, 2013). In addition to these pro-excitatory properties, hilar ectopic granule cells do receive increased tonic GABA current, which would be expected to decrease cellular excitability, although apparently not to sufficient levels to offset some of the abnormal excitability, such as bursting (Zhan and Nadler, 2009). Of interest, hilar ectopic granule cells are more likely to form abnormal dendrites, which are oriented away from the molecular layer (similar to hilar basal dendrites) and are more likely to contribute to mossy fiber sprouting than granule cells located appropriately within the granular layer (Cameron *et al.*, 2011; Pierce *et al.*, 2011; Scharfman and Pierce, 2012). While ectopic cells are best described in rodent epilepsy models, they also appear to be present in human temporal lobe epilepsy (Parent *et al.*, 2006).

Similar to mossy fiber sprouting and hilar basal dendrite formation, ectopic granule cells are derived from neural progenitor cells which are active after the epileptogenic brain injury (Figure 3) (Jessberger *et al.*, 2007; Walter *et al.*, 2007; Kron *et al.*, 2010). Interestingly, cells born before the insult, even very immature cells, do not appear to contribute to the ectopic cell population, perhaps suggesting that cell migration occurs very quickly following terminal cell division, and that once the cell has reached its correct location, its migration cannot be subsequently disrupted (Walter *et al.*, 2007).

'Normotopic' dentate granule cells

A key caveat that must be considered when interpreting these data is that not all newborn granule cells in the epileptic brain are equal. Morphological studies clearly demonstrate that this population is remarkably heterogeneous (Murphy *et al.*, 2011). Ectopically located cells, cells with basal dendrites, and cells with mossy fiber axon sprouting can be generated in concert with granule cells that appear morphologically normal; that is, cells with grossly normal apical dendritic trees that are correctly located in the granule cell body layer. These cells, termed 'normotopic' granule cells, exhibit physiological and anatomical changes which suggest they may play a protective role in the epileptic brain.

Using a viral-labeling approach to identify newborn cells, Jakubs and colleagues (2006) recorded excitatory postsynaptic currents (EPSCs) from normotopic newborn cells generated after electrically-induced *status epilepticus*. They found a decrease in spontaneous EPSCs among these cells relative to age-matched cells from control animals, indicating that the normotopic newborn granule cells receive less excitatory input within the epileptic brain. Consistent with the idea that some newborn granule cells may be less excitable, a study detailing the morphology of granule cells born up to one week before pilocarpine-induced *status epilepticus* demonstrated that the majority of normotopic granule cells exhibited reduced spines densities, although a subset (approximately 10%) had greater spine numbers (Murphy *et al.*, 2011). Similarly, six weeks following electrically-induced seizures, dendritic spines formed on newborn granule cells exhibited decreased protein levels of postsynaptic density 95 (PSD-95), a component of excitatory synapses, and increased expression of gephyrin, a scaffolding protein found at inhibitory synapses (Jackson *et al.*, 2012). Finally, while these studies suggest that normotopic granule cells may be protective, this may not be true for all epilepsy models.

The majority of normotopic granule cells examined by Jakubs and colleagues were morphologically normal, lacking basal dendrites or other gross pathologies; so whether physiological studies of normotopic cells with more abnormalities would produce different results is not known. Moreover, when investigators examined cells born after rapid kindling, a model which reduces seizures thresholds but does not produce epilepsy, newborn granule cells were found to receive increased excitatory input (Wood *et al.*, 2011). Together, these studies highlight the complexity of assessing granule cell function in epilepsy, with different populations of newborn cells making distinct, and potentially conflicting, contributions to dentate excitability.

Functional Consequences of Abnormal Adult-Generated Granule Cells in Epilepsy

It is unclear whether the acute surge of dentate granule cell proliferation following an epileptogenic insult is good or bad for the brain. Although evidence exists in support of a protective role for these cells, most data tends to favor a pro-epileptogenic role. Investigators have used a variety of approaches to assess the function of newborn granule cells in epilepsy, but in general these fall into two broad categories: (1) correlational studies and (2) approaches to directly manipulate the survival or integration of the new cells.

Correlational studies

If abnormal granule cells are epileptogenic, a logical prediction would be that animals with more abnormal granule cells will have more severe epilepsy. This prediction was tested recently using a genetic fate-mapping technique to assess anatomical abnormalities present among dentate granule cells born up to five weeks prior to pilocarpine-induced *status epilepticus* (Hester and Danzer, 2012). Animals were monitored continuously by video-EEG for one month to accurately assess seizure frequency. These studies revealed a positive correlation between seizure frequency and the extent of mossy fiber sprouting and the number of ectopically located granule cells. This study, however, only provides correlational data which is not necessarily indicative of causation. Nevertheless, the findings are consistent with the idea that abnormal granule cells may partially underlie the development of more frequent seizures following an epileptogenic brain insult.

Approaches to directly manipulate the survival or integration of the new cells

If abnormal granule cells are epileptogenic, then introducing abnormal cells into an otherwise healthy brain should cause epilepsy. Pun and colleagues (2012) were able to achieve this using tamoxifen-inducible Cre-lox technology to selectively delete the phosphatase and tensin homolog (PTEN) gene from neural progenitor cells in the postnatal rodent brain. PTEN negatively regulates mTOR; therefore, administration of tamoxifen leads to hyperactivation of the AKT-mTOR pathway in affected cells. This produced a mosaic within the dentate gyrus, with 10–25% of the entire population affected, while the remaining granule cells retained normal PTEN expression. PTEN knockout granule cells developed mossy fiber axon sprouts, basal dendrites, and occasionally migrated ectopically; similar to recently-generated granule cells in many animal models of temporal lobe epilepsy (Amiri *et al.*, 2012; Pun *et al.*, 2012). Strikingly, within about six weeks of gene deletion, animals began to exhibit spontaneous seizures which originated in the hippocampus and spread to the cortex. These data provide compelling evidence that abnormal granule cells are capable of causing epilepsy.

While abnormal granule cells appear to be sufficient to cause epilepsy, it does not necessarily indicate that these cells underlie spontaneous seizures in other epilepsy models. To more directly test the role of this cell population, several investigators have utilized anti-neurogenic strategies to prevent granule cell neurogenesis following an epileptogenic brain injury. To this end, Jung and colleagues (2004; 2006) used antimitotics to reduce neurogenesis following pilocarpine-induced *status epilepticus*. In their first study, cytosine-b-D-arabinofuranoside (AraC), a compound that ablates mitotically active neural progenitor cells, was infused into the left lateral ventricle for 14 days beginning the day prior to pilocarpine treatment. In their second study, celecoxib, a cyclooxygenase-2 inhibitor which prevents seizure-induced inflammatory responses and reduces neurogenesis, was administered as a dietary supplement every day beginning the day after pilocarpine treatment. Video monitoring revealed that animals receiving antimitotic treatments exhibited significantly fewer spontaneous seizures. These studies suggest that newborn dentate granule cells are epileptogenic following pilocarpine-induced *status epilepticus*; however, there are a few notable caveats. Firstly, blocking neurogenesis may provoke secondary changes in brain function which might inhibit seizures, even if the newborn cells play no direct role in epileptogenesis. Nonspecific drug effects might also play a role. Celecoxib, for example, has multiple effects on cellular processes including inhibition of seizure-induced proinflammatory responses (Seibert *et al.*, 1994), which may be important to epileptogenesis [for review see (Vezzani *et al.*, 2013)]. Finally, sole reliance on video monitoring further limits these findings, as non-convulsive seizures could have been missed. In a related study, Pekcec and colleagues (2008) used a different approach to inhibit neurogenesis and obtained different results. In this study, depolysialation of the neural cell adhesion molecule (NCAM) following self-sustained *status epilepticus* was used to reduce neurogenesis. Six weeks later, continuous video and EEG monitoring did not show any differences in seizure frequency, duration, or severity between treated and control animals. This study also included several notable caveats. Depolysialation of NCAM produced a very modest reduction in neurogenesis, leaving many newborn granule cells intact. Also, the treatment may have other unknown effects on this cell population which could have influenced seizure progression. One final caveat is that all three studies assessed the role of newborn granule cells born after an epileptogenic insult; however, studies indicate that recently-generated granule cells born up to five weeks prior to *status epilepticus* also contribute to anatomical abnormalities (Walter *et al.*, 2007; Kron *et al.*, 2010). Future studies targeting cells born before and after the insult should provide more definitive tests of the role recently-generated granule cells have upon epileptogenesis.

Conclusions

The mechanisms which underlie temporal lobe epileptogenesis remain obscure. In recent years, several studies have been conducted which suggest that recently-generated granule cells could play an important role in the disease. In animals many acute epileptogenic brain injuries lead to dramatic increases in dentate granule cell neurogenesis, and strikingly, many of these new cells integrate abnormally. These new cells sprout axons to the wrong targets, develop aberrant basal dendrites, and in the most extreme cases migrate to the wrong part of the hippocampus. Moreover, the abnormal cells can form recurrent excitatory connections which may impair the ability of dentate gyrus to limit the flow of excitatory information through the hippocampus. Despite anatomical evidence suggesting these new cells may be maladaptive, physiological studies have produce mixed results, with some studies finding the new cells to be more excitable and some studies finding less excitable cells. The discordant findings likely reflect the heterogeneous nature of newborn granule cells in the epileptic brain, with some new cells appearing strikingly abnormal, while others are similar to cells from control animals. Nonetheless, this heterogeneity complicates studies aimed at elucidating the net effect of the new cells, as neurogenesis may contribute both 'good' and 'bad' granule cells to the brain. Studies to manipulate granule cells in the normal and epileptic brain provide some additional support for a maladaptive role for the new cells. Selective PTEN deletion from hippocampal neural progenitor cells, which leads to the almost exclusive production of 'bad' granule cells, led to the development of a profound epilepsy syndrome; indicating that abnormal granule cells can cause epilepsy. Blocking granule cell neurogenesis after an epileptogenic insult, however, produced mixed findings, with some investigators observing a reduction in seizure frequency, while others reported no effect. These studies are still in their early stages, so future work with more selective techniques will be needed to allow investigators to untangle this complex story.

References

Acsády L, Káli S (2007) Models, structure, function: the transformation of cortical signals in the dentate gyrus. *Prog Brain Res* 163:577–599.

Acsády L, Kamondi A, Sík A, Freund T, Buzsáki G (1998) GABAergic cells are the major postsynaptic targets of mossy fibers in the rat hippocampus. *J Neurosci* 18(9):3386–3403.

Altman J, Bayer SA (1990a) Migration and distribution of two populations of hippocampal granule cell precursors during the perinatal and postnatal periods. *J Comp Neurol* 301(3):365–381.

Altman J, Bayer SA (1990b) Mosaic organization of the hippocampal neuroepithelium and the multiple germinal sources of dentate granule cells. *J Comp Neurol* 301(3):325–342.

Altman J, Das GD (1965) Autoradiographic and histological evidence of postnatal hippocampal neurogenesis in rats. *J Comp Neurol* 124(3): 319–335.

Amiri A, Cho W, Zhou J, Birnbaum SG, Sinton CM, McKay RM, Parada LF (2012) Pten deletion in adult hippocampal neural stem/progenitor cells causes cellular abnormalities and alters neurogenesis. *J Neurosci* 32(17):5880–5890.

Ang CW, Carlson GC, Coulter DA (2006) Massive and specific dysregulation of direct cortical input to the hippocampus in temporal lobe epilepsy. *J Neurosci* 26(46):11850–11856.

Austin JE, Buckmaster PS (2004) Recurrent excitation of granule cells with basal dendrites and low interneuron density and inhibitory postsynaptic current frequency in the dentate gyrus of macaque monkeys. *J Comp Neurol* 476(3):205–218.

Avanzi RD, Cavarsan CF, Santos JG Jr, Hamani C, Mello LE, Covolan L (2010) Basal dendrites are present in newly born dentate granule cells of young but not aged pilocarpine-treated chronic epileptic rats. *Neuroscience* 170(3):687–691.

Babb TL, Kupfer WR, Pretorius JK, Crandall PH, Levesque MF (1991) Synaptic reorganization by mossy fibers in human epileptic fascia dentata. *Neuroscience* 42(2):351–363.

Bayer SA (1980) Development of the hippocampal region in the rat. 1. Neurogenesis examined with 3H-thymidine autoradiography. *J Comp Neurol* 190(1):87–114.

Bayer SA, Yackel JW, Puri PS (1982) Neurons in the rat dentate gyrus granular layer substantially increase during juvenile and adult life. *Science* 216(4548):890–892.

Becker D, Willems LM, Vnencak M, Zahn N, Schuldt G, Jedlicka P, Maggio N, Deller T, Vlachos A (2012) Functional and structural properties of dentate granule cells with hilar basal dendrites in mouse entorhino-hippocampal slice cultures. *PLoS One* 7(11):e48500.

Bender RA, Dubé C, Gonzalaez-Vega R, Mina EW, Baram TZ (2003) Mossy fiber plasticity and enhanced hippocampal excitability, without hippo-campal cell loss or altered neurogenesis, in an animal model of prolonged febrile seizures. *Hippocampus* 13(3):399–412.

Behr J, Lyson KJ, Mody I (1998) Enhanced propagation of epileptiform activity through the kindled dentate gyrus. *J Neurophysiol* 79(4): 1726–1732.

Ben-Ari Y, Holmes GL (2006) Effects of seizures on developmental pro-cesses in the immature brain. *Lancet Neurol* 5(12):1055–1063.

Bengzon J, Kokaia Z, Elmér E, Nanobashvili A, Kokaia M, Lindvall O (1997) Apoptosis and proliferation of dentate gyrus neurons after single and intermittent limbic seizures. *Proc Natl Acad Sci U S A* 94(19): 10432–10437.

Bertram EH (2009) Temporal lobe epilepsy: where do the seizures really begin? *Epilepsy Behav* 14(suppl1):32–37.

Blümcke I, Schewe JC, Normann S, Brüstle O, Schramm J, Elger CE, Wiestler OD (2001) Increase of nestin-immunoreactive neural precur-sor cells in the dentate gyrus of pediatric patients with early-onset temporal lobe epilepsy. *Hippocampus* 11(3):311–321.

Bonde S, Ekdahl CT, Lindvall O (2006) Long-term neuronal replacement in adult rat hippocampus after status epilepticus despite chronic inflammation. *Eur J Neurosci* 23(4):965–974.

Buckmaster PS (2012) Mossy fiber sprouting in the dentate gyrus. In: Noebels JL, Avoli M, Rogawski MA, Olsen RW, Delgado-Escueta AV, editors. *Jasper's Basic Mechanisms of the Epilepsies* [Internet]. 4th edition. Bethesda (MD): National Center for Biotechnology Information (US).

Buckmaster PS, Dudek FE (1999) *In vivo* intracellular analysis of gran-ule cell axon reorganization in epileptic rats. *J Neurophysiol* 81(2): 712–721.

Buckmaster PS, Ingram EA, Wen X (2009) Inhibition of the mammalian target of rapamycin signaling pathway suppresses mossy fiber sprouting in a rodent model of temporal lobe epilepsy. *J Neurosci* 29(25): 8259–8269.

Buckmaster PS, Lew FH (2011) Rapamycin suppresses mossy fiber sprouting but not seizure frequency in a mouse model of temporal lobe epilepsy. *J Neurosci* 31(6):2337–2347.

Buss RR, Sun W, Oppenheim RW (2006) Adaptive roles of programmed cell death during nervous system development. *Annu Rev of Neurosci* 29:1–35.

Cameron MC, Zhan R, Nadler JV (2011) Morphologic integration of hilar ectopic granule cells into dentate circuitry in the pilocarpine model of temporal lobe epilepsy. *J Comp Neurol* 519(11):2175–2192.

Coras R, Siebzehnrubl FA, Pauli E, Huttner HB, Njunting M, Kobow K, Villmann C, Hahnen E, Neuhuber W, Weigel D, Buchfelder M, Stefan H, Beck H, Steindler DA, Blümcke I (2010) Low proliferation and differentiation capacities of adult hippocampal stem cells correlate with memory dysfunction in humans. *Brain* 133(11):3359–3372.

Covolan L, Ribeiro LT, Longo BM, Mello LE (2000) Cell damage and neurogenesis in the dentate granule cell layer of adult rats after pilocarpine- or kainate-induced status epilepticus. *Hippocampus* 10(2):169–180.

Crespel A, Rigau V, Coubes P, Rousset MC, de Bock F, Okano H, Baldy-Moulinier M, Bockaert J, Lerner-Natoli M (2005) Increased number of neural progenitors in human temporal lobe epilepsy. *Neurobiol Dis* 19(3):436–450.

da Silva AV, Houzel JC, Targas Yacubian EM, Carrete H Jr, Sakamoto AC, Priel MR, Martins HH, Oliveira I, Garzon E, Stavale JN, da Silva Centeno R, Machado H, Cavalheiro EA (2006) Dysmorphic neurons in patients with temporal lobe epilepsy. *Brain Res* 1072(1):200–207.

Dalla C, Bangasser DA, Edgecomb C, Shors TJ (2007) Neurogenesis and learning: Acquisition and asymptotic performance predict how many new cells survive in the hippocampus. *Neurobiol Learn Mem* 88(1): 143–148.

D'Alessio L, Konopka H, López EM, Seoane E, Consalvo D, Oddo S, Kochen S, López-Costa JJ (2010) Doublecortin (DCX) immunoreactivity in hippocampus of chronic refractory temporal lobe epilepsy patients with hippocampal sclerosis. *Seizure* 19(9):567–572.

Danzer SC (2012) Depression, stress, epilepsy and adult neurogenesis. *Exp Neurol* 233(1):22–32.

Dashtipour K, Tran PH, Okazaki MM, Nadler JV, Ribak CE (2001) Ultrastructural features and synaptic connections of hilar ectopic granule cells in the rat dentate gyrus are different from those of granule cells in the granule cell layer. *Brain Res* 890(2):261–271.

de Lanerolle NC, Kim JH, Robbins RJ, Spencer DD (1989) Hippocampal interneuron loss and plasticity in human temporal lobe epilepsy. *Brain Res* 495(2):387–395.

Deng W, Aimone JB, Gage FH (2010) New neurons and new memories: how does adult hippocampal neurogenesis affect learning and memory? *Nat Rev Neurosci* 11(5):339–350.

Dong H, Csernansky CA, Goico B, Csernansky JC (2003) Hippocampal neurogenesis follows kainic acid-induced apoptosis in neonatal rats. *J Neurosci* 23(5):1742–1749.

Dyhrfjeld-Johnsen J, Berdichevsky Y, Swiercz W, Sabolek H, Staley KJ (2010) Interictal spikes precede ictal discharges in an organotypic hippocampal slice culture model of epileptogenesis. *J Clin Neurophysiol* 27(6):418–424.

Eriksson PS, Perfilieva E, Björk-Eriksson T, Alborn AM, Nordborg C, Peterson DA, Gage FH (1998) Neurogenesis in the adult human hippocampus. *Nat Med* 4(11):1313–1317.

Frotscher M, Zimmer J (1983) Lesion-induced mossy fibers to the molecular layer of the rat fascia dentata: identification of postsynaptic granule cells by the Golgi-EM technique. *J Comp Neurol* 215(3): 299–311.

Giedd JN, Snell JW, Lange N, Rajapakse JC, Casey BJ, Kozuch PL, Vaituzis AC, Vauss YC, Hamburger SD, Kaysen D, Rapoport JL (1996) Quantitative magnetic resonance imaging of human brain development: ages 4–18. *Cerel Cortex* 6(4):551–560.

Gloveli T, Schmitz D, Heinemann U (1998) Interaction between superficial layers of the entorhinal cortex and the hippocampus in normal and epileptic temporal lobe. *Epilepsy Res* 32(1–2):183–193.

Gould E, Beylin A, Tanapat P, Reeves A, Shors TJ (1999) Learning enhances adult neurogenesis in the hippocampal formation. *Nat Neurosci* 2(3): 260–265.

Gutiérrez R, Heinemann U (2006) Co-existence of GABA and Glu in the hippocampal granule cells: implications for epilepsy. *Curr Top Med Chem* 6(10):975–978.

Gray WP, Sundstrom LE (1998) Kainic acid increases the proliferation of granule cell progenitors in the dentate gyrus of the adult rat. *Brain Res* 790(1–2):52–59.

Haas KZ, Sperber EF, Opanashuk LA, Stanton PK, Moshé SL (2001) Resistance of immature hippocampus to morphologic and physiologic alterations following status epilepticus or kindling. *Hippocampus* 11(6): 615–625.

Hairston IS, Little MT, Scanlon MD, Barakat MT, Palmer TD, Sapolsky RM, Heller HC (2005) Sleep restriction suppresses neurogenesis induced by hippocampus-dependent learning. *J Neurophysiol* 94(6):4224–4233.

Hattiangady B, Rao MS, Shetty AK (2004) Chronic temporal lobe epilepsy is associated with severely declined dentate neurogenesis in the adult hippocampus. *Neurobiol Dis* 17(3):473–490.

Hattiangady B, Shetty AK (2008) Implications of decreased hippocampal neurogenesis in chronic temporal lobe epilepsy. *Epilepsia* 49(supp5): 26–41.

Hattiangady B, Shetty AK (2010) Decreased neuronal differentiation of newly generated cells underlies reduced hippocampal neurogenesis in chronic temporal lobe epilepsy. *Hippocampus* 20(1):97–112.

Hauser WA (1994) The prevalence and incidence of convulsive disorders in children. *Epilepsia* 35(suppl 2):1–6.

Heinemann U, Beck H, Dreier JP, Ficker E, Stabel J, Zhang CL (1992) The dentate gyrus as a regulated gate for the propagation of epileptiform activity. *Epilepsy Res Suppl* 7:273–280.

Heng K, Haney MM, Buckmaster PS (2013) High-dose rapamycin blocks mossy fiber sprouting but not seizures in a mouse model of temporal lobe epilepsy. *Epilepsia* 54(9):1535–1541.

Henze DA, McMahon DB, Harris KM, Barrionuevo G (2002) Giant miniature EPSCs at the hippocampal mossy fiber to CA3 pyramidal cell synapse are monoquantal. *J Neurophysiol* 87(1):15–29.

Hester MS, Danzer SC (2013) Accumulation of abnormal adult-generated hippocampal granule cells predicts seizure frequency and severity. *J Neurosci* 33(21):8926–8936.

Holmes GL (2005) Effects of seizures on brain development: lessons from the laboratory. *Pediatr Neurol* 33(1):1–11.

Houser CR, Miyashiro JE, Swartz BE, Walsh GO, Rich JR, Delgado-Escueta AV (1990) Altered patterns of dynorphin immunoreactivity suggests mossy fiber reorganization in human hippocampal epilepsy. *J Neurosci* 10(1): 267–282.

Hsu D (2007) The dentate gyrus as a filter or gate: a look back and a look ahead. *Prog Brain Res* 163(1):601–613.

Huang X, Zhang H, Yang J, Wu J, McMahon J, Lin Y, Cao Z, Gruenthal M, Huang Y (2010) Pharmacological inhibition of the mammalian target of Rapamycin pathway suppresses acquired epilepsy. *Neurobiol Dis* 40(1):193–199.

Jabès A, Lavenex PB, Amaral DG, Lavenex P (2010) Quantitative analysis of postnatal neurogenesis and neuron number in the macaque monkey dentate gyrus. *Eur J Neurosci* 31(2):273–285.

Jackson J, Chugh D, Nilsson P, Wood J, Carlström, Lindvall O, Ekdahl CT (2012) Altered synaptic properties during integration of adult-born neurons following a seizure insult. *PLoS One* 7(4):e35557.

Jakubs K, Nanobashvili A, Bonde S, Ekdahl CT, Kokaia Z, Kokaia M, Lindvall O (2006) Environment matters: synaptic properties of neurons born in the epileptic adult brain develop to reduce excitability. *Neuron* 52(6):1047–1059.

Jessberger S, Zhao C, Toni N, Clemenson GD Jr, Li Y, Gage FH (2007) Seizure-associated, aberrant neurogenesis in adult rats characterized with retrovirus-mediated cell labeling. *J Neurosci* 27(35):9400–9407.

Jiruska P, Shtaya AB, Bodansky DM, Chang WC, Gray WP, Jefferys JG (2013) Dentate gyrus progenitor cell proliferation after the onset of spontaneous seizures in the tetanus toxin model of temporal lobe epilepsy. *Neurobiol Dis* 54:492–498.

Jones SP, Rahimi O, O'Boyle MP, Diaz DL, Claiborne BJ (2003) Maturation of granule cell dendrites after mossy fiber arrival in hippocampal field CA3. *Hippocampus* 13(3):413–427.

Jung KH, Chu K, Kim M, Jeong SW, Song YM, Lee ST, Kim JY, Lee SK, Roh JK (2004) Continuous cytosine-b-D-arabinofuranoside infusion reduces ectopic granule cells in adult rat hippocampus with attenuation of spontaneous recurrent seizures following pilocarpine-induced status epilepticus. *Eur J Neurosci* 19(12):3219–3226.

Jung KH, Chu K, Lee ST, Kim J, Sinn DI, Kim JM, Park DK, Lee JJ, Kim SU, Kim M, Lee SK, Roh JK (2006) Cyclooxygenase-2 inhibitor, celecoxib, inhibits the altered hippocampal neurogenesis with attenuation of spontaneous recurrent seizures following pilocarpine-induced status epilepticus. *Neurobiol Dis* 23(2):237–246.

Kanner AM (2008) Depression in epilepsy: a complex relation with unexpected consequences. *Curr Opin in Neurol* 21(2)190–194.

Kaplan MS and Hinds JW (1977) Neurogenesis in the adult rat: electron microscopic analysis of light radioautographs. *Science* 197(4308):1092–1094.

Kitabatake Y, Sailor KA, Ming GL, Song H (2007) Adult neurogenesis and hippocampal memory function: new cells, more plasticity, new memories? *Neurosurg Clin N Am* 18(1):105–113.

Kralic JE, Ledergerber DA, Fritschy JM (2005) Disruption of the neurogenic potential of the dentate gyrus in a mouse model of temporal lobe epilepsy with focal seizures. *Eur J Neurosci* 22(8):1916–1927.

Kron MM, Zhang H, Parent JM (2010) The developmental stage of dentate granule cells dictates their contribution to seizure-induced plasticity. *J Neurosci* 30(6):2051–2059.

Kuhn HG, Dickinson-Anson H, Gage FH (1996) Neurogenesis in the dentate gyrus of the adult rat: age-related decrease of neuronal progenitor proliferation. *J Neurosci* 16(6):2027–2033.

Kuruba R, Hattiangady B, Shetty AK (2009) Hippocampal neurogenesis and neural stem cells in temporal lobe epilepsy. *Epilepsy Behav* 14(suppl):65–73.

Lavenex P, Banta Lavenex P, Amaral DG (2007) Postnatal development of the primate hippocampal formation. *Dev Neurosci* 29(1–2):179–192.

Lawrence JJ, McBain CJ (2003) Interneuron diversity series: containing the detonation–feedforward inhibition in the CA3 hippocampus. *Trends Neurosci* 26(11):631–640.

Leuner B, Mendolia-Loffredo S, Kozorovitskiy Y, Samburg D, Gould E, Shors TJ (2004) Learning enhances the survival of new neurons beyond the time when the hippocampus is required for memory. *J Neurosci* 24(23):7477–7481.

Liu YW, Curtis MA, Gibbons HM, Mee EW, Bergin PS, Teoh HH, Connor B, Dragunow M, Faull RL (2008) Doublecortin expression in the normal and epileptic adult human brain. *Eur J Neurosci* 28(11):2254–2265.

Liu Z, Yang Y, Silveira DC, Sarkisian MR, Tandon P, Huang LT, Stafstrom CE, Holmes GL (1999) Consequences of recurrent seizures during early brain development. *Neuroscience* 92(4):1443–1454.

Madsen TM, Treschow A, Bengzon J, Bolwig TG, Lindvall O, Tingström A (2000) Increased neurogenesis in a model of electroconvulsive therapy. *Biol Psychiatry* 47(12):1043–1049.

Mathern GW, Leiphart JL, De Vera A, Adelson PD, Seki T, Neder L, Leite JP (2002) Seizures decrease postnatal neurogenesis and granule cell development in the human fascia dentata. *Epilepsia* 43(suppl 5):68–73.

McCabe BK, Silveira DC, Cilio MR, Cha BH, Liu X, Sogawa Y, Holmes GL (2001) Reduced neurogenesis after neonatal seizures. *J Neurosci* 21(6):2094–2103.

Mohapel P, Ekdahl CT, Lindvall O (2004) Status epilepticus severity influences the long-term outcome of neurogenesis in the adult dentate gyrus. *Neurobiol Dis* 15(2):196–205.

Murphy BL, Danzer SC (2011) Somatic translocation: a novel mechanism of granule cell dendritic dysmorphogenesis and dispersion. *J Neurosci* 31(8):2959–2964.

Murphy BL, Hofacer RD, Faulkner CN, Loepke AW, Danzer SC (2012) Abnormalities of granule cell dendritic structure are a prominent feature of the intrahippocampal model of epilepsy despite reduced postinjury neurogenesis. *Epilepsia* 53(5):908–921.

Murphy BL, Pun RY, Yin H, Faulkner CR, Loepke AW, Danzer SC (2011) Heterogeneous integration of adult-generated granule cells into the epileptic brain. *J Neurosci* 31(1):105–117.

Myers CE, Bermudez-Hernandez K, Scharfman HE (2013) The influence of ectopic migration of granule cells into the hilus on dentate gyrus-CA3 function. *PLoS One* 8(6):e68208.

Nadler JV, Perry BW, Cotman CW (1980) Selective reinnervation of hippocampal area CA1 and the fascia dentata after destruction of CA3-CA4 afferents with kainic acid. *Brain Res* 182(1):1–9.

Nadler JV (2003) The recurrent mossy fiber pathway of the epileptic brain. *Neurochem Res* 28(11):1649–1658.

Nakahara S, Tamura M, Matsuki N, Koyama R (2009) Neuronal hyperactivity sustains the basal dendrites of immature dentate granule cells: time-lapse confocal analysis using hippocampal slice cultures. *Hippocampus* 19(4):379–391.

Paradisi M, Fernández M, Del Vecchio G, Lizzo G, Marucci G, Giulioni M, Pozzati E, Antonelli T, Lanzoni G, Bagnara GP, Giardino L, Calzà L (2010) *Ex vivo* study of dentate gyrus neurogenesis in human pharmaco-resistant temporal lobe epilepsy. *Neuropathol Appl Neurobiol* 36(6):535–550.

Parent JM, Elliott RC, Pleasure SJ, Barbaro NM, Lowenstein DH (2006) Aberrant seizure-induced neurogenesis in experimental temporal lobe epilepsy. *Ann Neurol* 59(1):81–91.

Parent JM, Janumpalli S, McNamara JO, Lowenstein DH (1998) Increased dentate granule cell neurogenesis following amygdala kindling in the adult rat. *Neurosci Lett* 247(1):9–12.

Parent JM, Tada E, Fike JR, Lowenstein DH (1999) Inhibition of dentate granule cell neurogenesis with brain irradiation does not prevent seizure-induced mossy fiber synaptic reorganization in the rat. *J Neurosci* 19(11):4508–4519.

Parent JM, Yu TW, Leibowitz RT, Geschwind DH, Sloviter RS, Lowenstein DH (1997) Dentate granule cell neurogenesis is increased by seizures and contributes to aberrant network reorganization in the adult rat hippocampus. *J Neurosci* 17(10):3727–3738.

Pathak HR, Weissinger F, Terunuma M, Carlson GC, Hsu FC, Moss SJ, Coulter DA (2007) Disrupted dentate granule cell chloride regulation enhances synaptic excitability during development of temporal lobe epilepsy. *J Neurosci* 27(51):14012–14022.

Pekcec A, Fuest C, Mühlenhoff M, Gerardy-Schahn R, Potschka H (2008) Targeting epileptogenesis-associated induction of neurogenesis by enzymatic depolysialylation of NCAM counteracts spatial learning dysfunction but fails to impact epilepsy development. *J Neurochem* 105(2): 389–400.

Pierce JP, Melton J, Punsoni M, McCloskey DP, Scharfman HE (2005) Mossy fibers are the primary source of afferent input to ectopic granule cells that are born after pilocarpine-induced seizures. *Exp Neurol* 196(2):316–331.

Pierce JP, McCloskey DP, Scharfman HE (2011) Morphometry of hilar ectopic granule cells in the rat. *J Comp Neurol* 519(6):1196–1218.

Pun RY, Rolle IJ, LaSarge CL, Hosford BE, Rosen JM, Uhl JD, Schmeltzer SN, Faulkner C, Bronson SL, Murphy BL, Richards DA, Holland KD, Danzer SC (2012) Excessive activation of mTOR in postnatally generated granule cells is sufficient to cause epilepsy. *Neuron* 75(6):1022–1034.

Rao MS, Hattiangady B, Shetty AK (2008) Status epilepticus during old age is not associated with enhanced hippocampal neurogenesis. *Hippocampus* 28(9):931–944.

Ribak CE, Tran PH, Spigelman I, Okazaki MM, Nadler JV (2000) Status epilepticus-induced hilar basal dendrites on rodent granule cells contribute to recurrent excitatory circuitry. *J Comp Neurol* 428(2):240–253.

Ribak CE, Shapiro LA, Yan XX, Dashtipour K, Nadler JV, Obenaus A, Spigelman I, Buckmaster PS (2012) Seizure-induced formation of basal dendrites on granule cells of the rodent dentate gyrus. In: Noebels JL, Avoli M, Rogawski MA, Olsen RW, Delgado-Escueta AV, editors. *Jasper's Basic Mechanisms of the Epilepsies* [Internet]. 4th edition. Bethesda (MD): National Center for Biotechnology Information (US).

Sanchez RM, Jensen FE (2001) Maturational aspects of epilepsy mechanisms and consequences for the immature brain. *Epilepsia* 42(5):577–585.

Sankar R, Rho JM (2007) Do seizures affect the developing brain? Lessons from the laboratory. *J Child Neurol* 22(5 suppl):21–29.

Sankar R, Shin D, Liu H, Katsumori H, Wasterlain CG (2000) Granule cell neurogenesis after status epilepticus in the immature rat brain. *Epilepsia* 41 (suppl 6):53–56.

Sankar R, Shin DH, Liu H, Mazarati A, Pereira de Vasconcelos A, Wasterlain CG (1998) Patterns of status epilepticus-induced neuronal injury during development and long-term consequences. *J Neurosci* 18(20):8382–8393.

Scharfman HE (2007) The CA3 "backprojection" to the dentate gyrus. *Progs Brain Res* 163:627–637.

Scharfman HE, Goodman JH, Sollas AL (2000) Granule-like neurons at the hilar/CA3 border after status epilepticus and their synchrony with area CA3 pyramidal cells: functional implications of seizure induced neurogenesis. *J Neurosci* 20(16):6144–6158.

Scharfman HA, Myers CE (2013) Hilar mossy cells of the dentate gyrus: a historical perspective. *Front Neural Circuits* 6:1–17.

Scharfman HE, Pierce JP (2012) New insights into the role of hilar ectopic granule cells in the dentate gyrus based on quantitative anatomic analysis and three-dimensional reconstruction. *Epilepsia* 53 (suppl 1): 109–115.

Scharfman HE, Sollas AE, Berger RE, Goodman JH, Pierce JP (2003) Perforant path activation of ectopic granule cells that are born after pilocarpine-induced seizures. *Neuroscience* 121(4):1017–1029.

Scheibel ME, Crandall PH, Scheibel AB (1974) The hippocampal-dentate complex in temporal lobe epilepsy. *Epilepsia* 15(1):55–80.

Scott BW, Burnham WM (2006) Kindled seizures enhance young neuron survival in the adult rat dentate gyrus. *Acta Neuropathol* 111(4): 364–371.

Scott BW, Wojtowicz JM, Burnham WM (2000) Neurogenesis in the dentate gyrus of the rat following electroconvulsive shock seizures. *Expl Neurol* 165(2):231–236.

Schlessinger AR, Cowan WM, Gottlieb DI (1975) An autoradiographic study of the time of origin and the pattern of granule cell migration in the dentate gyrus of the rat. *J Comp Neurol* 159(2):149–175.

Seibert K, Zhang Y, Leahy K, Hauser S, Masferrer J, Perkins W, Lee L, Isakson P (1994) Pharmacological and biochemical demonstration of the role of cyclooxygenase 2 in inflammation and pain. *Proc Natl Acad Sci U S A* 91(25):12013–12017.

Seress L, Abrahám H, Tornóczky T, Kosztolányi G (2001) Cell formation in the human hippocampal formation from mid-gestation to the late postnatal period. *Neuroscience* 105(4):831–843.

Seress L, Mrzljak L (1987) Basal dendrites of granule cells are normal features of the fetal and adult dentate gyrus of both monkey and human hippocampal formations. *Brain Res* 405(1):169–174.

Seress L, Pokorny J (1981) Structure of the granular layer of the rat dentate gyrus. A light microscopic and Golgi study. *J Anat* 133(2): 181–195.

Shao LR, Dudek FE (2011) Repetitive perforant-path stimulation induced epileptiform bursts in minislices of dentate gyrus from rats with kainate-induced epilepsy. *J Neurophysiol* 105(2):522–527.

Shapiro LA, Ribak CE (2005) Integration of newly born dentate granule cells into adult brains: hypotheses based on normal and epileptic rodents. *Brain Res Brain Res Rev* 48(1):43–56.

Shapiro LA, Ribak CE (2006) Newly born dentate granule neurons after pilocarpine-induced epilepsy have hilar basal dendrites with immature synapses. *Epilepsy Res* 69(1):53–66.

Shapiro LA, Wang L, Upadhyaya P, Ribak CE (2011) Seizure-induced increased neurogenesis occurs in the dentate gyrus of aged Sprague-Dawley rats. *Aging Dis* 2(4):286–293.

Shi XY, Wang JW, Lei GF, Sun RP (2007) Morphological and behavioral consequences of recurrent seizures in neonatal rats are associated with glucocorticoid levels. *Neurosci Bull* 23(2):83–91.

Siebzehnrubl FA, Blümcke I (2008) Neurogenesis in the human hippocampus and its relevance to temporal lobe epilepsies. *Epilepsia* 49 (suppl 5): 55–65.

Silverstein FS, Jensen FE (2007) Neonatal seizures. *Ann Neurol* 62(2):112–120.

Sloviter RS (1992) Possible functional consequences of synaptic reorganization in the dentate gyrus of kainate-treated rats. *Neurosci Lett* 137(1): 91–96.

Sloviter RS (2006) Kainic acid-induced recurrent mossy fiber innervation of dentate gyrus inhibitory interneurons: possible anatomical substrate of granule cell hyperinhibition in chronically epileptic rats. *J Comp Neurol* 494(6):944–960.

Sperk G, Wieselthaler-Hölzl A, Pirker S, Tasan R, Strasser SS, Drexel M, Pifl C, Marschalek J, Ortler M, Trinka E, Heitmair-Wietzorrek K, Ciofi P, Feucht M, Baumgartner C, Czech T (2012) Glutamate decarboxylase 67 is expressed in hippocampal mossy fibers of temporal lobe epilepsy patients. *Hippocampus* 22(3):590–603.

Spigelman I, Yan XX, Obenaus A, Lee EY, Wasterlain CG, Ribak CE (1998) Dentate granule cells form novel basal dendrites in a rat model of temporal lobe epilepsy. *Neuroscience* 86(1):109–120.

Sutula T, Cascino G, Cavazos J, Parada I, Ramirez L (1989) Mossy fiber synaptic reorganization in the epileptic human temporal lobe. *Ann Neurol* 26(3):321–330.

Sutula TP, Dudek FE (2007) Unmasking a recurrent excitation generated by mossy fiber sprouting in the epileptic dentate gyrus: an emergent property of a complex system. *Prog Brain Res* 163(1): 541–563.

Tang H, Long H, Zeng C, Li Y, Bi F, Wang J, Qian H, Xiao B (2012) Rapamycin suppresses the recurrent excitatory circuits of dentate gyrus in a mouse model of temporal lobe epilepsy. *Biochem Biophys Res Commun* 420(1):199–204.

Tauck DL, Nadler JV (1985) Evidence of functional mossy fiber sprouting in hippocampal formation of kainic acid-treated rats. *J Neurosci* 5(4): 1016–1022.

Thind KK, Ribak CE, Buckmaster PS (2008) Synaptic input to dentate granule cell basal dendrites in a rat model of temporal lobe epilepsy. *J Comp Neurol* 509(2):190–202.

Urban NN, Henze DA, Barrionuevo G (2001) Revisiting the role of the hippocampal mossy fiber synapse. *Hippocampus* 11(4):408–417.

Vezzani A, Friedman A, Dingledine RJ (2013) The role of inflammation in epileptogenesis. *Neuropharmacology* 69:16–24.

von Campe G, Spencer DD, de Lanerolle NC (1997) Morphology of dentate granule cells in the human epileptogenic hippocampus. *Hippocampus* 7(5):472–488.

Walter C, Murphy BL, Pun RYK, Spieles-Engemann AI, Danzer SC (2007) Pilocarpine-induced seizures cause selective time-dependent changes to adult-generated hippocampal dentate granule cells. *J Neurosci* 27(28):7541–7552.

Wang L, Wang X, Yuan J, Xi Z, Xue T, Li Y, Xiao Z (2009) Nestin in the temporal neocortex of the intractable epilepsy patients. *Neurochem Res* 34(3):574–580.

Wood JC, Jackson JS, Jakubs K, Chapman KZ, Ekdahl CT, Kokaia Z, Kokaia M, Lindvall O (2011) Functional integration of new hippocampal neurons following insults to the adult brain is determined by characteristics of pathological environment. *Exp Neurol* 229(2):484–493.

Xiu-Yu S, Ruo-Peng S, Ji-Wen W (2007) Consequences of pilocarpine-induced recurrent seizures in neonatal rats. *Brain Dev* 29(3):157–163.

Zeng LH, Rensing NR, Wong M (2009) The mammalian target of rapamycin signaling pathway mediates epileptogenesis in a model of temporal lobe epilepsy. *J Neurosci* 29(21):6964–6972.

Zhan RZ, Nadler JV (2009) Enhanced tonic GABA current in normotopic and hilar ectopic dentate granule cells after pilocarpine-induced status epilepticus. *J Neurophysiol* 102(2):670–681.

Zhan RZ, Timofeeva O, Nadler JV (2010) High ratio of synaptic excitation to synaptic inhibition in hilar ectopic granule cells of pilocarpine-treated rats. *J Neurophysiol* 104(6):3293–3304.

Chapter 7

Endogenous Neural Stem Cell Response to Traumatic Brain Injury

Aminul I. Ahmed and William P. Gray

Traumatic Brain Injury (TBI) and its consequences are increasing despite the advancements in therapy. Clinical trials for TBI have largely been unsuccessful in producing a therapy that improves outcome, so interest has turned to the endogenous stem cell pool as a potential source to promote neuroprotection or even regeneration following TBI. Several rodent models have been used to recapitulate TBI *in vivo*, both in regions of known neurogenesis, including the subgranular zone of the dentate gyrus and the subventricular zone, and in areas traditionally regarded as non-neurogenic, such as the cerebral cortex. We discuss these responses and begin to detail the evidence of putative mechanisms that contribute to this increase in neurogenesis following injury. Finally, we touch upon progress of endogenous human stem cell studies in TBI.

Introduction

Traumatic Brain Injury — A public health concern: in patients under the age of 40, Traumatic Brain Injury (TBI) is the most significant cause of disability, and the World Health Organisation predicts that this is expected to grow over the next decade to become

191

the third leading cause of global mortality and disability (Hyder *et al.*, 2007; Maas *et al.*, 2008). In the UK, each year 135,000 patients are admitted to hospital with TBI and 15% of these are moderate or severe. Approximately half a million of these patients live with long-term disability. Similarly, in the USA, approximately 80,000 people per year sustain a TBI that results in a long-term disability, and the NIH estimates of people affected in the US alone amounts to over 3 million (Rose, 1999). The lifetime cost per patient is estimated at €170,000, with almost 90% attributable to indirect costs (Berg *et al.*, 2005). Some estimates indicate that TBI costs amount to €33 billion per year in Europe alone (Wittchen *et al.*, 2011). In recognition of this high cost to society, collaborations between the European Commission (EC) and the National Institutes of Health (NIH) were set up in 2011 to specifically advance clinical TBI research (Maas *et al.*, 2011). This focuses on promoting the use of international standards for TBI clinical data collection and a TBI patient registry. However, while this recognition of the impact of TBI has led to an increase in funding, little progress has been made in generating therapies that reduce or reverse the brain damage and currently there is no effective repair in humans (Okano, 2002; Aboody *et al.*, 2011). As a result, the potential for stem cells to aid the repair of the injured nervous system has become prominent in the goal to ameliorate the devastating consequences following TBI.

Interest in stem cells for therapy in TBI: 20 years ago a key paper demonstrated that the mammalian brain contains neural stem cells (NSCs) that have the capacity to self-renew and give rise to both neurons and glia (Reynolds and Weiss, 1992). NSCs have emerged as promising candidates to treat a number of neurodegenerative diseases although trials using exogenous stem cells have been somewhat disappointing with the exception of Parkinson's and Huntington's diseases. Subsequent interest has broadened towards harnessing endogenous stem cells for repair in many of these degenerative diseases and neurological insults including TBI. Although it is well established that following a TBI there is the formation of the glial scar, endogenous stem cells from the neurogenic niches contribute to scar formation. For instance, following a TBI in a rodent model, stem cells from the subventricular zone (SVZ) migrate out and contribute to the astroglial scar formation in the injured cortex (Salman *et al.*, 2004). Interestingly, quiescent precursor cells have been identified in non-permissive brain parenchyma including the adult cortex of rodents (Palmer *et al.*, 1999; Buffo *et al.*, 2008) and humans (Arsenijevic *et al.*, 2001; Richardson *et al.*, 2006) raising the intriguing possibility of repair in these regions initially thought to be non-neurogenic. This chapter focuses on endogenous stem cell activation in neurogenic regions following TBI. We also discuss TBI-induced neurogenesis in regions traditionally regarded as non-neurogenic, and chart the current experimental treatment strategies in reactivating neurogenesis following TBI. Finally, we discuss how this may translate to the clinical setting.

Brain Injury Models

While TBI is defined as damage secondary to an external force, the spectrum of the disease is highly variable. The primary injury, which is as a result of the force, includes rapid changes in speed, mechanical impacts, penetrations and blast injuries, and while the resulting pathophysiology is grouped as TBI, the spectrum includes contusion, hemorrhage and axonal shearing. The balance between these pathologies leads to a heterogeneous spectrum of TBI injuries from focal well-defined contusions to a more diffuse axonal injury. Complicating the process is the secondary injury as a result of the metabolic, cellular and excitotoxic events resulting in cell death and inflammation. Subsequent to this heterogeneity of injuries, animal TBI models have developed to replicate the wide spectrum of injuries seen. The obvious aim is to maintain a homogenous reproducible injury representative of one or several parts of the TBI spectrum seen in humans.

Four animal models have become established in *in vivo* models of TBI. These include those that are more diffuse in injury, such as the lateral fluid percussion injury (LFP), to the more localized in nature, such as the controlled cortical impact (CCI) model. These two have become widely accepted in the investigation of neurogenesis following TBI. The weight-drop impact acceleration injury and the blast injury models are less well used in the study of neurogenesis (Xiong *et al.*, 2013). Other models include several variations in the weight drop model that can be focal or diffuse and delivered to either an intact skull or through a craniotomy, and the optic nerve stretch model that is regarded as a focal injury model. Acceleration models, blast models and penetrating ballistic-like brain injury models aim to mimic a more diffuse injury (Xiong *et al.*, 2009, 2013).

The fluid percussion injury is widely accepted as a model of *in vivo* head injury (Dixon *et al.*, 1987). The injury is more diffuse in nature and results in a wide spectrum of neurological deficits. In rodents, the LFP combines a focal contusion coupled with a more diffuse subcortical injury. The LFP is delivered with a pendulum-induced pressure pulse in a reservoir of fluid. This device rests against the exposed dural surface, over which a craniotomy has been performed, and the pressure pulse is transmitted onto the dura and through the brain (Chirumamilla *et al.*, 2002). The second widely used injury model is the controlled cortical impact injury model in which a piston delivers a precise impact to the intact exposed dura. This causes a deformation in the underlying brain, resulting in cortical injury, hemorrhage and axonal injury. This injury model has the advantage of precise control of time, velocity, force and depth of injury, along with a reduction in the risk of rebound injury caused by a wave pulse. Thus it is regarded as a focused and controlled injury paradigm (Lighthall *et al.*, 1989).

The above injury models induce a significant change in the cellular environment. These injury paradigms have been associated with disruption of the blood brain barrier, activation of a robust inflammatory response, and upregulation of cytokines which accelerate this response (Morganti-Kossmann *et al.*, 2007). Moreover, astrocytes and microglia are activated and the resulting niche environment contains a mixture of both neurotoxic and neuroprotective cytokines. Indeed some of these cytokines have been shown to perform dual functions (Morganti-Kossmann *et al.*, 2007). While the two commonly used experimental paradigms, the CCI model and LFP aim to provide consistency in the injury between experiments, the nature of the models results in the inevitability of a combination of focal injuries (which dominate in the CCI model) and diffuse injuries (which dominate in the LFP model). Interestingly, in a rat model of moderate LFP injury, although evidence of axonal damage, including axonal swellings and synaptic loss, were observed in the acute phase, at 7 days ultrastructural analysis of the somata of these injured neurons was suggestive of repair (Singleton *et al.*, 2002). This indicates that endogenous cells have the potential to undergo anatomical repair under controlled experimental paradigms of TBI. Indeed, a stark degree of neuronal repair is seen in models of ischaemia-induced apoptosis (Nakatomi *et al.*, 2002; Bendel *et al.*, 2005) and chromophore-targeted apoptosis (Magavi *et al.*, 2000; Chen *et al.*, 2004). These demonstrate that an understanding of the injury niche may enable the rescue and restoration of neurons, following intervention. As a consequence, the endogenous stem and progenitor cells provide a potential target for these neuro-restorative interventions. Indeed, in TBI research, the stab injury model, in which a single penetrating stab incision is made into the cortex, aims to induce an attenuated inflammatory response, thus enabling the study of neuronal repair similar to those above (Buffo *et al.*, 2008; Sirko *et al.*, 2013).

Although, *in vivo* experiments have been the mainstay of assessing the response of endogenous stem cells following TBI, *in vitro* paradigms have served to complement current findings. These models have provided a reduction in cost, increased reproducibility, and ease of use following injury. The organotypic stretch injury (Morrison *et al.*, 2006) has an advantage in that it maintains cells in their original milieu allowing cell-cell interaction and local extracellular signaling events with the added advantage of ease of manipulation of the niche environment. With this in mind, we have developed an organotypic stretch injury paradigm where cortico-hippocampal slices are injured, and the subsequent environment can be manipulated and the neurogenic potential assessed (Ahmed *et al.*, 2012). Perhaps a reason why all these injury models investigating endogenous stem cells in TBI are still being used today is that while therapies aimed at neuroprotection have been widely investigated and have passed through clinical trials, the surprising headline fact is that there is currently no effective therapy that reduces or reverses the impact of TBI in humans (Okano, 2002; Aboody *et al.*, 2011). Hence, research into endogenous stem cells following TBI remains topical, and our understanding of the mechanisms following TBI in the two well-defined neurogenic niches, along with changes outside these niches, is the focus of this review.

Neurogenesis in the Hippocampus Following TBI

The evidence for an increase in neurogenesis in the hippocampus, and specifically the dentate gyrus, post-TBI is compelling. The initial papers used a combination of both CCI and LFP injury models, and primarily used Bromo-deoxyUridine (BrdU) to label newly proliferating cells. The first two papers were published in 2001 (Dash *et al.*, 2001; Kernie *et al.*, 2001). In the first paper, using the CCI injury model in adult mice, Kernie and colleagues (2001) administered BrdU for up to 7 days post-injury. Within 7 days, newly dividing cells co-localised with nestin (a putative stem/progenitor cell marker), with greater staining closer to the injury site. At 60 days post-injury, the number of proliferating cells in the ipsilateral dentate gyrus was 5-fold compared to uninjured controls, and in the contralateral dentate gyrus increased by 2-fold compared to controls. Proliferation around injury site was almost exclusively astrocytic, although within the granular layer, newly formed cells labeled calbindin suggesting that these cells were neuronal. Again using the CCI model, but in rats, Dash and colleagues (2001) demonstrated an increase in BrdU labeled cells peaking at 3 days following TBI, returning to baseline by 2 weeks. In the first few days, BrdU co-localised with the early neuronal marker TOAD-64. Similar to the findings of Kernie and colleagues, at 28 days, newly formed cells in the granular cell layer co-localised with calbindin suggestive of migration and subsequent integration (Dash *et al.*, 2001). Again in mice subjected to CCI, in which new cells were pulse-labeled either 1 or 2 weeks post-injury, an increase in cell proliferation in the dentate gyrus was observed at both time-points. After one month, there was a significant increase in newly formed neurons as detected by the mature neuronal marker NeuN (Yoshimura *et al.*, 2003). These studies demonstrate that in a focal injury model, cells in the dentate gyrus proliferate and can mature into newly formed neurons.

Several studies have utilized the LFP model to confirm similar observations in the rat. For example, following a moderate LFP injury, rats receiving either of BrdU or ^{3}H-thymidine at 2 days were sacrificed 1 day later. Quantification showed increased proliferation in the SGZ of the hippocampus although none of the cells expressed neural progenitor or neuronal markers at this early stage (Chirumamilla *et al.*, 2002). Similarly, again following LFP in rats, increased proliferation was observed in the SGZ two days after injury. After 10 days, BrdU and βIII-tubulin co-localisation was observed (Rice *et al.*, 2003). In a similar BrdU dosing regimen, following a LFP in rats, the proliferative effect of the injury was observed at 5 days, but had normalized to baseline levels by 35 days (Kleindienst *et al.*, 2005). In rats receiving a moderate LFP injury with BrdU dosing around the time of injury, newly formed mature neurons were observed at 2 weeks (Urrea *et al.*, 2007). From these studies, it is clear that the early administration of BrdU is key in identifying TBI-induced proliferation and neurogenesis. There is an observed increase in the number of proliferating cells, returning to baseline several weeks following injury.

As demonstrated above, the evidence for TBI-induced hippocampal neurogenesis has been persuasive. However, several studies reported that in their experimental paradigms, there was a reduction in injury-induced neurogenesis. For instance, following CCI injury in 2-month-old mice, BrdU was administered 1 week post-injury, and at 3 weeks a decrease in new neurons was observed on the ipsilateral side (Rola *et al.*, 2006). Similarly, following a moderate CCI in juvenile mice, BrdU was injected into the animals either 2 or 4 weeks before injury so as to label either immature or mature neurons. CCI resulted in a decrease in newly formed neurons, with a greater proportion of the immature neurons dying (Gao *et al.*, 2008). Interestingly, in a CCI model for adult rats, BrdU was administered for 7 days post-injury, however there was a reduction in the number of neuroblasts

(BrdU+PSA-NCAM+) compared to uninjured controls at 7 days (Shi *et al.*, 2013). In the above studies, this discrepancy in the observed failure in TBI-induced neurogenesis may be explained in two ways. Firstly, the dosing regimen of BrdU is important, since the first two studies failed to capture the key cellular proliferation within the first week post-injury. In the first study, BrdU was administered one week after injury, thereby labeling cells born after the initial injury phase. The next study labeled cells before the injury, thus capturing the response of newly formed neurons following injury. Secondly, the markers used, and therefore the cell type labeled, may influence the observations. In the third study, the authors used PSA-NCAM to label the neuroblasts, and the reduction may simply reflect an acceleration in proliferation and a shorter period of the cells in this immature state.

One of the limitations of using BrdU is the assumption that it labels proliferating cells only, and that cells undergoing repair, or dying cells attempting to repair (and hence also incorporate BrdU) are not significant. To overcome this, a transgenic approach was utilized in which cells expressed GFP under the nestin promoter (Yu *et al.*, 2008). Eight-week-old mice were subjected to a unilateral CCI. In the ipsilateral granular layer of hippocampus at 3 days, the number of GFP expressing early progenitors were increased, whereas doublecortin expressing late progenitors were decreased, indicative of this cell types vulnerability to the insult. Interestingly, on the contralateral side, both early and late progenitors were increased. Using an elegant transgenic approach in which early progenitors were ablated using ganciclovir, the authors demonstrated that the early progenitors were necessary for the TBI-induced neurogenesis (Yu *et al.*, 2008). Another key paper by the same group used a transgenic approach to determine that TBI-induced neurogenesis resulted in a functional improvement. Using tamoxifen-induced labelling of nestin expressing cells, a CCI injury tripled the number of new neurons in the dentate gyrus. Moreover, to determine whether these new CCI-induced neurons had any functional relevance, using a ganciclovir mediated ablation of dividing progenitors, the authors demonstrated a 4-week exposure to the anti-viral resulted in an approximately 90% reduction in injury-induced neurogenesis.

Importantly, while fear conditioning responses were unaffected by CCI nor reduced neurogenesis, testing using the hippocampus dependent Morris Water Maze (MWM) resulted in reduced performance in mice in which CCI-induced neurogenesis had been genetically ameliorated (Blaiss *et al.*, 2011). Age may influence the response to TBI, since LFP to juvenile 1-month-old rats compared to 3-month-old adult rats resulted in greater proliferation in juvenile rats. Furthermore, there was almost a doubling of new neurons in the juvenile SGZ compared to adult up to 28 days post-injury (Sun *et al.*, 2005).

While some of the above studies demonstrated morphological characteristics of the newly formed dentate gyrus neurons that were suggestive of integration, this has been demonstrated more definitively using tracer studies. These studies have provided evidence that these new neurons integrate with the Cornu Ammonis area 3 (CA3) pyramidal neurons. For instance, following the LFP in rats, fluorospheres injected into the CA3 retrogradely traced newly born neurons in the granular cell layer within the dentate gyrus indicative of integration at 2 weeks (Emery *et al.*, 2005). Similarly, at 10 weeks following injury, newly born neurons detectable in the granular cell layer contained Fluorogold, which had been injected into the CA3 region at 8 weeks post-injury, suggesting anatomical integration into the dentate gyrus (Sun *et al.*, 2007). Why does this neurogenesis and anatomical integration occur post-injury? Perhaps it helps to improve or compensate for the learning and memory deficits seen in the TBI population. This may be a consequence of a disruption of the continued neurogenesis in the hippocampus of humans (Eriksson *et al.*, 1998). Although, there is a note of caution since the increased neurogenesis may contribute to the increase in epilepsy observed in TBI patients (Kharatishvili and Pitkanen, 2010).

Neurogenesis in the Subventricular Zone (SVZ) Following TBI

The second of the well-defined neurogenic niches, the Subventricular Zone (SVZ), has also been characterised in its response following experimental TBI. The first evidence that cells proliferate in the SVZ following a traumatic injury used a stab injury model in rats. Following a stab wound to the cortex, and subsequent BrdU administration, the number of newly divided cells was increased in both the ipsi- and contralateral SVZ (Tzeng and Wu, 1999). In a later study, adult rats subjected to moderate LFP injury showed increased proliferation of cells within the SVZ at 48 hours. While this demonstrated injury-induced activation, there was no observed expression of astrocytic or neuronal markers (Chirumamilla *et al.*, 2002). Again in a LFP model in rats, there was an increase in proliferation in the sub-ependymal region in the first few days following injury. Similar to the first study, immunohistochemical staining did not show any new immature neurons in the SEZ, and in this example, cells were analyzed up to two week post-injury (Rice *et al.*, 2003). The apparent lack of immature neurons in both studies may have been in part due to the labeling regimen. In the first study, BrdU injections consisted of two intraperitoneal injection at 48 hours post-injury followed by sacrifice 24 hours later. In the second study, BrdU labeled cells early with four pulse injections followed by animal sacrifice within 24 hours after the first injection. In both cases, there may not have been sufficient time for differentiation of labeled cells into early neuronal or glial cells. Using peritoneal injections of BrdU, rats demonstrated increased proliferation of cells within the SVZ within 2 hours of LFP injury, although no evidence of co-localisation with NeuN was demonstrable (Urrea *et al.*, 2007), which is not surprising.

More recently, following either a mild or moderate CCI, adult mice showed an acute increase in cells proliferating in the SVZ. At one month post-injury, while the number of new cells were increased in the olfactory bulb, these was a decrease in the number of new neurons and this was associated with a deficit in olfactory avoidance behavior (Radomski *et al.*, 2013). These studies, while demonstrating an injury-induced proliferation, did not convincingly demonstrate the birth of new neurons, although one study did speculate that this may have been due to the 'fast migration' of these neuroblasts or neurons out of the SVZ into the rostral migratory stream.

Supporting this notion, following a CCI injury in mice, in which an increase in proliferation was seen at 3 days in the SVZ and the cortex, microbeads were injected into the lateral ventricle, allowing cells to endocytose the beads and thus use them as a marker of migration. Doublecortin/Microbead double-labelled cells, indicative of migrating neuroblasts, were seen towards the contusion cavity, the corpus callosum and sub-cortical regions (Ramaswamy *et al.*, 2005). Similarly, stem cells in the SVZ contribute to brain remodeling in the proximal region of a cortical contusion. Following CCI injury in mice, SVZ cells were labeled with intraventricular injection of DiO, and migrating cells were identified. These cells contribute to scar around injury site, with some expressing progenitor markers but not mature neuronal markers (Salman *et al.*, 2004). In an aspiration lesion of the mouse somatosensory cortex, although an increase in new neuroblasts were not observed in the SVZ (following a 5-day BrdU dosing regimen), the number of new cells in the corpus callosum was increased. Although not demonstrated, the authors suggest that these cells had migrated from the SVZ (Sundholm-Peters *et al.*, 2005). Why these cells migrate may be perhaps due to injury-induced trophic factors, which act as chemoattractants or the fact that the lesioned cortex may have connections with the SVZ leading to alteration in the niche environment. It is clear that TBI-induced cues exist, perhaps to encourage migration of progenitors leading to functional recovery and reorganization.

TBI-Induced Endogenous Cortical Neurogenesis

Under controlled experimental ablation paradigms, there is evidence of cortical neurogenesis in the rodent. Here, apoptosis is induced in an environment in which there is a minimal inflammatory response. For example, following chromophore-targeted apoptosis targeting the death of layer VI corticothalamic neurons, Magavi and colleagues (2000) used a combination of neuronal markers to demonstrate endogenous neurogenesis in the cortex. Following a similar targeted cell death, neuronal restoration is also observed in layer V corticospinal motor neurons, with cells extending axons into the cervical spine (Chen *et al.*, 2004). While, TBI-induced endogenous cortical neurogenesis *in vivo* is yet to be demonstrated, perhaps perturbed by the strong injury response, a landmark paper was published in 2008. Following a stab injury, which induces a more robust inflammatory response, mature protoplasmic reactive astrocytes (identified by genetic labelling) were isolated from the injured cerebral cortex and gave rise to stem cells capable of differentiating into neurons *in vitro* — where the local environmental inflammatory cues have been removed — but critically not *in vivo* (Buffo *et al.*, 2008). These cells have the capacity to differentiate, giving rise to neurons only following injury. This process, termed post-injury 'dedifferentiation' by the authors, suggests that mature cells of one lineage within the cerebral cortex are able to acquire stem/progenitor properties and then follow a different lineage pathway (Buffo *et al.*, 2008).

Our laboratory examined cortical neurogenesis using an *ex vivo* model of TBI using a rodent organotypic stretch injury model in which cortico-hippocampal slices are cultured on a deformable silicone membrane. Following a stretch TBI, cells in the normal juvenile brain are activated and lead to the formation of increased neurospheres only when cultured outside the cortical environment *in vitro*. Using slices from mice expressing a fluorescent reporter (eGFP) driven by the human Glial Fibrillary Acidic Protein (GFAP) promoter, we showed that GFAP positive cells account for the majority of neurospheres. These cells are multipotent but mechanisms underlying this process are largely unknown, although we identified sonic hedgehog (Shh) signalling as a candidate pathway (Ahmed *et al.*, 2012). Significantly, Shh signaling is upregulated in GFAP-expressing reactive astrocytes following a focal freeze injury to the cerebral cortex. Moreover, this expression contributes to an increase in the proliferation of a subset of progenitor cells (Amankulor *et al.*, 2009). Similarly, in an *in vivo* stab wound model, Shh is upregulated, peaking at 3 days post-injury. While activation of this pathway increased the number of injury-induced neurospheres generated from astrocytes, perhaps the most interesting finding was that even without injury — using an agonist of Shh signaling — the intact cortex was able to give rise to multipotent neurospheres (Sirko 2013). Therefore, this evidence provides a handle on some of the molecular cues that underpin the injury-activated response of cells to acquire stem cell-like properties.

Endogenous Repair Mechanisms

While the above evidence strongly supports the notion that endogenous neurogenesis is a real response in models of TBI, the size of this response remains modest, especially when compared to the glial response that results in the scar formation. The strategies to effect repair using endogenous stem or progenitor cells will require the manipulation of the proliferating cells towards a neurogenic fate, coupled with the alteration of the niche environment to support this. What are the mechanisms underlying injury-induced neurogenesis? While Shh signaling may be a potential factor in driving the injury-activated cells towards a neurogenic fate, other mechanisms undoubtedly contribute to this process. For instance, while glutamate and potassium chloride mediate toxicity in neurons, there is evidence of proliferation of immature cells (Shi *et al.*, 2007; Mattson, 2008). Furthermore, in a CCI model for TBI, mice deficient in the pro-apoptotic gene Bax, which is known to be upregulated following TBI, demonstrate an increase in nestin expressing progenitor cells in the dentate gyrus. This process depends, at least in part, on potassium channels (Shi *et al.*, 2007). In addition to the influence of intrinsic pro- and anti-apoptotic genes, cues in the injury niche leads to activation of the supporting glia, which include the microglia and astrocytes. Dissecting the mechanisms and the interplay between cell types in the injury milieu which may promote the proliferation and differentiation of stem or progenitor cells to a neuronal phenotype may be key to effect repair following TBI.

Vascular endothelial growth factor (VEGF), while seminal in angiogenesis following ischaemia, has emerged as an activator of neurogenesis in both the SGZ of the hippocampus and the SVZ (Jin *et al.*, 2002). In a closed head injury model in mice, VEGF was infused into the lateral ventricle for seven days and showed not only an increase in performance in the neurological severity score, but the size of the lesion was reduced. Moreover, the number of immature neurons was increased in the SVZ and the perilesional cortex. Perhaps more interestingly, the number of mature neurons was increased in the perilesional cortex, indicating not only a neuroprotective role for VEGF following trauma, but also perhaps a neurogenic role (Thau-Zuchman *et al.*, 2010). Nitric Oxide (NO) is also known to promote neurogenesis. In a CCI injury model in adult rats, The NO donor (Z)-1-[N-(2-aminoethyl)-N-(2-ammonioethyl) amino]diazen-1-ium-1,2-diolate (DETA/NONOate) was injected intraperitoneally for a week. Labeling experiments at one month demonstrated new cells in the SGZ of the dentate gyrus, striatum/ corpus callosum and the cortex, but not the SVZ, expressed the neuronal marker Hu. This was associated with a modest but significant functional recovery at 42 days as assessed by the modified neurological severity score (Lu *et al.*, 2003). 3-Hydroxy-3-methyglutaryl coenzyme A (HMG-CoA) reductase inhibitors (also known as statins) increase endothelium-derived NO production (Eto *et al.*, 2002). Moreover, following a CCI and either simvastatin or atorvastatin administration for two weeks, the number of newly born neurons in the ipsilateral dentate gyrus at one month is augmented. This was coupled with improvements in spatial learning deficits as assessed with the MWM for both statins (Lu *et al.*, 2007). This data indicates that manipulating components of vascular physiology can impact on the pool of injury activated cells, with a putative route to enhanced recovery.

Erythropoetin (EPO), which is central to haemopoetic progenitor cell maturation, has also emerged as a promoter of neurogenesis following TBI. In a CCI model of TBI in rats, recombinant EPO was first shown to reduce the volume of necrosis at the injury site (Brines *et al.*, 2000). In the same model, after a 2-week EPO administration, rats were sacrificed. Analysis of newly born neurons in the dentate gyrus demonstrated an increase in both ipsilateral and, to a lesser extent, the contralateral hippocampus. This was correlated with an increased performance in the MWM two weeks post-TBI (Lu *et al.*, 2005). In a shorter administration regimen of EPO, or a carbamylated EPO, up to 24 hours following CCI, both drugs increased performance in the MWM one month after injury. This was associated with an increase in cellular proliferation in the dentate gyrus, although no co-labelling was performed to determine the cell type of new proliferating cells. The authors postulate a mechanism through BDNF since levels were elevated in the ipsilateral brain (Mahmood *et al.*, 2007). Interestingly, the authors subsequently determined that the carbamylated EPO was able to promote a neuronal phenotype in SVZ derived neurospheres in mice, and this was mediated in part through Shh signaling (Wang *et al.*, 2007). In a follow-up study, they went on to investigate the effect of three intraperitoneal doses of EPO followed by analysis one month later. The number of newly born neurons was increased in both the dentate gyrus and, perhaps more interestingly, the perilesional cortex (termed the lesion boundary zone). While approximately 5% of BrdU positive cells in the perilesional cortex expressed NeuN in injured animals, with EPO administration this increased to around 20% (Xiong *et al.*, 2008). Similarly significant results, although less in magnitude, were also obtained with a single dose of EPO (Xiong *et al.*, 2010) with an optimal dose of 5000 units per kilogram of EPO (Meng *et al.*, 2011). While it is clear that in this experimental paradigm, EPO has the ability in rodents to increase the number of proliferating cells with a functional improvement as assessed by the MWM, it still remains to be determined whether clinical trials will demonstrate a benefit. Early trials with small numbers of patients suggest the case may not be simple, since initial data is not supportive of a benefit of EPO administration (Nirula *et al.*, 2010).

While epidermal growth factor (EGF) was initially shown to induce cell proliferation of adult mouse striatum *in vitro* (Reynolds and Weiss, 1992), it has emerged as a key factor in expanding neural stem cell proliferation *in vivo* (Gritti *et al.*, 1999). To investigate the effect of EGF administration following TBI, Sun and colleagues (Sun *et al.*, 2010) induced a LFP injury in adult rats followed by a 7-day administration of EGF directly into the ipsilateral ventricle. BrdU was administered for up to seven days. While EGF infusion increased the number of proliferating cells in the SGZ of the dentate gyrus and the SVZ at one week, by four weeks, in the SGZ the proliferative boost observed returned to baseline TBI only levels. At four weeks, the number of new neurons in the granular layer was reduced, whereas the number of new astrocytes were significantly increased, suggesting that the EGF infusion directed injury-induced stem/progenitor cells towards an astrocytic fate. Functionally, these animals performed better in the MWM task (Sun *et al.*, 2010). Therefore, in this experimental paradigm, EGF did not enhance neurogenesis although there was a functional improvement in hippocampus dependent performance. The mitogen fibroblast growth factor-2 (FGF-2) is also well established in maintaining cells in a stem/progenitor state (Richards *et al.*, 1992). Yoshimura and colleagues had previously shown that FGF-2 was necessary for seizure- or ischaemia-induced neurogenesis in the dentate gyrus but next sought to investigate the role of FGF-2 following a TBI. Using the CCI-injury model in FGF-2$^{-/-}$ mice, and BrdU administration one week after injury, knockout mice showed an attenuated injury-induced proliferation in the granular cell layer of the dentate gyrus one month after injury, paralleled with a reduction new neurons. Moreover, in mice with a viral vector induced overexpression of FGF2, following a CCI injury, increased proliferation along with an increase in newly labeled neurons was demonstrated in the granular cell layer at one month compared to control (Yoshimura *et al.*, 2003). In a separate study, FGF-2 was administered into the lateral ventricles of rats for one week after a LFP injury. The number of proliferating cells in both the SVZ and SGZ of the dentate gyrus was increased in the FGF-2 treated group, and at four weeks, this was still observed in the SGZ. The fate of newly generated cells did not alter with FGF-2 augmentation, suggesting that the increase in new neurons in the injured rat is secondary to an increase in the FGF-2-dependent proliferative response post-injury (Sun *et al.*, 2009). While the above evidence involves augmentation of various mitogens following injury, a more recent study examined the downstream effector of nerve growth factor signaling. The p75 neurotrophin receptor (P75^{NTR}) mediates the production of neuroblasts both in the SVZ and the hippocampus.

Given that in TBI, maintaining the new pool of neurons improves hippocampus dependent functional outcomes (Blaiss *et al.*, 2011), modulation of p75^{NTR} mediated signaling may exert similar benefits. Using an intranasal small molecule modulator of NGF binding to p75^{NTR}, in CCI-induced TBI in rats, the number of newly generated neuroblasts in the SGZ was increased compared to injury alone, with evidence suggesting that this was either through increased proliferation or cell survival. Interestingly, CCI reduced the number of immature neurons compared to uninjured controls. However, intranasal treatment with the p75^{NTR} modulator resulted in a greater increase in these cells than the control. Also, using the MWM, the injury-induced latency in the path length to the target was restored following p75^{NTR} modulator treatment. Unlike some of the studies above, the authors of this study reported a loss in early progenitors, which subsequently resulted in a long-term reduction of surviving neurons after CCI injury. The authors suggest that injury technique, species difference and BrdU dose and timing regimens may account for the difference (Shi *et al.*, 2013). The role of Transforming Growth Factor beta (TGFβ) dependent signaling was investigated following a CCI injury in 8-week-old mice. TGFβ signaling regulates neurogenesis in uninjured animals, although increased TGFβ may have opposing effects on neurogenesis (Battista *et al.*, 2006; Buckwalter *et al.*, 2006; Wachs *et al.*, 2006). How this may influence neurogenesis following TBI remains to be determined. One such factor that interacts with the intracellular transducers of TGFβ signaling, or the SMAD proteins, is Runt-related transcription factor-1 (Runx1). It is upregulated up to seven days post-TBI in both the SVZ and dentate gyrus as determined by mRNA and cellular expression. While most newly born Runx1 expressing cells were identified as microglia, a subpopulation expressed nestin in the dentate gyrus. Moreover, Runx1 expression was not seen with more mature neuronal markers suggesting expression with early proliferating NSCs. In the SVZ, nestin expressing cells also expressed Runx1 but were not BrdU positive. These cells were adjacent to doublecortin positive cells, and the expression was cytosolic rather than the nuclear nature in the dentate gyrus. While no function was attributable to the expression of Runx1, the authors suggest that the nuclear expression post-injury may alter proliferative effects in the dentate gyrus (Logan *et al.*, 2013).

From the evidence above, we are beginning to dissect the molecular cues that enhance post-TBI proliferation and neurogenesis, with Shh signaling, factors associated with angiogenesis and mitogens emerging as possible therapeutic targets. There are several targets in which a similar effect has been demonstrated, but where the evidence is limited to one or two papers. For example, S100β is an astrocyte specific mitogenic protein that is a well-established marker for mature astrocytes. Following an LFP in one study, intraventricular infusion of S100β continued for up to one week, with BrdU labeling at day 2. Infusion increased the number of proliferating cells in the SGZ at five days with an attenuation of this response by five weeks. In the injured hippocampus, newly born neurons were doubled following S100β infusion. Moreover, improved performance with the MWM correlated with an increase in this infusion-enhanced neurogenesis (Kleindienst *et al.*, 2005). Imipramine, a tricyclic antidepressant, has been shown to increase hippocampal neurogenesis following long-term administration (Santarelli *et al.*, 2003). Following a CCI injury in adult mice, imipramine was administered for up to four weeks after injury, with BrdU labelling in the first week. While injury or imipramine treatment alone increased the number of new proliferating cells in the hippocampus at four weeks, a combination of injury and imipramine treatment was additive. Newly born neurons in the granular zone of both the injured ipsilateral and uninjured contralateral hippocampus significantly increased following imipramine treatment. Using functional tests, the cognitive function was improved, but the motor function was unchanged (Han *et al.*, 2011).

The above is evidence of a rich number of putative therapeutics targets aimed at improving the neurogenic capacity within the first few weeks after injury (See Figure 1).

While much work at the basic and translational research level remains to be done, the fact that we have an idea of some of the

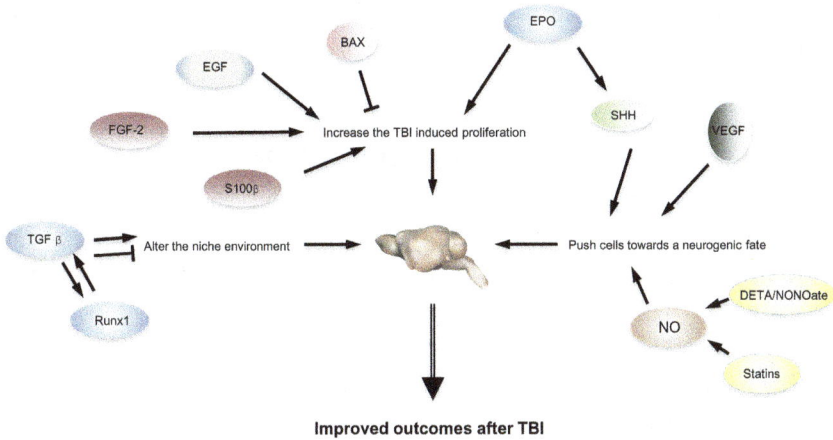

Figure 1. Endogenous repair mechanisms. Studies have demonstrated that several factors can alter the niche environment, promote cell proliferation and neurogenesis after TBI. The dissection and understanding of the interplay of these pathways is the first step in modulation of the injured brain to improve outcome.

potentially targetable signaling mechanisms which show an improvement in performance following TBI raises hope for this devastating injury.

Environmental Factors Influencing Repair Mechanisms

Age influences the potential for any post-TBI repair. Understanding the reasons underlying this age-dependent recovery could aid repair strategies. For instance, *in vitro* there is a watershed at postnatal day 10/11 after which the uninjured cortex does not give rise to neurospheres in culture (Laywell *et al.*, 2000), where the neurogenic potential of the cortex is lost and is only reactivated after an insult (Ahmed *et al.*, 2012). The juvenile rat (postnatal day 28) has a greater capacity for injury-induced neurogenesis in the hippocampus compared to the adult (3 months old). Following a LFP injury, younger rats show a more significant increase in the proliferation rate in the subgranular zone of the dentate gyrus compared to the adult. Moreover, when the fate of these cells was analyzed, there were more new neurons in the injured juvenile brain compared with the adult, and this correlated with a greater percentage of new astrocytes in the injured adult brain compared to the juvenile brain (Sun *et al.*, 2005). In a recent study, the authors started to postulate the mechanisms that may account for the age-related differences seen. Following LFP injury in Juvenile (28 days old) and adult (24 months old) mice, while there was an increase in number of cells undergoing apoptotic cell death, the magnitude of the cell death was increased in older animals. The dying cells in older mice were more likely to be mature neurons and this increase in death may in part be due an injury-induced increase in pro-apoptotic proteins (Sun *et al.*, 2013). Similarly, in the SVZ, over the period of one year, there is an age-dependent decrease in proliferation. However, a LFP injury results in proliferative rate returning to the levels seen in the younger adult (Chen *et al.*, 2003). The above authors have started to dissect the age-related differences that may account for the variability in the response seen (See Figure 2).

Human Studies

Clearly, for progression towards therapeutic intervention for TBI patients, an understanding of the pathophysiology, and any change

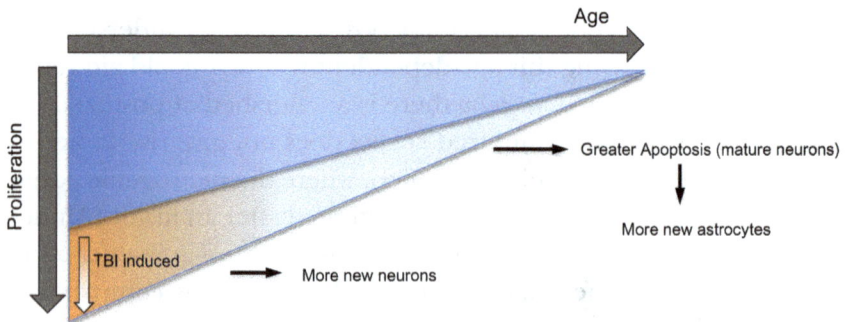

Figure 2. How age influences TBI induced neurogenesis in the hippocampus. With age, there is a decrease in the number of proliferating cells in the DG, and the aged rat has a lower capacity for injury induced proliferation and neurogenesis. In older animals, more mature neurons undergo apoptosis following TBI, resulting in a relative increase in astrocyte proliferation with age.

in injury-induced stem cell behavior in the neurogenic niches of these patients is important. Severe TBI patients present a challenge for any potential research study, especially due to sensitivities with the families of these patients and associated consent or assent issues during this difficult time. However, in the last few years, these challenges have been surmountable and a few reports have described histological findings in TBI tissue. In a recent report, 11 patients (with a median age of 57) underwent surgery for TBI and samples of perilesional tissue were taken during surgery. While the authors reported that early neural progenitors and immature neuronal markers were identified in normal uninjured cortex, the number of these cells was increased significantly in the perilesional cortex and these were associated with proliferating cells (Zheng *et al.*, 2013). In a recent study, post-mortem tissue in children who did not survive a TBI were compared to aged matched control patients. While doublecortin labeled cells were identified in both the hippocampus and SVZ with a concomitant decrease with age, there was no significant change in the number of these labeled cells in TBI patients (Taylor *et al.*, 2013). This may be in part due to the timing, since five of the six patients died within 24 hours. This may reflect the window of activation of potential precursors since our studies, along with others, demonstrate an optimal time-point of around three days for injury-induced activation, with 24 hours being far too soon for any observable response (Itoh *et al.*, 2005; Ahmed *et al.*, 2012). Several studies have isolated human neural stem/progenitor cells *in vitro*, using samples from surgical specimens, from the SVZ (Westerlund *et al.*, 2003; Moe *et al.*, 2005; Ayuso-Sacido *et al.*, 2008), the periventricular subependymal zone and the hippocampus (Kukekov *et al.*, 1999; Roy *et al.*, 2000). There are also quiescent precursors derived from the cortical parenchyma of both the frontal and temporal cortex of surgical patients (Arsenijevic *et al.*, 2001). Our experience of normal temporal cortical tissue indicates that in the presence of growth factors, multipotent spheres are generated and these are passagable for up to five or six passages (unpublished data). Following a severe TBI, in which two patients underwent emergency surgery, contused parenchymal tissue was dissociated and plated before being cultured in the presence of FGF-2. After several days in culture, more than half the cells expressed nestin and βIII tubulin in both patients (Richardson *et al.*, 2006). While the characteristics of the cells were not analyzed further, this demonstrates that tissue derived from TBI patients may have progenitor potential. If manipulation of stem cells to effect repair is to enter the mainstream, monitoring the fate of these cells would become important to correlate with any functional recovery. Short of performing post-mortem analyses, alternatives need to be established to monitor the progress of these cells *in vivo*. Magnetic resonance imaging may serve as a monitoring modality, and two papers address this in an intriguing way. In the first, Zhu and colleagues (2006) took contused tissue from a patient who suffered a severe head injury. After culturing *in vitro* to select a stem/progenitor population, cells were labeled with an iron oxide nanoparticle-containing agent and stereotactically injected back into the contused brain. In the first few weeks, an increase in signal intensity on magnetic resonance imaging (MRI) suggested that the cells had proliferated and migrated. However, by 7 weeks, this signal was lost, as the authors suggest, perhaps due to dilution of the signal secondary to cell proliferation (Zhu *et al.*, 2006). In the second paper, the authors characterized a metabolic biomarker specific to neural progenitor cells using magnetic resonance spectroscopy. Using this method, they demonstrated that the level of activity of the biomarker in the hippocampus reduced with age. Adult patients had a reduced signal compared with adolescents and much more so compared to preadolescents (Manganas *et al.*, 2007). We are therefore arming ourselves with the knowledge and tools to investigate whether stem cell manipulation following TBI results in a recovery both at the anatomical and functional level in our patients. This promises to be an exciting period in TBI research in the forthcoming years.

Conclusion

While this early research shows promise in harnessing endogenous stem cells for repair, there remain many challenges. Once such challenge is the heterogenic nature of the injury itself. A proportion of patients sustain a diffuse axonal injury. This translates to a large volume of injury that may in itself present a challenge for any targeted pharmacological delivery or intervention. On the other hand, focal injuries may represent hostile niche environments, with an abundance of inflammatory mediators, which are anti-neurogenic (Ekdahl *et al.*, 2003). It is clear that while progress has been made in understanding the biological and pathological determinants of TBI-induced neurogenesis, progress towards ameliorating the consequences of TBI and improving outcome remain elusive. The availability of human tissue for research has been fundamental in our understanding of neural stem cell biology, and for progress in this field, the usage of this tissue, especially of human TBI tissue remains key. While there are challenges in obtaining appropriate contused tissue from neurosurgical resection, the streamlining of many university and hospital policies towards generic research from tissue of all patients may aid this. Until this time, our understanding of the mechanisms that influence and define post-TBI neurogenesis and the potential for neurogenesis will undoubtedly continue in our rodent studies.

References

Aboody K, Capela A, Niazi N, Stern JH, Temple S (2011) Translating stem cell studies to the clinic for CNS repair: current state of the art and the need for a Rosetta Stone. *Neuron* 70:597–613.

Ahmed AI, Shtaya AB, Zaben MJ, Owens EV, Kiecker C, Gray WP (2012) Endogenous GFAP-positive neural stem/progenitor cells in the postnatal mouse cortex are activated following traumatic brain injury *Neurotrauma* 29:828–842.

Amankulor NM, Hambardzumyan D, Pyonteck SM, Becher OJ, Joyce JA, Holland EC (2009) Sonic hedgehog pathway activation is induced by acute brain injury and regulated by injury-related inflammation. *J Neurosci* 29:10299–10308.

Arsenijevic Y, Villemure JG, Brunet JF, Bloch JJ, Deglon N, Kostic C, Zurn A, Aebischer P (2001) Isolation of multipotent neural precursors residing in the cortex of the adult human brain. *Exp Neurol* 170:48–62.

Ayuso-Sacido A, Roy NS, Schwartz TH, Greenfield JP, Boockvar JA (2008) Long-term expansion of adult human brain subventricular zone precursors. *Neurosurgery* 62:223–229; discussion 229–231.

Battista D, Ferrari CC, Gage FH, Pitossi FJ (2006) Neurogenic niche modulation by activated microglia: transforming growth factor beta increases neurogenesis in the adult dentate gyrus. *Eur J Neurosci* 23:83–93.

Bendel O, Bueters T, von Euler M, Ove Ogren S, Sandin J, von Euler G (2005) Reappearance of hippocampal CA1 neurons after ischemia is associated with recovery of learning and memory. *J Cereb Blood Flow Metab* 25:1586–1595.

Berg J, Tagliaferri F, Servadei F (2005) Cost of trauma in Europe. *Eur J Neurol* 12 Suppl 1:85–90.

Blaiss CA, Yu TS, Zhang G, Chen J, Dimchev G, Parada LF, Powell CM, Kernie SG (2011) Temporally specified genetic ablation of neurogenesis impairs cognitive recovery after traumatic brain injury. *J Neurosci* 31:4906–4916.

Brines ML, Ghezzi P, Keenan S, Agnello D, de Lanerolle NC, Cerami C, Itri LM, Cerami A (2000) Erythropoietin crosses the blood-brain barrier to protect against experimental brain injury. *Proc Natl Acad Sci U S A* 97:10526–10531.

Buckwalter MS, Yamane M, Coleman BS, Ormerod BK, Chin JT, Palmer T, Wyss-Coray T (2006) Chronically increased transforming growth factor-beta1 strongly inhibits hippocampal neurogenesis in aged mice. *Am J Pathol* 169:154–164.

Buffo A, Rite I, Tripathi P, Lepier A, Colak D, Horn AP, Mori T, Gotz M (2008) Origin and progeny of reactive gliosis: A source of multipotent cells in the injured brain. *Proc Natl Acad Sci U S A* 105:3581–3586.

Chen J, Magavi SS, Macklis JD (2004) Neurogenesis of corticospinal motor neurons extending spinal projections in adult mice. *Proc Natl Acad Sci U S A* 101:16357–16362.

Chen XH, Iwata A, Nonaka M, Browne KD, Smith DH (2003) Neurogenesis and glial proliferation persist for at least one year in the subventricular zone following brain trauma in rats. *J Neurotrauma* 20:623–631.

Chirumamilla S, Sun D, Bullock MR, Colello RJ (2002) Traumatic brain injury induced cell proliferation in the adult mammalian central nervous system. *J Neurotrauma* 19:693–703.

Dash PK, Mach SA, Moore AN (2001) Enhanced neurogenesis in the rodent hippocampus following traumatic brain injury. *J Neurosci Res* 63:313–319.

Dixon CE, Lyeth BG, Povlishock JT, Findling RL, Hamm RJ, Marmarou A, Young HF, Hayes RL (1987) A fluid percussion model of experimental brain injury in the rat. *J Neurosurg* 67:110–119.

Ekdahl CT, Claasen JH, Bonde S, Kokaia Z, Lindvall O (2003) Inflammation is detrimental for neurogenesis in adult brain. Proc Natl Acad Sci U S A 100:13632–13637.

Emery DL, Fulp CT, Saatman KE, Schutz C, Neugebauer E, McIntosh TK (2005) Newly born granule cells in the dentate gyrus rapidly extend axons into the hippocampal CA3 region following experimental brain injury. *J Neurotrauma* 22:978–988.

Eriksson PS, Perfilieva E, Bjork-Eriksson T, Alborn AM, Nordborg C, Peterson DA, Gage FH (1998) Neurogenesis in the adult human hippocampus. *Nat Med* 4:1313–1317.

Eto M, Kozai T, Cosentino F, Joch H, Luscher TF (2002) Statin prevents tissue factor expression in human endothelial cells: role of Rho/Rho-kinase and Akt pathways. *Circulation* 105:1756–1759.

Gao X, Deng-Bryant Y, Cho W, Carrico KM, Hall ED, Chen J (2008) Selective death of newborn neurons in hippocampal dentate gyrus following moderate experimental traumatic brain injury. *J Neurosci Res* 86:2258–2270.

Gritti A, Frolichsthal-Schoeller P, Galli R, Parati EA, Cova L, Pagano SF, Bjornson CR, Vescovi AL (1999) Epidermal and fibroblast growth factors behave as mitogenic regulators for a single multipotent stem cell-like population from the subventricular region of the adult mouse forebrain. *J Neurosci* 19:3287–3297.

Han X, Tong J, Zhang J, Farahvar A, Wang E, Yang J, Samadani U, Smith DH, Huang JH (2011) Imipramine treatment improves cognitive outcome associated with enhanced hippocampal neurogenesis after traumatic brain injury in mice. *J Neurotrauma* 28: 995–1007.

Hyder AA, Wunderlich CA, Puvanachandra P, Gururaj G, Kobusingye OC (2007) The impact of traumatic brain injuries: a global perspective. *NeuroRehabilitation* 22:341–353.

Itoh T, Satou T, Hashimoto S, Ito H (2005) Isolation of neural stem cells from damaged rat cerebral cortex after traumatic brain injury. *Neuroreport* 16:1687–1691.

Jin K, Zhu Y, Sun Y, Mao XO, Xie L, Greenberg DA (2002) Vascular endothelial growth factor (VEGF) stimulates neurogenesis *in vitro* and *in vivo*. *Proc Natl Acad Sci U S A* 99:11946–11950.

Kernie SG, Erwin TM, Parada LF (2001) Brain remodeling due to neuronal and astrocytic proliferation after controlled cortical injury in mice. *J Neurosci Res* 66:317–326.

Kharatishvili I, Pitkanen A (2010) Posttraumatic epilepsy. *Curr Opin Neurol* 23:183–188.

Kleindienst A, McGinn MJ, Harvey HB, Colello RJ, Hamm RJ, Bullock MR (2005) Enhanced hippocampal neurogenesis by intraventricular S100B infusion is associated with improved cognitive recovery after traumatic brain injury. *J Neurotrauma* 22:645–655.

Kukekov VG, Laywell ED, Suslov O, Davies K, Scheffler B, Thomas LB, O'Brien TF, Kusakabe M, Steindler DA (1999) Multipotent stem/progenitor cells with similar properties arise from two neurogenic regions of adult human brain. *Exp Neurol* 156:333–344.

Laywell ED, Rakic P, Kukekov VG, Holland EC, Steindler DA (2000) Identification of a multipotent astrocytic stem cell in the immature and adult mouse brain. *Proc Natl Acad Sci U S A* 97:13883–13888.

Lighthall JW, Dixon CE, Anderson TE (1989) Experimental models of brain injury. *J Neurotrauma* 6:83–97.

Logan TT, Villapol S, Symes AJ (2013) TGF-beta superfamily gene expression and induction of the Runx1 transcription factor in adult neurogenic regions after brain injury. *PLoS One* 8:e59250.

Lu D, Mahmood A, Zhang R, Copp M (2003) Upregulation of neurogenesis and reduction in functional deficits following administration of DEtA/NONOate, a nitric oxide donor, after traumatic brain injury in rats. *J Neurosurg* 99:351–361.

Lu D, Mahmood A, Qu C, Goussev A, Schallert T, Chopp M (2005) Erythropoietin enhances neurogenesis and restores spatial memory in rats after traumatic brain injury. *J Neurotrauma* 22:1011–1017.

Lu D, Qu C, Goussev A, Jiang H, Lu C, Schallert T, Mahmood A, Chen J, Li Y, Chopp M (2007) Statins increase neurogenesis in the dentate gyrus, reduce delayed neuronal death in the hippocampal CA3 region, and improve spatial learning in rat after traumatic brain injury. *J Neurotrauma* 24:1132–1146.

Maas AI, Stocchetti N, Bullock R (2008) Moderate and severe traumatic brain injury in adults. *Lancet Neurol* 7:728–741.

Maas AI, Menon DK, Lingsma HF, Pineda JA, Sandel ME, Manley GT (2011) Re-orientation of Clinical Research in Traumatic Brain Injury: Report of an International Workshop on Comparative Effectiveness Research. *J Neurotrauma* 29:32–46.

Magavi SS, Leavitt BR, Macklis JD (2000) Induction of neurogenesis in the neocortex of adult mice. *Nature* 405:951–955.

Mahmood A, Lu D, Qu C, Goussev A, Zhang ZG, Lu C, Chopp M (2007) Treatment of traumatic brain injury in rats with erythropoietin and carbamylated erythropoietin. *J Neurosurg* 107:392–397.

Manganas LN, Zhang X, Li Y, Hazel RD, Smith SD, Wagshul ME, Henn F, Benveniste H, Djuric PM, Enikolopov G, Maletic-Savatic M (2007) Magnetic resonance spectroscopy identifies neural progenitor cells in the live human brain. *Science* 318:980–985.

Mattson MP (2008) Glutamate and neurotrophic factors in neuronal plasticity and disease. *Ann N Y Acad Sci* 1144:97–112.

Meng Y, Xiong Y, Mahmood A, Zhang Y, Qu C, Chopp M (2011) Dose-dependent neurorestorative effects of delayed treatment of traumatic brain injury with recombinant human erythropoietin in rats. *J Neurosurg* 115:550–560.

Moe MC, Varghese M, Danilov AI, Westerlund U, Ramm-Pettersen J, Brundin L, Svensson M, Berg-Johnsen J, Langmoen IA (2005) Multipotent progenitor cells from the adult human brain: neurophysiological differentiation to mature neurons. *Brain* 128:2189–2199.

Morganti-Kossmann MC, Satgunaseelan L, Bye N, Kossmann T (2007) Modulation of immune response by head injury. *Injury* 38:1392–1400.

Morrison B, 3rd, Cater HL, Benham CD, Sundstrom LE (2006) An in vitro model of traumatic brain injury utilising two-dimensional stretch of organotypic hippocampal slice cultures. *J Neurosci Methods* 150:192–201.

Nakatomi H, Kuriu T, Okabe S, Yamamoto S, Hatano O, Kawahara N, Tamura A, Kirino T, Nakafuku M (2002) Regeneration of hippocampal pyramidal neurons after ischemic brain injury by recruitment of endogenous neural progenitors. *Cell* 110:429–441.

Nirula R, Diaz-Arrastia R, Brasel K, Weigelt JA, Waxman K (2010) Safety and efficacy of erythropoietin in traumatic brain injury patients: a pilot randomized trial. *Crit Care Res Pract* 2010.

Okano H (2002) Stem cell biology of the central nervous system. *J Neurosci Res* 69:698–707.

Palmer TD, Markakis EA, Willhoite AR, Safar F, Gage FH (1999) Fibroblast growth factor-2 activates a latent neurogenic program in neural stem cells from diverse regions of the adult CNS. *J Neurosci* 19:8487–8497.

Radomski KL, Zhou Q, Yi KJ, Doughty ML (2013) Cortical contusion injury disrupts olfactory bulb neurogenesis in adult mice. *BMC Neurosci* 14:142.

Ramaswamy S, Goings GE, Soderstrom KE, Szele FG, Kozlowski DA (2005) Cellular proliferation and migration following a controlled cortical impact in the mouse. *Brain Res* 1053:38–53.

Reynolds BA, Weiss S (1992) Generation of neurons and astrocytes from isolated cells of the adult mammalian central nervous system. *Science* 255:1707–1710.

Rice AC, Khaldi A, Harvey HB, Salman NJ, White F, Fillmore H, Bullock MR (2003) Proliferation and neuronal differentiation of mitotically active cells following traumatic brain injury. *Exp Neurol* 183:406–417.

Richards LJ, Kilpatrick TJ, Bartlett PF (1992) *De novo* generation of neuronal cells from the adult mouse brain. *Proc Natl Acad Sci U S A* 89:8591–8595.

Richardson RM, Holloway KL, Bullock MR, Broaddus WC, Fillmore HL (2006) Isolation of neuronal progenitor cells from the adult human neocortex. *Acta Neurochir (Wien)* 148:773–777.

Rola R, Mizumatsu S, Otsuka S, Morhardt DR, Noble-Haeusslein LJ, Fishman K, Potts MB, Fike JR (2006) Alterations in hippocampal neurogenesis following traumatic brain injury in mice. *Exp Neurol* 202: 189–199.

Rose VL (1999) NIH issues consensus statement on the rehabilitation of persons with traumatic brain injury. *Am Family Physician* 59:1051–1053.

Roy NS, Wang S, Jiang L, Kang J, Benraiss A, Harrison-Restelli C, Fraser RA, Couldwell WT, Kawaguchi A, Okano H, Nedergaard M, Goldman SA (2000) *In vitro* neurogenesis by progenitor cells isolated from the adult human hippocampus. *Nat Med* 6:271–277.

Salman H, Ghosh P, Kernie SG (2004) Subventricular zone neural stem cells remodel the brain following traumatic injury in adult mice. *J Neurotrauma* 21:283–292.

Santarelli L, Saxe M, Gross C, Surget A, Battaglia F, Dulawa S, Weisstaub N, Lee J, Duman R, Arancio O, Belzung C, Hen R (2003) Requirement of hippocampal neurogenesis for the behavioral effects of antidepressants. *Science* 301:805–809.

Shi J, Longo FM, Massa SM (2013) A small molecule p75(NTR) ligand protects neurogenesis after traumatic brain injury. *Stem Cells* 31:2561–2574.

Shi J, Miles DK, Orr BA, Massa SM, Kernie SG (2007) Injury-induced neurogenesis in Bax-deficient mice: evidence for regulation by voltage-gated potassium channels. *Eur J Neurosci* 25:3499–3512.

Singleton RH, Zhu J, Stone JR, Povlishock JT (2002) Traumatically induced axotomy adjacent to the soma does not result in acute neuronal death. *J Neurosci* 22:791–802.

Sirko S *et al.* (2013) Reactive glia in the injured brain acquire stem cell properties in response to sonic hedgehog glia. *Cell Stem Cell* 12:426–439.

Sun D, McGinn MJ, Zhou Z, Harvey HB, Bullock MR, Colello RJ (2007) Anatomical integration of newly generated dentate granule neurons following traumatic brain injury in adult rats and its association to cognitive recovery. *Exp Neurol* 204:264–272.

Sun D, McGinn M, Hankins JE, Mays KM, Rolfe A, Colello RJ (2013) Aging- and injury-related differential apoptotic response in the dentate gyrus of the hippocampus in rats following brain trauma. *Front Aging Neurosci* 5:95.

Sun D, Colello RJ, Daugherty WP, Kwon TH, McGinn MJ, Harvey HB, Bullock MR (2005) Cell proliferation and neuronal differentiation in the dentate gyrus in juvenile and adult rats following traumatic brain injury. *J Neurotrauma* 22:95–105.

Sun D, Bullock MR, McGinn MJ, Zhou Z, Altememi N, Hagood S, Hamm R, Colello RJ (2009) Basic fibroblast growth factor-enhanced neurogenesis contributes to cognitive recovery in rats following traumatic brain injury. *Exp Neurol* 216:56-65.

Sun D, Bullock MR, Altememi N, Zhou Z, Hagood S, Rolfe A, McGinn MJ, Hamm R, Colello RJ (2010) The effect of epidermal growth factor in the injured brain after trauma in rats. *J Neurotrauma* 27:923–938.

Sundholm-Peters NL, Yang HK, Goings GE, Walker AS, Szele FG (2005) Subventricular zone neuroblasts emigrate toward cortical lesions. *J Neuropathol Exp Neurol* 64:1089–1100.

Taylor SR, Smith C, Harris BT, Costine BA, Duhaime AC (2013) Maturation-dependent response of neurogenesis after traumatic brain injury in children. *J Neurosurg Pediatr* 12:545–554.

Thau-Zuchman O, Shohami E, Alexandrovich AG, Leker RR (2010) Vascular endothelial growth factor increases neurogenesis after traumatic brain injury. *J Cerebral Blood Flow Metab* 30:1008–1016.

Tzeng SF, Wu JP (1999) Responses of microglia and neural progenitors to mechanical brain injury. *Neuroreport* 10:2287–2292.

Urrea C, Castellanos DA, Sagen J, Tsoulfas P, Bramlett HM, Dietrich WD (2007) Widespread cellular proliferation and focal neurogenesis after traumatic brain injury in the rat. *Restor Neurol Neurosci* 25:65–76.

Wachs FP, Winner B, Couillard-Despres S, Schiller T, Aigner R, Winkler J, Bogdahn U, Aigner L (2006) Transforming growth factor-beta1 is a negative modulator of adult neurogenesis. *J Neuropathol Exp Neurol* 65:358–370.

Wang L, Zhang ZG, Gregg SR, Zhang RL, Jiao Z, LeTourneau Y, Liu X, Feng Y, Gerwien J, Torup L, Leist M, Noguchi CT, Chen ZY, Chopp M (2007) The Sonic hedgehog pathway mediates carbamylated erythropoietin-enhanced proliferation and differentiation of adult neural progenitor cells. *J Biol Chem* 282:32462–32470.

Westerlund U, Moe MC, Varghese M, Berg-Johnsen J, Ohlsson M, Langmoen IA, Svensson M (2003) Stem cells from the adult human brain develop into functional neurons in culture. *Exp Cell Res* 289:378–383.

Wittchen HU, Jacobi F, Rehm J, Gustavsson A, Svensson M, Jonsson B, Olesen J, Allgulander C, Alonso J, Faravelli C, Fratiglioni L, Jennum P, Lieb R, Maercker A, van Os J, Preisig M, Salvador-Carulla L, Simon R, Steinhausen HC (2011) The size and burden of mental disorders and other disorders of the brain in Europe 2010. *Eur Neuropsychopharmacol* 21:655–679.

Xiong Y, Mahmood A, Chopp M (2009) Emerging treatments for traumatic brain injury. *Exp Opin Emerg Drugs* 14:67–84.

Xiong Y, Mahmood A, Chopp M (2013) Animal models of traumatic brain injury. *Nat Rev Neurosci* 14:128–142.

Xiong Y, Lu D, Qu C, Goussev A, Schallert T, Mahmood A, Chopp M (2008) Effects of erythropoietin on reducing brain damage and improving functional outcome after traumatic brain injury in mice. *J Neurosurg* 109:510–521.

Xiong Y, Mahmood A, Meng Y, Zhang Y, Qu C, Schallert T, Chopp M (2010) Delayed administration of erythropoietin reducing hippocampal cell loss, enhancing angiogenesis and neurogenesis, and improving functional outcome following traumatic brain injury in rats: comparison of treatment with single and triple dose. *J Neurosurg* 113:598–608.

Yoshimura S, Teramoto T, Whalen MJ, Irizarry MC, Takagi Y, Qiu J, Harada J, Waeber C, Breakefield XO, Moskowitz MA (2003) FGF-2 regulates neurogenesis and degeneration in the dentate gyrus after traumatic brain injury in mice. *J Clin Invest* 112:1202–1210.

Yu TS, Zhang G, Liebl DJ, Kernie SG (2008) Traumatic brain injury-induced hippocampal neurogenesis requires activation of early nestin-expressing progenitors. *J Neurosci* 28:12901–12912.

Zheng W, ZhuGe Q, Zhong M, Chen G, Shao B, Wang H, Mao X, Xie L, Jin K (2013) Neurogenesis in adult human brain after traumatic brain injury. *J Neurotrauma* 30:1872–1880.

Zhu J, Zhou L, XingWu F (2006) Tracking neural stem cells in patients with brain trauma. *New Eng J Med* 355:2376–2378.

Chapter 8

Neural Stem Cells in Alzheimer's Disease

Orly Lazarov

Neural stem cells exist in the adult mammalian brain in discrete niches throughout life. Increasing evidence suggests that neural stem cells play a role in hippocampal plasticity and hippocampus-dependent learning and memory. Interestingly, recent studies suggest that neurogenesis is impaired in Alzheimer's disease. Alzheimer's disease is a progressive neurodegenerative characterized by memory loss and cognitive decline. In support of that, proteins linked to familial Alzheimer's disease regulate neurogenesis. This chapter will discuss the contribution of neurogenesis to hippocampal plasticity, and consider a possible role for neurogenesis in the development of cognitive deficits in Alzheimer's disease and possibly in other neurodegenerative diseases characterized by loss of memory.

Introduction

Once thought to be restricted to embryogenesis and the post-natal period, neurogenesis is now known to occur throughout life. Neural stem cells (NSC) have unique characteristics, exhibiting unlimited self-renewal and continuously producing new neurons and glia in the subventricular zone (SVZ), beneath the walls of the lateral ventricles, and in the subgranular layer (SGL) of the dentate gyrus (DG)

(Alvarez-Buylla and Lim, 2004; Lie *et al.*, 2004). In the hippocampus, newly differentiating neural progenitor cells (NPC) migrate out of the SGL to populate the granular cell layer of the DG (GCL). Thus, the DG consists of younger and older excitatory neurons in an age range of 4 weeks to the age of the organism. These neurons incorporate in the GCL, which receives input from the entorhinal cortex (EC) via the lateral and medial perforant pathway (PP) and send their axons via the mossy fiber pathway to the CA3 region (van Praag *et al.*, 2002; Ming and Song, 2005; Zhao *et al.*, 2006). Thus, the DG is a main 'entry point' into hippocampal circuitry, and is well positioned to contribute to hippocampal function, such as learning and memory. Increasing evidence suggests that neurogenesis regulates hippocampal function and plasticity [for review, (Aimone *et al.*, 2010, 2011; Aimone and Gage, 2011)]. In the DG, they play a crucial role in the formation of new episodic memories by transforming similar events into discrete non-overlapping representations, a process known as 'pattern separation' (Treves *et al.*, 2008; Sahay *et al.*, 2011). Enhanced neurogenesis using different methodologies, such as environmental enrichment (Kempermann *et al.*, 1997), running (van Praag *et al.*, 1999), different strains of mice (Kempermann and Gage, 2002), and genetic manipulation (Zhao *et al.*, 2003; Saxe *et al.*, 2006; Shimazu *et al.*, 2006; Zhang *et al.*, 2008), correlates with enhanced performance in learning and memory tasks. On the other hand, depletion of neurogenesis using several manipulations, such as stress paradigms (Lemaire *et al.*, 2000), irradiation (Madsen *et al.*, 2003; Rola *et al.*, 2004), DNA methylating agents (Shors *et al.*, 2002; Imayoshi *et al.*, 2008) or aged rats [For review see (Bizon and Gallagher, 2005)], correlates with impairment in hippocampus-dependent memory tasks. Computational models suggest that new neurons may provide protection against memory interference when similar items are presented (Becker, 2005; Wiskott *et al.*, 2006). An alternative theory suggests that due to the increased excitability of newly-formed neurons and their tendency to undergo more readily long-term potentiation, they may be a means by which memories are temporally organized (Aimone *et al.*, 2006). Other studies suggest a role for neurogenesis in acquisition of new memories (Kee *et al.*, 2007). Taken together, these studies suggest that hippocampal neurogenesis plays important roles in numerous aspects of hippocampus-dependent learning and memory.

Importantly, the generation of new neurons is a critical contributor to synaptic plasticity in the adult brain. During their maturation into neurons, neural progenitor cells undergo many changes that affect the involved circuitry. As soon as they develop their dendritic tree towards the outer molecular layer of the DG and their axons towards the CA3 region, neural progenitor cells start to be functionally involved in the hippocampal circuitry. They differ from fully mature neurons in several important characteristics, such as their membrane resistance, activation threshold and capacitance (Ge *et al.*, 2006; Markwardt *et al.*, 2009). Thus, they affect the circuitry in ways that fully mature neurons are incapable of. By the completion of their maturation, however, they are essentially indistinguishable from other fully mature neurons (Laplagne *et al.*, 2006). Neurogenesis has additional effects on the brain. For example, NPC express neurotrophins, such as brain-derived neurotrophic factor (BDNF) that exert high level of plasticity (Chen *et al.*, 2001; Shirayama *et al.*, 2002). Lastly, neurogenesis responds to brain insult, injury and disease (Lazarov and Marr, 2010; Lazarov *et al.*, 2010). Thus, hippocampal neurogenesis has important roles in the maintenance of hippocampal circuitry and their function in learning and memory.

Numerous studies in different mouse models suggest that the rate of neurogenesis in the DG declines with age (Seki and Arai, 1995; Kuhn *et al.*, 1996; Tropepe *et al.*, 1997; Kempermann *et al.*, 1998; Kempermann *et al.*, 2002; Demars *et al.*, 2013), raising the possibility that reduced neurogenesis may, at least in part, account for impaired learning and memory and cognitive deterioration in the elderly and may enhance vulnerability to Alzheimer's disease (AD), the most prevalent form of cognitive impairment in the elderly [for review, see (Demars *et al.*, 2010)]. Recent evidence suggests that neurogenesis is deficient as early as 2–3 months of age in mouse models of familial AD (Demars *et al.*, 2010), suggesting that neurogenesis may play a role in AD. This chapter will outline the evidence about the fate of neurogenesis in aging and its role in AD, discuss the changes neurogenesis may undergo with disease progression, the role of proteins linked to Alzheimer's disease in neurogenesis, and finally outline some future directions in research.

Hippocampal Neurogenesis, Brain Plasticity and Cognition in the Aging Brain

Numerous studies in rodent models have suggested that the rate of neurogenesis in both SVZ and DG declines with age, raising the possibility that reduced neurogenesis may account for, at least in part, impaired learning and memory and cognitive deterioration in the elderly (Seki and Arai, 1995; Kuhn *et al.*, 1996; Tropepe *et al.*, 1997; Kempermann *et al.*, 1998; Kempermann *et al.*, 2002). In the aging brain, levels of neurogenesis are reduced in both the subventricular zone (SVZ) (Mirich *et al.*, 2002; Shook *et al.*, 2012) and subgranular layer (SGL) (Kuhn *et al.*, 1996; Cameron and McKay, 1999; Bernal and Peterson, 2004; Bondolfi *et al.*, 2004; Kronenberg *et al.*, 2006; Ben Abdallah *et al.*, 2010; Encinas *et al.*, 2011; Miranda *et al.*, 2012). Importantly, the decline in neurogenesis takes place long before aging. In mice, it takes place throughout adulthood and proceeds into aging. Thus, a dramatic decline in neurogenesis takes place at the age of 7–9 months, compared to mice at 2 months of age, while further decrease takes place by the age of 20 months (Demars *et al.*, 2013). This decline is characterized by reduced numbers of fast proliferating NPC (type II cells in the SGL and type C cells in the SVZ), but no decline in the number of NSC. There is about 80% reduction in neuroblasts during the transition from young adult (2 months) to mid-age (7–9 months) in mice (Demars *et al.*, 2013), and a similar reduction from adult (4 months) to older (12 months) age in rats (Kuhn *et al.*, 1996; Nacher *et al.*, 2003; Rao *et al.*, 2006). After this period of dramatic reductions, the rate of decline is substantially reduced (Rao *et al.*, 2006) though number of cells continues to decline (Demars *et al.*, 2013). A quantitative inter- and intra-species comparison among rodents, carnivores, and primates suggest an exponential decline in NPC proliferation that is independent on lifespan, but is chronologically equal (Amrein *et al.*, 2011).

The cause of neurogenic decline in the aging brain remains somewhat controversial. Some studies argue that the proliferation of NPC and their maturation declines with age (Kuhn *et al.*, 1996; Heine *et al.*, 2004; Rao *et al.*, 2006; Morgenstern *et al.*, 2008). Others suggest that this decline is not due to alterations in the length of the cell cycle of NPC in the SGL (Olariu *et al.*, 2007). Another study suggests that neurogenic decline is due to the disappearance of NSC by their conversion into mature hippocampal astrocytes (Encinas *et al.*, 2011). Upregulation of bone morphogenetic protein (BMP) signaling or downregulation of its antagonists may underlie age-linked reduced self-renewal of NSC leading to the decline in neurogenesis (Bonaguidi *et al.*, 2008). Other groups have argued that the rate of proliferation does not decline with aging, but the cells may exhibit increased quiescence that may be attributed to a decline in the vascular niche (Hattiangady and Shetty, 2008). Notably, comparative quantitative analysis of gene expression in the young and old rat DG reveals that the expression level of most genes playing a role in NPC proliferation and differentiation is comparable (Shetty *et al.*, 2013). Despite the ongoing debate about the mechanism, it is apparent that the neurogenic niche undergoes changes associated with aging that have the potential to underlie neurogenic decline (Ahlenius *et al.*, 2009; Villeda *et al.*, 2011; Miranda *et al.*, 2012). For instance, the expression of many growth factors and their receptors that are integral to neurogenic processes peak during development and decline in expression thereafter [for review, see (Klempin and Kempermann, 2007)]. These findings raise the possibility that reduced neurogenesis may, at least in part, account for impaired learning and memory and cognitive deterioration in the elderly (Seki and Arai, 1995; Kuhn *et al.*, 1996; Tropepe *et al.*, 1997; Kempermann *et al.*, 1998; Kempermann *et al.*, 2002) and may enhance vulnerability to AD [for review, see (Lazarov and Marr, 2010)].

An important debate is over the fate of neurogenesis during the human lifespan. Lack of techniques for the detection of neural stem cells in live humans makes this investigation challenging. An age-dependent decline in expression of proliferation factors in the human hippocampus suggests a decline in the number of proliferating NPC as a function of age (Knoth *et al.*, 2010). Expression of neurogenic markers that are used in rodents for the detection of NPC, such as DCX, are present in the human SGL throughout life. However, the number of DCX decreases as a function of age (Knoth *et al.*, 2010). Assessment of the extent of hippocampal neurogenesis throughout the human lifespan using nuclear levels of ^{14}C reveals that hippocampal neurogenesis declines dramatically in the first year of life with only a modest decline thereafter (Spalding *et al.*, 2013). For a detailed overview of recent literature concerning neurogenesis in the human brain, see (Lazarov and Marr, 2013). Some interesting observations support hippocampal alterations as a function of age in rodents and humans. For example, changes have been noted in the volume of the molecular layer of the DG, with the medial layer thinning and the inner layer showing increased volume with age (Rapp *et al.*, 1999). This may simply reflect fewer connections from the entorhinal cortex (medial layer) and a greater level of connection with CA3 of the hippocampus. Similar reorganizations may occur in humans. Studies in adult and elderly people with similar cognitive function have shown reduced activity by fMRI in the medial temporal regions while an increase in activity was found in the parietal and prefrontal cortex with age (Burgmans *et al.*, 2010). The development of new experimental tools for the detection of neurogenesis in the human brain would advance our understanding of the age-linked alterations in neurogenesis, as well as of the association between cognitive function and neurogenesis.

Cognitive Consequences of Reduced Neurogenesis with Age

Some of the difficulty in investigating the role of adult hippocampal neurogenesis in learning and memory stems from an incomplete understanding of the role of the DG in these processes. Nevertheless, decline in neurogenesis has been shown to manifest in deficits in olfactory function and hippocampal-dependent learning and memory (Bizon *et al.*, 2004; Enwere *et al.*, 2004; Dupret *et al.*, 2008). Specifically, interventions in the neurogenic areas, such as irradiation, cytostatic or cytotoxic agents, as well as transgenic approaches for the depletion of neurogenesis have produced deficits in learning/memory (Shors *et al.*, 2001; Winocur *et al.*, 2006; Dupret *et al.*, 2008; Imayoshi *et al.*, 2008; Kim *et al.*, 2008). Suppression of neurogenesis produced deficits in hippocampal-dependent learning while not affecting other cognitive domains (Zhang *et al.*, 2008). A more recent study used both irradiation and genetic ablation of NSC and found that acquisition of avoidance behavior of a shock zone was unimpaired; however, the ability to then adapt and learn the location after changing shock location was impaired (Burghardt *et al.*, 2012; Denny *et al.*, 2012). Irradiated mice were impaired in the rotating shock location test only if their initial training was in a fixed shock location. Taken together, this shows that neurogenesis plays a significant role in affecting the ability to distinguish between multiple similar memories.

The connection of neurogenesis to cognition is also supported by the general observation that both hippocampal-dependent memory performance and neurogenesis decline with age. However, currently, the link between neurogenesis and learning/memory with aging appears to be correlative at best. Intra-group comparisons show clear positive correlations between cognitive function and neurogenesis. While performance in hippocampal-dependent learning is clearly reduced with age, the correlation with levels of residual neurogenesis becomes more complicated [reviewed in (Couillard-Despres and Aigner, 2011)]. The extent of neuroblast formation along with survival and differentiation is correlated with age-dependent learning/memory in rats (Drapeau *et al.*, 2003; Driscoll *et al.*, 2006). However, other studies have found that neurogenesis is not correlated or is inversely correlated with memory performance in aged rats (Bizon and Gallagher, 2003; Merrill *et al.*, 2003; Bizon *et al.*, 2004). It is noteworthy that chronic reductions in neurogenesis compromises the morphology and function of other hippocampal areas, such as CA3 (Schloesser *et al.*, 2013), or other brain regions. Importantly, neither in rodents nor in humans, it is not clear whether the exchange rate or the ratio of new neurons to old neurons changes as a function of age. In future experiments, it would be important to determine the neurogenic parameter(s) that reflect age-dependent reduction in neurogenesis and that correlates with cognitive decline.

Alzheimer's Disease and Hippocampal Neurogenesis

AD is the most prevalent cause of dementia in adults. Affected individuals experience progressive memory loss and impaired cognition. As the disease progresses, loss of memory and impaired acquisition of new information interfere with executive decisions, problem solving, recall accuracy and language retrieval to a degree that severely interferes with daily activities. This stage is generally referred to as dementia. Neurons in specific brain areas, such as, the entorhinal cortex and the hippocampus, exhibit high vulnerability, leading to neuronal death. The parahippocampal regions are the earliest to be affected (Braak stages I and II). In particular, the entorhino-hippocampal circuit exhibits an early and significant neuropathology (Figure 1).

Neuropathology in this region correlates significantly with degree of cognitive dysfunction. As the disease progresses, neurons in other brain areas are affected. Aging is the greatest risk factor for AD, and the vast majority of affected individual experience the sporadic, late onset form of the disease. Rare, familial, early-onset autosomal dominant forms of Alzheimer's disease (FAD) are caused by mutations in genes encoding amyloid precursor protein (APP), presenilin-1 (PS1) and presenilin-2 (PS2). PS play a central role in the function of the aspartyl protease γ-secretase complex that cleaves numerous membrane proteins intramembranously [(De Strooper, 2003); for review, see (Selkoe and Wolfe, 2007)]. The neuropathological hallmarks of the disease are senile plaques and neurofibrillary tangles throughout the cerebral cortex and hippocampal formation, and loss of neurons in these specific brain areas [For review, see (Price *et al.*, 1998)]. Senile plaques are composed of dystrophic neuritis surrounding extracellular aggregates of Aβ peptides. Aβ peptides are liberated from APP by the concerted action of BACE 1 and γ-secretase [For review, see (Selkoe, 2001)]. Numerous mouse models have been generated. Most of these models express one or more human mutation in APP and or PS1. The combination and level of

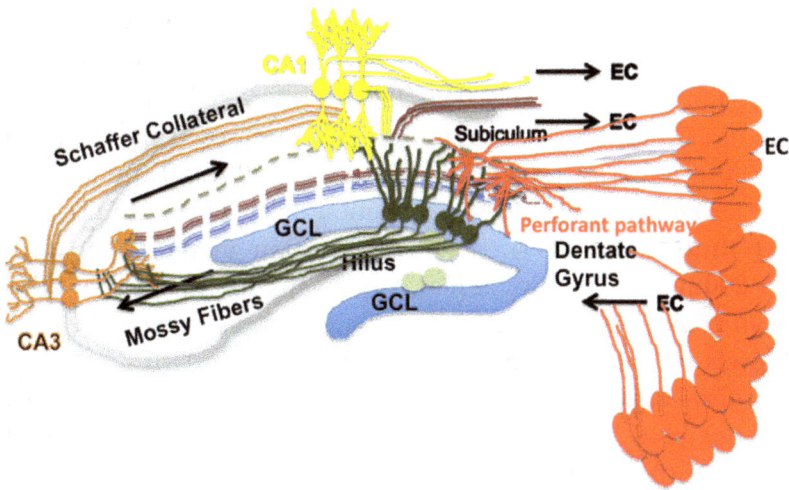

Figure 1. Vulnerable areas in Alzheimer's and the hippocampal neurogenic niche. The entorhinal cortex and the hippocampus are the primary brain regions exhibiting early neuropathology and neuronal loss. Particularly vulnerable is layer II of the entorhinal cortex. Neurons in layer II of the entorhinal cortex project to the dentate gyrus through the perforant pathways and form synapses with granular neurons in the dentate gyrus, including newly integrated neurons that migrated from the subgranular layer. Thus, the dentate gyrus is a main 'entry point' into hippocampal circuitry and thus is well positioned to contribute to hippocampus-dependent learning and memory. New and older neurons in the granular layer project to the CA3 region through the mossy fiber path. In turn, CA3 neurons convey information to the CA1 through the Schaffer collateral pathways into the subiculum and back to the entorhinal cortex.

symptoms exhibited by these mouse models vary, and currently, there is no mouse model that faithfully mimics the human disease [for review, see (Ashe and Zahs, 2010)]. That said, mouse models of FAD are a valuable tool for the understanding of molecular signaling and cellular processes in the disease.

Hippocampal memory

Progressive loss of hippocampus-dependent memory and cognitive decline are the fundamental characteristics of AD. FAD-linked transgenic mice exhibit impairments in learning and memory paradigms [For review, see (Ashe, 2001)], including, acquisition of long-term spatial memory (Chapman *et al.*, 1999; Janus *et al.*, 2000; Morgan *et al.*, 2000; Arendash *et al.*, 2001a; Chishti *et al.*, 2001; Dewachter *et al.*, 2002; Dineley *et al.*, 2002; Trinchese *et al.*, 2004), spatial reversal learning, utilization of spatial working memory (Chapman *et al.*, 1999; Morgan *et al.*, 2000; Arendash *et al.*, 2001a; Trinchese *et al.*, 2004; Jankowsky *et al.*, 2005), acquisition of social recognition memory (Ohno *et al.*, 2004), object recognition memory (Dewachter *et al.*, 2002), and contextual fear conditioning (Dineley *et al.*, 2002). In some cases, the severity of the impairment has been correlated to Aβ levels in the brains of individual mice (Arendash *et al.*, 2001b; Gordon *et al.*, 2001; Puolivali *et al.*, 2002), or levels of oligomeric Aβ [(Billings *et al.*, 2005; Cleary *et al.*, 2005; Billings *et al.*, 2007); for review, see (Ashe, 2006)]. Nevertheless, it becomes apparently clear that while some studies report a correlation between extent of neurofibrillary tangles and cognitive level, there is lack of correlation between cognitive performance and levels of amyloid deposition. In fact, the mechanisms underlying memory impairments are largely elusive. Increasing evidence suggests the contribution of impaired hippocampal neurogenesis to memory deficits (Yamasaki *et al.*, 2007).

Several studies suggest a correlation between impaired neurogenesis and learning and memory deficits in transgenic mice harboring FAD-linked PS1 variants or in mice with conditional ablation of PSEN1. Most of these studies are confined to hippocampal neurogenesis. Using conditional knockout mice in which PS1 is knocked out in the forebrain, Feng and colleagues show that lack of PS1 reduced enrichment-induced proliferation of NSC as well as enrichment-induced increase in number of newly formed neurons. Learning and memory behavioral tests did not show increased learning in mice that experienced enriched environmental conditions. However, a significant increase in contextual freezing response was observed in the PS1 conditional KO mice using a learning-enrichment-retrieval paradigm for fear conditioning, suggesting that neurogenesis may play a role in the periodic clearance of outdated memory traces (Feng *et al.*, 2001). In a different study, Janus and colleagues did not observe deficits in spatial memory in transgenic mice expressing FAD-linked PS1M146L or L268V using the Morris water maze test (Janus *et al.*, 2000). Wang and colleagues report deficits in hippocampal associative learning, as measured by performance in contextual fear conditioning, accompanied by reduced hippocampal neurogenesis, in FAD-linked PS1M146V KI mice (Wang *et al.*, 2004). Using similar PS1M146V KI mice, Sun and colleagues observed deficits in hippocampal spatial memory 3 and 9 months of age (Sun *et al.*, 2005). Yu and colleagues report subtle deficits in spatial learning and memory in PS1 conditional KO in which expression of PS1 is eliminated in excitatory neurons of the brain (Yu *et al.*, 2001). Conditional PS null mice lacking both PS1 and PS2 in the brain exhibit significant deficits in hippocampal spatial and associative memory and long-term potentiation, followed by progressive neurodegeneration (Saura *et al.*, 2005).

Olfaction memory

In humans, a decrease in olfactory function appears to be one of the earliest markers of possible AD (Albers *et al.*, 2006). Deficits in olfactory sensitivity, odor discrimination, and odor identification are common and appear early in disease progression (Warner *et al.*, 1986; Serby, 1987; Kesslak *et al.*, 1988; Bacon *et al.*, 1998). Indeed, clinical tests of olfactory sensitivity and olfactory discrimination abilityare in use to predict the stage of AD pathology (Suzuki *et al.*, 2004; Wilson *et al.*, 2007). In addition to the clinical relevance of olfaction to AD, the olfactory system has two significant advantages for studies of learning and memory (Larson and Sieprawska, 2002). First, primary olfactory cortex, the target of the first brain processing stage for smell, the olfactory bulb, is directly and densely connected to three learning-related forebrain structures: the hippocampus via the lateral entorhinal cortex, the amygdala, and the prefrontal cortex (Lynch, 1986; Shipley *et al.*, 1995). The olfactory-hippocampal circuit represents the most direct path for experiential stimuli to reach the hippocampus. Second, the olfactory system is highly developed in rodents and mice readily learn dozens of odor-reward associations and remember them for weeks

(Larson and Sieprawska, 2002). It is also the case that rodents exhibit other important memory phenomena when olfactory cues guide behavior (Slotnick, 2001); these include development of learning sets (Slotnick and Katz, 1974; Slotnick, 2001), serial inference (Dusek and Eichenbaum, 1997), paired-associate learning (Bunsey and Eichenbaum, 1993), and working memory (Otto and Eichenbaum, 1992; Young *et al.*, 2007).

In spite of the importance of olfaction memory and its relevance to AD, information concerning olfactory function in transgenic mice, the effect of FAD mutations on olfaction memory and its association with neurogenesis in the SVZ is scarce.

Neurogenesis in AD

Examination of the brains of FAD mice reveals that neurogenesis is impaired early in life in FAD mice, preceding hallmarks and cognitive deficits(Demars *et al.*, 2010). Specifically, adecline in both proliferative capacity of NPC and in early neuronal differentiation takes place in the SGL and SVZ of FAD-linked APPswe/PS1ΔE9 mice as early as two months of age (Demars *et al.*, 2010). Early neurogenic impairments were detected in other models of FAD, such as 3XTg-AD mice (Rodriguez, 2008; Hamilton, 2010; Kuttner, In Preparation), PS1M146V mice (Wang *et al.*, 2004), PS1P117L (Wen *et al.*, 2004), APP23 mice (Hartl *et al.*, 2008) and PS2APP (Poirier *et al.*, 2010), preceding the hallmarks of the disease and cognitive deficits, as well as following neurodegeneration in conditional PS1/PS2KO (Chen *et al.*, 2008), later in life in APP/PS1KI (Zhang *et al.*, 2007a), APPswe/PS1ΔE9 (Taniuchi *et al.*, 2007; Verret *et al.*, 2007), 3XTg-AD (Blanchard *et al.*, 2010), APPswe/PS1L166P and APP23 mutant (Ermini *et al.*, 2008) and at multiple time points in Tg2576 (APPswe) mice (Dong *et al.*, 2004; Krezymon *et al.*, 2013). Impairments were also found in conditional PS1KO (Feng *et al.*, 2001), PS1ΔE9 and PS1M146L mutant following environmental enrichment (Choi *et al.*, 2008). However, some controversy exists concerning the fate of neurogenesis in mutant APP mice with some studies reporting increased (Jin *et al.*, 2004; Lopez-Toledano and Shelanski, 2007; Gan *et al.*, 2008; Mirochnic *et al.*, 2009) or decreased (Haughey *et al.*, 2002; Dong *et al.*, 2004; Donovan *et al.*, 2006) proliferation and survival of BrdU+ cells in the SGL of these mice [see our review, (Lazarov and Marr, 2010)]. This might be explained by the differential level of soluble APPα,β (sAPPα,β) produced in these models. Recent studies suggest that both APPα,β regulate NPC proliferation (Demars *et al.*, 2011). Interestingly, in culture conditions, differences between the effect of APPα,β on neurogenesis are conflicting. Below, we discuss the evidence concerning the role of APPα,β in adult neurogenesis.

An important issue to keep in mind when examining neurogenesis and reviewing the evidence, is the age of the mice, their gender and the level of pathology. AD is a progressive disease, and it is reasonable to assume that neurogenesis will get altered at different stages of pathology, thus, yielding an apparent outcome in different studies. In addition, females exhibit greater extent of pathology and an earlier onset. Notably, not all animal models used in these studies equally exhibit the same course of AD neuropathology and this controversy calls for further investigation of the role of APP in neurogenesis.

Many of the molecular players in AD are also modulators of neurogenesis. Therefore, it is not surprising that these sets of processes influence each other [reviewed in (Lazarov and Marr, 2010; Lazarov *et al.*, 2010)]. The most prominent players are presenilin-1 (PS1) and soluble amyloid precursor protein α (sAPPα). PS1 regulates NPC differentiation (Gadadhar *et al.*, 2011) while sAPPα regulates NPC proliferation (Caille *et al.*, 2004; Gakhar-Koppole *et al.*, 2008; Rohe *et al.*, 2008; Demars *et al.*, 2011; Demars *et al.*, 2013). The role of these players in neurogenesis is discussed in detail in the next paragraphs. α-secretase activities (primarily the ADAM proteases) that produce the sAPPα product from APP also cleave important substrates like Notch-1 and components of EGF signaling. Furthermore, certain ADAM family members (TACE, ADAM21) are expressed in the SVZ (Yang *et al.*, 2005, 2006; Katakowski *et al.*, 2007). Thus, mutations associated with AD that alter the production of these metabolites or the activities of their processing enzymes can also alter neurogenesis.

There is a limited number of somewhat contradictory studies addressing the role of neurogenesis in the human disease using post-mortem tissue. In fact, the role of neurogenesis in AD is still a matter of some debate, mainly because of lack of experimental tool for the detection of human neurogenesis.

Molecular Signals in Familial Alzheimer's Disease Regulate Neurogenesis

Presenilin-1 regulates neural progenitor cell differentiation

PS1 has increasingly been considered an appealing signal in fundamental neurogenic pathways. Regulated intramembrane proteolysis (RIP) of numerous molecules implicated in neurogenesis, such as the receptor tyrosine kinases ErbB4 (Ni *et al.*, 2001; Sardi *et al.*, 2006), IGF-1R (McElroy *et al.*, 2007) and insulin receptor (Kasuga *et al.*, 2007), as well as of the neurogenic signals Notch1 (De Strooper *et al.*, 1999), L1 (Maretzky *et al.*, 2005b) and E-cadherin (Marambaud *et al.*, 2002) is catalyzed by PS1/γ-secretase. Notably, following ErbB4 activation and PS1/γ-secretase-dependent cleavage in neural stem cells, the C'-terminus of ErbB4 forms a complex that undergoes nuclear translocation, binds the promoters of the astrocytic genes GFAP and S100β, leading to inhibition of their differentiation into astrocytes (Sardi *et al.*, 2006). Recent evidence suggests that PS1/γ-secretase acts as a tumor suppressor in epithelia and that epidermal growth factor receptor (EGFR) levels inversely correlate with PS1/γ-secretase activity (Li *et al.*, 2007; Zhang *et al.*, 2007b). Intriguingly, EGFR signaling plays a major role in regulation of neural stem proliferation, migration and survival [For review, see (Ayuso-Sacido *et al.*, 2006)]. In that regard, soluble APP is reported to act on EGF-responsive progenitor cells in the SVZ (Caille *et al.*, 2004; Demars *et al.*, 2013). PS1 is further implicated in the Wnt/β-catenin signaling pathway (Tesco *et al.*, 1998; Maretzky *et al.*, 2005a) that regulates adult hippocampal neurogenesis (Lie *et al.*, 2005). The first indication that PS1 may play a role in neurogenesis has been provided by experiments in mice with genomic deletions of

PSEN1 exhibiting severely abnormal somitogenic and neurogenic processes in the brain (Shen *et al.*, 1997; Wong *et al.*, 1997). These mice die in late embryogenesis. This has hampered further studies of the role of PS1 in a natural brain setting in postnatal life.

Some studies in transgenic mice harboring FAD-linked PS1 variants reveal that expression of FAD-linked mutant PS1P117L (Wen *et al.*, 2004), PS1M146V (Wang *et al.*, 2004) or conditional ablation of PS1 in the forebrain (Feng *et al.*, 2001) induce impaired hippocampal neurogenesis. Other studies suggest that expression of FAD-linked PS1A246E enhances proliferation of progenitor cells in the adult DG (Chevallier *et al.*, 2005). Conditional ablation of PS1 in the forebrain and knock out of PS2 in adult mice (PS1/PS2 KO mice) induces massive neurodegeneration in the cortex and hippocampus. Neurodegeneration is accompanied by induced cell proliferation in the SGL. However, most of these newly formed cells do not survive (Chen *et al.*, 2008).

There is some disadvantage in the use of FAD-linked PS1 transgenic mice for the examination of neurogenesis — a set of processes that take place postnatally in restricted brain areas with a unique population of dividing progenitor cells, as transgenes are expressed in a ubiquitously, nonspecific manner. Lack or dysfunction of PS1 in mature neurons in the brain may induce processes that may alter neurogenesis indirectly (Chen *et al.*, 2008). Studies injecting lentiviral vectors coexpress siRNA for silencing PS1 into neurogenic areas reveal that NPC proliferation dramatically decreases, while differentiation is increased (Gadadhar *et al.*, 2011), suggesting that in the adult brain, PS1 regulates the differentiation of adult NPC in a γ-secretase dependent manner (Gadadhar *et al.*, 2011), thus FAD-linked mutant PS1 variants are likely to impair neurogenesis, probably via compromised Notch, β-catenin or the β-catenin/Wnt signaling (Gadadhar *et al.*, 2011) (Figure 2). Yet, this should be determined in future experiments in models in which expression of mutant PS1 is exclusively in NPC.

sAPP regulates neural progenitor proliferation

Soluble amyloid precursor protein α (sAPPα) is a proteolytic product of amyloid precursor protein (APP), a ubiquitously expressed type I glycoprotein. Mutations in *APP* cause FAD and upregulate the production ratio of certain beta-amyloid (Aβ) species. Alternatively, APP is cleaved in a non-amyloidogenic pathway, in which Aβ is not formed, but rather, sAPPα is liberated following α-secretase cleavage of APP [for review, see (Thinakaran and Koo, 2008)]. The function of sAPPα generated by the non-amyloidogenic pathway, is not fully understood. Likewise, the identity of α-secretase is not fully elucidated. Members of the 'a disintegrin and metalloproteinase' (ADAM) family ADAM10 (Lammich *et al.*, 1999), ADAM17 [TACE; (Buxbaum *et al.*, 1998; Lammich *et al.*, 1999; Asai *et al.*, 2003; Postina *et al.*, 2004)], as well as aspartyl protease beta-site APP cleaving enzyme 2 [BACE2 (Yan *et al.*, 2001)] exhibit α-secretase activity (Buxbaum *et al.*, 1998; Asai *et al.*, 2003). In the central nervous system, increase in APP expression during development overlaps with neuronal differentiation (Hung *et al.*, 1992). Nevertheless, the physiological role(s) of APP and APP metabolites remains largely unknown.

A crystal structure of the amino terminal of sAPPα reveals a domain that is similar to cysteine-rich growth factors, suggesting that sAPPα may act as a potential ligand for growth factor receptors (Rossjohn *et al.*, 1999), (Figure 2). Specifically, the crystal structure of sAPPα (APP28–123, residues 28–123) suggests that the overall fold of the APP N-terminal domain can be classified as mainly β, a fold that includes a number of cysteine-rich growth factors [such as epidermal growth factor (EGF), tumor necrosis factor (TNF) and nerve growth factor (NGF)]. In addition, APP, like a number of growth factors such as midkine19, hepatocyte growth factor (HGF) and vascular endothelial growth factor (VEGF), possess disulfide-bonded, β-hairpin loops implicated in proteoglycan binding (Rossjohn *et al.*, 1999). sAPPα has been shown to exhibit trophic and proliferative properties in fibroblasts (Saitoh *et al.*, 1989), thyroid epithelial cells (Pietrzik *et al.*, 1998) and embryonic stem cells (Ohsawa *et al.*, 1999). EGF responsive neural progenitor cell (NPCs) in the subventricular zone (SVZ) have been shown to have binding sites for sAPP (Caille *et al.*, 2004). Deficiency of the sortilin-related receptor with type-A repeats (SORLA) results in enhancement of sAPP production, ERK stimulation and increased proliferation

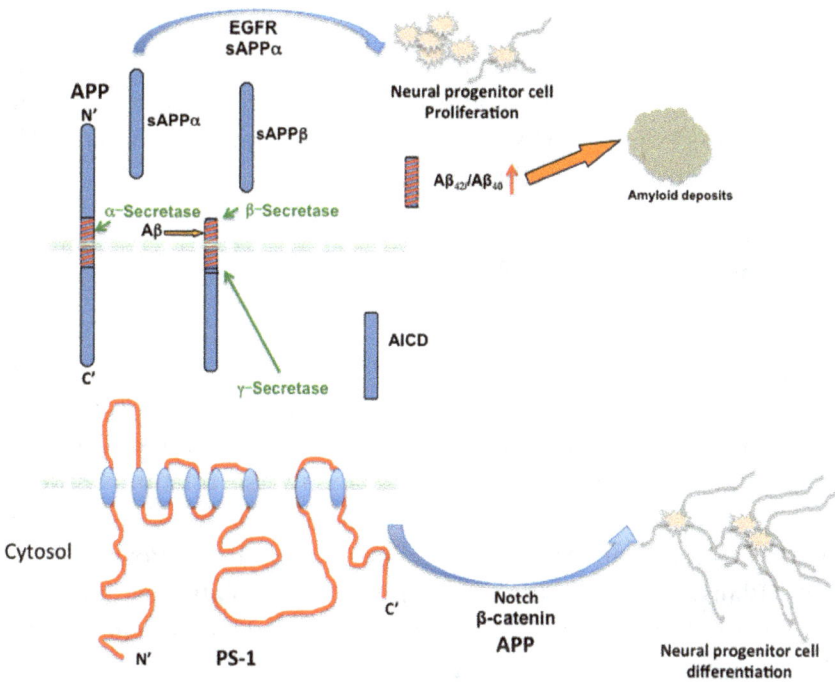

Figure 2.   Genes linked to familial Alzheimer's disease regulate neurogenesis-Mutations in amyloid precursor protein (APP), presenilin1,2 (PS1,2) cause familial Alzheimer's disease. APP can be cleaved by the amyloidogenic or the non-amyloidogenic pathways. In the nonamyloidogenic pathway, cleavage by α-secretase yields sAPPα that regulates neural progenitor cell proliferation. PS are the catalytic core of γ-secretase that cleaves APP. PS1 regulates neural progenitor cell differentiation through notch, β-catenin and epidermal growth factor receptor (EGFR).

and survival of NPCs in both the SVZ and subgranular layer of the dentate gyrus (SGL) (Rohe *et al.*, 2008).

Importantly, the production of sAPPα by α-secretase processing is essential for the proliferation of NPCs derived from the adult mouse brain(Demars *et al.*, 2011). Inhibition of NPC proliferation by MMP inhibitors could be rescued by the addition of recombinant sAPPα (Demars *et al.*, 2011), suggesting that sAPPα is sufficient for the induction of NPC proliferation.Recent studies show that injection of sAPPα into the SVZ of adult mice enhances NPC proliferation (Demars *et al.*, 2013) (Figure 2). It is not fully understood what directs APP molecules to be cleaved on the cell membrane and yield mostly sAPPα, or reinternalized and get cleaved by the amyloido-genic pathway. Nevertheless, it becomes apparently clear that the latter takes over during AD and probably many years prior to the disease. Interestingly, ADAM10 level is reduced in the brains of AD patients (Bernstein *et al.*, 2003).

Environmental Factors, Neurogenesis and Alzheimer's Disease

Learning and exercising are proving to be invaluable in supporting and maintaining our minds and bodies in a healthy state (Fratiglioni *et al.*, 2004). Numerous studies report the benefits of physical activity in the elderly. These studies suggest an inverse relation between exercise and physical dysfunction, cardiovascular disorders, mortal-ity, depression, and cognitive decline (Leon, 1985; Powell *et al.*, 1986; Blair *et al.*, 1989; Blumenthal *et al.*, 1991; Paffenbarger *et al.*, 1995; Churchill *et al.*, 2002; Lord *et al.*, 2003; Colcombe *et al.*, 2004b; Colcombe *et al.*, 2004a; Lytle *et al.*, 2004; Taylor *et al.*, 2004). It has become increasingly clear that this attitude and lifestyle may also prevent aging-related diseases, such as AD (Larson and Wang, 2004; Larson *et al.*, 2006). A large number of epidemiologic studies consist-ently report a reduced risk of cognitive decline and dementia associ-ated with physical activity(PAGAC, 2008; Chodzko-Zajko *et al.*, 2009; Hamer and Chida, 2009). In addition, studies support the conclu-sion that extent of education and high mental activity throughout life correlates with reduced risk for AD (Stern *et al.*, 1994; Snowdon *et al.*, 1996; Evans *et al.*, 1997; Letenneur *et al.*, 1999; Friedland *et al.*, 2001; Wilson *et al.*, 2002). Thus, epidemiologic studies suggest that cognitive stimulation and physical activity may reduce the risk of cognitive decline and dementia.

Behavioral studies in animal models of AD are an invaluable tool that have been providing significant insight into these crucial questions. Specifically, the beneficial effects of 'enriched' or 'complex' environments (EE) on synaptic plasticity and cognitive function in relation to AD are noteworthy (Lazarov *et al.*, 2005; Hu *et al.*, 2010; Hu *et al.*, 2013). A consensus seems to emerge that experience in enriched environmental conditions results in greater level of plasticity (Herring *et al.*, 2009), increased neurogenesis (Lazarov *et al.*, 2005; Wolf *et al.*, 2006; Herring *et al.*, 2009; Hu *et al.*, 2010) and reduced tau pathology (Billings *et al.*, 2007; Hu *et al.*, 2010). Importantly, experience of FAD-linked transgenic mice in EE rescues impaired neurogenesis in these mice (Hu *et al.*, 2010). These results open up an interesting array of questions concerning the association between the signals provided by the environment, enhanced neurogenesis and the level of pathology in the brains of these mice. Experiments in the future should investigate whether upregulation of neurogenesis plays a role in enrichment-induced reduced neuropathology, and whether upregulation of neurogenesis is a prerequisite or a contributor to enhanced cognitive function or to the attenuation of cognitive decline in AD.

Summary

Increasing evidence in mouse models of AD suggests that hippocampal neurogenesis plays a role in the development of AD, and in cognitive deficits in particular. The important role of neurogenesis in hippocampal function and plasticity is increasingly acknowledged. New neurons incorporate in the dentate gyrus, where critical information from the entorhinal cortex is received and conveyed in a feedback and feed-forward manner into other hippocampal regions. The hippocampal formation is essential for learning and memory and neuropathology in the entorhinal cortex and hippocampus plays a major role in cognitive deficits in AD. Numerous studies in animal models of FAD suggest that neurogenesis is altered in the disease, and that critical molecular signals play a role in both AD and regulation of neurogenesis. Future experiments using greater spatial and temporal specificity of molecular signals for the examination of neurogenesis, will provide valuable information concerning the role of neurogenesis in AD. Lastly, future development of experimental tools for the detection of neurogenesis in humans will be crucial for the understanding of the role of neurogenesis in the human disease.

References

Ahlenius H, Visan V, Kokaia M, Lindvall O, Kokaia Z (2009) Neural stem and progenitor cells retain their potential for proliferation and differentiation into functional neurons despite lower number in aged brain. *J Neurosci* 29:4408–4419.

Aimone JB, Gage FH (2011) Modeling new neuron function: a history of using computational neuroscience to study adult neurogenesis. *Eur J Neurosci* 33:1160–1169.

Aimone JB, Wiles J, Gage FH (2006) Potential role for adult neurogenesis in the encoding of time in new memories. *Nat Neurosci* 9:723–727.

Aimone JB, Deng W, Gage FH (2010) Adult neurogenesis: integrating theories and separating functions. *Trends Cogn Sci* 14:325–337.

Aimone JB, Deng W, Gage FH (2011) Resolving new memories: a critical look at the dentate gyrus, adult neurogenesis, and pattern separation. *Neuron* 70:589–596.

Albers MW, Tabert MH, Devanand DP (2006) Olfactory dysfunction as a predictor of neurodegenerative disease. *Curr Neurol Neurosci Rep* 6: 379–386.

Alvarez-Buylla A, Lim DA (2004) For the long run: maintaining germinal niches in the adult brain. *Neuron* 41:683–686.

Amrein I, Isler K, Lipp HP (2011) Comparing adult hippocampal neurogenesis in mammalian species and orders: influence of chronological age and life history stage. *Eur J Neurosci* 34:978–987.

Arendash GW, King DL, Gordon MN, Morgan D, Hatcher JM, Hope CE, Diamond DM (2001a) Progressive, age-related behavioral impairments in transgenic mice carrying both mutant amyloid precursor protein and presenilin-1 transgenes. *Brain Res* 891:42–53.

Arendash GW, Gordon MN, Diamond DM, Austin LA, Hatcher JM, Jantzen P, DiCarlo G, Wilcock D, Morgan D (2001b) Behavioral assessment of Alzheimer's transgenic mice following long-term Abeta vaccination: task specificity and correlations between Abeta deposition and spatial memory. *DNA Cell Biol* 20:737–744.

Asai M, Hattori C, Szabo B, Sasagawa N, Maruyama K, Tanuma S, Ishiura S (2003) Putative function of ADAM9, ADAM10, and ADAM17 as APP alpha-secretase. *Biochem Biophys Res Commun* 301:231–235.

Ashe KH (2001) Learning and memory in transgenic mice modeling Alzheimer's disease. *Learn Mem* 8:301–308.

Ashe KH (2006) In search of the molecular basis of memory loss in Alzheimer disease. *Alzheimer Dis Assoc Disord* 20:200–201.

Ashe KH, Zahs KR (2010) Probing the biology of Alzheimer's disease in mice. *Neuron* 66:631–645.

Ayuso-Sacido A, Graham C, Greenfield JP, Boockvar JA (2006) The duality of epidermal growth factor receptor (EGFR) signaling and neural stem cell phenotype: cell enhancer or cell transformer? *Curr Stem Cell Res Ther* 1:387–394.

Bacon AW, Bondi MW, Salmon DP, Murphy C (1998) Very early changes in olfactory functioning due to Alzheimer's disease and the role of apolipoprotein E in olfaction. *Ann N Y Acad Sci* 855:723–731.

Becker S (2005) A computational principle for hippocampal learning and neurogenesis. *Hippocampus* 15:722–738.

Ben Abdallah NM, Slomianka L, Vyssotski AL, Lipp HP (2010) Early age-related changes in adult hippocampal neurogenesis in C57 mice. *Neurobiol Aging* 31:151–161.

Bernal GM, Peterson DA (2004) Neural stem cells as therapeutic agents for age-related brain repair. *Aging Cell* 3:345–351.

Bernstein HG, Bukowska A, Krell D, Bogerts B, Ansorge S, Lendeckel U (2003) Comparative localization of ADAMs 10 and 15 in human cerebral cortex normal aging, Alzheimer disease and Down syndrome. *J Neurocytol* 32:153–160.

Billings LM, Green KN, McGaugh JL, LaFerla FM (2007) Learning decreases Abeta*56 and tau pathology and ameliorates behavioral decline in 3xTg-AD mice. *J Neurosci* 27:751–761.

Billings LM, Oddo S, Green KN, McGaugh JL, LaFerla FM (2005) Intraneuronal Abeta causes the onset of early Alzheimer's disease-related cognitive deficits in transgenic mice. *Neuron* 45:675–688.

Bizon JL, Gallagher M (2003) Production of new cells in the rat dentate gyrus over the lifespan: relation to cognitive decline. *Eur J Neurosci* 18:215–219.

Bizon JL, Gallagher M (2005) More is less: neurogenesis and age-related cognitive decline in Long-Evans rats. *Sci Aging Knowledge Environ* 2005:re2.

Bizon JL, Lee HJ, Gallagher M (2004) Neurogenesis in a rat model of age-related cognitive decline. *Aging Cell* 3:227–234.

Blair SN, Kohl HW, 3rd, Paffenbarger RS, Jr., Clark DG, Cooper KH, Gibbons LW (1989) Physical fitness and all-cause mortality. A prospective study of healthy men and women. *Jama* 262:2395–2401.

Blanchard J, Wanka L, Tung YC, Cardenas-Aguayo Mdel C, LaFerla FM, Iqbal K, Grundke-Iqbal I (2010) Pharmacologic reversal of neurogenic and neuroplastic abnormalities and cognitive impairments without affecting Abeta and tau pathologies in 3xTg-AD mice. *Acta Neuropathol* 120:605–621.

Blumenthal JA, Emery CF, Madden DJ, Coleman RE, Riddle MW, Schniebolk S, Cobb FR, Sullivan MJ, Higginbotham MB (1991) Effects of exercise training on cardiorespiratory function in men and women older than 60 years of age. *Am J Cardiol* 67:633–639.

Bonaguidi MA, Peng CY, McGuire T, Falciglia G, Gobeske KT, Czeisler C, Kessler JA (2008) Noggin expands neural stem cells in the adult hippocampus. *J Neurosci* 28:9194–9204.

Bondolfi L, Ermini F, Long JM, Ingram DK, Jucker M (2004) Impact of age and caloric restriction on neurogenesis in the dentate gyrus of C57BL/6 mice. *Neurobiol Aging* 25:333–340.

Bunsey M, Eichenbaum H (1993) Critical role of the parahippocampal region for paired-associate learning in rats. *Behav Neurosci* 107:740–747.

Burghardt NS, Park EH, Hen R, Fenton AA (2012) Adult-born hippocampal neurons promote cognitive flexibility in mice. *Hippocampus* 22: 1795–1808.

Burgmans S, van Boxtel MP, Vuurman EF, Evers EA, Jolles J (2010) Increased neural activation during picture encoding and retrieval in 60-year-olds compared to 20-year-olds. *Neuropsychologia* 48:2188–2197.

Buxbaum JD, Liu KN, Luo Y, Slack JL, Stocking KL, Peschon JJ, Johnson RS, Castner BJ, Cerretti DP, Black RA (1998) Evidence that tumor necrosis factor alpha converting enzyme is involved in regulated alpha-secretase cleavage of the Alzheimer amyloid protein precursor. *J Biol Chem* 273: 27765–27767.

Caille I, Allinquant B, Dupont E, Bouillot C, Langer A, Muller U, Prochiantz A (2004) Soluble form of amyloid precursor protein regulates proliferation of progenitors in the adult subventricular zone. *Development* 131: 2173–2181.

Cameron HA, McKay RD (1999) Restoring production of hippocampal neurons in old age. *Nat Neurosci* 2:894–897.

Chapman PF, White GL, Jones MW, Cooper-Blacketer D, Marshall VJ, Irizarry M, Younkin L, Good MA, Bliss TV, Hyman BT, Younkin SG, Hsiao KK (1999) Impaired synaptic plasticity and learning in aged amyloid precursor protein transgenic mice. *Nat Neurosci* 2:271–276.

Chen AC, Shirayama Y, Shin KH, Neve RL, Duman RS (2001) Expression of the cAMP response element binding protein (CREB) in hippocampus produces an antidepressant effect. *Biol Psychiatry* 49:753–762.

Chen Q, Nakajima A, Choi SH, Xiong X, Sisodia SS, Tang YP (2008) Adult neurogenesis is functionally associated with AD-like neurodegeneration. *Neurobiol Dis* 29:316–326.

Chevallier NL, Soriano S, Kang DE, Masliah E, Hu G, Koo EH (2005) Perturbed neurogenesis in the adult hippocampus associated with presenilin-1 A246E mutation. *Am J Pathol* 167:151–159.

Chishti MA *et al.* (2001) Early-onset amyloid deposition and cognitive deficits in transgenic mice expressing a double mutant form of amyloid precursor protein 695. *J Biol Chem* 276:21562–21570.

Chodzko-Zajko WJ, Proctor DN, Fiatarone Singh MA, Minson CT, Nigg CR, Salem GJ, Skinner JS (2009) American College of Sports Medicine position stand. Exercise and physical activity for older adults. *Med Sci Sports Exerc* 41:1510–1530.

Choi SH, Veeraraghavalu K, Lazarov O, Marler S, Ransohoff RM, Ramirez JM, Sisodia SS (2008) Non-cell-autonomous effects of presenilin 1 variants on enrichment-mediated hippocampal progenitor cell proliferation and differentiation. *Neuron* 59:568–580.

Churchill JD, Galvez R, Colcombe S, Swain RA, Kramer AF, Greenough WT (2002) Exercise, experience and the aging brain. *Neurobiol Aging* 23:941–955.

Cleary JP, Walsh DM, Hofmeister JJ, Shankar GM, Kuskowski MA, Selkoe DJ, Ashe KH (2005) Natural oligomers of the amyloid-beta protein specifically disrupt cognitive function. *Nat Neurosci* 8:79–84.

Colcombe SJ, Kramer AF, McAuley E, Erickson KI, Scalf P (2004a) Neurocognitive aging and cardiovascular fitness: recent findings and future directions. *J Mol Neurosci* 24:9–14.

Colcombe SJ, Kramer AF, Erickson KI, Scalf P, McAuley E, Cohen NJ, Webb A, Jerome GJ, Marquez DX, Elavsky S (2004b) Cardiovascular fitness, cortical plasticity, and aging. *Proc Natl Acad Sci U S A* 101:3316–3321.

Couillard-Despres S, Aigner L (2011) *In vivo* imaging of adult neurogenesis. *Eur J Neurosci* 33:1037–1044.

De Strooper B (2003) Aph-1, Pen-2, and Nicastrin with Presenilin Generate an Active gamma-Secretase Complex. *Neuron* 38:9–12.

De Strooper B, Annaert W, Cupers P, Saftig P, Craessaerts K, Mumm JS, Schroeter EH, Schrijvers V, Wolfe MS, Ray WJ, Goate A, Kopan R

(1999) A presenilin-1-dependent gamma-secretase-like protease mediates release of Notch intracellular domain [see comments]. *Nature* 398:518–522.

Demars M, Hu YS, Gadadhar A, Lazarov O (2010) Impaired neurogenesis is an early event in the etiology of familial Alzheimer's disease in transgenic mice. *J Neurosci Res* 88:2103–2117.

Demars MP, Bartholomew A, Strakova Z, Lazarov O (2011) Soluble amyloid precursor protein: a novel proliferation factor of adult progenitor cells of ectodermal and mesodermal origin. *Stem Cell Res Ther* 2:36.

Demars MP, Hollands C, Zhao KD, Lazarov O (2013) Soluble amyloid precursor protein-alpha rescues age-linked decline in neural progenitor cell proliferation. *Neurobiol Aging* 34:2431–2440.

Denny CA, Burghardt NS, Schachter DM, Hen R, Drew MR (2012) 4- to 6-week-old adult-born hippocampal neurons influence novelty-evoked exploration and contextual fear conditioning. *Hippocampus* 22:1188–1201.

Dewachter I, Reverse D, Caluwaerts N, Ris L, Kuiperi C, Van den Haute C, Spittaels K, Umans L, Serneels L, Thiry E, Moechars D, Mercken M, Godaux E, Van Leuven F (2002) Neuronal deficiency of presenilin 1 inhibits amyloid plaque formation and corrects hippocampal long-term potentiation but not a cognitive defect of amyloid precursor protein [V717I] transgenic mice. *J Neurosci* 22:3445–3453.

Dineley KT, Xia X, Bui D, Sweatt JD, Zheng H (2002) Accelerated plaque accumulation, associative learning deficits, and up-regulation of alpha 7 nicotinic receptor protein in transgenic mice co-expressing mutant human presenilin 1 and amyloid precursor proteins. *J Biol Chem* 277: 22768–22780.

Dong H, Goico B, Martin M, Csernansky CA, Bertchume A, Csernansky JG (2004) Modulation of hippocampal cell proliferation, memory, and amyloid plaque deposition in APPsw (Tg2576) mutant mice by isolation stress. *Neuroscience* 127:601–609.

Donovan MH, Yazdani U, Norris RD, Games D, German DC, Eisch AJ (2006) Decreased adult hippocampal neurogenesis in the PDAPP mouse model of Alzheimer's disease. *J Comp Neurol* 495:70–83.

Drapeau E, Mayo W, Aurousseau C, Le Moal M, Piazza PV, Abrous DN (2003) Spatial memory performances of aged rats in the water maze predict levels of hippocampal neurogenesis. *Proc Natl Acad Sci U S A* 100:14385–14390.

Driscoll I, Howard SR, Stone JC, Monfils MH, Tomanek B, Brooks WM, Sutherland RJ (2006) The aging hippocampus: a multi-level analysis in the rat. *Neuroscience* 139:1173–1185.

Dupret D, Revest JM, Koehl M, Ichas F, De Giorgi F, Costet P, Abrous DN, Piazza PV (2008) Spatial relational memory requires hippocampal adult neurogenesis. *PLoS One* 3:e1959.

Dusek JA, Eichenbaum H (1997) The hippocampus and memory for orderly stimulus relations. *Proc Natl Acad Sci U S A* 94:7109–7114.

Encinas JM, Michurina TV, Peunova N, Park JH, Tordo J, Peterson DA, Fishell G, Koulakov A, Enikolopov G (2011) Division-coupled astrocytic differentiation and age-related depletion of neural stem cells in the adult hippocampus. *Cell Stem Cell* 8:566–579.

Enwere E, Shingo T, Gregg C, Fujikawa H, Ohta S, Weiss S (2004) Aging results in reduced epidermal growth factor receptor signaling, diminished olfactory neurogenesis, and deficits in fine olfactory discrimination. *J Neurosci* 24:8354–8365.

Ermini FV, Grathwohl S, Radde R, Yamaguchi M, Staufenbiel M, Palmer TD, Jucker M (2008) Neurogenesis and alterations of neural stem cells in mouse models of cerebral amyloidosis. *Am J Pathol* 172:1520–1528.

Evans DA, Hebert LE, Beckett LA, Scherr PA, Albert MS, Chown MJ, Pilgrim DM, Taylor JO (1997) Education and other measures of socioeconomic status and risk of incident Alzheimer disease in a defined population of older persons. *Arch Neurol* 54:1399–1405.

Feng R, Rampon C, Tang YP, Shrom D, Jin J, Kyin M, Sopher B, Miller MW, Ware CB, Martin GM, Kim SH, Langdon RB, Sisodia SS, Tsien JZ (2001) Deficient neurogenesis in forebrain-specific presenilin-1 knockout mice is associated with reduced clearance of hippocampal memory traces. *Neuron* 32:911–926.

Fratiglioni L, Paillard-Borg S, Winblad B (2004) An active and socially integrated lifestyle in late life might protect against dementia. *Lancet Neurol* 3:343–353.

Friedland RP, Fritsch T, Smyth KA, Koss E, Lerner AJ, Chen CH, Petot GJ, Debanne SM (2001) Patients with Alzheimer's disease have reduced activities in midlife compared with healthy control-group members. *Proc Natl Acad Sci U S A* 98:3440–3445.

Gadadhar A, Marr RA, Lazarov O (2011) Presenilin-1 regulates neural progenitor cell differentiation in the adult brain. *J Neurosci* 31:2615–2623.

Gakhar-Koppole N, Hundeshagen P, Mandl C, Weyer SW, Allinquant B, Muller U, Ciccolini F (2008) Activity requires soluble amyloid precursor protein alpha to promote neurite outgrowth in neural stem cell-derived neurons via activation of the MAPK pathway. *Eur J Neurosci* 28:871–882.

Gan L, Qiao S, Lan X, Chi L, Luo C, Lien L, Yan Liu Q, Liu R (2008) Neurogenic responses to amyloid-beta plaques in the brain of Alzheimer's disease-like transgenic (pPDGF-APPSw,Ind) mice. *Neurobiol Dis* 29:71–80.

Ge S, Goh EL, Sailor KA, Kitabatake Y, Ming GL, Song H (2006) GABA regulates synaptic integration of newly generated neurons in the adult brain. *Nature* 439:589–593.

Gordon MN, King DL, Diamond DM, Jantzen PT, Boyett KV, Hope CE, Hatcher JM, DiCarlo G, Gottschall WP, Morgan D, Arendash GW (2001) Correlation between cognitive deficits and Abeta deposits in transgenic APP+PS1 mice. *Neurobiol Aging* 22:377–385.

Hamer M, Chida Y (2009) Physical activity and risk of neurodegenerative disease: a systematic review of prospective evidence. *Psychol Med* 39: 3–11.

Hartl D, Rohe M, Mao L, Staufenbiel M, Zabel C, Klose J (2008) Impairment of adolescent hippocampal plasticity in a mouse model for Alzheimer's disease precedes disease phenotype. *PLoS One* 3:e2759.

Hattiangady B, Shetty AK (2008) Aging does not alter the number or phenotype of putative stem/progenitor cells in the neurogenic region of the hippocampus. *Neurobiol Aging* 29:129–147.

Haughey NJ, Nath A, Chan SL, Borchard AC, Rao MS, Mattson MP (2002) Disruption of neurogenesis by amyloid beta-peptide, and perturbed neural progenitor cell homeostasis, in models of Alzheimer's disease. *J Neurochem* 83:1509–1524.

Heine VM, Maslam S, Joels M, Lucassen PJ (2004) Prominent decline of newborn cell proliferation, differentiation, and apoptosis in the aging dentate gyrus, in absence of an age-related hypothalamus-pituitary-adrenal axis activation. *Neurobiol Aging* 25:361–375.

Herring A, Ambree O, Tomm M, Habermann H, Sachser N, Paulus W, Keyvani K (2009) Environmental enrichment enhances cellular plasticity in transgenic mice with Alzheimer-like pathology. *Exp Neurol* 216: 184–192.

Hu YS, Long N, Pigino G, Brady ST, Lazarov O (2013) Molecular mechanisms of environmental enrichment: impairments in Akt/GSK3beta, neurotrophin-3 and CREB signaling. *PLoS One* 8:e64460.

Hu YS, Xu P, Pigino G, Brady ST, Larson J, Lazarov O (2010) Complex environment experience rescues impaired neurogenesis, enhances synaptic plasticity, and attenuates neuropathology in familial Alzheimer's disease-linked APPswe/PS1{Delta}E9 mice. *Faseb J* 24:1667–1681.

Hung AY, Koo EH, Haass C, Selkoe DJ (1992) Increased expression of beta-amyloid precursor protein during neuronal differentiation is not accompanied by secretory cleavage. *Proc Natl Acad Sci U S A* 89:9439–9443.

Imayoshi I, Sakamoto M, Ohtsuka T, Takao K, Miyakawa T, Yamaguchi M, Mori K, Ikeda T, Itohara S, Kageyama R (2008) Roles of continuous neurogenesis in the structural and functional integrity of the adult forebrain. *Nat Neurosci* 11:1153–1161.

Jankowsky JL, Melnikova T, Fadale DJ, Xu GM, Slunt HH, Gonzales V, Younkin LH, Younkin SG, Borchelt DR, Savonenko AV (2005) Environmental enrichment mitigates cognitive deficits in a mouse model of Alzheimer's disease. *J Neurosci* 25:5217–5224.

Janus C, D'Amelio S, Amitay O, Chishti MA, Strome R, Fraser P, Carlson GA, Roder JC, St George-Hyslop P, Westaway D (2000) Spatial learning in transgenic mice expressing human presenilin 1 (PS1) transgenes. *Neurobiol Aging* 21:541–549.

Jin K, Galvan V, Xie L, Mao XO, Gorostiza OF, Bredesen DE, Greenberg DA (2004) Enhanced neurogenesis in Alzheimer's disease transgenic (PDGF-APPSw,Ind) mice. *Proc Natl Acad Sci U S A* 101:13363–13367.

Kasuga K, Kaneko H, Nishizawa M, Onodera O, Ikeuchi T (2007) Generation of intracellular domain of insulin receptor tyrosine kinase by gamma-secretase. *Biochem Biophys Res Commun* 360:90–96.

Katakowski M, Chen J, Zhang ZG, Santra M, Wang Y, Chopp M (2007) Stroke-induced subventricular zone proliferation is promoted by tumor necrosis factor-alpha-converting enzyme protease activity. *J Cereb Blood Flow Metab* 27:669–678.

Kee N, Teixeira CM, Wang AH, Frankland PW (2007) Preferential incorporation of adult-generated granule cells into spatial memory networks in the dentate gyrus. *Nat Neurosci* 10:355–362.

Kempermann G, Gage FH (2002) Genetic determinants of adult hippocampal neurogenesis correlate with acquisition, but not probe trial performance, in the water maze task. *Eur J Neurosci* 16:129–136.

Kempermann G, Kuhn HG, Gage FH (1997) More hippocampal neurons in adult mice living in an enriched environment. *Nature* 386:493–495.

Kempermann G, Kuhn HG, Gage FH (1998) Experience-induced neurogenesis in the senescent dentate gyrus. *J Neurosci* 18:3206–3212.

Kempermann G, Gast D, Gage FH (2002) Neuroplasticity in old age: sustained fivefold induction of hippocampal neurogenesis by long-term environmental enrichment. *Ann Neurol* 52:135–143.

Kesslak JP, Cotman CW, Chui HC, Van den Noort S, Fang H, Pfeffer R, Lynch G (1988) Olfactory tests as possible probes for detecting and monitoring Alzheimer's disease. *Neurobiol Aging* 9:399–403.

Kim JS, Lee HJ, Kim JC, Kang SS, Bae CS, Shin T, Jin JK, Kim SH, Wang H, Moon C (2008) Transient impairment of hippocampus-dependent learning and memory in relatively low-dose of acute radiation syndrome is associated with inhibition of hippocampal neurogenesis. *J Radiat Res* 49:517–526.

Klempin F, Kempermann G (2007) Adult hippocampal neurogenesis and aging. *Eur Arch Psychiatry Clin Neurosci* 257:271–280.

Knoth R, Singec I, Ditter M, Pantazis G, Capetian P, Meyer RP, Horvat V, Volk B, Kempermann G (2010) Murine features of neurogenesis in the human hippocampus across the lifespan from 0 to 100 years. *PLoS One* 5:e8809.

Krezymon A, Richetin K, Halley H, Roybon L, Lassalle JM, Frances B, Verret L, Rampon C (2013) Modifications of hippocampal circuits and early disruption of adult neurogenesis in the tg2576 mouse model of Alzheimer's disease. *PLoS One* 8:e76497.

Kronenberg G, Bick-Sander A, Bunk E, Wolf C, Ehninger D, Kempermann G (2006) Physical exercise prevents age-related decline in precursor cell activity in the mouse dentate gyrus. *Neurobiol Aging* 27:1505–1513.

Kuhn HG, Dickinson-Anson H, Gage FH (1996) Neurogenesis in the dentate gyrus of the adult rat: age-related decrease of neuronal progenitor proliferation. *J Neurosci* 16:2027–2033.

Lammich S, Kojro E, Postina R, Gilbert S, Pfeiffer R, Jasionowski M, Haass C, Fahrenholz F (1999) Constitutive and regulated alpha-secretase cleavage of Alzheimer's amyloid precursor protein by a disintegrin metalloprotease. *Proc Natl Acad Sci U S A* 96:3922–3927.

Laplagne DA, Esposito MS, Piatti VC, Morgenstern NA, Zhao C, van Praag H, Gage FH, Schinder AF (2006) Functional convergence of neurons generated in the developing and adult hippocampus. *PLoS Biol* 4: e409.

Larson EB, Wang L (2004) Exercise, aging, and Alzheimer disease. *Alzheimer Dis Assoc Disord* 18:54–56.

Larson EB, Wang L, Bowen JD, McCormick WC, Teri L, Crane P, Kukull W (2006) Exercise is associated with reduced risk for incident dementia among persons 65 years of age and older. *Ann Intern Med* 144:73–81.

Larson J, Sieprawska D (2002) Automated study of simultaneous-cue olfactory discrimination learning in adult mice. *Behav Neurosci* 116: 588–599.

Lazarov O, Marr RA (2010) Neurogenesis and Alzheimer's disease: At the crossroads. *Exp Neurol* 223:267–281.

Lazarov O, Marr RA (2013) Of mice and men: neurogenesis, cognition and Alzheimer's disease. *Front Aging Neurosci* 5:43.

Lazarov O, Mattson MP, Peterson DA, Pimplikar SW, van Praag H (2010) When neurogenesis encounters aging and disease. *Trends Neurosci* 33:569–579.

Lazarov O, Robinson J, Tang YP, Hairston IS, Korade-Mirnics Z, Lee VM, Hersh LB, Sapolsky RM, Mirnics K, Sisodia SS (2005) Environmental enrichment reduces Abeta levels and amyloid deposition in transgenic mice. *Cell* 120:701–713.

Lemaire V, Koehl M, Le Moal M, Abrous DN (2000) Prenatal stress produces learning deficits associated with an inhibition of neurogenesis in the hippocampus. *Proc Natl Acad Sci U S A* 97:11032–11037.

Leon AS (1985) Physical activity levels and coronary heart disease. Analysis of epidemiologic and supporting studies. *Med Clin North Am* 69:3–20.

Letenneur L, Gilleron V, Commenges D, Helmer C, Orgogozo JM, Dartigues JF (1999) Are sex and educational level independent predictors of dementia and Alzheimer's disease? Incidence data from the PAQUID project. *J Neurol Neurosurg Psychiatry* 66:177–183.

Li T, Wen H, Brayton C, Das P, Smithson LA, Fauq A, Fan X, Crain BJ, Price DL, Golde TE, Eberhart CG, Wong PC (2007) EGFR and notch pathways participate in the tumor suppressor function of gamma-secretase. *J Biol Chem* 282:32264–32273.

Lie DC, Song H, Colamarino SA, Ming GL, Gage FH (2004) Neurogenesis in the adult brain: new strategies for central nervous system diseases. *Annu Rev Pharmacol Toxicol* 44:399–421.

Lie DC, Colamarino SA, Song HJ, Desire L, Mira H, Consiglio A, Lein ES, Jessberger S, Lansford H, Dearie AR, Gage FH (2005) Wnt signalling regulates adult hippocampal neurogenesis. *Nature* 437:1370–1375.

Lopez-Toledano MA, Shelanski ML (2007) Increased neurogenesis in young transgenic mice overexpressing human APP (Sw, Ind). *J Alzheimers Dis* 12:229–240.

Lord SR, Castell S, Corcoran J, Dayhew J, Matters B, Shan A, Williams P (2003) The effect of group exercise on physical functioning and falls in frail older people living in retirement villages: a randomized, controlled trial. *J Am Geriatr Soc* 51:1685–1692.

Lynch G (1986) *Synapses, Circuits, and the Beginnings of Memory*, MIT Press, Cambridge, MA.

Lytle ME, Vander Bilt J, Pandav RS, Dodge HH, Ganguli M (2004) Exercise level and cognitive decline: the MoVIES project. *Alzheimer Dis Assoc Disord* 18:57–64.

Madsen TM, Kristjansen PE, Bolwig TG, Wortwein G (2003) Arrested neuronal proliferation and impaired hippocampal function following fractionated brain irradiation in the adult rat. *Neuroscience* 119:635–642.

Marambaud P, Shioi J, Serban G, Georgakopoulos A, Sarner S, Nagy V, Baki L, Wen P, Efthimiopoulos S, Shao Z, Wisniewski T, Robakis NK (2002) A presenilin-1/gamma-secretase cleavage releases the E-cadherin intracellular domain and regulates disassembly of adherens junctions. *Embo J* 21:1948–1956.

Maretzky T, Reiss K, Ludwig A, Buchholz J, Scholz F, Proksch E, de Strooper B, Hartmann D, Saftig P (2005a) ADAM10 mediates E-cadherin shedding and regulates epithelial cell-cell adhesion, migration, and beta-catenin translocation. *Proc Natl Acad Sci U S A* 102: 9182–9187.

Maretzky T, Schulte M, Ludwig A, Rose-John S, Blobel C, Hartmann D, Altevogt P, Saftig P, Reiss K (2005b) L1 is sequentially processed by two differently activated metalloproteases and presenilin/gamma-secretase and regulates neural cell adhesion, cell migration, and neurite outgrowth. *Mol Cell Biol* 25:9040–9053.

Markwardt SJ, Wadiche JI, Overstreet-Wadiche LS (2009) Input-specific GABAergic signaling to newborn neurons in adult dentate gyrus. *J Neurosci* 29:15063–15072.

McElroy B, Powell JC, McCarthy JV (2007) The insulin-like growth factor 1 (IGF-1) receptor is a substrate for gamma-secretase-mediated intramembrane proteolysis. *Biochem Biophys Res Commun* 358:1136–1141.

Merrill DA, Karim R, Darraq M, Chiba AA, Tuszynski MH (2003) Hippocampal cell genesis does not correlate with spatial learning ability in aged rats. *J Comp Neurol* 459:201–207.

Ming GL, Song H (2005) Adult neurogenesis in the mammalian central nervous system. *Annu Rev Neurosci* 28:223–250.

Miranda CJ, Braun L, Jiang Y, Hester ME, Zhang L, Riolo M, Wang H, Rao M, Altura RA, Kaspar BK (2012) Aging brain microenvironment decreases hippocampal neurogenesis through Wnt-mediated survivin signaling. *Aging Cell* 11:542–552.

Mirich JM, Williams NC, Berlau DJ, Brunjes PC (2002) Comparative study of aging in the mouse olfactory bulb. *J Comp Neurol* 454:361–372.

Mirochnic S, Wolf S, Staufenbiel M, Kempermann G (2009) Age effects on the regulation of adult hippocampal neurogenesis by physical activity and environmental enrichment in the APP23 mouse model of Alzheimer disease. *Hippocampus* 19:1008–1018.

Morgan D, Diamond DM, Gottschall PE, Ugen KE, Dickey C, Hardy J, Duff K, Jantzen P, DiCarlo G, Wilcock D, Connor K, Hatcher J, Hope C, Gordon M, Arendash GW (2000) A beta peptide vaccination prevents memory loss in an animal model of Alzheimer's disease. *Nature* 408: 982–985.

Morgenstern NA, Lombardi G, Schinder AF (2008) Newborn granule cells in the ageing dentate gyrus. *J Physiol* 586:3751–3757.

Nacher J, Alonso-Llosa G, Rosell DR, McEwen BS (2003) NMDA receptor antagonist treatment increases the production of new neurons in the aged rat hippocampus. *Neurobiol Aging* 24:273–284.

Ni CY, Murphy MP, Golde TE, Carpenter G (2001) gamma -Secretase cleavage and nuclear localization of ErbB-4 receptor tyrosine kinase. *Science* 294:2179–2181.

Ohno M, Sametsky EA, Younkin LH, Oakley H, Younkin SG, Citron M, Vassar R, Disterhoft JF (2004) BACE1 deficiency rescues memory deficits and cholinergic dysfunction in a mouse model of Alzheimer's disease. *Neuron* 41:27–33.

Ohsawa I, Takamura C, Morimoto T, Ishiguro M, Kohsaka S (1999) Amino-terminal region of secreted form of amyloid precursor protein stimulates proliferation of neural stem cells. *Eur J Neurosci* 11: 1907–1913.

Olariu A, Cleaver KM, Cameron HA (2007) Decreased neurogenesis in aged rats results from loss of granule cell precursors without lengthening of the cell cycle. *J Comp Neurol* 501:659–667.

Otto T, Eichenbaum H (1992) Complementary roles of the orbital prefrontal cortex and the perirhinal-entorhinal cortices in an odor-guided delayed-nonmatching-to-sample task. *Behav Neurosci* 106:762–775.

Paffenbarger RS, Jr., Wing AL, Hyde RT (1995) Physical activity as an index of heart attack risk in college alumni. 1978. *Am J Epidemiol* 142:889–903; discussion 887–888.

PAGAC PAGAC (2008) *Physical Activity Guidelines Advisory Committee Report.* Washington, DC US Department of Health and Human Services: G8–23.

Pietrzik CU, Hoffmann J, Stober K, Chen CY, Bauer C, Otero DA, Roch JM, Herzog V (1998) From differentiation to proliferation: the secretory amyloid precursor protein as a local mediator of growth in thyroid epithelial cells. *Proc Natl Acad Sci U S A* 95:1770–1775.

Poirier R, Veltman I, Pflimlin MC, Knoflach F, Metzger F (2010) Enhanced dentate gyrus synaptic plasticity but reduced neurogenesis in a mouse model of amyloidosis. *Neurobiol Dis* 40:386–393.

Postina R, Schroeder A, Dewachter I, Bohl J, Schmitt U, Kojro E, Prinzen C, Endres K, Hiemke C, Blessing M, Flamez P, Dequenne A, Godaux E, van Leuven F, Fahrenholz F (2004) A disintegrin-metalloproteinase prevents amyloid plaque formation and hippocampal defects in an Alzheimer disease mouse model. *J Clin Invest* 113:1456–1464.

Powell KE, Spain KG, Christenson GM, Mollenkamp MP (1986) The status of the 1990 objectives for physical fitness and exercise. *Public Health Rep* 101:15–21.

Price DL, Tanzi RE, Borchelt DR, Sisodia SS (1998) Alzheimer's disease: genetic studies and transgenic models. *Annu Rev Genet* 32:461–493.

Puolivali J, Wang J, Heikkinen T, Heikkila M, Tapiola T, van Groen T, Tanila H (2002) Hippocampal A beta 42 levels correlate with spatial memory deficit in APP and PS1 double transgenic mice. *Neurobiol Dis* 9:339–347.

Rao MS, Hattiangady B, Shetty AK (2006) The window and mechanisms of major age-related decline in the production of new neurons within the dentate gyrus of the hippocampus. *Aging Cell* 5:545–558.

Rapp PR, Stack EC, Gallagher M (1999) Morphometric studies of the aged hippocampus: I. Volumetric analysis in behaviorally characterized rats. *J Comp Neurol* 403:459–470.

Rohe M, Carlo AS, Breyhan H, Sporbert A, Militz D, Schmidt V, Wozny C, Harmeier A, Erdmann B, Bales KR, Wolf S, Kempermann G, Paul SM, Schmitz D, Bayer TA, Willnow TE, Andersen OM (2008) Sortilin-related Receptor with A-type Repeats (SORLA) Affects the Amyloid Precursor Protein-dependent Stimulation of ERK Signaling and Adult Neurogenesis. *J Biol Chem* 283:14826–14834.

Rola R, Raber J, Rizk A, Otsuka S, VandenBerg SR, Morhardt DR, Fike JR (2004) Radiation-induced impairment of hippocampal neurogenesis is associated with cognitive deficits in young mice. *Exp Neurol* 188: 316–330.

Rossjohn J, Cappai R, Feil SC, Henry A, McKinstry WJ, Galatis D, Hesse L, Multhaup G, Beyreuther K, Masters CL, Parker MW (1999) Crystal structure of the N-terminal, growth factor-like domain of Alzheimer amyloid precursor protein. *Nat Struct Biol* 6:327–331.

Sahay A, Wilson DA, Hen R (2011) Pattern separation: a common function for new neurons in hippocampus and olfactory bulb. *Neuron* 70: 582–588.

Saitoh T, Sundsmo M, Roch JM, Kimura N, Cole G, Schubert D, Oltersdorf T, Schenk DB (1989) Secreted form of amyloid beta protein precursor is involved in the growth regulation of fibroblasts. *Cell* 58:615–622.

Sardi SP, Murtie J, Koirala S, Patten BA, Corfas G (2006) Presenilin-dependent ErbB4 nuclear signaling regulates the timing of astrogenesis in the developing brain. *Cell* 127:185–197.

Saura CA, Chen G, Malkani S, Choi SY, Takahashi RH, Zhang D, Gouras GK, Kirkwood A, Morris RG, Shen J (2005) Conditional inactivation of presenilin 1 prevents amyloid accumulation and temporarily rescues contextual and spatial working memory impairments in amyloid precursor protein transgenic mice. *J Neurosci* 25:6755–6764.

Saxe MD, Battaglia F, Wang JW, Malleret G, David DJ, Monckton JE, Garcia AD, Sofroniew MV, Kandel ER, Santarelli L, Hen R, Drew MR (2006) Ablation of hippocampal neurogenesis impairs contextual fear conditioning and synaptic plasticity in the dentate gyrus. *Proc Natl Acad Sci U S A* 103:17501–17506.

Schloesser RJ, Jimenez DV, Hardy NF, Paredes D, Catlow BJ, Manji HK, McKay RD, Martinowich K (2013) Atrophy of pyramidal neurons and increased stress-induced glutamate levels in CA3 following chronic suppression of adult neurogenesis. *Brain Struct Funct* 219:1139–1148.

Seki T, Arai Y (1995) Age-related production of new granule cells in the adult dentate gyrus. *Neuroreport* 6:2479–2482.

Selkoe DJ (2001) Alzheimer's disease: genes, proteins, and therapy. *Physiol Rev* 81:741–766.

Selkoe DJ, Wolfe MS (2007) Presenilin: running with scissors in the membrane. *Cell* 131:215–221.

Serby M (1987) Olfactory deficits in Alzheimer's disease. *J Neural Transm Suppl* 24:69–77.

Shen J, Bronson RT, Chen DF, Xia W, Selkoe DJ, Tonegawa S (1997) Skeletal and CNS defects in Presenilin-1-deficient mice. *Cell* 89:629–639.

Shetty GA, Hattiangady B, Shetty AK (2013) Neural stem cell- and neurogenesis-related gene expression profiles in the young and aged dentate gyrus. *Age (Dordr)* 35:2165–2176.

Shimazu K, Zhao M, Sakata K, Akbarian S, Bates B, Jaenisch R, Lu B (2006) NT-3 facilitates hippocampal plasticity and learning and memory by regulating neurogenesis. *Learn Mem* 13:307–315.

Shipley MT, McLean JH, Ennis M (1995) Olfactory system. In: Paxinos,G. (Ed.), *The Rat Nervous System,* Academic Press, San Diego, pp. 899–826.

Shirayama Y, Chen AC, Nakagawa S, Russell DS, Duman RS (2002) Brain-derived neurotrophic factor produces antidepressant effects in behavioral models of depression. *J Neurosci* 22:3251–3261.

Shook BA, Manz DH, Peters JJ, Kang S, Conover JC (2012) Spatiotemporal changes to the subventricular zone stem cell pool through aging. *J Neurosci* 32:6947–6956.

Shors TJ, Townsend DA, Zhao M, Kozorovitskiy Y, Gould E (2002) Neurogenesis may relate to some but not all types of hippocampal-dependent learning. *Hippocampus* 12:578–584.

Shors TJ, Miesegaes G, Beylin A, Zhao M, Rydel T, Gould E (2001) Neurogenesis in the adult is involved in the formation of trace memories. *Nature* 410:372–376.

Slotnick B (2001) Animal cognition and the rat olfactory system. *Trends Cogn Sci* 5:216–222.

Slotnick BM, Katz HM (1974) Olfactory learning-set formation in rats. *Science* 185:796–798.

Snowdon DA, Kemper SJ, Mortimer JA, Greiner LH, Wekstein DR, Markesbery WR (1996) Linguistic ability in early life and cognitive function and Alzheimer's disease in late life. Findings from the Nun Study. *Jama* 275:528–532.

Spalding KL, Bergmann O, Alkass K, Bernard S, Salehpour M, Huttner HB, Bostrom E, Westerlund I, Vial C, Buchholz BA, Possnert G, Mash DC, Druid H, Frisen J (2013) Dynamics of hippocampal neurogenesis in adult humans. *Cell* 153:1219–1227.

Stern Y, Gurland B, Tatemichi TK, Tang MX, Wilder D, Mayeux R (1994) Influence of education and occupation on the incidence of Alzheimer's disease. *Jama* 271:1004–1010.

Sun X, Beglopoulos V, Mattson MP, Shen J (2005) Hippocampal spatial memory impairments caused by the familial Alzheimer's disease-linked presenilin 1 M146V mutation. *Neurodegener Dis* 2:6–15.

Suzuki Y, Yamamoto S, Umegaki H, Onishi J, Mogi N, Fujishiro H, Iguchi A (2004) Smell identification test as an indicator for cognitive impairment in Alzheimer's disease. *Int J Geriatr Psychiatry* 19:727–733.

Taniuchi N, Niidome T, Goto Y, Akaike A, Kihara T, Sugimoto H (2007) Decreased proliferation of hippocampal progenitor cells in APPswe/PS1dE9 transgenic mice. *Neuroreport* 18:1801–1805.

Taylor AH, Cable NT, Faulkner G, Hillsdon M, Narici M, Van Der Bij AK (2004) Physical activity and older adults: a review of health benefits and the effectiveness of interventions. *J Sports Sci* 22:703–725.

Tesco G, Kim TW, Diehlmann A, Beyreuther K, Tanzi RE (1998) Abrogation of the presenilin 1/beta-catenin interaction and preservation of the heterodimeric presenilin 1 complex following caspase activation. *J Biol Chem* 273:33909–33914.

Thinakaran G, Koo EH (2008) Amyloid precursor protein trafficking, processing, and function. *J Biol Chem* 283:29615–29619.

Treves A, Tashiro A, Witter MP, Moser EI (2008) What is the mammalian dentate gyrus good for? *Neuroscience* 154:1155–1172.

Trinchese F, Liu S, Battaglia F, Walter S, Mathews PM, Arancio O (2004) Progressive age-related development of Alzheimer-like pathology in APP/PS1 mice. *Ann Neurol* 55:801–814.

Tropepe V, Craig CG, Morshead CM, van der Kooy D (1997) Transforming growth factor-alpha null and senescent mice show decreased neural progenitor cell proliferation in the forebrain subependyma. *J Neurosci* 17:7850–7859.

van Praag H, Christie BR, Sejnowski TJ, Gage FH (1999) Running enhances neurogenesis, learning, and long-term potentiation in mice. *Proc Natl Acad Sci U S A* 96:13427–13431.

van Praag H, Schinder AF, Christie BR, Toni N, Palmer TD, Gage FH (2002) Functional neurogenesis in the adult hippocampus. *Nature* 415:1030–1034.

Verret L, Jankowsky JL, Xu GM, Borchelt DR, Rampon C (2007) Alzheimer's-type amyloidosis in transgenic mice impairs survival of newborn neurons derived from adult hippocampal neurogenesis. *J Neurosci* 27:6771–6780.

Villeda SA *et al.* (2011) The ageing systemic milieu negatively regulates neurogenesis and cognitive function. *Nature* 477:90–94.

Wang R, Dineley KT, Sweatt JD, Zheng H (2004) Presenilin 1 familial Alzheimer's disease mutation leads to defective associative learning and impaired adult neurogenesis. *Neuroscience* 126:305–312.

Warner MD, Peabody CA, Flattery JJ, Tinklenberg JR (1986) Olfactory deficits and Alzheimer's disease. *Biol Psychiatry* 21:116–118.

Wen PH, Hof PR, Chen X, Gluck K, Austin G, Younkin SG, Younkin LH, DeGasperi R, Gama Sosa MA, Robakis NK, Haroutunian V, Elder GA (2004) The presenilin-1 familial Alzheimer disease mutant P117L impairs neurogenesis in the hippocampus of adult mice. *Exp Neurol* 188:224–237.

Wilson RS, Arnold SE, Schneider JA, Tang Y, Bennett DA (2007) The relationship between cerebral Alzheimer's disease pathology and odour identification in old age. *J Neurol Neurosurg Psychiatry* 78:30–35.

Wilson RS, Bennett DA, Bienias JL, Aggarwal NT, Mendes De Leon CF, Morris MC, Schneider JA, Evans DA (2002) Cognitive activity and incident AD in a population-based sample of older persons. *Neurology* 59:1910–1914.

Winocur G, Wojtowicz JM, Sekeres M, Snyder JS, Wang S (2006) Inhibition of neurogenesis interferes with hippocampus-dependent memory function. *Hippocampus* 16:296–304.

Wiskott L, Rasch MJ, Kempermann G (2006) A functional hypothesis for adult hippocampal neurogenesis: avoidance of catastrophic interference in the dentate gyrus. *Hippocampus* 16:329–343.

Wolf SA, Kronenberg G, Lehmann K, Blankenship A, Overall R, Staufenbiel M, Kempermann G (2006) Cognitive and Physical Activity Differently Modulate Disease Progression in the Amyloid Precursor Protein (APP)-23 Model of Alzheimer's Disease. *Biol Psychiatry* 60:1314–1323.

Wong PC, Zheng H, Chen H, Becher MW, Sirinathsinghji DJ, Trumbauer ME, Chen HY, Price DL, Van der Ploeg LH, Sisodia SS (1997) Presenilin 1 is required for Notch1 and Dll1 expression in the paraxial mesoderm. *Nature* 387:288–292.

Yamasaki TR, Blurton-Jones M, Morrissette DA, Kitazawa M, Oddo S, LaFerla FM (2007) Neural stem cells improve memory in an inducible mouse model of neuronal loss. *J Neurosci* 27:11925–11933.

Yan R, Munzner JB, Shuck ME, Bienkowski MJ (2001) BACE2 functions as an alternative alpha-secretase in cells. *J Biol Chem* 276:34019–34027.

Yang P, Baker KA, Hagg T (2005) A disintegrin and metalloprotease 21 (ADAM21) is associated with neurogenesis and axonal growth in developing and adult rodent CNS. *J Comp Neurol* 490:163–179.

Yang P, Baker KA, Hagg T (2006) The ADAMs family: coordinators of nervous system development, plasticity and repair. *Prog Neurobiol* 79:73–94.

Young JW, Kerr LE, Kelly JS, Marston HM, Spratt C, Finlayson K, Sharkey J (2007) The odour span task: A novel paradigm for assessing working memory in mice. *Neuropharmacology* 52:634–645.

Yu H, Saura CA, Choi SY, Sun LD, Yang X, Handler M, Kawarabayashi T, Younkin L, Fedeles B, Wilson MA, Younkin S, Kandel ER, Kirkwood A, Shen J (2001) APP processing and synaptic plasticity in presenilin-1 conditional knockout mice. *Neuron* 31:713–726.

Zhang C, McNeil E, Dressler L, Siman R (2007a) Long-lasting impairment in hippocampal neurogenesis associated with amyloid deposition in a knock-in mouse model of familial Alzheimer's disease. *Exp Neurol* 204: 77–87.

Zhang CL, Zou Y, He W, Gage FH, Evans RM (2008) A role for adult TLX-positive neural stem cells in learning and behaviour. *Nature* 451: 1004–1007.

Zhang YW, Wang R, Liu Q, Zhang H, Liao FF, Xu H (2007b) Presenilin/gamma-secretase-dependent processing of beta-amyloid precursor protein regulates EGF receptor expression. *Proc Natl Acad Sci U S A* 104: 10613–10618.

Zhao X, Ueba T, Christie BR, Barkho B, McConnell MJ, Nakashima K, Lein ES, Eadie BD, Willhoite AR, Muotri AR, Summers RG, Chun J, Lee KF, Gage FH (2003) Mice lacking methyl-CpG binding protein 1 have deficits in adult neurogenesis and hippocampal function. *Proc Natl Acad Sci U S A* 100:6777–6782.

Zhao Z, Sun P, Chauhan N, Kaur J, Hill MD, Papadakis M, Buchan AM (2006) Neuroprotection and neurogenesis: modulation of cornus ammonis 1 neuronal survival after transient forebrain ischemia by prior fimbria-fornix deafferentation. *Neuroscience* 140:219–226.

Chapter 9

Roles of Neural Stem Cells in Alcohol Use Disorders

Jennifer L. Wagner, Emily A. Barton, Chelsea R. Geil,
J. Leigh Leasure, and Kimberly Nixon

Alcohol use disorders remain a major public health issue with exorbitant costs to the individual, families, and society. Excessive alcohol drinking, the defining characteristic of an alcohol use disorder, results in cognitive, behavioral and neurological dysfunction, some of which may recover with abstinence. Both the dysfunction as well as recovery may be the result of alcohol-induced effects on neural stem cells. This chapter will discuss the detrimental effects of alcohol intoxication and dependence on neural stem cells and adult neurogenesis, as well as the even lesser known effects on adult gliogenesis. Furthermore, reactive increases in neural stem cell proliferation and neurogenesis have been observed in abstinence from alcohol dependence. Thus, neural stem cells have many roles in alcoholism, whether contributing to the neuropathology or self-repair mechanisms in abstinence. Either way, as neural stem cells contribute to hippocampal integrity, a better understanding of the effects of alcohol on neural stem cells could lead to novel treatment options to prevent or reverse alcoholic neuropathology.

Introduction

The discovery that the mammalian brain is capable of generating newborn neurons throughout life has changed the way we think about the mechanisms, causes and treatment of psychiatric and neurodegenerative conditions such as the alcohol use disorders (AUDs; Eisch, 2002). This change in viewpoint is especially true for AUDs because excessive alcohol consumption is preferentially neurotoxic to these same regions that contain neural stem cells (NSCs) and are permissive to adult neurogenesis. This chapter defines the AUDs and their common neurological sequelae, then reviews the potential role that NSCs may have in alcohol-induced neurodegeneration during alcohol intoxication and/or dependence, but also in the promotion of self-repair and recovery mechanisms in abstinence.

Alcohol Use Disorders and Neurological Deficits

The compulsive use of alcohol, or alcoholism, remains one of the world's major public health issues. In the United States alone, 8.5% of the population meets diagnostic criteria for an AUD (Grant *et al.*, 2007), which is characterized by: (1) compulsion to take the drug; (2) loss of control over intake; and (3) a negative emotional state in the absence of the drug (Koob and Volkow, 2010). Compulsion to seek alcohol, and loss of control over its intake, may stem from dysfunction in prefrontal cortical behavioral control circuits, which can no longer control mesolimbic reward system drive (Baler and Volkow, 2006; Wilcox *et al.*, 2014). Alcohol damages frontal cortices, which have primary roles in executive function, working memory, and other cognitive functions, but also damages limbic regions, which are receiving new attention because of their direct inputs to frontal cortices [reviewed in (Crews and Nixon, 2009)]. For example, the hippocampus was thought to be solely involved in learning and memory (Eichenbaum, 2004) and therefore it was believed that its role in substance use disorders involved formation of context-dependent drug memories [reviewed in (Geil *et al.*, 2014; Hyman *et al.*, 2006)]. However, compelling evidence has built a case for hippocampal involvement in drug seeking, and even relapse, primarily through its interconnections with frontal cortices and mesolimbic reward systems (Belujon and Grace, 2011; Godsil *et al.*, 2013). Indeed, glutamatergic efferents from the hippocampus to the prefrontal cortex are implicated in executive function and working memory (Godsil *et al.*, 2013), which has led to the hypothesis that disruptions in the hippocampus could subsequently underlie impairments in these "cortical" functions. Therefore, understanding what factors contribute to alcohol-induced degeneration in the hippocampus and frontal cortices are critical to our understanding of how AUDs develop.

Excessive alcohol consumption results in a wide array of neuropsychological deficits, though the frontal cortices and associated behaviors appear to be particularly susceptible (Crews and Nixon, 2009; Parsons, 1993; Sullivan and Pfefferbaum, 2005). Interestingly, many of these impairments are subserved by the hippocampus either directly or indirectly, as discussed above (Chanraud *et al.*, 2007; Ozsoy *et al.*, 2013; Parsons, 1993).

Post-mortem tissue and imaging technology have provided evidence of neurodegeneration associated with heavy alcohol exposure (Harper, 1985; 2009; Pfefferbaum *et al.*, 1992; Sullivan and Pfefferbaum, 2005). Collectively, such studies show that the hippocampus and cerebral cortex are among the most alcohol-vulnerable gray matter structures.[1] Historically, the data on human hippocampal neurodegeneration has been quite mixed: reports vary as to whether volume loss occurs in either the right, left, or both hippocampi, and whether degeneration was due to white matter or gray matter loss (Agartz *et al.*, 1999; Bengochea and Gonzalo, 1990; Harding *et al.*, 1997; Laakso *et al.*, 2000; Sullivan *et al.*, 1995). As well, one group reported astroglial loss was the major contributor to hippocampal neurodegeneration (Korbo, 1999). More

---

[1]Alcohol has significant neurotoxic effects on the cerebellum that results in clinically distinct ataxia in severe AUDs. The cerebellum, however, lacks a well-accepted neural stem cell population and therefore including its pathology in this discussion is outside the scope of this chapter.

recently, however, several groups have shown hippocampal neuro-degeneration (Beresford *et al.*, 2006; De Bellis *et al.*, 2000; Nagel *et al.*, 2005; Ozsoy *et al.*, 2013) and specifically hippocampal grey matter degeneration in humans with AUDs (Chanraud *et al.*, 2007; Mechtcheriakov *et al.*, 2007).

Animal models have been essential for teasing apart the discrepancies in the human literature. In fact, animal research produced direct evidence that alcohol is neurotoxic to hippocampal structure and function (Riley and Walker, 1978; Walker *et al.*, 1980). For example, chronic ethanol liquid diet reduces dentate gyrus and pyramidal cell number as well as dendritic branching in both populations, all of which contribute to hippocampal volume loss (Riley and Walker, 1978; Walker *et al.*, 1980). Striking neurodegeneration (Collins *et al.*, 1996) has been observed in a four-day model of alcohol dependence with high-blood ethanol concentrations characteristic of binge-pattern drinking; whereas evidence of perturbation can be observed with as little as 24 hours of binge-like exposure (Hayes *et al.*, 2013). In sum, the recent human data when coupled with animal models support that the hippocampus is highly susceptible to ethanol neurotoxicity.

Although some of the discrepancies in the human hippocampal pathology literature can be explained away by the technological limitations of the time, the idea that hippocampal neurogenesis contributes to recovery in abstinence was not considered because of the former dogma that neurons were not born or replaced in adulthood. Other plastic processes such as dendritic expansion (Cadete-Leite *et al.*, 1988), recovery of synapse number (Lukoyanov *et al.*, 2000), and spine density (King, 1988) were assumed to account for recovery of volume loss, but the contribution of these events has always seemed inadequate to explain the recovery of such significant volume loss. Furthermore, it seems more than coincidental that brain regions with populations of NSCs overlap with the regions that appear to recover with abstinence (Armstrong and Barker, 2001; Nixon, 2006). The fact that many alcoholics recover brain mass in abstinence is consistent with the idea that NSCs could regenerate or repopulate some portions of the CNS and contribute to recovery of the associated circuits.

Neural Stem Cells and Adult Neurogenesis and Gliogenesis

Adult neurogenesis or gliogenesis describe the proliferation, differentiation into a neuron or glia, migration, and incorporation of newborn cells into cellular networks. Although gliogenesis occurs widely throughout the brain, the adult mammalian brain has two regions that contain NSCs and are permissive to adult neurogenesis under normal conditions: (1) the subventricular zone (SVZ), which generates cells that migrate and incorporate into the olfactory bulb (Alvarez-Buylla and Lois, 1995); and (2) the subgranular zone (SGZ) of the dentate gyrus, which generates cells that join the network of the hippocampal formation (Palmer *et al.*, 1997). These multipotent, proliferating NSCs, by definition, are not fate restricted and thus are able to differentiate into neurons, astrocytes or oligodendrocytes, although more than 80% of NSCs generated in the SGZ go on to adopt a neuronal fate (Brown *et al.*, 2003). The majority of the remaining adult-born cells mature into astroglia (Cameron *et al.*, 1993). Although much evidence exists that these newborn neurons integrate into the hippocampal circuitry as dentate gyrus granule cells (Gould *et al.*, 1999), the function of these new neurons remains an active area of investigation (Kempermann, 2008; Lacar *et al.*, 2014; Shors *et al.*, 2001). Given their location and role in maintaining the structure of the hippocampus, new neurons are thought to be involved in learning and memory (Aimone *et al.*, 2006; Imayoshi *et al.*, 2008; Shors *et al.*, 2012) [see also (Snyder and Cameron, 2012) for review]. In rodents, SVZ neurogenesis appears to play a role in olfaction (Breton-Provencher *et al.*, 2009); however recent work has led to doubt about a homologous population in adult humans (Sanai *et al.*, 2011). As these debates are chapters unto themselves, this chapter focuses primarily on hippocampal adult neurogenesis. A population of hippocampal NSCs is well accepted in humans (Eriksson *et al.*, 1998) and hippocampal degeneration and recovery in AUDs supports the existence of such a plastic process.

Neural Stem Cells in Alcoholic Neurodegeneration

Alcohol and neurogenesis

Numerous reviews have described early work reporting the effects of alcohol on adult NSC and neurogenesis (Crews *et al.*, 2003; Nixon, 2006; Nixon *et al.*, 2010). Reports have shown consistently that alcohol inhibits adult neurogenesis, at least when neurogenesis truly has been examined (and not cell proliferation). The mechanism of this inhibition is where things get interesting. To begin in reverse order of the four mechanistic components of neurogenesis, alcohol's effects on cell survival clearly contribute to alcohol inhibition of adult neurogenesis (Herrera *et al.*, 2003; Nixon and Crews, 2002). Alcohol is also a well-described neurotoxin and developing cells may be particularly susceptible to alcohol toxicity (Crews and Nixon; 2009; Goodlett and Johnson, 1999). By estimating putative newborn cell survival with BrdU pulse-chase technology, the duration of alcohol exposure appears to be a major factor in whether alcohol impacts the survival of newborn cells independently of its effects on cell proliferation (Nixon and Crews, 2002). Next, few studies have reported or observed any effect of alcohol on differentiation or new cell migration in adult models. In addition, these studies did not examine differentiation per se, but merely which cell population was dividing. A handful of studies in models of Fetal Alcohol Syndrome, however, have reported a potential effect of alcohol on cell differentiation (Marcussen *et al.*, 1994; Vangipuram and Lyman, 2010; Zhou *et al.*, 2011). While altered cell migration is a major factor in fetal alcohol spectrum disorders (Charness *et al.*, 1994), nothing has been reported to date or observed, even upon examination of new neuron location in adult or adolescent models. Again, that does not mean alcohol does not have these effects in adult neurogenesis, but the effects either have not been striking enough or experiments were not designed to test this question specifically. Finally, alcohol's effects on NSC proliferation are where the field is most interesting. Therefore, this section integrates the more recent work on alcohol and NSC proliferation in an attempt to reconcile these seemingly divergent reports.

Since the original findings that ethanol reduced cell proliferation as a mechanism of reducing adult neurogenesis (Nixon and Crews, 2002), evidence continues to build that alcohol-induced effects on NSC proliferation may be dose-dependent or blood ethanol concentration-dependent [reports from 2002–2006 reviewed in (Nixon, 2006)]. More recent reports continue to support that ethanol intoxication dose- or blood ethanol concentration-dependently decreases the number of dividing cells in the SGZ of the dentate gyrus and SVZ (Campbell *et al.*, 2014; Contet *et al.*, 2013; Hansson *et al.*, 2010; Richardson *et al.*, 2009; Taffe *et al.*, 2010) [see also (Geil *et al.*, 2014) for review]. The devil is really in the details, as these findings below initially seem divergent until one examines, the differences in exposures, timing of analysis, blood alcohol levels and markers used; only then some consistencies do emerge. Acutely, alcohol intoxication reduces the number of cells in the S-phase of the cell cycle as labeled by BrdU (Crews *et al.*, 2006; Jang *et al.*, 2002; Nixon and Crews, 2002), which is consistent with its anti-proliferative effect in many cell populations as well as in development (Cook *et al.*, 1990) [see (Luo and Miller, 1998) for review]. In exposure models that are more chronic, there is clearly some threshold or dose-dependency of blood alcohol concentration above which cell proliferation is decreased. The concept of a threshold best explains the divergent findings from a few chronic exposure studies where low doses or low blood alcohol levels either increased (Aberg *et al.*, 2005; Pawlak *et al.*, 2002), or had no effect on dentate gyrus cell proliferation (Campbell *et al.*, 2014; Crews *et al.*, 2006; Jang *et al.*, 2002). It is of note that in studies where little to no effect of alcohol was seen on cell proliferation, the experiments were conducted in mice with voluntary drinking exposure that typically results in only moderate blood ethanol concentrations [18–24 mg%; e.g. (Aberg *et al.*, 2005; Campbell *et al.*, 2014)]. Therefore, alcohol effects on NSC proliferation in the SGZ appear to be dose-dependent but those cells may also be sensitive to the duration of exposure.

Although alcohol can arrest the cell cycle in other cell populations, which is likely the case with these acute exposures, alcohol may also reduce the number of cells that are actively cycling [i.e. Ki67-positive (+), the well-accepted marker for cells that are actively dividing (Scholzen and Gerdes, 2000; Crews *et al.*, 2006)]. Alcohol may either keep NSCs in quiescence (G_0) or kill dividing cells. The latter has been suggested in several studies where alcohol intoxication is separated in time from tissue harvesting (Contet *et al.*, 2013; Ehlers *et al.*, 2013; Hanson *et al.*, 2010; Taffe *et al.*, 2010). It is also important to note that persistent reductions in the actively cycling pool, typically measured as the number Ki67+ cells, only seems to occur in more chronic exposure models. For example, following four days of binge-like exposure, there is little evidence for a persistent decrease in NSC proliferation as the number of BrdU+ cells returns to control levels for a few days after alcohol exposure and before "reactive neurogenesis" is observed (McClain *et al.*, 2013; Nixon and Crews, 2004). These data, however, still leave the question as to whether it is a reduction in the number of cycling cells or some effect on the cell cycle. Either mechanism is plausible and supported by literature, but requires a time intensive assay of the cell cycle. Thus, exploring the effect of alcohol on the NSC cycle remains a critical gap in our knowledge.

Across the adult neurogenesis/neural stem cell literature in general, only a few groups have employed multiple approaches or even endogenous markers in order to address the mechanism by which a drug affects adult neurogenesis. For example, adolescent rats immediately following their last dose of ethanol in a 4-day binge model have reduced BrdU+ cells due to an acceleration of the cell cycle (McClain *et al.*, 2011; Morris *et al.*, 2010). This discovery only emerged when the endogenous cell cycle marker, Ki67, was observed to not be reduced following ethanol exposure despite reductions in BrdU at proliferation and 'survival' time points (Morris *et al.*, 2010). Therefore, these data suggest that exposure to acute or short durations of high peak blood alcohol levels may impact the cell cycle to have a net effect of decreasing adult neurogenesis, while longer, chronic exposures to moderate (125–250 mg%; Contet *et al.*, 2013; Richardson *et al.*, 2009) and high (>250%; McClain *et al.*, 2011) blood alcohol levels may permanently reduce the number of proliferating cells.

Studies of the effects of alcohol on NSCs in the SVZ are few, perhaps due in part to the decreased relevance of this region to the human condition, especially when compared to the ease of translation of hippocampal deficits between animal models of AUDs and human alcoholics. Although some have reported similar populations of newborn cells in the adult human brain (Bedard and Parent, 2004), others have not (Sanai *et al.*, 2011). Effects across models are more consistent for the SVZ, both the short, 4-day binge model in adolescent rats (Crews *et al.*, 2006) and chronic voluntary drinking in mice (Crews *et al.*, 2004b) resulted in a decrease in the number of proliferating cells (BrdU+ cells). Furthermore, recent work has directly examined this effect and shown that voluntary moderate alcohol intake in mice decreases NSC proliferation in the SVZ without altering the NSC pool or its capacity to form neurospheres (Campbell *et al.*, 2014). Similar to the hippocampus, chronic exposure results in an enduring suppression of proliferation in the SVZ using a high-dose, dependence-inducing model of chronic alcohol-vapor in rats (Hansson *et al.*, 2010). Intriguingly, this study found that dentate gyrus neurogenesis recovered within three weeks in these animals, whereas SVZ neurogenesis did not rebound. This effect was purportedly due to the depletion of the NSC pool, illustrated by a deficit in SOX2-expressing cells that persisted at least three weeks (Hansson *et al.*, 2010). A postmortem study of human alcoholic brain has failed to find differences in "proliferation" in the SVZ compared to normal controls (Sutherland *et al.*, 2013). Although the authors of this study described their results as a lack of difference in cell proliferation between alcoholics and normal controls (Sutherland *et al.*, 2013), the markers chosen in this study, proliferating cell nuclear antigen (PCNA) and Ki67, do not support that conclusion. PCNA is not specific to the cell cycle and may be induced by DNA repair or cell death, both of which occur in alcoholism (Wang, 2014). Ki67 identifies cells in the active portion of the cell cycle, therefore it merely suggests that the actively dividing pool of NSCs is not different between alcoholics and normal controls, which is identical to previous reports in SVZ in rats (Campbell *et al.*, 2014), as well as the SGZ in adolescent rats (Morris *et al.*, 2010).

Additional work is critically needed to determine whether cell proliferation is impacted in the human brain similar to what has been reported in animal models.

Alcohol and gliogenesis

It is abundantly clear that alcohol intoxication diminishes cell proliferation in the brain. The focus, historically, has been on neurogenesis, and the concern that alcohol suppresses the normal creation, survival and maturation of neurons, contributing ultimately to alcohol-induced neurodegeneration (Morris *et al.*, 2010; Nixon, 2006; Nixon and Crews, 2002). However, neurons are not the only brain cells that are generated throughout the life of the brain. Glia, specifically macroglia (astroglia, oligodendroglia) are also continuously generated, and represent a crucial support network for neurons. A great deal is known about the effects of alcohol on NSCs and neurogenesis. Comparably little, however, is known about the effects of alcohol on gliogenesis.

The importance of glia for neuronal health

Neurons exist within a supportive system of glial cells (see Figure 1). Glial cells have a diverse range of functions, including releasing neurotrophins, monitoring and cleaning the neural microenvironment, aiding in communication, and providing metabolic support to neurons (Barzilai, 2011; Streit, 2002, 2005; Streit and Xue, 2009). In essence, glia are a supportive system necessary for sustaining neuronal health and proper functioning. Thus, glial function determines the overall state of the neuronal environment (Banker, 1980; Giaume *et al.*, 2007; Wagner *et al.*, 2006), meaning when the glial support system fails, neuronal health breaks down. This idea has been elegantly stated by Barzilai (2011), "Brain pathology, is, to a very great extent, a pathology of glia: the outcome and the scale of neurological deficit is dependent on the degree of dysfunction of glial cells."

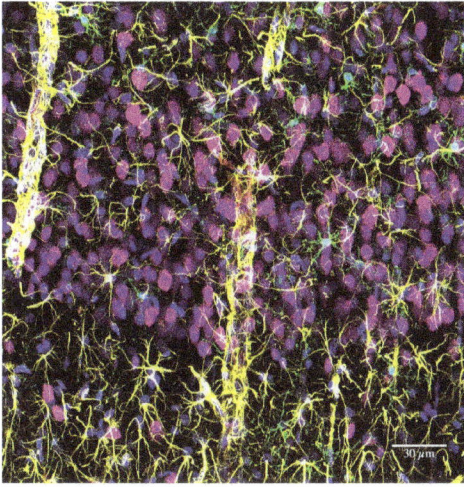

Figure 1. Multi-channel confocal image showing neurons (pink) amidst glia and vasculature. Blood vessels are visible in red, astrocyte arbors in yellow and microglial cells in green. Scale bar = 30 μm.

Alcohol and gliogenesis

Alcohol effects on gliogenesis have largely been studied in the context of developmental exposure. For example, radial glia, which act as both neural precursor cells and guides for migrating neurons, show a marked sensitivity to developmental ethanol exposure. Exposure to ethanol during development causes radial glia morphological defects, delayed neuronal migration, and decreased numbers of neuroblasts (Aronne *et al.*, 2011). Alcohol effects on radial glia in turn impact cortical astrocyte development — chronic ethanol exposure during rat embryogenesis delays the differentiation of radial glia cells into astrocytes and significantly disrupts astrogliogenesis (Rubert *et al.*, 2006; Valles *et al.*, 1997; Vemuri and Chetty, 2005). Additionally, chronic ethanol consumption during gestation causes significant damage to cortical astrocyte progenitor cells and alters astrocyte growth and cytoskeleton formation (Guerri *et al.*, 1990). Oligodendrocyte precursor cells are also sensitive to developmental alcohol exposure (Godin *et al.*, 2011).

While it is clear that early exposure to alcohol is detrimental to glial cell development and proliferation, much less is known about the effects of alcohol on gliogenesis in the adult brain. Given the importance of glia for neuronal health and function, they represent appealing therapeutic targets; especially since, unlike neurons; they are generated in all regions of the adult brain, throughout the lifespan. Moreover, in neurogenic regions, gliogenesis and neurogenesis occur concurrently and are tightly linked [for review see (Morrens *et al.*, 2012)]. To illustrate, astrocytes are produced alongside neurons in neurogenic regions of the adult brain. Mature, postmitotic astrocytes emerge from precursor cells (Encinas *et al.*, 2011; Kuhn *et al.*, 1996; Suh *et al.*, 2007). Thus, its profound suppressive effect on cell genesis means that alcohol has the power to influence astrocyte numbers.

Alcohol has well-documented effects on glia in human alcoholic brain as well as animal models of alcoholism (Harper, 1985; Korbo, 1999; Miguel-Hidalgo *et al.*, 2002; Rintala *et al.*, 2001; Sullivan *et al.*, 1996) with few disagreements (Dlugos and Pentney, 2001; Fabricius *et al.*, 2007). Indeed, some suggest that glia may be more sensitive to alcohol toxicity than neurons, which leads to the similar conclusion of Barzilai above: glial pathology could be the primary basis of alcoholic neuropathology (Harper and Krill, 1990; Korbo, 1999; Miguel-Hidalgo *et al.*, 2002). Alcohol has been shown, also, to affect cell proliferation in non-neurogenic regions of the brain. Cell proliferation in non-neurogenic regions is assumed to reflect production of glia, and evidence from a rodent model of alcohol dependence indicates that cell genesis in the cortex is permanently suppressed (Richardson *et al.*, 2009). Oligodendrocytes emerge from oligodendrocyte precursor cells [for review, see (Morrens *et al.*, 2012)]. Given the prominent white matter loss seen in alcoholics (Pfefferbaum, 1996; Sullivan and Pfefferbaum, 2005), alcohol would be expected to have marked effects on generation of oligodendrocytes. Indeed, it has recently been demonstrated that chronic intermittent ethanol exposure diminishes the proliferative activity of oligodendrocyte precursor cells in the medial prefrontal cortex (Kim *et al.*, 2014).

To summarize, what evidence is available strongly indicates a profound suppressive effect of alcohol on gliogenesis in corticolimbic brain regions. It is likely that this deficit in available glial support contributes to alcohol effects on both neurogenesis and neuronal function. However, on the positive side, this means that promoting the health of glia, which are continuously generated throughout the entire brain during the lifespan, represents a viable means by which to promote health in the normal brain, and recovery in the damaged brain.

Potential Role of Neural Stem Cells in Recovery from Alcoholism

The alcoholic's brain and behavior can recover, at least partially, with sustained abstinence, which supports that some type of plastic mechanism exists that aids in recovery of neural function (Carlen *et al.*, 1978; Fein *et al.*, 2006; Pfefferbaum *et al.*, 1995; Sullivan *et al.*, 2000a, b). There are many possible mechanisms of this recovery as glia proliferate and regenerate after damage, while axons and dendrites may extend and elaborate to produce new synapses (Cadete-Leite *et al.*, 1988; King, 1988; Lukoyanov *et al.*, 2000). Indeed, many have assumed that recovery from alcoholic neurodegeneration was primarily glial in nature (Harper, 1998). Although this is likely the case in non-neurogenic regions, in neurogenic regions such as the hippocampus, the ability of NSC to self-repair or repopulate the dentate gyrus must be considered (Armstrong and Barker, 2001). Moreover, adult neurogenesis can be enhanced through manipulations of environment, behavior, and certain drugs, which highlights possible means to induce the repair and recovery of neurogenic regions such as the hippocampus (Kozorovitskiy and Gould, 2003; Ming and Song, 2011).

Reactive neurogenesis: a mechanism of self-repair?

In many models of brain insult, including traumatic brain injury, seizure, ischemia, excitotoxic lesions, and AUD, there is a compensatory response in NSC proliferation referred to as reactive neurogenesis (Dash *et al.*, 2001; Gould and Tanapat, 1997; Jin *et al.*, 2001; Nixon and Crews, 2004; Parent *et al.*, 1997). Certainly, excessive alcohol exposure is a significant insult to the brain, resulting in cell death and degeneration (Collins *et al.*, 1996; Kelso *et al.*, 2011; Obernier *et al.*, 2002; Walker *et al.*, 1980). As such, reactive increases in NSC proliferation have been observed after either chronic vapor or drinking and especially in an acutely damaging 4-day binge model (Hansson *et al.*, 2010; He *et al.*, 2005; Nixon and Crews, 2004). Specifically, seven days after binge alcohol exposure there is an increase in NSC proliferation which drives a subsequent increase in neurogenesis as measured by both endogenous markers such as doublecortin, but also the gold standard pulse and chase with BrdU, co-labeled with the neuron-specific marker, NeuN (McClain *et al.*, 2013; Nixon and Crews, 2004). Interestingly, this burst in proliferation is transient; NSC proliferation returns to normal by 10 days of exposure (unpublished observations; Nixon *et al.*, 2008). Thus far, reactive neurogenesis is associated with the recovery of dentate gyrus granule cell number at a month in abstinence in male Sprague-Dawley rats (unpublished observations), but not female Long-Evans rats (Maynard and Leasure, 2013). Although the literature suggests that alcohol-induced reactive proliferation may act as a mechanism of hippocampal self-repair, many questions remain about whether cells born during this event develop and integrate normally (Parent and Lowenstein, 2002; Turnley *et al.*, 2014). Studies are needed also to determine whether neurons born during reactive neurogenesis mature and function normally, survive long-term, and/or contribute to recovery. Although it is reasonable to presume that reactive neurogenesis contributes to some level of regeneration, the extent of that repair may be limited (Turnley *et al.*, 2014). As mentioned above, in female Long Evans rats, a decrement in the number of hippocampal granule cells was recently reported at 35 days in abstinence, though long-term time points have not been explored (Maynard and Leasure, 2013). It is possible that rates of adult neurogenesis need to normalize in order for dentate gyrus cell number to also fully normalize

(Mandyam and Koob, 2012). This idea implies that functional recovery will only be observed months after abstinence.

Manipulating NSC for brain repair

Many groups have speculated about the therapeutic potential of endogenous NSCs in hippocampal-related disorders (Taylor *et al.*, 2013). As increases in neurogenesis are associated with improvements in learning and memory (Gould *et al.*, 1999; van Praag *et al.*, 1999), there have been a host of studies which have identified behaviors, environments, and drugs that can promote adult neurogenesis (and notably gliogenesis as well) and potentially enhance cognition (Ming and Song, 2011; Taylor *et al.*, 2013). Thus, exploiting the pool of quiescent progenitor cells may represent a resource for repairing alcohol-induced hippocampal damage.

One means of promoting neurogenesis that has been explored in alcohol-induced neurodegeneration is voluntary exercise (Crews *et al.*, 2004; Leasure and Nixon, 2010; Maynard and Leasure, 2013). In contrast to alcohol, which damages the brain, exercise enhances brain health (Cotman *et al.*, 2007; Gomez-Pinilla *et al.*, 2008; Hillman *et al.*, 2008). One of the neural benefits of exercise is an increase in the availability of neurotrophic factors (Gomez-Pinilla *et al.*, 1997; Gomez-Pinilla *et al.*, 2008; Vaynman and Gomez-Pinilla, 2005; Vaynman *et al.*, 2004). It is possible that the reason that post-binge hippocampal self-repair is incomplete is that there is insufficient trophic support available to both heal mature granule neurons damaged by alcohol and sustain the development of those generated post-binge. We therefore asked the question whether these self-repair attempts could be augmented by voluntary exercise by giving animals access to exercise for 28 days beginning one week post-binge. We found that the volume of the dentate gyrus in binged, exercised animals was identical to that of non-binged controls (Maynard and Leasure, 2013). Though the evidence is only correlative, this upholds the idea that neurotrophic support is necessary in order to heal the alcohol-damaged hippocampus, and that exercise is a useful method to augment trophic support.

Conclusions

In conclusion, NSCs play a variety of roles in the alcoholic brain. Moderate to high dose binge-like and chronic exposures reduce the proliferation of neural stem cells and impact survival of newborn neurons to reduce neurogenesis. Conversely, upon abstinence, reactive neurogenesis may serve to repopulate the damaged dentate gyrus, but studies are needed to determine whether these cells are in fact an adaptive form of recovery. In both cases, little is known about the mechanism of these effects. Therefore, significant gaps in our knowledge of alcohol effects on NSC remain. A better understanding of how alcohol affects NSCs could lead to the identification of novel pharmacological targets for the prevention or treatment of alcoholic neuropathology.

Acknowledgements

The authors and authors' work are supported by the National Institute of Alcohol Abuse and Alcoholism R01AA016959 (KN), R21AA021260 (JLL), F31AA023459 (CRG), and the National Institute of Drug Abuse T32DA016176 (CRG).

References

Aberg E, Hofstetter C, Olson L, Brene, S (2005) Moderate ethanol consumption increases hippocampal cell proliferation and neurogenesis in the adult mouse. *Int J Neuropsychopharmacol* 8:557–567.

Agartz I, Momenan R, Rawlings RR, Kerich MJ, Hommer DW (1999) Hippocampal volume in patients with alcohol dependence. *Arch Gen Psychiatry* 56:356–363.

Aimone JB, Wiles J, Gage FH (2006) Potential role for adult neurogenesis in the encoding of time in new memories. *Nat Neurosci* 9: 723–727.

Alvarez-Buylla A, Lois C (1995) Neuronal stem cells in the brain of adult vertebrates. *Stem Cells* 13:263–272.

Armstrong RJ, Barker RA (2001) Neurodegeneration: a failure of neuroregeneration? *Lancet* 358:1174–1176.

Aronne MP, Guadagnoli T, Fontanet P, Evrard SG, Brusco A (2011) Effects of prenatal ethanol exposure on rat brain radial glia and neuroblast migration. *Exp Neurol* 229:364–371.

Baler RD, Volkow ND (2006) Drug addiction: the neurobiology of disrupted self-control. *Trends Mol Med* 12:559–566.

Banker GA (1980) Trophic interactions between astroglial cells and hippocampal neurons in culture. *Science* 209:809–810.

Barzilai A (2011) The neuro-glial-vascular interrelations in genomic instability symptoms. *Mech Ageing Dev* 132:395–404.

Bedard A, Parent A (2004) Evidence of newly generated neurons in the human olfactory bulb. *Brain Res Dev Brain Res* 151:159–168.

Belujon P, Grace AA (2011) Hippocampus, amygdala, and stress: interacting systems that affect susceptibility to addiction. *Ann N Y Acad Sci* 1216:114–121.

Bengochea O, Gonzalo LM (1990) Effect of chronic alcoholism on the human hippocampus. *Histol Histopathol* 5:349–357.

Beresford TP, Arciniegas DB, Alfers J, Clapp L, Martin B, Du, Y, Liu D, Shen D, Davatzikos C (2006) Hippocampus volume loss due to chronic heavy drinking. *Alcohol Clin Exp Res* 30:1866–1870.

Breton-Provencher V, Lemasson M, Peralta MR 3rd, Saghatelyan A (2009) Interneurons produced in adulthood are required for the normal functioning of the olfactory bulb network and for the execution of selected olfactory behaviors. *J Neurosci* 29:15245–15257.

Brown JP, Couillard-Despres S, Cooper-Kuhn CM, Winkler J, Aigner L, Kuhn HG (2003) Transient expression of doublecortin during adult neurogenesis. *J Comp Neurol* 467:1–10.

Cadete-Leite A, Tavares MA, Uylings HBM, Paula-Barbosa MM (1988) Granule cell loss and dendritic regrowth in the hippocampal dentate gyrus of the rat after chronic alcohol consumption. *Brain Research* 473:1–14.

Cameron H A, Woolley CS, Gould E (1993) Adrenal steroid receptor immunoreactivity in cells born in the adult rat dentate gyrus. *Brain Research* 611:342–346.

Campbell JC, Stipcevic T, Flores RE, Perry C, Kippin TE (2014) Alcohol exposure inhibits adult neural stem cell proliferation. *Exp Brain Res* 232:2775–2784.

Carlen PL, Wortzman G, Holgate RC, Wilkinson DA, Rankin JC (1978) Reversible cerebral atrophy in recently abstinent chronic alcoholics measured by computed tomography scans. *Science* 200:1076–1078.

Chanraud S, Martelli C, Delain F, Kostogianni N, Douaud G, Aubin HJ, Reynaud M, Martinot JL (2007) Brain morphometry and cognitive performance in detoxified alcohol-dependents with preserved psychosocial functioning. *Neuropsychopharmacology* 32:429–438.

Charness ME, Safran RM, Perides G (1994) Ethanol inhibits neural cell-cell adhesion. *J Biol Chem* 269:9304–9309.

Collins MA, Corse TD, Neafsey EJ (1996) Neuronal degeneration in rat cerebrocortical and olfactory regions during subchronic "binge" intoxication with ethanol: possible explanation for olfactory deficits in alcoholics. *Alcohol Clin Exp Res* 20:284–292.

Contet C, Kim A, Le D, Iyengar SK, Kotzebue RW, Yuan CJ, Kieffer BL, Mandyam CD (2013) mu-Opioid receptors mediate the effects of chronic ethanol binge drinking on the hippocampal neurogenic niche. *Addict Biol* 19:770–780.

Cook RT, Keiner JA, Yen A (1990) Ethanol causes accelerated G1 arrest in differentiating HL-60 cells. *Alcohol Clin Exp Res* 14:695–703.

Cotman CW, Berchtold NC, Christie LA (2007) Exercise builds brain health: key roles of growth factor cascades and inflammation. *Trends Neurosci* 30:464–472.

Crews F, Nixon K, Kim D, Joseph J, Shukitt-Hale B, Qin L, Zou J (2006) BHT blocks NF-kappaB activation and ethanol-induced brain damage. *Alcohol Clin Exp Res* 30:1938–1949.

Crews FT, Collins MA, Dlugos C, Littleton J, Wilkins L, Neafsey EJ, Pentney R, Snell LD, Tabakoff B, Zou J, Noronha A (2004a) Alcohol-induced neurodegeneration: when, where and why? *Alcohol Clin Exp Res* 28: 350–364.

Crews FT, Mdzinarishvili A, Kim D, He J, Nixon K (2006) Neurogenesis in adolescent brain is potently inhibited by ethanol. *Neuroscience* 137: 437–445.

Crews FT, Miller MW, Ma W, Nixon K, Zawada WM, Zakhari S (2003) Neural stem cells and alcohol. *Alcohol Clin Exp Res* 27:324–335.

Crews FT, Nixon K (2009) Mechanisms of neurodegeneration and regeneration in alcoholism. *Alcohol Alcohol* 44:115–127.

Crews FT, Nixon K, Wilkie ME (2004b) Exercise reverses ethanol inhibition of neural stem cell proliferation. *Alcohol* 33:63–71.

Dash PK, Mach SA, Moore AN (2001) Enhanced neurogenesis in the rodent hippocampus following traumatic brain injury. *J Neurosci Res* 63:313–319.

De Bellis MD, Clark DB, Beers SR, Soloff PH, Boring AM, Hall J, Kersh A, Keshavan MS (2000) Hippocampal volume in adolescent-onset alcohol use disorders. *Am J Psychiatry* 157:737–744.

Dlugos CA, Pentney RJ (2001) Quantitative immunocytochemistry of glia in the cerebellar cortex of old ethanol-fed rats. *Alcohol* 23:63–69.

Ehlers CL, Liu W, Wills DN, Crews FT (2013) Periadolescent ethanol vapor exposure persistently reduces measures of hippocampal neurogenesis that are associated with behavioral outcomes in adulthood. *Neuroscience* 244:1–15.

Eichenbaum H (2004) Hippocampus: cognitive processes and neural representations that underlie declarative memory. *Neuron* 44:109–120.

Eisch AJ (2002) Adult neurogenesis: implications for psychiatry. *Prog Brain Res* 138:315–342.

Encinas JM, Michurina TV, Peunova N, Park JH, Tordo J, Peterson DA, Fishell G, Koulakov A, Enikolopov, G (2011) Division-coupled astrocytic differentiation and age-related depletion of neural stem cells in the adult hippocampus. *Cell Stem Cell* 8:566–579.

Eriksson PS, Perfilieva E, Bjork-Eriksson T, Alborn AM, Nordborg C, Peterson DA, Gage FH (1998) Neurogenesis in the adult human hippocampus. *Nat Med* 4:1313–1317.

Fabricius K, Pakkenberg H, Pakkenberg B (2007) No changes in neocortical cell volumes or glial cell numbers in chronic alcoholic subjects compared to control subjects. *Alcohol Alcohol* 42:400–406.

Fein G, Torres J, Price LJ, Di Sclafani V (2006) Cognitive performance in long-term abstinent alcoholic individuals. *Alcohol Clin Exp Res* 30: 1538–1544.

Geil CR, Hayes DM, McClain JA, Liput DJ, Marshall SA, Chen KY, Nixon K (2014) Alcohol and adult hippocampal neurogenesis: Promiscuous drug, wanton effects. *Prog Neuro-Psychopharm Biol Psych* 54C:103–113.

Giaume C, Kirchhoff F, Matute C, Reichenbach A, Verkhratsky A (2007) Glia: the fulcrum of brain diseases. *Cell Death Differ* 14:1324–1335.

Godin EA, Dehart DB, Parnell SE, O'Leary-Moore SK, Sulik KK (2011) Ventromedian forebrain dysgenesis follows early prenatal ethanol exposure in mice. *Neurotoxicol Teratol* 33:231–239.

Godsil BP, Kiss JP, Spedding M, Jay TM (2013) The hippocampal-prefrontal pathway: the weak link in psychiatric disorders? *Eur Neuropsychopharmacol* 23:1165–1181.

Gomez-Pinilla F, Dao L, So V (1997) Physical exercise induces FGF-2 and its mRNA in the hippocampus. *Brain Res* 764:1–8.

Gomez-Pinilla F, Vaynman S, Ying Z (2008) Brain-derived neurotrophic factor functions as a metabotrophin to mediate the effects of exercise on cognition. *Eur J Neurosci* 28:2278–2287.

Goodlett CR, Johnson TB (1999) Temporal windows of vulnerability within the third trimester equivalent: Why "knowing when" matters. In: *Alcohol and Alcoholism: Effects on Brain Development* (Hannigan JH, Spear LP, Spear NE, Goodlett CR eds.), pp. 1–16. New Jersey: Lawrence Erlbaum Associates.

Gould E, Beylin A, Tanapat P, Reeves A, Shors TJ (1999) Learning enhances adult neurogenesis in the hippocampal formation. *Nat Neurosci* 2: 260–265.

Gould E, Tanapat P (1997) Lesion-induced proliferation of neuronal progenitors in the dentate gyrus of the adult rat. *Neuroscience* 80: 427–436.

Grant BF, Harford TC, Muthen BO, Yi HY, Hasin DS, Stinson FS (2007) DSM-IV alcohol dependence and abuse: further evidence of validity in the general population. *Drug Alcohol Depend* 86:154–166.

Guerri C, Saez R, Sancho-Tello M, Martin de Aquilera E, Renau-Piqueras J (1990) Ethanol alters astrocyte development: a study of critical periods using primary cultures. *Neurochem Res* 15:559–565.

Hanson KL, Medina KL, Nagel BJ, Spadoni AD, Gorlick A, Tapert SF (2010) Hippocampal volumes in adolescents with and without a family history of alcoholism. *Am J Drug Alcohol Abuse* 36:161–167.

Hansson AC, Nixon K, Rimondini R, Damadzic R, Sommer WH, Eskay R, Crews FT, Heilig, M (2010) Long-term suppression of forebrain neurogenesis and loss of neuronal progenitor cells following prolonged alcohol dependence in rats. *Int J Neuropsychopharmacol* 13: 583–593.

Harding AJ, Wong A, Svoboda M, Kril JJ, Halliday GM (1997) Chronic alcohol consumption does not cause hippocampal neuron loss in humans. *Hippocampus* 7:78–87.

Harper C (1985). Brain atrophy in chronic alcoholic patients: a quantitative pathological study. *J Neurol Neurosurg Psychiatry* 48:211–217.

Harper C (1998) The neuropathology of alcohol-specific brain damage, or does alcohol damage the brain? *J Neuropathol Exp Neurol* 57:101–110.

Harper C (2009) The neuropathology of alcohol-related brain damage. *Alcohol Alcohol* 44:136–140.

Harper CB, Krill JJ (1990) Neuropathology of alcoholism. *Alcohol* 25: 207–216.

Hayes DM, Deeny MA, Shaner CA, Nixon K (2013) Determining the threshold for alcohol-induced brain damage: New evidence with gliosis markers. *Alcohol Clin Exp Res* 37:425–434.

He J, Nixon K, Shetty AK, Crews FT (2005) Chronic alcohol exposure reduces hippocampal neurogenesis and dendritic growth of newborn neurons. *Eur J Neurosci* 21:2711–2720.

Herrera DG, Yague AG, Johnsen-Soriano S, Bosch-Morell F, Collado-Morente L, Muriach M, Romero FJ, Garcia-Verdugo JM (2003) Selective impairment of hippocampal neurogenesis by chronic alcoholism: protective effects of an antioxidant. *Proc Natl Acad Sci U S A* 100: 7919–7924.

Hillman CH, Erickson KI, Kramer AF (2008) Be smart, exercise your heart: exercise effects on brain and cognition. *Nat Rev Neurosci* 9:58–65.

Hyman SE, Malenka RC, Nestler EJ (2006) Neural mechanisms of addiction: the role of reward-related learning and memory. *Annu Rev Neurosci* 29:565–598.

Imayoshi I, Sakamoto M, Ohtsuka T, Takao K, Miyakawa T, Yamaguchi M, Mori K, Ikeda T, Itohara S, Kageyama R (2008) Roles of continuous neurogenesis in the structural and functional integrity of the adult forebrain. *Nat Neurosci* 11:1153–1161.

Jang MH, Shin MC, Jung SB, Lee TH, Bahn GH, Kwon YK, Kim EH, Kim CJ (2002) Alcohol and nicotine reduce cell proliferation and enhance apoptosis in dentate gyrus. *Neuroreport* 13:1509–1513.

Jang MH, Shin MC, Kim EH, Kim CJ (2002) Acute alcohol intoxication decreases cell proliferation and nitric oxide synthase expression in dentate gyrus of rats. *Toxicol Lett* 133: 255–262.

Jin K, Minami M, Lan JQ, Mao XO, Batteur S, Simon RP, Greenberg DA (2001) Neurogenesis in dentate subgranular zone and rostral subventricular zone after focal cerebral ischemia in the rat. *Proc Natl Acad Sci U S A* 98:4710–4715.

Kelso ML, Liput DJ, Eaves DW, Nixon K (2011) Upregulated vimentin suggests new areas of neurodegeneration in a model of an alcohol use disorder. *Neuroscience* 197:381–393.

Kempermann G (2008) The neurogenic reserve hypothesis: what is adult hippocampal neurogenesis good for? *Trends Neurosci* 31:163–169.

Kim A, Zamora-Martinez ER, Edwards S, Mandyam CD (2014) Structural reorganization of pyramidal neurons in the medial prefrontal cortex of alcohol dependent rats is associated with altered glial plasticity. *Brain Struct Funct* In press.

King MA (1988) Alterations and recovery of dendritic spine density in rat hippocampus following long-term ethanol ingestion. *Brain Res* 459: 381–385.

Koob GF, Volkow ND (2010) Neurocircuitry of addiction. *Neuropsychopharmacology* 35:217–238.

Korbo L (1999) Glial cell loss in the hippocampus of alcoholics. *Alcohol Clin Exp Res* 23:164–168.

Kozorovitskiy Y, Gould E (2003) Adult neurogenesis: a mechanism for brain repair? *J Clin Exp Neuropsychol* 25:721–732.

Kuhn HG, Dickinson-Anson H, Gage FH (1996) Neurogenesis in the dentate gyrus of the adult rat: age-related decrease of neuronal progenitor proliferation. *J Neurosci* 16:2027–2033.

Laakso MP, Vaurio O, Savolainen L, Repo E, Soininen H, Aronen HJ, Tiihonen J (2000) A volumetric MRI study of the hippocampus in type 1 and 2 alcoholism. *Behav Brain Res* 109:177–186.

Lacar B, Parylak SL, Vadodaria KC, Sarkar A, Gage FH (2014) Increasing the resolution of the adult neurogenesis picture. *F1000Prime Rep* 6:8.

Leasure JL, Nixon K (2010) Exercise neuroprotection in a rat model of binge alcohol consumption. *Alcohol Clin Exp Res* 34:404–414.

Lukoyanov NV, Brandao F, Cadete-Leite A, Madeira MD, Paula-Barbosa MM (2000) Synaptic reorganization in the hippocampal formation of alcohol-fed rats may compensate for functional deficits related to neuronal loss. *Alcohol* 20:139–148.

Luo J, Miller MW (1998) Growth factor-mediated neural proliferation: target of ethanol toxicity. *Brain Res Brain Res Rev* 27:157–167.

Mandyam CD, Koob GF (2012) The addicted brain craves new neurons: putative role for adult-born progenitors in promoting recovery. *Trends Neurosci* 35:250–260.

Marcussen BL, Goodlett CR, Mahoney JC, West JR (1994) Developing rat Purkinje cells are more vulnerable to alcohol-induced depletion during differentiation than during neurogenesis. *Alcohol* 11:147–156.

Maynard ME, Leasure JL (2013) Exercise enhances hippocampal recovery following binge ethanol exposure. *PLoS One* 8:e76644.

McClain JA, Hayes DM, Morris SA, Nixon K (2011) Adolescent binge alcohol exposure alters hippocampal progenitor cell proliferation in rats: effects on cell cycle kinetics. *J Comp Neurol* 519:2697–2710.

McClain JA, Morris SA, Marshall SA, Nixon K (2013) Ectopic hippocampal neurogenesis in adolescent male rats following alcohol dependence. *Addict Biol* 19:687–699.

Mechtcheriakov S, Brenneis C, Egger K, Koppelstaetter F, Schocke M, Marksteiner J (2007) A widespread distinct pattern of cerebral atrophy in patients with alcohol addiction revealed by voxel-based morphometry. *J Neurol Neurosurg Psychiatry* 78:610–614.

Miguel-Hidalgo JJ, Wei J, Andrew M, Overholser JC, Jurjus G, Stockmeier CA, Rajkowska G (2002) Glia pathology in the prefrontal cortex in alcohol dependence with and without depressive symptoms. *Biol Psychiatry* 52:1121–1133.

Ming GL, Song H (2011) Adult neurogenesis in the mammalian brain: significant answers and significant questions. *Neuron* 70:687–702.

Morrens J, Van Den Broeck W, Kempermann G (2012) Glial cells in adult neurogenesis. *Glia* 60:159–174.

Morris SA, Eaves DW, Smith AR, Nixon K (2010) Alcohol inhibition of neurogenesis: a mechanism of hippocampal neurodegeneration in an adolescent alcohol abuse model. *Hippocampus* 20:596–607.

Nagel BJ, Schweinsburg AD, Phan V, Tapert, SF (2005) Reduced hippocampal volume among adolescents with alcohol use disorders without psychiatric comorbidity. *Psychiatry Res* 139:181–190.

Nixon K (2006) Alcohol and adult neurogenesis: roles in neurodegeneration and recovery in chronic alcoholism. *Hippocampus* 16:287–295.

Nixon K, Crews FT (2002) Binge ethanol exposure decreases neurogenesis in adult rat hippocampus. *J Neurochem* 83:1087–1093.

Nixon K, Crews FT (2004) Temporally specific burst in cell proliferation increases hippocampal neurogenesis in protracted abstinence from alcohol. *J Neurosci* 24:9714–9722.

Nixon K, Kim DH, Potts EN, He J, Crews FT (2008) Distinct cell proliferation events during abstinence after alcohol dependence: microglia proliferation precedes neurogenesis. *Neurobiol Dis* 31:218–229.

Nixon K, Morris SA, Liput DJ, Kelso ML (2010) Roles of neural stem cells and adult neurogenesis in adolescent alcohol use disorders. *Alcohol* 44:39–56.

Obernier JA, Bouldin TW, Crews FT (2002) Binge ethanol exposure in adult rats causes necrotic cell death. *Alcohol Clin Exp Res* 26:547–557.

Ozsoy S, Durak AC, Esel E (2013) Hippocampal volumes and cognitive functions in adult alcoholic patients with adolescent-onset. *Alcohol* 47:9–14.

Palmer TD, Takahashi J, Gage FH (1997) The adult rat hippocampus contains primordial neural stem cells. *Mol Cell Neurosci* 8:389–404.

Parent JM, Lowenstein DH (2002) Seizure-induced neurogenesis: are more new neurons good for an adult brain? *Prog Brain Res* 135:121–131.

Parent JM, Yu TW, Leibowitz RT, Geschwind DH, Sloviter RS, Lowenstein DH (1997) Dentate granule cell neurogenesis is increased by seizures and contributes to aberrant network reorganization in the adult rat hippocampus. *J Neurosci* 17:3727–3738.

Parsons OA (1993) Impaired neuropsychological cognitive functioning in sober alcoholics. In: *Alcohol-Induced Brain Damage: NIAAA Research Monograph No. 22* (Hunt WA, Nixon SJ eds.), pp. 173–194. Rockville, MD: National Institutes of Health.

Pawlak R, Skrzypiec A, Sulkowski S, Buczko, W (2002) Ethanol-induced neurotoxicity is counterbalanced by increased cell proliferation in mouse dentate gyrus. *Neurosci Lett* 327:83–86.

Pfefferbaum A (1996) Thinning of the corpus callosum in older alcoholic men: a magnetic resonance imaging study. *Alcohol Clin Exp Res* 20:752–757.

Pfefferbaum A, Lim KO, Zipursky RB, Mathalon DH, Rosenbloom MJ, Lane B, Ha CN, Sullivan, EV (1992) Brain gray and white matter volume loss accelerates with aging in chronic alcoholics: a quantitative MRI study. *Alcohol Clin Exp Res* 16:1078–1089.

Pfefferbaum A, Sullivan EV, Mathalon DH, Shear PK, Rosenbloom MJ, Lim KO (1995) Longitudinal changes in magnetic resonance imaging brain volumes in abstinent and relapsed alcoholics. *Alcohol Clin Exp Res* 19:1177–1191.

Richardson HN, Chan SH, Crawford EF, Lee YK, Funk CK, Koob GF, Mandyam CD (2009) Permanent impairment of birth and survival of cortical and hippocampal proliferating cells following excessive drinking during alcohol dependence. *Neurobiol Dis* 36:1–10.

Riley JN, Walker DW (1978) Morphological alterations in hippocampus after long-term alcohol consumption in mice. *Science* 201:646–648.

Rintala J, Jaatinen P, Kiianmaa K, Riikonen J, Kemppainen O, Sarviharju M, Hervonen A (2001) Dose-dependent decrease in glial fibrillary acidic protein-immunoreactivity in rat cerebellum after lifelong ethanol consumption. *Alcohol* 23:1–8.

Rubert G, Minana R, Pascual M, Guerri C (2006) Ethanol exposure during embryogenesis decreases the radial glial progenitorpool and affects the generation of neurons and astrocytes. *J Neurosci Res* 84:483–496.

Sanai N, Nguyen T, Ihrie RA, Mirzadeh Z, Tsai HH, Wong M, Gupta N, Berger MS, Huang E, Garcia-Verdugo JM, Rowitch DH, Alvarez-Buylla A (2011) Corridors of migrating neurons in the human brain and their decline during infancy. *Nature* 478:382–386.

Scholzen T, Gerdes J (2000) The Ki-67 protein: from the known and the unknown. *J Cell Physiol* 182:311–322.

Shors TJ, Anderson ML, Curlik DM 2nd, Nokia MS (2012) Use it or lose it: how neurogenesis keeps the brain fit for learning. *Behav Brain Res* 227:450–458.

Shors TJ, Miesegaes G, Beylin A, Zhao M, Rydel T, Gould E (2001) Neurogenesis in the adult is involved in the formation of trace memories. *Nature* 410:372–376.

Snyder JS, Cameron HA (2012) Could adult hippocampal neurogenesis be relevant for human behavior? *Behav Brain Res* 227:384–390.

Streit WJ (2002) Microglia as neuroprotective, immunocompetent cells of the CNS. *Glia* 40:133–139.

Streit WJ (2005) Microglia and neuroprotection: implications for Alzheimer's disease. *Brain Res Brain Res Rev* 48:234–239.

Streit WJ, Xue QS, (2009) Life and death of microglia. *J Neuroimmune Pharmacol* 4:371–379.

Suh H, Consiglio A, Ray J, Sawai T, D'Amour KA, Gage FH (2007) *In vivo* fate analysis reveals the multipotent and self-renewal capacities of Sox2+ neural stem cells in the adult hippocampus. *Cell Stem Cell* 1:515–528.

Sullivan EV, Marsh L, Mathalon DH, Lim KO, Pfefferbaum A (1995) Anterior hippocampal volume deficits in nonamnesic, aging chronic alcoholics. *Alcohol Clin Exp Res* 19:110–122.

Sullivan EV, Marsh L, Mathalon DH, Lim KO, Pfefferbaum A (1996) Relationship between alcohol withdrawal seizures and temporal lobe white matter volume deficits. *Alcohol Clin Exp Res* 20:348–354.

Sullivan EV, Pfefferbaum A (2005) Neurocircuitry in alcoholism: a substrate of disruption and repair. *Psychopharmacology* 180:583–594.

Sullivan EV, Rosenbloom MJ, Lim KO, Pfefferbaum A (2000) Longitudinal changes in cognition, gait, and balance in abstinent and relapsed alcoholic men: relationships to changes in brain structure. *Neuropsychology* 14:178–188.

Sullivan EV, Rosenbloom MJ, Pfefferbaum A (2000) Pattern of motor and cognitive deficits in detoxified alcoholic men. *Alcohol Clin Exp Res* 24:611–621.

Sutherland GT, Sheahan PJ, Matthews J, Dennis CV, Sheedy DS, McCrossin T, Curtis MA, Kril JJ (2013) The effects of chronic alcoholism on cell proliferation in the human brain. *Exp Neurol* 247:9–18.

Taffe MA, Kotzebue RW, Crean RD, Crawford EF, Edwards S, Mandyam CD (2010) Long-lasting reduction in hippocampal neurogenesis by alcohol consumption in adolescent nonhuman primates. *Proc Natl Acad Sci U S A* 107:11104–11109.

Taylor CJ, Jhaveri DJ, Bartlett PF (2013) The therapeutic potential of endogenous hippocampal stem cells for the treatment of neurological disorders. *Front Cell Neurosci* 7:5.

Turnley AM, Basrai HS, Christie KJ (2014) Is integration and survival of newborn neurons the bottleneck for effective neural repair by endogenous neural precursor cells? *Front Neurosci* 8:29.

Valles S, Pitarch J, Renau-Piqueras J, Guerri C (1997) Ethanol exposure affects glial fibrillary acidic protein gene expression and transcription during rat brain development. *J Neurochem* 69:2484–2493.

van Praag H, Christie BR, Sejnowski TJ, Gage FH (1999) Running enhances neurogenesis, learning, and long-term potentiation in mice. *Proc Natl Acad Sci U S A* 96:13427–13431.

Vangipuram SD, Lyman WD (2010) Ethanol alters cell fate of fetal human brain-derived stem and progenitor cells. *Alcohol Clin Exp Res* 34:1574–1583.

Vaynman S, Gomez-Pinilla F (2005) License to run: exercise impacts functional plasticity in the intact and injured central nervous system by using neurotrophins. *Neurorehabil Neural Repair* 19:283–295.

Vaynman S, Ying Z, Gomez-Pinilla F (2004) Hippocampal BDNF mediates the efficacy of exercise on synaptic plasticity and cognition. *Eur J Neurosci* 20:2580–2590.

Vemuri MC, Chetty CS (2005) Alcohol impairs astrogliogenesis by stem cells in rodent neurospheres. *Neurochem Int* 47:129–135.

Wagner B, Natarajan A, Grunaug S, Kroismayr R, Wagner EF, Sibilia M (2006) Neuronal survival depends on EGFR signaling in cortical but not midbrain astrocytes. *EMBO J* 25:752–762.

Walker DW, Barnes DE, Zornetzer SF, Hunter BE, Kubanis P (1980) Neuronal loss in hippocampus induced by prolonged ethanol consumption in rats. *Science* 209:711–713.

Wang SC (2014) PCNA: a silent housekeeper or a potential therapeutic target? *Trends Pharmacol Sci* 35:178–186.

Wilcox CE, Dekonenko CJ, Mayer AR, Bogenschutz MP, Turner JA (2014) Cognitive control in alcohol use disorder: deficits and clinical relevance. *Rev Neurosci* 25:1–24.

Zhou FC, Balaraman Y, Teng M, Liu Y, Singh RP, Nephew KP (2011) Alcohol alters DNA methylation patterns and inhibits neural stem cell differentiation. *Alcohol Clin Exp Res* 35:735–746.

Chapter 10

Neural Stem Cells in Methamphetamine Addiction

Chitra D. Mandyam

The need for effective treatments for addiction and dependence to the illicit stimulant methamphetamine in primary care settings is increasing, yet no effective medications have been FDA-approved to reduce dependence (NIDA, 2006, 2010, 2011). Medication development to treat methamphetamine addiction, particularly the relapse stage of addiction, could revolutionize methamphetamine addiction treatment. In this context, preclinical studies demonstrate that the hippocampus is a brain region that affects relapse to drug-seeking behaviors, and clinical studies demonstrate that methamphetamine addicts show altered hippocampal response, volume and morphology and enhanced hippocampal neurotoxicity. Therefore, it appears that methamphetamine disrupts normal functioning in the hippocampus and this disruption enhances relapse in methamphetamine addicts. This chapter will highlight the role of neurogenesis in the adult mammalian hippocampus in regulating and maintaining hippocampal networking and function. This chapter will also discuss the emerging role of hippocampal neurogenesis in relapse to methamphetamine-seeking behavior in preclinical models of methamphetamine addiction. Additionally, normalization of methamphetamine-impaired hippocampal function by reversing the maladaptive neuroplasticity during abstinence may help reduce the vulnerability to relapse and aid recovery in methamphetamine addicts.

Introduction

Definition of addiction, the stages of addiction and animal models of addiction

Broadly defined, addiction is one of many disorders that involve impulsivity and compulsivity. The impulsive and compulsive phases of addiction can be grouped into three stages: (1) binge/prolonged intoxication; (2) withdrawal neutral/negative affect; and (3) preoccupation/anticipation (craving). The last stage of the addiction cycle describes a key element of relapse in humans and therefore defines addiction as a chronic relapsing disorder (Koob and Volkow, 2010). Relapse to drug-seeking behavior has been a challenging area for neuroscientists, causing it to become one of the lesser-studied aspects of addiction. Understanding the neuroplastic changes that underlie the relapse stage of addiction can help generate better treatment options. This chapter focuses on the clinically relevant rodent self-administration model of addiction and relapse and considers novel evidence that implicates neural progenitors in the phenomenology of drug abuse.

Animal models of addiction and craving

Clinically defined, addiction or substance dependence involves the loss of behavioral control over drug-taking and drug-seeking. The limited use of drugs with the potential for abuse is distinct from escalated drug use and the materialization of a chronic drug-dependent state (Koob and Le Moal, 1997). Addiction-like behavior has been demonstrated in rodent models of intravenous drug self-administration, in which rodents are trained to self-administer drugs by pressing a lever for an intravenous drug infusion in an operant conditioning chamber (Ahmed and Koob, 1998). Therefore, intravenous drug self-administration with intermittent

(1 hr biweekly), limited (1 hr daily), or long (extended; > 4 hr daily) access has significant clinical relevance by illustrating a range of different drug-seeking behaviors (Mandyam *et al.*, 2007). An increase in drug availability or a history of drug intake has been shown to accelerate the development of dependence in humans (Kramer *et al.*, 1967; Gawin and Ellinwood, 1989). In rats, extended access to drugs of abuse, including cocaine, methamphetamine, nicotine, heroin, and alcohol, produce an escalation of drug self-administration, suggesting compulsive drug intake and therefore reflecting dependence-like behavior. Animal models of escalation, therefore, may provide a useful approach to understanding the neurobiological mechanisms responsible for the transition from limited drug use to compulsive intake and may represent a particularly suitable model for testing the hypothesis that alterations in adult brain plasticity induced by the drug are partially responsible for addictive behavior (Ahmed and Koob, 1998).

The reinstatement of drug-seeking behavior in rats is widely used as a model of craving to mimic the relapse stage of addiction in human addicts (Shaham *et al.*, 2003) and is used extensively to uncover the key brain regions, brain circuitry, neurotransmitters, and neuromodulators associated with reinstatement behavior. The paradigm extinguishes learned self-administration behavior by explicitly not rewarding the animal after a lever press and tests the ability of a priming stimulus to reinstate drug-seeking behavior, which is measured by lever pressing in the operant chamber (Shalev *et al.*, 2002). The stimuli can be cues previously paired with drug self-administration (cue priming) or acute noncontingent exposure to the drug (which is usually delivered to the rat by the experimenter; i.e., drug priming) or context (spatial location) where the drug was self-administered. The drug-seeking reinstatement model can be used to measure repeated operant behavior to mimic an addict's drug-response pattern (McFarland and Kalivas, 2001) and mimic high rates of relapse (McFarland and Kalivas, 2001; Rogers *et al.*, 2008). Thus, the intravenous self-administration model of drug exposure appears to be the best suited for studying the neural mechanisms of relapse.

Reward and relapse circuitry in the adult brain

The reward and relapse circuitry in the adult mammalian brain has been delineated based on multiple groundbreaking studies performed in rodent models of acute and chronic reinforcement schedules and reinstatement to drug-seeking behavior (Shaham *et al.*, 2003). The key brain regions implicated in the acute reinforcing actions of drugs of abuse include, but are not limited to, the nucleus accumbens, amygdala, and ventral tegmental area (Koob and Volkow, 2010). Release of the neurotransmitter dopamine in these regions is considered to be significantly modulated by various drugs of abuse, particularly psychostimulants, such as cocaine, methamphetamine, and nicotine, to produce their rewarding effects. Furthermore, there is evidence that neurotransmitters other than dopamine may also play a significant role in the rewarding effects of drugs of abuse. For example, the nucleus accumbens is tactically situated in the brain such that it receives inputs from several other brain regions, including the medial prefrontal cortex and hippocampal regions (Koob and Volkow, 2010). Notably, the neurotransmitter glutamate from the medial prefrontal cortex and hippocampus regulates dopamine release from the nucleus accumbens and ventral tegmental area, suggesting that drugs of abuse dysregulate prefrontocortical and hippocampal neurocircuitry and may partially contribute to the enhanced dopamine release from the mesolimbic dopamine pathway (Taepavarapruk *et al.*, 2000; Floresco *et al.*, 2001a; Floresco *et al.*, 2001b). Altogether, it appears that several brain regions which receive connections from the limbic system play critical roles in the acute reinforcing effects of drugs of abuse (Koob and Volkow, 2010).

The key brain regions implicated in the reinstatement of drug-seeking behavior include, but are not limited to, the medial prefrontal cortex, nucleus accumbens, bed nucleus of the stria terminalis, central nucleus of the amygdala, basolateral amygdala, hippocampal regions, and ventral tegmental area (Shaham *et al.*, 2003; Koob and Volkow, 2010). The ventral striatum, a terminal projection of the neural connections from the ventral tegmental area to prefrontal cortex, and the nucleus accumbens are considered focal points for reward and reinstatement of drug-seeking behavior (Koob and Volkow, 2010). Most importantly, it is believed that the release of the neurotransmitters dopamine, glutamate, and corticotropin-releasing factor in key brain regions associated with relapse are essential for the behavioral effects of the drug (Koob, 1999; Knackstedt and Kalivas, 2009).

To add to the existing theories on addiction, one recent discovery about the adult mammalian brain that is potentially important for addiction research is the ability of the brain to continuously generate new progenitors throughout adulthood. Broadly defined, progenitors are progeny of stem cells that are characterized by limited self-renewal and can survive and mature into differentiating cells, such as neurons and glia in the brain. The discovery (Messier and Leblond, 1960; Altman, 1969) and eventual acceptance (Eriksson *et al.*, 1998; Gould *et al.*, 1999b; Manganas *et al.*, 2007) of adult-generated progenitors that mature into neurons or glial cells has spurred substantial investigation of the proliferative capacity of brain regions such as the hippocampus. New emerging correlative data suggests that the phenomena of adult neurogenesis in the hippocampus may contribute to the resistance of some aspects of drug taking and acquisition of drug seeking. Therefore, to appreciate the promising role of adult hippocampal progenitors in the plasticity of addiction and relapse, this chapter focuses on the hippocampal neurogenesis and its contribution to methamphetamine-taking and the reinstatement of methamphetamine-seeking behavior.

Neurogenesis in the hippocampus in adulthood

Adult neurogenesis occurs in a discrete region in the hippocampus, namely the subgranular zone, situated on the border of the granule cell layer and hilus of the dentate gyrus (Figure 1). Adult neurogenesis plays an important role in maintaining hippocampal plasticity. The process of neurogenesis involves stem-like precursor cells (type 1 cells) that proliferate into preneuronal progenitors (type 2 and type 3), which in turn differentiate into immature neurons and

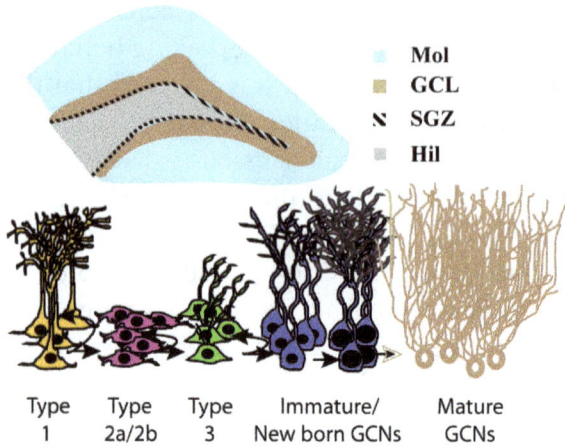

Figure 1.   Neurogenesis occurs in the subgranular zone of the hippocampus. DG, dentate gyrus; GCL, granule cell layer; Mol, molecular layer; SGZ, subgranular zone; Hil, hilus. Schematic representation of the coronal view of the hippocampus region; magnification of the DG region in a coronal view −3.6 mm from bregma indicating the subregions of the DG and highlighting the neurogenic region; GCL in tan and SGZ as the hatched area. Stages of adult hippocampal neurogenesis are indicated below the schematic of the coronal view of the hippocampus. In the DG, type 1 putative stem-like cells are slowly dividing and rarely label with the commonly used exogenous mitotic marker 5-bromo-2′-deoxyuridine (BrdU) but can be identified via morphology and staining for nestin/GFAP/Sox2. BrdU will label rapidly dividing type 2 and some type 3 cells. Type 3 cells mature and differentiate into immature granule cell neurons (GCNs) and migrate a short distance into the granule cell layer to become granule cell neurons and integrate into the hippocampal circuitry.

eventually mature into granule cell neurons (Kempermann *et al.*, 2004; Abrous *et al.*, 2005) (Figure 1). A large proportion (> 80%) of hippocampal progenitors migrate a short distance to become granule cell neurons in the dentate gyrus (Kaplan and Hinds, 1977; Hastings *et al.*, 2001), and there is evidence demonstrating functional incorporation of the newly born neurons in the dentate gyrus (Gould *et al.*, 1999a; Shors *et al.*, 2002; Aimone *et al.*, 2006). For example, dentate gyrus neurogenesis has been implicated in the maintenance of hippocampal networking (Aimone *et al.*, 2006; Clark *et al.*, 2012; Lacefield *et al.*, 2012) and assists with certain behaviors that depend on the hippocampus (Feng *et al.*, 2001;

Deisseroth *et al.*, 2004; Schmidt-Hieber *et al.*, 2004; Kim *et al.*, 2012) and is critical for encoding new information by facilitating the formation of new memories that assist with hippocampus-dependent behaviors (McHugh *et al.*, 2007; Bakker *et al.*, 2008; Clelland *et al.*, 2009; Aimone *et al.*, 2011; Sahay *et al.*, 2011). Reinforcing doses of several illicit drugs decrease hippocampal neurogenesis (Mandyam and Koob, 2012) and this data suggests that the normalization of drug-impaired neurogenesis during withdrawal may help reverse altered hippocampal neuroplasticity during protracted abstinence. Ultimately, this may help reduce the vulnerability to relapse and aid recovery.

Methamphetamine addiction and impact on society

The burden of methamphetamine abuse is increasing in the United States; available SAMHSA reports show 8% of all drug/alcohol treatment admissions involve methamphetamine and treatment studies report frequent relapses to methamphetamine-seeking among those that are trying to quit (2008). Furthermore, methamphetamine abuse takes emotional and financial tolls on society, cutting across ages, races, ethnicities, and genders. It increases mortality, morbidity, and economic costs. Therefore, successfully reducing risk behaviors, such as methamphetamine abuse, can potentially result in large public health gains (WHO, 1980; USPSTF, 2008).

According to the recent reports from the National Institutes on Drug abuse (NIDA) and others, there are a few really successful treatments for methamphetamine addiction (NIDA, 2006; Gonzales *et al.*, 2010; NIDA, 2010, 2011). For example, the best treatment is the behavioral treatment approach (Matrix model); however, behavioral therapies are associated with lower beneficial effects on maintaining an individual's abstinence as well as drug cravings elicited by drug-related context and cues. Therefore, NIDA is currently conducting research on creating a medication that may treat methamphetamine addiction, particularly the relapse (preoccupation/anticipation) stage of addiction.

Methamphetamine Produces Neurotoxicity in the Striatum

Studies over the past four decades have conceptualized that methamphetamine produces significant toxicity in the striatum, and that the neurotoxicity is responsible for the addictive properties of the drug. For example, methamphetamine-induced striatal neurotoxicity results from: (1) excessive dopamine production and release; (2) enhanced reactive oxygen species and reactive nitrogen species; and (3) compromised mitochondrial function. Specifically in the striatum, methamphetamine causes excessive dopamine release into the synaptic cleft along with enhanced dopamine concentration inside the presynpatic terminal. These pharmacological activities are due to methamphetamine's actions on dopamine transporters, vesicular monoamine transporters and tyrosine hydroxylase (Fleckenstein *et al.*, 2007; Ares-Santos *et al.*, 2013). The accumulation of intracellular dopamine promotes formation of dopamine-associated reactive oxygen species and reactive nitrogen species (nitric oxide and peroxynitrite), resulting in persistent neurotoxicity (Itzhak, 1997; Itzhak *et al.*, 1998; Itzhak *et al.*, 1999; Fleckenstein *et al.*, 2000; Itzhak *et al.*, 2000; Fleckenstein and Hanson, 2003; Itzhak *et al.*, 2004; Yamamoto and Bankson, 2005; Eyerman and Yamamoto, 2007; Wang *et al.*, 2008; Zhu *et al.*, 2009; Shiba *et al.*, 2011; Wang and Angulo, 2011). Accumulation of nitric oxide by methamphetamine is associated with inactivity of cytochrome c oxidase (complex IV) and release of cytochrome c indicating compromised mitochondrial function (Burrows *et al.*, 2000; Deng *et al.*, 2002). Methamphetamine also increases mitochondria-dependent pro-apoptotic proteins, decreases mitochondria-dependent anti-apoptotic proteins, and causes damage to the endoplasmic reticulum, all of which lead to neuronal death (Deng *et al.*, 2002; Jayanthi *et al.*, 2004). These studies suggest that progressive increases in the intake of methamphetamine over extended access schedules of reinforcement lead to persistent neuroadaptive changes in the striatum which may be critical for the acute rewarding effects of the psychostimulant, and the transition to compulsive use (Everitt *et al.*, 2008). However, it has been argued that the activation of the striatal system is not necessarily critical for the emergence of the relapse/preoccupation anticipation stage of addiction, suggesting the activation of multiple brain regions, particularly, the hippocampus, is critical to the recruitment of relapse circuitry in methamphetamine addiction (Koob and Volkow, 2010).

Methamphetamine exposure alters structure and behaviors dependent on the hippocampus and alters functional plasticity of hippocampal neurons

Clinical studies demonstrate profound deficits in executive function, declarative memory, and impulsivity in methamphetamine addicts, indicating impaired behavioral and cognitive responses that are dependent on the frontal cortex and the hippocampus (Thompson *et al.*, 2004; Price *et al.*, 2011; Weber *et al.*, 2012). Human imaging studies show reduced frontal cortical, hippocampal and amygdala volume, particularly gray matter volume in these regions, and decreased frontal cortical and hippocampal response in chronic methamphetamine users (Thompson *et al.*, 2004; Kim *et al.*, 2010; Schwartz *et al.*, 2010; Daumann *et al.*, 2011; Nakama *et al.*, 2011; Orikabe *et al.*, 2011; Morales *et al.*, 2012), indicating maladaptive cortical and hippocampal networking in methamphetamine-exposed individuals. Postmortem analysis in human brain tissue confirms that chronic methamphetamine use produces neurotoxicity in the hippocampus (Kitamura, 2009; Kitamura *et al.*, 2010), which suggests an association between hippocampal dysfunction and hippocampal toxicity in methamphetamine addicts.

The behavioral deficits observed in methamphetamine addicts have been demonstrated in preclinical models of binge methamphetamine exposure and methamphetamine self-administration with extended access to the drug, where methamphetamine exposure produces cognitive dysfunction and memory impairments dependent on the hippocampus (Itoh *et al.*, 1984; Yoshikawa *et al.*, 1991; Yamamoto, 1997; Friedman *et al.*, 1998; Rogers *et al.*, 2008; Recinto *et al.*, 2012). Neurodegeneration and neurotoxicity in the hippocampus are also observed in animal models of binge methamphetamine exposure and methamphetamine self-administration, suggesting a positive correlation between methamphetamine-induced toxicity and methamphetamine-induced behavioral deficits (Commins and Seiden, 1986; Eisch *et al.*, 1996; Schmued and Bowyer, 1997; Mandyam *et al.*, 2008). Additional mechanistic studies show that methamphetamine exposure alters the functional plasticity of hippocampal neurons. For example, acute methamphetamine treatment and systemic methamphetamine treatment reduces long-term potentiation of CA1 pyramidal neurons through activation of D1 receptors and increases baseline excitatory synaptic transmission (Onaivi *et al.*, 2002; Swant *et al.*, 2010). In the dentate gyrus specifically, acute methamphetamine exposure also reduces excitability of dentate gyrus neurons, whereas, repeated exposure to methamphetamine increases excitability of dentate gyrus neurons (Criado *et al.*, 2000). These studies demonstrate that methamphetamine exposure (via experimenter delivered paradigms) produces synaptic maladaptation in the hippocampus that may mediate some of the addiction behaviors dependent on the hippocampus. These electrophysiological studies also suggest that altered plasticity of CA1 neurons and granule cell neurons in the dentate gyrus may be mediated by methamphetamine's effects on neurogenesis in the dentate gyrus. This is because several studies suggest bi-directional interactions between long-term potentiation and dentate gyrus neurogenesis. Neurogenesis contributes to long-term potentiation induction (van Praag *et al.*, 1999; Derrick *et al.*, 2000; Snyder *et al.*, 2001; Farmer *et al.*, 2004) and, conversely, long-term potentiation induction promotes dentate gyrus neurogenesis (Chun *et al.*, 2006; Chun *et al.*, 2009). Because newly born granule cell neurons in the dentate gyrus of the hippocampus modulate the processing of the overall tone of dentate gyrus activity and maintain hippocampal networking (Lacefield *et al.*, 2012), reduced long-term potentiation and enhanced excitability of dentate gyrus neurons by methamphetamine may be assisted by the reduced survival of newly born granule cell neurons.

In this context, emerging studies in adult rats self-administering methamphetamine under extended access conditions demonstrated that methamphetamine self-administration with extended access to the drug altered hippocampal neuroplasticity by reducing dentate gyrus neurogenesis, and these effects were relative to the amount of methamphetamine consumed (Mandyam *et al.*, 2008; Yuan *et al.*, 2011). Furthermore, withdrawal from methamphetamine self-administration produced compensatory changes in dentate gyrus neurogenesis (i.e., the aberrant survival of newly born neurons, born after methamphetamine self-administration), and the hypothesis is that these changes in the hippocampus during withdrawal may regulate relapse to methamphetamine-seeking (Recinto *et al.*, 2012). These findings have allowed the identification and validation of a novel target for drug discovery for treating the relapse stage of methamphetamine addiction. The concluding topics in the chapter will therefore discuss the cellular mechanisms underlying methamphetamine-induced reduction in hippocampal neurogenesis and will suggest possible future directions to determine the functional significance of hippocampal neurogenesis in methamphetamine addiction.

Methamphetamine self-administration regulates developmental stages of hippocampal neurogenesis

Recent evidence has shown that some aspects of hippocampal neurogenesis could be involved in the altered neuroplasticity that underlies methamphetamine addiction. Experimenter-delivered (Hildebrandt *et al.*, 1999; Teuchert-Noodt *et al.*, 2000; Kochman *et al.*, 2009) and clinically relevant models of intravenous self-administration (Mandyam *et al.*, 2008; Yuan *et al.*, 2011; Recinto *et al.*, 2012; Engelmann *et al.*, 2013) of methamphetamine in rodents negatively impact the proliferation and survival of adult hippocampal neural progenitors. Experimenter-delivered and self-administered methamphetamine intake produces hippocampal cell death (Schmued and Bowyer, 1997; Mandyam *et al.*, 2008), signifying a potential role for hippocampal cell death in methamphetamine addiction. Thus, while there is preliminary evidence supporting the devastating effects of methamphetamine on adult hippocampal neuroplasticity, little information exists on the mechanisms underlying these effects.

Some important advances have been made to determine the mechanisms underlying methamphetamine-induced inhibition of hippocampal neurogenesis. For example, in rats given one hour access (short access), or six hour access (long access), of methamphetamine per day for four or thirteen days (4 days, 13 days) it has been demonstrated that different durations of access alter distinct aspects of cell cycle dynamics and stages of neuronal development (Yuan *et al.*, 2011). Long access methamphetamine self-administration (4 days, 13 days) decreased net proliferation (as assessed by Ki-67 labeling) and proliferation of *S*-phase progenitors (as assessed by 5-chloro-2′-deoxyuridine (CldU) labeling]. Exogenous mitotic markers are incorporated into DNA during the synthesis-(*S*)-phase of the cell cycle of actively dividing progenitors in the brain such as CldU. Ki-67 is expressed in cells during all phases of the cell cycle (*S*, *G2*, *M*, and *G1*) (Scholzen and Gerdes, 2000), whereas CldU is only incorporated into the cells during the *S*-phase of the cell cycle (Eisch and Mandyam, 2004). Therefore, reduced Ki-67 cells and CldU cells in long access animals suggest that the decreased progenitor pool is due to fewer cells in the *S*-phase. Short access methamphetamine self-administration (13 days) does not alter net proliferation and reduces proliferation of *S*-phase progenitors, suggesting that proliferating cells are probably arrested in the *G1* phase of the cell cycle (Morris *et al.*, 2009). Additionally, methamphetamine-induced inhibition of proliferation is not due to a shortened *S*-phase, but due to reduced pool of neural progenitors that could be produced by arresting cells in the *G1* phase, followed by killing cells in the *G1* phase or G_1/S checkpoint of the cell cycle (Yuan *et al.*, 2011).

In addition to exploring the effects of methamphetamine self-administration on the cell cycle dynamics of proliferating cells, the effects of methamphetamine on the development of Ki-67 labeled cells have been investigated (Mandyam *et al.*, 2008, Yuan *et al.*, 2011). Ki-67 is a transcription factor expressed in a heterogeneous population of proliferating progenitor cells in the subgranular zone, and Ki-67 labeling can be used to identify distinct neural developmental stages (namely type1/2a/2b/3) of proliferating progenitors (Filippov *et al.*, 2003; Kronenberg *et al.*, 2003; Steiner *et al.*, 2006; Taffe *et al.*, 2010). Four days to two weeks of methamphetamine exposure via self-administration produces activation of proliferating type1 radial glia-like stem cells and inhibition of proliferating type2a preneuronal neuroblasts (Yuan *et al.*, 2011). Six weeks of methamphetamine self-administration produces an inhibition of several cell types, namely, intermediate/ early neuronal type2b/3 cell types and inhibits hippocampal neurogenesis (Figure 2) (Mandyam *et al.*, 2008). These interesting findings add to the growing literature showing that the preneuronal stages of a proliferating cell influences its response to stimuli (Tashiro *et al.*, 2007; Arguello *et al.*, 2008). In summary, these observations suggest that certain neuromodulatory effects in the brain are perhaps more sensitive to the amount and duration of daily methamphetamine intake and confirm that higher amounts and greater duration of methamphetamine intake produce more pronounced effects on neuroplastic events that are affected by addiction.

Withdrawal from methamphetamine self-administration regulates hippocampal neurogenesis

Mechanistic studies demonstrate that the hippocampus plays a role in relapse to methamphetamine seeking (Hiranita *et al.*, 2006). Withdrawal from methamphetamine self-administration enhances methamphetamine-seeking following priming in animals given extended access (but not limited access) to methamphetamine self-administration, suggesting that the magnitude of methamphetamine-seeking is directly related to the amount of intake during prolonged methamphetamine self-administration (Yan *et al.*, 2007; Rogers *et al.*, 2008; Recinto *et al.*, 2012). Furthermore, enhanced methamphetamine seeking following withdrawal correlated with increases in the survival of hippocampal neural progenitors and the neuronal activation (assessed by expression of immediate early genes; e.g. cFos) of hippocampal granule cell neurons (Recinto *et al.*, 2012), suggesting that adult hippocampal neurogenesis may impact hippocampal function in

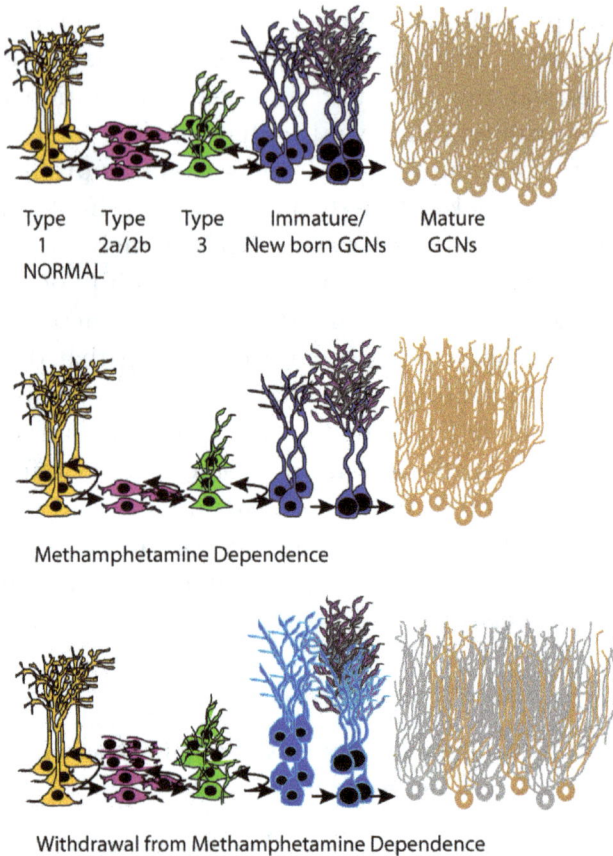

Figure. 2 Schematic of methamphetamine dependence-induced inhibition of neurogenesis and withdrawal from methamphetamine dependence-induced aberrant survival of new born granule cell neurons in the dentate gyrus of the hippocampus. Top panel shows the normal levels of cells in each stage of neurogenesis: proliferation (pink cells), maturation (green cells) differentiation (blue cells) and survival (tan cells). Middle panel shows methamphetamine dependence-induced reduction in the levels of proliferation (type 2 and 3 cells), maturation (type 3 cells) differentiation and survival. Bottom panel shows withdrawal-induced increase in proliferation, maturation and aberrant survival of cells born during withdrawal (distinguished by gray cells).

general and relapse in particular (Noonan *et al.*, 2008; Garcia-Fuster *et al.*, 2011; Deschaux *et al.*, 2012).

Some recent advances have been made to determine the cellular mechanisms underlying withdrawal-induced aberrant survival of newly born cells in the dentate gyrus in animals that self-administered methamphetamine. For example, in long access rats, protracted withdrawal increased proliferation, reflected by increased number of Ki-67 cells compared with acute withdrawal and drug naïve controls (Figure 2). The enhanced proliferation (increases above naïve controls) could not be attributable to a compensatory effect (i.e., decreased cell death) that might have occurred for the decreased population of progenitors (2 h BrdU cells) during self-administration (Recinto *et al.*, 2012). Alternatively, the modulation of the cell division of progenitors, such as the increased rate of symmetric division, or enhanced survival of progenitors could be responsible for the aberrant neurogenesis during protracted withdrawal after methamphetamine (or cocaine) self-administration (Noonan *et al.*, 2008; Deschaux *et al.*, 2012; Recinto *et al.*, 2012). This withdrawal-specific effect in methamphetamine (and cocaine) rats is worth noting because this maladaptive change could function to return the homeostasis of granule cell neuron turnover, or incubate drug, and drug-context associations relating to drug seeking (Vorel *et al.*, 2001; Hiranita *et al.*, 2006; Rademacher *et al.*, 2006; Shen *et al.*, 2006; Zhou and Zhu, 2006; Lasseter *et al.*, 2010; Noonan *et al.*, 2010; Luo *et al.*, 2011; Deschaux *et al.*, 2012; Recinto *et al.*, 2012). However, further functional exploration of this putative enhanced survival is warranted, as well as identification of other neuroadaptations during protracted withdrawal that may regulate the hippocampus and hippocampus-dependent relapse behavior (Tani *et al.*, 2001; Hiranita *et al.*, 2006; Zhou and Zhu, 2006; Lasseter *et al.*, 2010; Noonan *et al.*, 2010; Garcia-Fuster *et al.*, 2011).

Acknowledgements

Preparation of this chapter was supported by funds from the National Institute on Drug Abuse (DA034140), National Institute on Alcohol Abuse and Alcoholism (AA020098 and AA006420), and the Alcoholic Beverage Medical Research Foundation. I would like to thank McKenzie Fannon for her editorial assistance.

References

Abrous DN, Koehl M, Le Moal M (2005) Adult neurogenesis: from precursors to network and physiology. *Physiol Rev* 85:523–569.

Ahmed SH, Koob GF (1998) Transition from moderate to excessive drug intake: change in hedonic set point. *Science* 282:298–300.

Aimone JB, Deng W, Gage FH (2011) Resolving new memories: a critical look at the dentate gyrus, adult neurogenesis, and pattern separation. *Neuron* 70:589–596.

Aimone JB, Wiles J, Gage FH (2006) Potential role for adult neurogenesis in the encoding of time in new memories. *Nat Neurosci* 9:723–727.

Altman J (1969) Autoradiographic and histological studies of postnatal neurogenesis. 3. Dating the time of production and onset of differentiation of cerebellar microneurons in rats. *J Comp Neurol* 136: 269–293.

Ares-Santos S, Granado N, Moratalla R (2013) The role of dopamine receptors in the neurotoxicity of methamphetamine. *J Intern Med* 273:437–453.

Arguello AA, Harburg GC, Schonborn JR, Mandyam CD, Yamaguchi M, Eisch AJ (2008) Time course of morphine's effects on adult hippocampal subgranular zone reveals preferential inhibition of cells in S phase of the cell cycle and a subpopulation of immature neurons. *Neuroscience* 157:70–79.

Bakker A, Kirwan CB, Miller M, Stark CE (2008) Pattern separation in the human hippocampal CA3 and dentate gyrus. *Science* 319:1640–1642.

Burrows KB, Gudelsky G, Yamamoto BK (2000) Rapid and transient inhibition of mitochondrial function following methamphetamine or 3,4-methylenedioxymethamphetamine administration. *Eur J Pharmacol* 398:11–18.

Chun SK, Sun W, Jung MW (2009) LTD induction suppresses LTP-induced hippocampal adult neurogenesis. *Neuroreport* 20:1279–1283.

Chun SK, Sun W, Park JJ, Jung MW (2006) Enhanced proliferation of progenitor cells following long-term potentiation induction in the rat dentate gyrus. *Neurobiol Learn Mem* 86:322–329.

Clark PJ, Bhattacharya TK, Miller DS, Kohman RA, DeYoung EK, Rhodes JS (2012) New neurons generated from running are broadly recruited into neuronal activation associated with three different hippocampus-involved tasks. *Hippocampus* 22:1860–1867.

Clelland CD, Choi M, Romberg C, Clemenson GD, Jr., Fragniere A, Tyers P, Jessberger S, Saksida LM, Barker RA, Gage FH, Bussey TJ (2009) A functional role for adult hippocampal neurogenesis in spatial pattern separation. *Science* 325:210–213.

Commins DL, Seiden LS (1986) alpha-Methyltyrosine blocks methylamphetamine-induced degeneration in the rat somatosensory cortex. *Brain Res* 365:15–20.

Criado JR, Gombart LM, Huitron-Resendiz S, Henriksen SJ (2000) Neuroadaptations in dentate gyrus function following repeated methamphetamine administration. *Synapse* 37:163–166.

Daumann J, Koester P, Becker B, Wagner D, Imperati D, Gouzoulis-Mayfrank E, Tittgemeyer M (2011) Medial prefrontal gray matter volume reductions in users of amphetamine-type stimulants revealed by combined tract-based spatial statistics and voxel-based morphometry. *Neuroimage* 54:794–801.

Deisseroth K, Singla S, Toda H, Monje M, Palmer TD, Malenka RC (2004) Excitation-neurogenesis coupling in adult neural stem/progenitor cells. *Neuron* 42:535–552.

Deng X, Cai NS, McCoy MT, Chen W, Trush MA, Cadet JL (2002) Methamphetamine induces apoptosis in an immortalized rat striatal cell line by activating the mitochondrial cell death pathway. *Neuropharmacology* 42:837–845.

Derrick BE, York AD, Martinez JL, Jr (2000) Increased granule cell neurogenesis in the adult dentate gyrus following mossy fiber stimulation sufficient to induce long-term potentiation. *Brain Res* 857:300–307.

Deschaux O, Vendruscolo LF, Schlosburg JE, Diaz-Aguilar L, Yuan CJ, Sobieraj JC, George O, Koob GF, Mandyam CD (2012) Hippocampal neurogenesis protects against cocaine-primed relapse. *Addict Biol.*

Eisch AJ, Mandyam CD (2004) Beyond BrdU: Basic and clinical implications for analysis of endogenous cell cycle proteins. *Progress Stem Cell Res* Nova Science Publishers Inc.

Eisch AJ, O'Dell SJ, Marshall JF (1996) Striatal and cortical NMDA receptors are altered by a neurotoxic regimen of methamphetamine. *Synapse* 22:217–225.

Engelmann AJ, Aparicio MB, Kim A, Sobieraj JC, Yuan CJ, Grant Y, Mandyam CD (2013) Chronic wheel running reduces maladaptive patterns of methamphetamine intake: regulation by attenuation of methamphetamine-induced neuronal nitric oxide synthase. *Brain Struct Funct.*

Eriksson PS, Perfilieva E, Bjork-Eriksson T, Alborn AM, Nordborg C, Peterson DA, Gage FH (1998) Neurogenesis in the adult human hippocampus. *Nat Med* 4:1313–1317.

Everitt BJ, Belin D, Economidou D, Pelloux Y, Dalley JW, Robbins TW (2008) Review. Neural mechanisms underlying the vulnerability to develop compulsive drug-seeking habits and addiction. *Philos Trans R Soc Lond B Biol Sci* 363:3125–3135.

Eyerman DJ, Yamamoto BK (2007) A rapid oxidation and persistent decrease in the vesicular monoamine transporter 2 after methamphetamine. *J Neurochem* 103:1219–1227.

Farmer J, Zhao X, van Praag H, Wodtke K, Gage FH, Christie BR (2004) Effects of voluntary exercise on synaptic plasticity and gene expression in the dentate gyrus of adult male Sprague-Dawley rats *in vivo*. *Neuroscience* 124:71–79.

Feng R, Rampon C, Tang YP, Shrom D, Jin J, Kyin M, Sopher B, Miller MW, Ware CB, Martin GM, Kim SH, Langdon RB, Sisodia SS, Tsien JZ (2001) Deficient neurogenesis in forebrain-specific presenilin-1 knockout mice is associated with reduced clearance of hippocampal memory traces. *Neuron* 32:911–926.

Filippov V, Kronenberg G, Pivneva T, Reuter K, Steiner B, Wang LP, Yamaguchi M, Kettenmann H, Kempermann G (2003) Subpopulation of nestin-expressing progenitor cells in the adult murine hippocampus shows electrophysiological and morphological characteristics of astrocytes. *Mol Cell Neurosci* 23:373–382.

Fleckenstein AE, Gibb JW, Hanson GR (2000) Differential effects of stimulants on monoaminergic transporters: pharmacological consequences and implications for neurotoxicity. *Eur J Pharmacol* 406:1–13.

Fleckenstein AE, Hanson GR (2003) Impact of psychostimulants on vesicular monoamine transporter function. *Eur J Pharmacol* 479:283–289.

Fleckenstein AE, Volz TJ, Riddle EL, Gibb JW, Hanson GR (2007) New insights into the mechanism of action of amphetamines. *Annu Rev Pharmacol Toxicol* 47:681–698.

Floresco SB, Blaha CD, Yang CR, Phillips AG (2001a) Modulation of hippocampal and amygdalar-evoked activity of nucleus accumbens neurons by dopamine: cellular mechanisms of input selection. *J Neurosci* 21:2851–2860.

Floresco SB, Todd CL, Grace AA (2001b) Glutamatergic afferents from the hippocampus to the nucleus accumbens regulate activity of ventral tegmental area dopamine neurons. *J Neurosci* 21:4915–4922.

Friedman SD, Castaneda E, Hodge GK (1998) Long-term monoamine depletion, differential recovery, and subtle behavioral impairment following methamphetamine-induced neurotoxicity. *Pharmacol Biochem Behav* 61:35–44.

Garcia-Fuster MJ, Flagel SB, Mahmood ST, Mayo LM, Thompson RC, Watson SJ, Akil H (2011) Decreased proliferation of adult hippocampal stem cells during cocaine withdrawal: possible role of the cell fate regulator FADD. *Neuropsychopharmacology.*

Gawin FH, Ellinwood EH, Jr (1989) Cocaine dependence. *Annu Rev Med* 40:149–161.

Gonzales R, Mooney L, Rawson RA (2010) The methamphetamine problem in the United States. *Annu Rev Public Health* 31:385–398.

Gould E, Beylin A, Tanapat P, Reeves A, Shors TJ (1999a) Learning enhances adult neurogenesis in the hippocampal formation. *Nat Neurosci* 2:260–265.

Gould E, Reeves AJ, Fallah M, Tanapat P, Gross CG, Fuchs E (1999b) Hippocampal neurogenesis in adult Old World primates. *Proc Nat Acad Sci U S A* 96:5263–5267.

Hastings NB, Tanapat P, Gould E (2001) Neurogenesis in the adult mammalian brain. *Clin Neurosci Res* 1:175–182.

Hildebrandt K, Teuchert-Noodt G, Dawirs RR (1999) A single neonatal dose of methamphetamine suppresses dentate granule cell proliferation in adult gerbils which is restored to control values by acute doses of haloperidol. *J Neural Transm* 106:549–558.

Hiranita T, Nawata Y, Sakimura K, Anggadiredja K, Yamamoto T (2006) Suppression of methamphetamine-seeking behavior by nicotinic agonists. *Proc Natl Acad Sci U S A* 103:8523–8527.

Itoh K, Fukumori R, Suzuki Y (1984) Effect of methamphetamine on the locomotor activity in the 6-OHDA dorsal hippocampus lesioned rat. *Life Sci* 34:827–833.

Itzhak Y (1997) Modulation of cocaine- and methamphetamine-induced behavioral sensitization by inhibition of brain nitric oxide synthase. *J Pharmacol Exp Ther* 282:521–527.

Itzhak Y, Anderson KL, Ali SF (2004) Differential response of nNOS knockout mice to MDMA ("ecstasy")- and methamphetamine-induced psychomotor sensitization and neurotoxicity. *Ann N Y Acad Sci* 1025:119–128.

Itzhak Y, Gandia C, Huang PL, Ali SF (1998) Resistance of neuronal nitric oxide synthase-deficient mice to methamphetamine-induced dopaminergic neurotoxicity. *J Pharmacol Exp Ther* 284:1040–1047.

Itzhak Y, Martin JL, Ali SF (1999) Methamphetamine- and 1-methyl-4-phenyl-1,2,3, 6-tetrahydropyridine-induced dopaminergic neurotoxicity in inducible nitric oxide synthase-deficient mice. *Synapse* 34:305–312.

Itzhak Y, Martin JL, Ali SF (2000) Comparison between the role of the neuronal and inducible nitric oxide synthase in methamphetamine-induced neurotoxicity and sensitization. *Ann N Y Acad Sci* 914:104–111.

Jayanthi S, Deng X, Noailles PA, Ladenheim B, Cadet JL (2004) Methamphetamine induces neuronal apoptosis via cross-talks between endoplasmic reticulum and mitochondria-dependent death cascades. *FASEB J* 18:238–251.

Kaplan MS, Hinds JW (1977) Neurogenesis in the adult rat: electron microscopic analysis of light radioautographs. *Science* 197:1092–1094.

Kempermann G, Jessberger S, Steiner B, Kronenberg G (2004) Milestones of neuronal development in the adult hippocampus. *Trends Neurosci* 27:447–452.

Kim WR, Christian K, Ming GL, Song H (2012) Time-dependent involvement of adult-born dentate granule cells in behavior. *Behav Brain Res* 227:470–479.

Kim YT, Lee JJ, Song HJ, Kim JH, Kwon DH, Kim MN, Yoo DS, Lee HJ, Kim HJ, Chang Y (2010) Alterations in cortical activity of male methamphetamine abusers performing an empathy task: fMRI study. *Hum Psychopharmacol* 25:63–70.

Kitamura O (2009) Detection of methamphetamine neurotoxicity in forensic autopsy cases. *Leg Med (Tokyo)* 11 Suppl 1:S63–65.

Kitamura O, Takeichi T, Wang EL, Tokunaga I, Ishigami A, Kubo S (2010) Microglial and astrocytic changes in the striatum of methamphetamine abusers. *Leg Med (Tokyo)* 12:57–62.

Knackstedt LA, Kalivas PW (2009) Glutamate and reinstatement. *Curr Opin Pharmacol* 9:59–64.

Kochman LJ, Fornal CA, Jacobs BL (2009) Suppression of hippocampal cell proliferation by short-term stimulant drug administration in adult rats. *Eur J Neurosci* 29:2157–2165.

Koob GF (1999) Stress, corticotropin-releasing factor, and drug addiction. *Ann N Y Acad Sci* 897:27–45.

Koob GF, Le Moal M (1997) Drug abuse: hedonic homeostatic dysregulation. *Science* 278:52–58.

Koob GF, Volkow ND (2010) Neurocircuitry of addiction. *Neuropsychopharmacology* 35:217–238.

Kramer JC, Fischman VS, Littlefield DC (1967) Amphetamine abuse. Pattern and effects of high doses taken intravenously. *Jama* 201:305–309.

Kronenberg G, Reuter K, Steiner B, Brandt MD, Jessberger S, Yamaguchi M, Kempermann G (2003) Subpopulations of proliferating cells of the adult hippocampus respond differently to physiologic neurogenic stimuli. *J Comp Neurol* 467:455–463.

Lacefield CO, Itskov V, Reardon T, Hen R, Gordon JA (2012) Effects of adult-generated granule cells on coordinated network activity in the dentate gyrus. *Hippocampus* 22:106–116.

Lasseter HC, Xie X, Ramirez DR, Fuchs RA (2010) Sub-region specific contribution of the ventral hippocampus to drug context-induced reinstatement of cocaine-seeking behavior in rats. *Neuroscience* 171: 830–839.

Luo AH, Tahsili-Fahadan P, Wise RA, Lupica CR, Aston-Jones G (2011) Linking context with reward: a functional circuit from hippocampal CA3 to ventral tegmental area. *Science* 333:353–357.

Mandyam CD, Koob GF (2012) The addicted brain craves new neurons: putative role for adult-born progenitors in promoting recovery. *Trends Neurosci* 35:250–260.

Mandyam CD, Wee S, Crawford EF, Eisch AJ, Richardson HN, Koob GF (2008) Varied access to intravenous methamphetamine self-administration differentially alters adult hippocampal neurogenesis. *Biol Psychiatry* 64:958–965.

Mandyam CD, Wee S, Eisch AJ, Richardson HN, Koob GF (2007) Methamphetamine self-administration and voluntary exercise have opposing effects on medial prefrontal cortex gliogenesis. *J Neurosci* 27:11442–11450.

Manganas LN, Zhang X, Li Y, Hazel RD, Smith SD, Wagshul ME, Henn F, Benveniste H, Djuric PM, Enikolopov G, Maletic-Savatic M (2007) Magnetic resonance spectroscopy identifies neural progenitor cells in the live human brain. *Science* 318:980–985.

McFarland K, Kalivas PW (2001) The circuitry mediating cocaine-induced reinstatement of drug-seeking behavior. *J Neurosci* 21:8655–8663.

McHugh TJ, Jones MW, Quinn JJ, Balthasar N, Coppari R, Elmquist JK, Lowell BB, Fanselow MS, Wilson MA, Tonegawa S (2007) Dentate gyrus NMDA receptors mediate rapid pattern separation in the hippocampal network. *Science* 317:94–99.

Messier B, Leblond CP (1960) Cell proliferation and migration as revealed by radioautography after injection of thymidine-H3 into male rats and mice. *Am J Anat* 106:247–285.

Morales AM, Lee B, Hellemann G, O'Neill J, London ED (2012) Gray-matter volume in methamphetamine dependence: cigarette smoking and changes with abstinence from methamphetamine. *Drug Alcohol Depend* 125:230–238.

Morris SA, Eaves DW, Smith AR, Nixon K (2009) Alcohol inhibition of neurogenesis: A mechanism of hippocampal neurodegeneration in an adolescent alcohol abuse model. *Hippocampus.*

Nakama H, Chang L, Fein G, Shimotsu R, Jiang CS, Ernst T (2011) Methamphetamine users show greater than normal age-related cortical gray matter loss. *Addiction* 106:1474–1483.

NIDA (2006) Research reports: Methamphetamine abuse and addiction. *The Science of Drug Abuse and Addiction.*

NIDA (2010) Drug Facts: Methamphetamine. *The Science of Drug Abuse and Addiction.*

NIDA (2011) Topics in brief: methamphetamine addiction: progress, but need to remain vigilant. *The Science of Drug Abuse and Addiction.*

Noonan MA, Bulin SE, Fuller DC, Eisch AJ (2010) Reduction of adult hippocampal neurogenesis confers vulnerability in an animal model of cocaine addiction. *J Neurosci* 30:304–315.

Noonan MA, Choi KH, Self DW, Eisch AJ (2008) Withdrawal from cocaine self-administration normalizes deficits in proliferation and enhances maturity of adult-generated hippocampal neurons. *J Neurosci* 28: 2516–2526.

Onaivi ES, Ali SF, Chirwa SS, Zwiller J, Thiriet N, Akinshola BE, Ishiguro H (2002) Ibogaine signals addiction genes and methamphetamine alteration of long-term potentiation. *Ann N Y Acad Sci* 965:28–46.

Orikabe L, Yamasue H, Inoue H, Takayanagi Y, Mozue Y, Sudo Y, Ishii T, Itokawa M, Suzuki M, Kurachi M, Okazaki Y, Kasai K (2011) Reduced amygdala and hippocampal volumes in patients with methamphetamine psychosis. *Schizophr Res* 132:183–189.

Price KL, DeSantis SM, Simpson AN, Tolliver BK, McRae-Clark AL, Saladin ME, Baker NL, Wagner MT, Brady KT (2011) The impact of clinical and demographic variables on cognitive performance in methamphetamine-dependent individuals in rural South Carolina. *Am J Addict* 20:447–455.

Rademacher DJ, Kovacs B, Shen F, Napier TC, Meredith GE (2006) The neural substrates of amphetamine conditioned place preference: implications for the formation of conditioned stimulus-reward associations. *Eur J Neurosci* 24:2089–2097.

Recinto P, Samant AR, Chavez G, Kim A, Yuan CJ, Soleiman M, Grant Y, Edwards S, Wee S, Koob GF, George O, Mandyam CD (2012) Levels of neural progenitors in the hippocampus predict memory impairment and relapse to drug seeking as a function of excessive methamphetamine self-administration. *Neuropsychopharmacology* 37:1275–1287.

Rogers JL, De Santis S, See RE (2008) Extended methamphetamine self-administration enhances reinstatement of drug seeking and impairs novel object recognition in rats. *Psychopharmacology* Berl) 199:615–624.

Sahay A, Scobie KN, Hill AS, O'Carroll CM, Kheirbek MA, Burghardt NS, Fenton AA, Dranovsky A, Hen R (2011) Increasing adult hippocampal neurogenesis is sufficient to improve pattern separation. *Nature* 472:466–470.

SAMHSA (2008) Results from the 2007 National Survey on Drug Use and Health: Detailed Tables. Substance Abuse and Mental Health Services Administration, Office of Applied Studies.

Schmidt-Hieber C, Jonas P, Bischofberger J (2004) Enhanced synaptic plasticity in newly generated granule cells of the adult hippocampus. *Nature* 429:184–187.

Schmued LC, Bowyer JF (1997) Methamphetamine exposure can produce neuronal degeneration in mouse hippocampal remnants. *Brain Res* 759:135–140.

Scholzen T, Gerdes J (2000) The Ki-67 protein: from the known and the unknown. *J Cell Physiol* 182:311–322.

Schwartz DL, Mitchell AD, Lahna DL, Luber HS, Huckans MS, Mitchell SH, Hoffman WF (2010) Global and local morphometric differences in recently abstinent methamphetamine-dependent individuals. *Neuroimage* 50:1392–1401.

Shaham Y, Shalev U, Lu L, De Wit H, Stewart J (2003) The reinstatement model of drug relapse: history, methodology and major findings. *Psychopharmacology (Berl)* 168:3–20.

Shalev U, Grimm JW, Shaham Y (2002) Neurobiology of relapse to heroin and cocaine seeking: a review. *Pharmacol Rev* 54:1–42.

Shen F, Meredith GE, Napier TC (2006) Amphetamine-induced place preference and conditioned motor sensitization requires activation of tyrosine kinase receptors in the hippocampus. *J Neurosci* 26:11041–11051.

Shiba T, Yamato M, Kudo W, Watanabe T, Utsumi H, Yamada K (2011) *In vivo* imaging of mitochondrial function in methamphetamine-treated rats. *Neuroimage* 57:866–872.

Shors TJ, Townsend DA, Zhao M, Kozorovitskiy Y, Gould E (2002) Neurogenesis may relate to some but not all types of hippocampal-dependent learning. *Hippocampus* 12:578–584.

Snyder JS, Kee N, Wojtowicz JM (2001) Effects of adult neurogenesis on synaptic plasticity in the rat dentate gyrus. *J Neurophysiol* 85:2423–2431.

Steiner B, Klempin F, Wang L, Kott M, Kettenmann H, Kempermann G (2006) Type-2 cells as link between glial and neuronal lineage in adult hippocampal neurogenesis. *Glia* 54:805–814.

Swant J, Chirwa S, Stanwood G, Khoshbouei H (2010) Methamphetamine reduces LTP and increases baseline synaptic transmission in the CA1 region of mouse hippocampus. *PLoS ONE* 5:e11382.

Taepavarapruk P, Floresco SB, Phillips AG (2000) Hyperlocomotion and increased dopamine efflux in the rat nucleus accumbens evoked by electrical stimulation of the ventral subiculum: role of ionotropic glutamate and dopamine D1 receptors. *Psychopharmacology (Berl)* 151:242–251.

Taffe MA, Kotzebue RW, Crean RD, Crawford EF, Edwards S, Mandyam CD (2010) Long-lasting reduction in hippocampal neurogenesis by alcohol consumption in adolescent nonhuman primates. *Proc Natl Acad Sci U S A* 107:11104–11109.

Tani K, Iyo M, Matsumoto H, Kawai M, Suzuki K, Iwata Y, Won T, Tsukamoto T, Sekine Y, Sakanoue M, Hashimoto K, Ohashi Y, Takei N, Mori N (2001) The effects of dentate granule cell destruction on behavioural activity and Fos protein expression induced by systemic methamphetamine in rats. *Br J Pharmacol* 134:1411–1418.

Tashiro A, Makino H, Gage FH (2007) Experience-specific functional modification of the dentate gyrus through adult neurogenesis: a critical period during an immature stage. *J Neurosci* 27:3252–3259.

Teuchert-Noodt G, Dawirs RR, Hildebrandt K (2000) Adult treatment with methamphetamine transiently decreases dentate granule cell proliferation in the gerbil hippocampus. *J Neural Transm* 107:133–143.

Thompson PM, Hayashi KM, Simon SL, Geaga JA, Hong MS, Sui Y, Lee JY, Toga AW, Ling W, London ED (2004) Structural abnormalities in the brains of human subjects who use methamphetamine. *J Neurosci* 24:6028–6036.

USPSTF (2008) Screening for illicit drug use.

van Praag H, Christie BR, Sejnowski TJ, Gage FH (1999) Running enhances neurogenesis, learning, and long-term potentiation in mice. *Proc Natl Acad Sci U S A* 96:13427–13431.

Vorel SR, Liu X, Hayes RJ, Spector JA, Gardner EL (2001) Relapse to cocaine-seeking after hippocampal theta burst stimulation. *Science* 292:1175–1178.

Wang J, Angulo JA (2011) Synergism between methamphetamine and the neuropeptide substance P on the production of nitric oxide in the striatum of mice. *Brain Res* 1369:131–139.

Wang J, Xu W, Ali SF, Angulo JA (2008) Connection between the striatal neurokinin-1 receptor and nitric oxide formation during methamphetamine exposure. *Ann N Y Acad Sci* 1139:164–171.

Weber E, Blackstone K, Iudicello JE, Morgan EE, Grant I, Moore DJ, Woods SP (2012) Neurocognitive deficits are associated with unemployment in chronic methamphetamine users. *Drug Alcohol Depend* 125:146–153.

WHO (1980).

Yamamoto BK, Bankson MG (2005) Amphetamine neurotoxicity: cause and consequence of oxidative stress. *Crit Rev Neurobiol* 17:87–117.

Yamamoto J (1997) Cortical and hippocampal EEG power spectra in animal models of schizophrenia produced with methamphetamine, cocaine, and phencyclidine. *Psychopharmacology (Berl)* 131:379–387.

Yan Y, Yamada K, Nitta A, Nabeshima T (2007) Transient drug-primed but persistent cue-induced reinstatement of extinguished methamphetamine-seeking behavior in mice. *Behav Brain Res* 177:261–268.

Yoshikawa T, Shibuya H, Kaneno S, Toru M (1991) Blockade of behavioral sensitization to methamphetamine by lesion of hippocampo-accumbal pathway. *Life Sci* 48:1325–1332.

Yuan CJ, Quiocho JM, Kim A, Wee S, Mandyam CD (2011) Extended access methamphetamine decreases immature neurons in the hippocampus which results from loss and altered development of neural progenitors without altered dynamics of the S-phase of the cell cycle. *Pharmacol Biochem Behav* 100:98–108.

Zhou LF, Zhu YP (2006) Changes of CREB in rat hippocampus, prefrontal cortex and nucleus accumbens during three phases of morphine induced conditioned place preference in rats. *J Zhejiang Univ Sci B* 7:107–113.

Zhu J, Xu W, Wang J, Ali SF, Angulo JA (2009) The neurokinin-1 receptor modulates the methamphetamine-induced striatal apoptosis and nitric oxide formation in mice. *J Neurochem* 111:656–668.

Chapter 11

Studies on Developmental Exposures to Anesthetic Agents and Stem Cell Derived Models

Fang Liu, Merle G. Paule, Tucker A. Patterson,
Cheng Wang, and William Slikker, Jr.

Because of obvious concerns, it is not possible to thoroughly explore the adverse effects of anesthetics in human infants and children. Nor is it possible to obtain relevant dose response and time-course data of anesthetic-induced neural damage and associated behavioral deficits in humans. However, the availability of stem cell-derived models, especially human embryonic neural stem cells (NSCs), along with their capacity for proliferation and their potential for differentiation, has provided an invaluable tool to examine the etiology of neurotoxicity and underlying mechanisms associated with developmental exposure to general pediatric anesthetic agents. Understanding such mechanisms will also help identify avenues of protection or prevention.

Introduction

Concerns have been raised that the effects of anesthetic drugs on the central nervous system (CNS) may result in long-term impairment after surgery or general anesthesia in humans. The field of anesthesia-related toxicology has employed multiple scientific disciplines in attempts to identify the basic characteristics of the anesthetic agents that may result in harmful, acute and/or chronic effects on the nervous system. Such characteristics continue to be defined at the molecular, biochemical, cellular, physiological and functional levels. It is now well known that the developing nervous system can vary dramatically in susceptibility to neurotoxic insults depending on the stage of development. Because of the complexity and temporal features underlying developmental neurotoxicity, this area of study may benefit greatly from the use of stem cell models.

Stem cell biology and/or models, in the context of toxicological insult, might provide an important structure around which information can be arrayed in the form of a biological model. The goals of applying stem cell-based approaches to developmental toxicology are to predict the functional outcomes of stimuli using integral *in vitro* models that allow for the directional and quantitative descriptions of responses at the cellular and molecular levels. The stimuli eliciting such responses may be environmental alterations, exposures to drugs or other chemicals, general anesthetics or infectious agents. Specifically, the utilization of stem cell models in exploring issues relevant to developmental anesthetic-induced brain damage has the potential to advance our understanding of brain-related biological processes, including those critical for normal processes such as neural plasticity, as well as those associated with the expression of toxicity (Keirstead *et al.*, 2005; Li *et al.*, 2005; Lamba *et al.*, 2006; Lee *et al.*, 2006; Kang *et al.*, 2007).

Pre-Clinical Findings on Anesthetic-Induced Developmental Neurotoxicity

As early as in 1974, in response to the concern that anesthesiologists and operating room nurses may suffer from occupational exposure to anesthetics, especially when they are pregnant, Quimby *et al.* (Quimby *et al.*, 1974) treated rats at different ages with a trace amount of halothane (10 ppm) and found that the rats were vulnerable to halothane during early development: 10 ppm halothane was sufficient to cause behavioral deficits, neuronal degeneration and abnormal synaptic networking, whereas the adult rats were not affected. No general concern was raised regarding the consequences of developmental anesthetic exposure until the end of the last century when Ikonomidou *et al.* (Ikonomidou *et al.*, 1999) reported an N-methyl-D-aspartate (NMDA) receptor antagonist caused extensive neurodegeneration in the developing rat brain. Pre-clinical studies from other groups confirmed their findings and extended the observations to the effects of GABA$_A$ receptor agonists, another category of general anesthetics (Jevtovic-Todorovic *et al.*, 2003; Wang *et al.*, 2003; Fredriksson *et al.*, 2004; Scallet *et al.*, 2004; Fredriksson *et al.*, 2007; Slikker *et al.*, 2007; Kahraman *et al.*, 2008; Satomoto *et al.*, 2009; Istaphanous *et al.*, 2011; Paule *et al.*, 2011; Creeley *et al.*, 2013).

Subsequent studies further defined anesthetic-induced effects with various findings, in addition to apoptotic neurodegeneration. For example, researchers from Vutskits' group performed a series of experiments evaluating the effect of anesthetics on synaptogenesis (De Roo *et al.*, 2009; Briner *et al.*, 2010; Briner *et al.*, 2011). They found some anesthetics significantly interfered with synaptogenesis after a 2-hr exposure, when no cell death was observed. Consequently, abnormal synaptogenesis may affect circuit assembly in the developing brain (Briner *et al.*, 2010). Animal experiments by another group (Zhu *et al.*, 2010) showed daily isoflurane exposure for 35 minutes for four successive days impaired object recognition and reversal learning in young, but not adult animals. The scientists found that the memory deficit in young animals was paralleled by a decrease in the hippocampal stem cell pool and reduced neurogenesis. The group did not further explore the mechanisms by which reduced neurogenesis was induced, but they did not observe increased cell death of progenitors or neurons in the hippocampus, which could contribute to reduced neurogenesis. Their findings indicated another possible neurotoxic effect the anesthetics possess.

In recent years, there are substantially increased publications examining the potential impact of anesthetics on the developing brain, which advance our understanding on how and why anesthetics cause developmental neurotoxicity. It has been suggested that increased reactive oxygen species (ROS) generation plays a critical role in anesthetic-induced developmental neurotoxicity (Zou *et al.*, 2008; Boscolo *et al.*, 2012; Liu *et al.*, 2013). Evaluated by the production of fluorescent DCF, it was shown that treatment with nitrous oxide (N_2O) and isoflurane for 6 hr significantly increased ROS generation in postnatal day (PND) 7 rat subiculum. This effect was effectively attenuated by an ROS scavenger, EUK-134 (Boscolo *et al.*, 2012). Studies from Wang's group indicated an anti-oxidant, L-carnitine's protective effects on anesthetic-induced toxic effects in the developing brain (Wang *et al.*, 2000, Zou *et al.*, 2008, Liu *et al.*, 2013), indirectly demonstrated the roles of ROS generation. These data also suggest a promising role of anti-oxidants in reducing/minimizing anesthetic-induced neurotoxicity.

Neurotrophic factors are a family of proteins that can regulate neuronal cell survival, which include nerve growth factor (NGF), brain derived neurotrophic factor (BDNF), neurotrophin-3, and -4/5, etc. (Skaper, 2012). It has shown that BDNF can either promote neuronal survival or cause neuronal apoptosis by binding to tropomyosin receptor kinase B or p75 neurotrophic receptor (p75[NTR]) (Lee *et al.*, 2001; Pang *et al.*, 2004). Head *et al.* (2009) managed to attenuate isoflurane-induced neuronal apoptosis in the neonatal CNS by inhibiting p75[NTR], indicating another pathway through which anesthetics (e.g., isoflurane) cause neuronal apoptosis.

Frequently used anesthetics either block NMDA-receptors or potentiate γ-aminobutyric acid (GABA)-receptors, Wang and his colleagues (Wang *et al.*, 1999; Wang *et al.*, 2000; Wang *et al.*, 2005a; Wang *et al.*, 2005b; Wang *et al.*, 2006; Slikker *et al.*, 2007; Liu *et al.*, 2013) have evaluated the roles of NMDA-receptors in ketamine or phencyclidine (PCP)-induced neuronal cell death, using multiple methods and experimental models. The group found the neurons that had been exposed to ketamine or PCP expressed higher levels of NMDA-receptors. They, therefore, hypothesize that the up-regulation of NMDA-receptors is a compensatory response of neurons whose

NMDA-receptors have been blocked by ketamine or PCP. After the anesthetic agent was eliminated from the plasma and brain, the NMDA-receptor antagonists' effects were diminished. The neurons bearing the up-regulated NMDA receptors will be more vulnerable to the excitotoxic effects of endogenous glutamate by allowing more Ca^{2+} influx through the activated NMDA receptors, followed by increased ROS generation and cell death (Slikker *et al.*, 2007).

While experimental studies imply potential clinical relevance, their extrapolation to clinical practice is not practical because of the obvious differences between human patients and animal models. For example, experimental animals were generally dosed much higher than human to achieve a surgical plane of anesthesia; secondly, the animal models did not have confounding factors as human patients do, such as surgery stimuli or concomitant illnesses. In addition, it is difficult to accurately match the developmental stages of an animal model to human, even non-human primates have a significantly shorter CNS development period compared with human.

Each year, there are approximate 6 million children receiving anesthesia in the USA (DeFrances *et al.*, 2007). Among them, 1.5 million are below 12 months of age (Sun, 2010). An estimated 2% of pregnant women in North America undergo anesthesia during their pregnancy for surgery that is not related to delivery (Bai *et al.*, 2013a). Hence, exposure to anesthesia during development is not rare. It has become a public concern whether general anesthetics are detrimental to the developing brain.

Clinical Studies on the Potential Adverse Effects of Anesthetics on Developing CNS

The United States Food and Drug Administration Anesthetic and Life Support Drugs Advisory Committee met in March 2007 to discuss the growing body of knowledge about the neurotoxicity of anesthetic and sedative drugs in juvenile animals and the implications of these data for children exposed to those agents. Although there were not sufficient data to support direct extrapolation of the findings from animals to humans, the committee participants agreed that strategies were needed to assess the impact of the drugs on the developing brain in order to provide appropriate guidance regarding the clinical use of these drugs and address public concerns.

Human studies are therefore necessary. In fact, it has been many years since an initial report indicating potential impact of anesthesia on behavior changes in children (Eckenhoff, 1953). Dr. Eckenhoff pointed out a correlation of anesthesia with personality changes in 612 children who underwent otolaryngological operations. Among these children, 17% of them showed personality changes; and the younger the child, the more likely they were to develop personality changes (Eckenhoff, 1953).

Due to multiple limitations, till now there are no prospective studies evaluating the impact of anesthetics on young children. In recent years a few retrospective studies have emerged (Loepke and Soriano, 2008; Bartels *et al.*, 2009; DiMaggio *et al.*, 2009; Wilder *et al.*, 2009), with mixed implication of anesthesia-related neurotoxicity. For example, Bartel *et al.* (2009) evaluated the cognitive functions of 1,143 monozygotic twin pairs who received anesthesia before age 3 and found they showed lower educational achievement scores and significantly more cognitive problems than twins who were not exposed to anesthesia. However, they also found that the unexposed co-twin from discordant pairs did not differ from their exposed co-twin. Therefore, they concluded there was no evidence for a causal relationship between anesthesia administration and later learning-related outcomes, at least in the sample they studied. Although there were questions concerning the methods and analysis conducted in Bartel's study, the consensus is the use of twin studies has great potential to advance our knowledge surrounding the issue of anesthetic neurotoxicity in children (Flick *et al.*, 2009). Later, Hansen *et al.* (2011) compared the academic performance of adolescents who had inguinal hernia surgery prior to 1 year of age with a randomly selected 5% population of age-matched cohorts in Denmark. After adjusting some confounding factors the researchers concluded that the hernia repair in infancy, accompanied with relatively short anesthetic exposure, did not significantly affect academic performance during adolescence.

However, some studies conclude a negative impact of early exposure to anesthetics on children. An analysis of a retrospective cohort study from DiMaggio *et al.* (2009) evaluated behavioral and developmental disorders in 383 children who received inguinal hernia surgery before 3 years of age and compared the results with those from 5,050 age-matched children with no history of hernia-repair prior to age 3. Their analysis indicated a significant relevance of anesthesia and surgery of hernia repair under age 3 to increased risk of behavioral/developmental disorders. Another study from the same group (DiMaggio *et al.*, 2011) evaluated the behavioral/ developmental disorders in 10,450 siblings, 304 of them were exposed to anesthetics before 3 years of age and 10,146 children were not exposed. The results also suggested children younger than 3 who received anesthesia for surgeries were more likely to have developmental and behavioral disorders compared with their siblings who did not undergo surgery. In line with these two studies, a study from Ing *et al.* (2012) implied that exposure to anesthesia under age 3 increased the risk of developing language and abstract reasoning deficits by age 10, confining the outcome to a specific domain.

Some data suggested that the earlier a child receives general anesthesia, the more vulnerable the child is to anesthetics. A population-based birth cohort study by Warner's group (Wilder *et al.*, 2009), which included 5,357 children, demonstrated that multiple exposures to anesthesia before age 4 was a significant risk factor for the later development of learning disabilities in children, while a single anesthetic treatment was not. As the authors stated, although it was not clear whether exposure to anesthesia itself contributed to the development of learning disabilities in children who had more than one treatment with anesthesia, or the need for multiple treatments of anesthesia indicated other unidentified confounding factors that contributed to learning disabilities, their results implied the possibility of potential adverse effects of repeated anesthetic exposures on the developing CNS. The same group further analyzed the data and concluded that repeated exposure to anesthesia during surgery before age 2 was a significant risk factor for developing learning disabilities (Flick *et al.*, 2011). Later, the group related the development of Attention-Deficit/Hyperactivity Disorder (ADHD) to multiple general anesthesia exposure before age 2, even after adjusting for comorbidities (Sprung *et al.*, 2012).

Although researchers interpreted their results with great caution, there are limitations to the methods that were employed. Various confounding factors cannot be excluded from the indicated neurotoxicity, which limited the significance of these observations. Currently, there are some on-going studies, such as Pediatric Anesthesia and NeuroDevelopment Assessment (PANDA) (Sun, 2010), etc., which aim at providing more informative evidence that can add to the body of knowledge surrounding the important topic of the long-term neurodevelopmental effects of anesthesia and surgery in infants and young children.

Challenges We are Facing

A well-controlled human study would undoubtedly provide more convincing evidence compared to animal studies. However, legal and ethical issues, the complexity and diversity of pediatric anesthesia, the lack of standard criteria to assess the consequence of anesthesia, and the loss of follow-up during studies, etc., make a comprehensive human study quite challenging.

Until recently, most pre-clinical studies focused on anesthetic-induced cell death in the developing brain during the growth spurt period, when it is the most vulnerable. Although neuronal cell death is the major pathological finding, some other changes in neural biological processes, such as neural cell proliferation, migration and differentiation, etc., may also play critical roles in anesthetic-induced deficits. Currently, it is not practical to monitor such effects of anesthetics on the CNS in infants and children. To bridge this gap, NSCs, especially human embryonic NSCs, along with their capacity for proliferation and their potential for differentiation, may be a feasible model.

Application of NSC Models to Evaluate Anesthetic-Induced Neurotoxicity During Development

The advances in our knowledge of stem cell biology have made stem cells a potential therapy for some diseases, and an emerging *in vitro* model to test drugs and chemicals for developmental toxicity. Additionally, application of NSC models in developmental neurotoxicity has been an invaluable tool for testing the potential of anesthetic-induced neurotoxicity.

During development NSCs are the sources of neurons, astrocytes and oligodendrocytes in the CNS, owing to their ability to self-renew and be multipotent. The self-renewal of NSCs is characterized by two different types of cell divisions: symmetric and asymmetric. Symmetric cell division refers to the generation of two daughter cells that have same fate; while through asymmetric cell division, only one daughter cell remains the same as the mother cell, the other does not, being more differentiated. Symmetric cell renewal precedes the asymmetric one, generating enough amounts of NSCs for development of the CNS. Asymmetric cell divisions give rise to more differentiated neural cells, such as progenitor cells, or even neurons (Gotz and Huttner, 2005). Various factors may contribute to determining the fates of NSCs and control the transition from neural proliferation to differentiation. Therefore, development of embryonic NSC-based models could recapitulate CNS development *in vitro*, distinguish roles of some specific factors during the development process, and evaluate whether anesthetics may change the growth rate of NSCs or limit the types and numbers of cells they may eventually become.

Establishment of NSC models

It has been shown that by embryonic day 17, most cells that are destined to become cerebral cortical neurons are generated in rodent (Parnavelas, 1999; Levers *et al.*, 2001). To test how anesthetics affect NSCs (or neural progenitor cells) and neurogenesis, NSCs could be harvested from the cortex of Sprague-Dawley rat brain between embryonic day 14 to 16 (Liu *et al.*, 2014). The harvested brain tissues were triturated with a fire-polished Pasteur pipette to dissociate the cells in ice-cold Hank's solution without Ca^{2+} or Mg^{2+}. The dissociated cells were washed with serum-free medium by centrifugation ($200 \times g$, 10 min), and cultured in serum-free medium supplemented with N-2, growth factors [e.g. basic fibroblast growth factor (bFGF); epidermal growth factor (EGF); and platelet-derived growth factor (PDGF)], and neurotrophin-3 at a cell density of $3–5 \times 10^5$/ml in 25 ml flasks for proliferation in a humidified cell culture incubator at 37°C with 5% CO_2. The cells grew in the form of spheres in flasks. They were then collected, physically separated into single cells by aspiration and transferred to culture dishes. The culture dishes were coated with poly-lysine, which is absorbed to the culture surface to increase the positive charge of the surface, therefore enhancing electrostatic interaction between culture dish surface and cell membrane to help cells attach. The undifferentiated cells kept proliferating and they were ready for experiments.

The NSCs could be characterized using NSC specific markers (such as nestin and SOX2). Nestin is one of the intermediate filaments, a widely employed neural stem marker. It has been demonstrated that most stem cells or progenitor cells expressing nestin are actively engaged in proliferation during early development (Wiese *et al.*, 2004). SOX proteins are expressed in many tissues during development. SOX2 is expressed in embryonic and adult NSCs, and its expression lasts until the cells differentiate, rendering SOX2 a marker of NSCs (Thiel, 2013). Previous data showed that the majority of the cells, both in the periphery and the center of spheres, are nestin and SOX2 positive (Figure 1). The NSC proliferation could be determined using the 5-ethynyl-2′-deoxyruidine (EdU) incorporation assay. EdU is a nucleoside analog of thymidine. It can be incorporated in newly synthesized DNA, thus it is used to assess cellular proliferation. The rat NSCs showed an active proliferation status as indicated by numerous EdU-positive stained nuclei.

Potential adverse effects of anesthetics on NSCs

This review presents an overview of representative general anesthetics — primarily propofol — as examples of how NSCs can

Immunocytochemical Staining
(Rat Embryonic Neural Stem Cells)

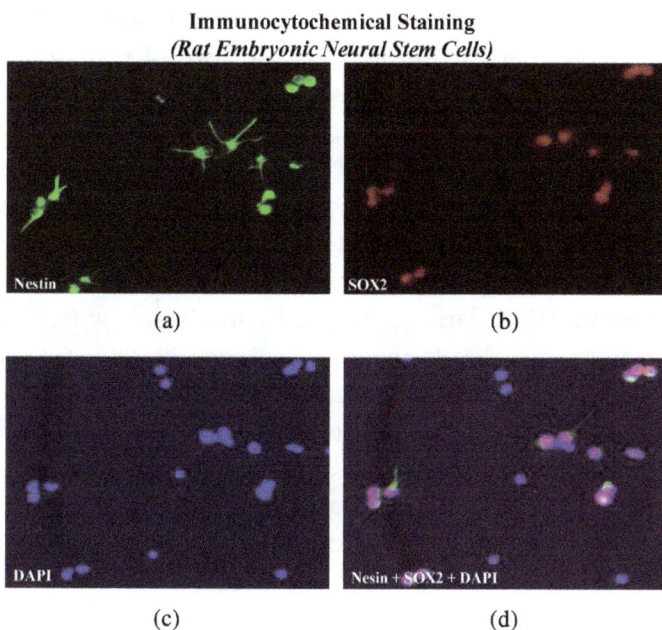

Figure 1. Photographs of rat embryonic NSC culture on DIV-8 (20x). (a) shows nestin immunostaining (green fluorescence); (b)indicates SOX2 staining (rhodamine) and (c) illustrates the DAPI staining (nuclear staining in blue, a dye for total nuclei). (d) is a merged picture of a, b, and c.

be valuable in identifying the doses and time course over which the individual drug produces damages and/or protects NSCs and cells differentiated from them, changes their proliferation rate, and alters their fates (differentiation into neurons, oligodendrocytes and astrocytes) *in vitro*. Here, a strategy of the use of embryonic NSC cultures for monitoring potential adverse effects of anesthetics (e.g., propofol) on NSC expansion, proliferation, differentiation and receptor functions has been defined (Liu *et al.*, 2014).

To study the vulnerability of NSCs to anesthetic-induced toxicity, lactate dehydrogenase (LDH) release and MTT [3-(4,5-dimethylthiazole-2-yl)-2,5-diphenyltetrazolium bromide] assays were utilized. Higher LDH release from cells suggests the rupture of cell membrane integrity, while decreased MTT uptake implies mitochondrial damage and dysfunctions. Propofol exposure resulted in a dose-dependent reduction of NSC viability, as indicated by a significant decrease of mitochondrial metabolism of MTT into formazon. However, a clinically relevant dose of propofol did not significantly increase LDH release. These observations indicated propofol may have caused a higher rate of apoptosis in NSCs. Propofol-induced apoptosis was confirmed by an enzyme-linked immunosorbant assay (ELISA) assay (Cell Death ELISA assay) and FITC-annexin V -propidium iodide (PI) staining (Figure 2).

In the developing brain, nuclear genome and mitochondrial genomes incur DNA damage, primarily mediated by free radicals. During embryonic development, accelerated DNA transactions, which support rapid cell proliferation, may even further jeopardize the integrity of DNA. To investigate whether oxidative DNA damage could be induced by propofol exposure, an 8-hydroxy-2'-deoxy-guanosine (8-oxo-dG) ELISA assay was utilized (Liu *et al.*, 2014), which determined levels of 8-ox-dG and its analogs in the culture medium. 8-ox-dG is used as a biomarker for oxidative DNA damage. In this study, NSC cultures were exposed to propofol at a clinically relevant concentration (50 µM) for 24 hr. Propofol remarkably increased oxidative DNA damage as evidenced by significant increases in 8-oxo-dG expression, and no significant effects were detected in cultures exposed to propofol (50 µM) for either 3 or 6 hr.

Given the importance of NSC proliferation in neurogenesis and developmental toxicity, it was necessary to examine whether enhanced NSC damage after propofol exposure could be associated with interruptions in the cell division cycle and relevant mechanisms. In the same study (Liu *et al.*, 2014), NSC proliferation was determined using a commercially available EdU incorporation assay. After a 24-hr exposure to propofol (50 µM), the number of dividing cells was substantially decreased compared to controls, suggesting a decrease in NSC proliferation. In this study, the impaired proliferation rate and enhanced cell death were attenuated by acetyl-L-carnitine. These data strongly suggest propofol can initially cause oxidative mitochondrial damage and dysfunction, and subsequently affect neural stem cell proliferation by slowing down or even stopping the cell cycle, and finally enhancing the damage of NSCs.

(a)

(b)

(c)

(d)

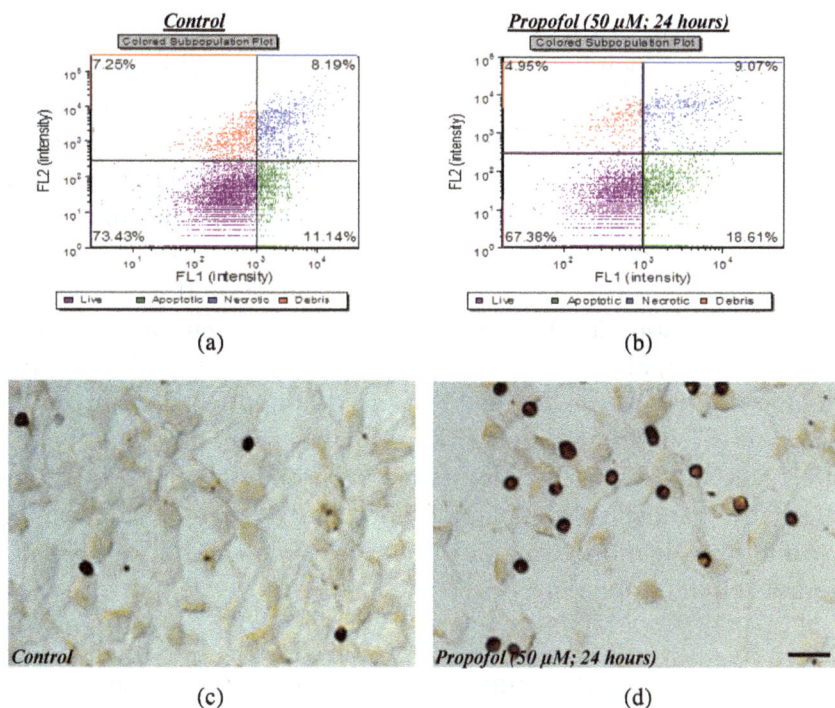

Figure 2. Propofol-induced NSC toxicity. Representative scatter plots (a and b) indicate the live cells in violet, apoptotic cells in green (FITC annexin-V staining) and necrotic cells in blue (propidium iodide staining). Compared with controls (a), propofol (50 µM) exposure for 24 hr (b) resulted in an increase in apoptosis and a reduction in live cells. However, no significant effect was observed for necrotic cells. (c and d) show the representative photographs of the TUNEL assay. Only a few TUNEL-positive cells were observed in the control culture (c), however, numerous darkly stained TUNEL-positive cells exhibiting typical nuclear condensation indicative of enhanced apoptosis were observed in propofol-treated culture (d). Cited from (Liu *et al.*, 2014).

Similarly, another study by Culley *et al.* (2011) also utilized embryonic NSCs from SD rats to evaluate isoflurane's effects. After exposure to different doses (0.7, 1.4, or 2.8%) of isoflurane for 6 hr, enhanced NSC damage was not detected, but a substantial reduction of NSC proliferation was observed. In addition, 24 hr after isoflurane exposure a significantly decreased number of NSCs was detected compared with controls (Culley *et al.*, 2011). Notably, a

15–20% decrease in neurogenesis *in vivo* was sufficient to impair hippocampal-dependent memory in rodents (Imayoshi *et al.*, 2008). Therefore, the reduced NSC proliferation may underlie the impaired neurogenesis/neurologic development *in vivo* (Culley *et al.*, 2011).

Based on these recent studies (Culley *et al.*, 2011; Liu *et al.*, 2014), it is consistently observed that different anesthetics and different exposure durations have different impacts on NSCs. Moreover, the effects of anesthetics on NSCs can be far beyond NSC viability and proliferation that have been observed. As mentioned earlier, anesthetics may also affect neural cell migration, differentiation, and change the types of cells the NSCs are destined to, etc. Currently, many research groups are working on assessing how anesthetics affect NSC differentiation. NSC-based *in vitro* models may serve as an alternative parallel to animal experiments, which can reduce animal use and provide more dynamic observations while mimicking *in vivo* neural cell development.

Human embryonic NSCs and neural induction from human embryonic stem (ES) and induced pluripotent stem (iPS) cells

There is always the question of whether the findings from animals or animal-derived models can mirror those in human. With the emergence of commercially available human embryonic NSCs, a promising alternative exists for evaluating the impact of anesthetics on the developing human CNS. The commercial human embryonic NSCs are primarily from cortical and/or hippocampal areas of fetal brain. Again, human embryonic NSC features can be verified using NSC markers such as nestin, SOX1, 2, etc. In the human body, oxygen concentrations vary from 1% to 10%. For example, oxygen concentrations range from 0.5% to 7% in the brain. This lower oxygen environment supports hypoxia-inducible factor 1α (HIF1α) to facilitate signal transduction pathways that promote self-renewal and inhibit NSC differentiation or apoptosis (Panchision, 2009). Therefore, cultures of human NSCs in low oxygen (5%) help maintain their active proliferative state and minimize their spontaneous differentiation. Under such *in vitro* conditions, similar to the embryonic NSCs of rodents, human NSCs should perfectly exhibit their capability of proliferation and potential to differentiate into different lineages of neurons, astrocytes and oligodendrocytes. Actually, our preliminary observations (unpublished data) have indicated that well-enriched human NSCs and differentiated neurons (differentiated from the same human NSCs) are quite sensitive to prolonged anesthetic (e.g. ketamine) exposure.

Meanwhile, a recent human NSC study (Bai *et al.*, 2013b) reported a remarkable increase in NSC proliferation rate after a 6-hr exposure to ketamine, but no enhanced NSC death was observed even after a 24-hr ketamine exposure. However, after 24-hr ketamine exposure (100 µM), typical apoptotic features/enhanced apoptosis and mitochondria damage were detected from the differentiated neurons, and those neurons were differentiated from the same human embryonic NSCs. Consistently, these data suggest that pediatric sedative/anesthesia-induced neurotoxicity depends on the amounts (doses) given, durations of the exposure, routes of administration, the receptor sub-type activated, and the stages of the neural development at the time of exposure. These contributors can help identify thresholds of exposure for producing neurotoxicity in the developing nervous system. There are yet many questions to answer before the findings of pediatric drug-induced neurotoxicity observed *in vitro* can be correlated to the effects in human.

Despite the fact that data generated from human NSCs and human ES cells are more relevant, ethical and moral concerns limit their sources and applications. In 2006, Takahashi and Yamanaka established the first iPS cell model that had almost the same pluripotency as ES cells (Takahashi and Yamanaka, 2006). The discovery of iPS cells may circumvent those concerns. The discovery also provides a possibility to generate iPS cells using somatic cells from any one, either a healthy person or a patient with a specific disease. Like ES cells, iPS cells can be induced to various cell types, including neural cells, which can be further differentiate to neurons, astrocytes and oligodendrocytes. Although scientists have found some discrepancies between human ES cells and iPS cells (Feng *et al.*, 2010; Hu *et al.*, 2010), the vast available sources for generating iPS cells, especially generation of patient-specific stem cells from iPS cells, such as NSCs, can facilitate studies of human neurological disorders and patient-specific therapy. In the meantime, iPS cells are becoming a valuable tool for drug development and toxicological studies, such as developmental neurotoxicity studies. Therefore, utilization of human iPS cells to evaluate the effects of anesthetics on the developing CNS is promising.

Application Outlook

From 2007, the National Research Council has advocated the use of *in vitro* systems and pathway analysis for toxicological studies (National Research Council, 2007). NSCs, especially human NSCs, could fit well into the advocacy and be used in evaluating the impacts of anesthetics on the developing CNS before the concerns can be cleared by any clinical studies.

A variety of NSCs have now been identified, many of which differ from each other in their ability to differentiation, their responses to cytokines, and their surface antigen characteristics. By studying NSC induction and development, we can identify the various factors that stimulate or inhibit their differentiation and the requirements of these cells and their offspring for survival and optimal function. While NSCs show good potential in neurotoxicity studies, variability exists. It is critical to establish reliable, stable and reproducible *in vitro* NSC models for quality control and consistency. As mentioned, control of oxygen concentration in the culture environment can be more critical to stem cells than cell lines. A low-oxygen environment is favorable for NSC culture.

While NSC models are valuable tools for neuroscience, in general, and for preclinical research in particular, they also hold great promise for clinical use in the treatment of neurodegenerative diseases and neurological disorders. There are, however, some limitations for their use in evaluating aspects of developmental neurotoxicity. One of the main concerns surrounding the use of the current two-dimensional (2D) NSC cultures is the lack of three-dementional (3D) structure that more closely resembles actual *in vivo* microenvironments which include extracellular matrices, adhesion junctions, etc. In addition, the utilization of digestive enzymes, such as trypsin and papain, during NSC isolation and harvest may significantly alter their surface antigen characteristics, thus, rendering them different from *in vivo* cells.

On the other hand, recent advances in technology and our understanding of stem cell biology and neuroscience have opened up new avenues of research for detecting developmental neurotoxicity. Currently, 3D culture systems are generally available and using such systems, cell growth, migration, connectivity and more naturalistic structures and environments can be optimally supported and studied. Additionally, mechanical trituration in calcium- and magnesium-free isolation buffer using fire-polished Pasteur pipettes instead of digestive enzymes may result in more physiologically-relevant, less disruptive dissociating conditions and, thus, higher quality cell cultures.

NSCs have become a promising tool for neurotoxicity studies. *In vitro* neurotoxicity tests using NSCs are currently evolving. Similar to their promise for therapeutic purposes, there remains significant uncertainty to define before the roles of NSCs become explicit in toxicological studies and regulatory science.

Disclaimer: This document has been reviewed in accordance with United States Food and Drug Administration (FDA) policy and approved for publication. Approval does not signify that the contents necessarily reflect the position or opinions of the FDA. The findings and conclusions in this report are those of the authors and do not necessarily represent the views of the FDA.

Competing Interests:

No external funding and no competing interests declared.

References

Bai X, Twaroski D, Bosnjak ZJ (2013a) Modeling anesthetic developmental neurotoxicity using human stem cells. *Semin Cardiothorac Vasc Anesth* 17:276–287.

Bai X, Yan Y, Canfield S, Muravyeva MY, Kikuchi C, Zaja I, Corbett JA, Bosnjak ZJ (2013b) Ketamine enhances human neural stem cell proliferation and induces neuronal apoptosis via reactive oxygen species-mediated mitochondrial pathway. *Anesth Analg* 116:869–880.

Bartels M, Althoff RR, Boomsma DI (2009) Anesthesia and cognitive performance in children: no evidence for a causal relationship. *Twin Res Hum Genet* 12:246–253.

Boscolo A, Starr JA, Sanchez V, Lunardi N, DiGruccio MR, Ori C, Erisir A, Trimmer P, Bennett J, Jevtovic-Todorovic V (2012) The abolishment of anesthesia-induced cognitive impairment by timely protection of mitochondria in the developing rat brain: the importance of free oxygen radicals and mitochondrial integrity. *Neurobiol Dis* 45:1031–1041.

Briner A, De Roo M, Dayer A, Muller D, Habre W, Vutskits L (2010) Volatile anesthetics rapidly increase dendritic spine density in the rat medial prefrontal cortex during synaptogenesis. *Anesthesiology* 112:546–556.

Briner A, Nikonenko I, De Roo M, Dayer A, Muller D, Vutskits L (2011) Developmental Stage-dependent persistent impact of propofol anesthesia on dendritic spines in the rat medial prefrontal cortex. *Anesthesiology* 115:282–293.

Creeley C, Dikranian K, Dissen G, Martin L, Olney J, Brambrink A (2013) Propofol-induced apoptosis of neurones and oligodendrocytes in fetal and neonatal rhesus macaque brain. *Br J Anaesth* 110 Suppl 1:i29–38.

Culley DJ, Boyd JD, Palanisamy A, Xie Z, Kojima K, Vacanti CA, Tanzi RE, Crosby G (2011) Isoflurane decreases self-renewal capacity of rat cultured neural stem cells. *Anesthesiology* 115:754–763.

De Roo M, Klauser P, Briner A, Nikonenko I, Mendez P, Dayer A, Kiss JZ, Muller D, Vutskits L (2009) Anesthetics rapidly promote synaptogenesis during a critical period of brain development. *PLoS One* 4:e7043.

DeFrances CJ, Cullen KA, Kozak LJ (2007) National Hospital Discharge Survey: 2005 annual summary with detailed diagnosis and procedure data. *Vital Health Stat* 13:1–209.

DiMaggio C, Sun LS, Kakavouli A, Byrne MW, Li G (2009) A retrospective cohort study of the association of anesthesia and hernia repair surgery with behavioral and developmental disorders in young children. *J Neurosurg Anesthesiol* 21:286–291.

DiMaggio C, Sun LS, Li G (2011) Early childhood exposure to anesthesia and risk of developmental and behavioral disorders in a sibling birth cohort. *Anesth Analg* 113:1143–1151.

Eckenhoff JE (1953) Relationship of anesthesia to postoperative personality changes in children. *AMA Am J Dis Child* 86:587–591.

Feng Q, Lu SJ, Klimanskaya I, Gomes I, Kim D, Chung Y, Honig GR, Kim KS, Lanza R (2010) Hemangioblastic derivatives from human induced pluripotent stem cells exhibit limited expansion and early senescence. *Stem Cells* 28:704–712.

Flick RP, Katusic SK, Colligan RC, Wilder RT, Voigt RG, Olson MD, Sprung J, Weaver AL, Schroeder DR, Warner DO (2011) Cognitive and behavioral outcomes after early exposure to anesthesia and surgery. *Pediatrics* 128:e1053–1061.

Flick RP, Wilder RT, Sprung J, Katusic SK, Voigt R, Colligan R, Schroeder DR, Weaver AL, Warner DO (2009) Anesthesia and cognitive performance in children: no evidence for a causal relationship. Are the conclusions justified by the data? Response to Bartels *et al.*, 2009. *Twin Res Hum Genet* 12:611–612; discussion 613–614.

Fredriksson A, Archer T, Alm H, Gordh T, Eriksson P (2004) Neurofunctional deficits and potentiated apoptosis by neonatal NMDA antagonist administration. *Behav Brain Res* 153:367–376.

Fredriksson A, Ponten E, Gordh T, Eriksson P (2007) Neonatal exposure to a combination of N-methyl-D-aspartate and gamma-aminobutyric acid type A receptor anesthetic agents potentiates apoptotic neurodegeneration and persistent behavioral deficits. *Anesthesiology* 107:427–436.

Gotz M, Huttner WB (2005) The cell biology of neurogenesis. *Nat Rev Mol Cell Biol* 6:777–788.

Hansen TG, Pedersen JK, Henneberg SW, Pedersen DA, Murray JC, Morton NS, Christensen K (2011) Academic performance in adolescence after inguinal hernia repair in infancy: a nationwide cohort study. *Anesthesiology* 114:1076–1085.

Head BP, Patel HH, Niesman IR, Drummond JC, Roth DM, Patel PM (2009) Inhibition of p75 neurotrophin receptor attenuates isoflurane-mediated neuronal apoptosis in the neonatal central nervous system. *Anesthesiology* 110:813–825.

Hu BY, Weick JP, Yu J, Ma LX, Zhang XQ, Thomson JA, Zhang SC (2010) Neural differentiation of human induced pluripotent stem cells follows developmental principles but with variable potency. *Proc Natl Acad Sci U S A* 107:4335–4340.

Ikonomidou C, Bosch F, Miksa M, Bittigau P, Vockler J, Dikranian K, Tenkova TI, Stefovska V, Turski L, Olney JW (1999) Blockade of NMDA receptors and apoptotic neurodegeneration in the developing brain. *Science* 283:70–74.

Imayoshi I, Sakamoto M, Ohtsuka T, Takao K, Miyakawa T, Yamaguchi M, Mori K, Ikeda T, Itohara S, Kageyama R (2008) Roles of continuous neurogenesis in the structural and functional integrity of the adult forebrain. *Nat Neurosci* 11:1153–1161.

Ing C, DiMaggio C, Whitehouse A, Hegarty MK, Brady J, von Ungern-Sternberg BS, Davidson A, Wood AJ, Li G, Sun LS (2012) Long-term differences in language and cognitive function after childhood exposure to anesthesia. *Pediatrics* 130:e476–485.

Istaphanous GK, Howard J, Nan X, Hughes EA, McCann JC, McAuliffe JJ, Danzer SC, Loepke AW (2011) Comparison of the neuroapoptotic properties of equipotent anesthetic concentrations of desflurane, isoflurane, or sevoflurane in neonatal mice. *Anesthesiology* 114: 578–587.

Jevtovic-Todorovic V, Hartman RE, Izumi Y, Benshoff ND, Dikranian K, Zorumski CF, Olney JW, Wozniak DF (2003) Early exposure to common anesthetic agents causes widespread neurodegeneration in the developing rat brain and persistent learning deficits. *J Neurosci* 23:876–882.

Kahraman S, Zup SL, McCarthy MM, Fiskum G (2008) GABAergic mechanism of propofol toxicity in immature neurons. *J Neurosurg Anesthesiol* 20:233–240.

Kang SM, Cho MS, Seo H, Yoon CJ, Oh SK, Choi YM, Kim DW (2007) Efficient induction of oligodendrocytes from human embryonic stem cells. *Stem Cells* 25:419–424.

Keirstead HS, Nistor G, Bernal G, Totoiu M, Cloutier F, Sharp K, Steward O (2005) Human embryonic stem cell-derived oligodendrocyte progenitor cell transplants remyelinate and restore locomotion after spinal cord injury. *J Neurosci* 25:4694–4705.

Lamba DA, Karl MO, Ware CB, Reh TA (2006) Efficient generation of retinal progenitor cells from human embryonic stem cells. *Proc Natl Acad Sci U S A* 103:12769–12774.

Lee DS, Yu K, Rho JY, Lee E, Han JS, Koo DB, Cho YS, Kim J, Lee KK, Han YM (2006) Cyclopamine treatment of human embryonic stem cells followed by culture in human astrocyte medium promotes differentiation into nestin- and GFAP-expressing astrocytic lineage. *Life Sci* 80:154–159.

Lee R, Kermani P, Teng KK, Hempstead BL (2001) Regulation of cell survival by secreted proneurotrophins. *Science* 294:1945–1948.

Levers TE, Edgar JM, Price DJ (2001) The fates of cells generated at the end of neurogenesis in developing mouse cortex. *J Neurobiol* 48: 265–277.

Li XJ, Du ZW, Zarnowska ED, Pankratz M, Hansen LO, Pearce RA, Zhang SC (2005) Specification of motoneurons from human embryonic stem cells. *Nat Biotechnol* 23:215–221.

Liu F, Patterson TA, Sadovova N, Zhang X, Liu S, Zou X, Hanig JP, Paule MG, Slikker W, Jr., Wang C (2013) Ketamine-induced neuronal damage and altered N-methyl-D-aspartate receptor function in rat primary forebrain culture. *Toxicol Sci* 131:548–557.

Liu F, Rainosek SW, Sadovova N, Fogle CM, Patterson TA, Hanig JP, Paule MG, Slikker W, Jr., Wang C (2014) Protective effect of acetyl-l-carnitine on propofol-induced toxicity in embryonic neural stem cells. *Neurotoxicology* 42C:49–57.

Loepke AW, Soriano SG (2008) An assessment of the effects of general anesthetics on developing brain structure and neurocognitive function. *Anesth Analg* 106:1681–1707.

National Research Council (2007) *Toxicity Testing in the 21st Century: A Vision and a Strategy.* Washington, D.C

Panchision DM (2009) The role of oxygen in regulating neural stem cells in development and disease. *J Cell Physiol* 220:562–568.

Pang PT, Teng HK, Zaitsev E, Woo NT, Sakata K, Zhen S, Teng KK, Yung WH, Hempstead BL, Lu B (2004) Cleavage of proBDNF by tPA/plasmin is essential for long-term hippocampal plasticity. *Science* 306:487–491.

Parnavelas JG (1999) Glial cell lineages in the rat cerebral cortex. *Exp Neurol* 156:418–429.

Paule MG, Li M, Allen RR, Liu F, Zou X, Hotchkiss C, Hanig JP, Patterson TA, Slikker W, Jr., Wang C (2011) Ketamine anesthesia during the first week of life can cause long-lasting cognitive deficits in rhesus monkeys. *Neurotoxicol Teratol* 33:220–230.

Quimby KL, Aschkenase LJ, Bowman RE, Katz J, Chang LW (1974) Enduring learning deficits and cerebral synaptic malformation from exposure to 10 parts of halothane per million. *Science* 185:625–627.

Satomoto M, Satoh Y, Terui K, Miyao H, Takishima K, Ito M, Imaki J (2009) Neonatal exposure to sevoflurane induces abnormal social behaviors and deficits in fear conditioning in mice. *Anesthesiology* 110:628–637.

Scallet AC, Schmued LC, Slikker W, Jr., Grunberg N, Faustino PJ, Davis H, Lester D, Pine PS, Sistare F, Hanig JP (2004) Developmental neurotoxicity of ketamine: morphometric confirmation, exposure parameters, and multiple fluorescent labeling of apoptotic neurons. *Toxicol Sci* 81:364–370.

Skaper SD (2012) *The Neurotrophic Factors: Methods and Protocols. Springer.*

Slikker W, Jr., Zou X, Hotchkiss CE, Divine RL, Sadovova N, Twaddle NC, Doerge DR, Scallet AC, Patterson TA, Hanig JP, Paule MG, Wang C (2007) Ketamine-induced neuronal cell death in the perinatal rhesus monkey. *Toxicol Sci* 98:145–158.

Sprung J, Flick RP, Katusic SK, Colligan RC, Barbaresi WJ, Bojanic K, Welch TL, Olson MD, Hanson AC, Schroeder DR, Wilder RT, Warner DO (2012) Attention-deficit/hyperactivity disorder after early exposure to procedures requiring general anesthesia. *Mayo Clin Proc* 87:120–129.

Sun L (2010) Early childhood general anaesthesia exposure and neuro-cognitive development. *Br J Anaesth* 105 Suppl 1:i61–68.

Takahashi K, Yamanaka S (2006) Induction of pluripotent stem cells from mouse embryonic and adult fibroblast cultures by defined factors. *Cell* 126:663–676.

Thiel G (2013) How Sox2 maintains neural stem cell identity. *Biochem J* 450:e1–2.

Wang C, Fridley J, Johnson KM (2005a) The role of NMDA receptor upregulation in phencyclidine-induced cortical apoptosis in organotypic culture. *Biochem Pharmacol* 69:1373–1383.

Wang C, Kaufmann JA, Sanchez-Ross MG, Johnson KM (2000) Mechanisms of N-methyl-D-aspartate-induced apoptosis in phencyclidine-treated cultured forebrain neurons. *J Pharmacol Exp Ther* 294:287–295.

Wang C, McInnis J, West JB, Bao J, Anastasio N, Guidry JA, Ye Y, Salvemini D, Johnson KM (2003) Blockade of phencyclidine-induced cortical apoptosis and deficits in prepulse inhibition by M40403, a superoxide dismutase mimetic. *J Pharmacol Exp Ther* 304:266–271.

Wang C, Sadovova N, Fu X, Schmued L, Scallet A, Hanig J, Slikker W (2005b) The role of the N-methyl-D-aspartate receptor in ketamine-induced apoptosis in rat forebrain culture. *Neuroscience* 132:967–977.

Wang C, Sadovova N, Hotchkiss C, Fu X, Scallet AC, Patterson TA, Hanig J, Paule MG, Slikker W, Jr. (2006) Blockade of N-methyl-D-aspartate receptors by ketamine produces loss of postnatal day 3 monkey frontal cortical neurons in culture. *Toxicol Sci* 91:192–201.

Wang C, Showalter VM, Hillman GR, Johnson KM (1999) Chronic phency-clidine increases NMDA receptor NR1 subunit mRNA in rat forebrain. *J Neurosci Res* 55:762–769.

Wiese C, Rolletschek A, Kania G, Blyszczuk P, Tarasov KV, Tarasova Y, Wersto RP, Boheler KR, Wobus AM (2004) Nestin expression — a property of multi-lineage progenitor cells? *Cell Mol Life Sci* 61:2510–2522.

Wilder RT, Flick RP, Sprung J, Katusic SK, Barbaresi WJ, Mickelson C, Gleich SJ, Schroeder DR, Weaver AL, Warner DO (2009) Early exposure to anesthesia and learning disabilities in a population-based birth cohort. *Anesthesiology* 110:796–804.

Zhu C, Gao J, Karlsson N, Li Q, Zhang Y, Huang Z, Li H, Kuhn HG, Blomgren K (2010) Isoflurane anesthesia induced persistent, progressive memory impairment, caused a loss of neural stem cells, and reduced neurogenesis in young, but not adult, rodents. *J Cereb Blood Flow Metab* 30:1017–1030.

Zou X, Sadovova N, Patterson TA, Divine RL, Hotchkiss CE, Ali SF, Hanig JP, Paule MG, Slikker W, Jr., Wang C (2008) The effects of L-carnitine on the combination of, inhalation anesthetic-induced developmental, neuronal apoptosis in the rat frontal cortex. *Neuroscience* 151: 1053–1065.

Chapter 12

Induced Neurogenesis as a Mechanism for Adult Central Nervous System Regeneration

Derek K. Smith, Wenze Niu, and Chun-Li Zhang

The multipotent neural stem cell (NSC), a fundamental regulator of human central nervous system development and maintenance, has garnered much interest as a candidate for regeneration after neural injury. The restricted localization of these cells in the adult brain and spinal cord provides neural tissues with only a limited potential for self-regeneration following traumatic injury or degeneration. Therefore, state-of-the-art research is utilizing the principles of NSC differentiation to induce neurogenesis in non-neurogenic cells and tissues. Recent advances in cell fate reprogramming have enabled the *in vitro* induction of NSCs and numerous subtype-specific neurons from post-mitotic terminally-differentiated cells. The molecular insights from these studies laid the groundwork for *in vivo* reprogramming of resident glial cells in models of injury and neurodegenerative disease. Proof-of-principle *in vivo* studies have demonstrated the induction of neuroblasts and mature neurons with the potential to survive and integrate into neuronal circuits in a functionally meaningful manner. Here, we briefly highlight recent advances in NSC- and neurogenesis-inspired cell identity reprogramming methods and the current challenges facing the clinical relevance of these methodologies.

Introduction

The broad goal of regenerative medicine is to identify methods that treat injury or disease through the regeneration of damaged tissue. This concept is of particular value with respect to the central nervous system (CNS), which retains a limited capacity for self-regeneration in adulthood. In recent years, cell fate reprogramming has catapulted to the forefront of regenerative research and is widely regarded as one of the most promising techniques for engineering patient-specific CNS cell therapies. As a rapidly evolving technology, cell identity reprogramming still faces many barriers to clinical implementation. In this chapter, we will highlight how the fundamental principles of adult neural stem cell (NSC) differentiation have informed the refinement of *in vitro* and *in vivo* reprogramming methodologies, as well as, recent advances poised to translate this technology from the laboratory to the clinic.

Neurogenesis in the adult CNS

The human nervous system is an intricate network of diverse cell types that function cooperatively to process and relay information throughout the body. In the earliest stages of CNS development, the neural plate folds into the neural tube to establish the birthplace of all CNS-derived cell types. A precise cascade of signaling molecules then patterns the developing CNS by modulating the activity of transcription factors that specify distinct neuronal lineages (Hevner, 2006). This fine-tuning induces NSC populations to generate billions of neurons throughout early neurogenesis (Götz and Huttner, 2005). As the CNS matures, neurogenesis slows and non-neurogenic cell populations begin to predominate the adult brain and spinal cord.

Neurogenesis is localized to two defined regions in the adult brain, the subgranular zone (SGZ) of the dentate gyrus and the subventricular zone (SVZ) of the lateral ventricles (Eriksson *et al.*, 1998; Alvarez-Buylla and García-Verdugo, 2002; Hsieh, 2012). In the SGZ, slow-dividing NSCs expressing glial fibrillary acidic protein (GFAP) and nestin give rise to transit-amplifying progenitor cells.

These early nestin-expressing progenitors gradually mature into doublecortin-positive neuroblasts. The immature neurons derived from these neuroblasts differentiate into glutamatergic granule neurons. In a mechanism independent of SGZ neurogenesis, SVZ radial glial cells generate self-renewing NSCs that pass through a transit-amplifying state before becoming neuroblasts. These neuroblasts primarily differentiate into GABAergic inhibitory interneurons and migrate into the olfactory bulb. While neurogenesis in these adult brain regions has been well established, the limited presence of quiescent multipotent progenitors resident to the central canal of the adult spinal cord remains under scrutiny (Weiss *et al.*, 1996; Panayiotou and Malas, 2013).

This neurogenic potential endows the adult CNS with a limited capacity for self-regeneration following traumatic injury and neuro-degeneration. However, while new neurons can be generated in response to trauma, the migration, survival, and integration of these adult-born neurons is often inadequate for complete functional recovery (Panayiotou and Malas, 2013; Ming and Song, 2005). Therefore, insight into the underlying mechanisms of adult NSC maintenance and neurogenesis, as well as, the factors specifying subtype-specific neurons from these progenitors is imperative to the development of regenerative therapies targeting neural trauma.

Traumatic injury in the adult CNS

The intricate architecture of the neuronal circuits permeating the adult brain and spinal cord permits a precise regulation of homeo-static, motor, and cognitive functions. While this complexity affords an unparalleled level of biological sophistication, any disruption in this interconnected network by traumatic brain injury (TBI) or spinal cord injury (SCI) has far-reaching, often detrimental, functional consequences. TBI and SCI can be loosely parsed into two distinct classifications: (1) focal insult resulting from a high-impact force, impalement or ischemic stroke and (2) diffuse insult resulting from gradual neurodegeneration or chronic disease. The scope of this chapter will be limited to focal TBI and SCI; although, the later described reprogramming methodologies find application in both focal and diffuse injury models.

Acute focal TBI and SCI result in severe neural tissue damage and can be accompanied by a local breakdown of blood–brain barrier (BBB) integrity (Abbott *et al.*, 2006; Burda and Sofroniew, 2014). Cytokine and chemokine secreting hematogenous cells infiltrate the lesion site through this perforation in the BBB. The extracellular signaling molecules secreted from these hematogenous cells, damaged or dead neurons, and local reactive glia trigger microgliosis (Raivich *et al.*, 1999; Streit *et al.*, 1999). Early responding microglia rapidly migrate into the lesion site, phagocytose cell debris, and release proinflammatory signaling molecules. A concurrent migration of NG2-positive oligodendrocyte precursor cells (NG2-OPC) toward the lesion site is also observed (Nishiyama *et al.*, 2009; Hughes *et al.*, 2013). Astrocytes resident to the affected region exhibit hypertrophy, swollen end feet due to the disruption of BBB neurovascular units, and respond to diverse injury-signaling factors with the induction of astrogliosis (Zhang *et al.*, 2010; Sofroniew, 2009; Gadea *et al.*, 2008; Sirko *et al.*, 2013). In the days following injury, reactive astrocytes populate the perimeter of the damaged region forming a glial scar (Sofroniew and Vinters, 2010; Wanner *et al.*, 2013). Concomitantly, proliferating fibroblasts populate the lesion core and modify the extracellular matrix to establish a fibrotic scar directly over the outer-facing layer of reactive astrocytes (Göritz *et al.*, 2011; Soderblom *et al.*, 2013). This layered structure seals the interior BBB perforation to isolate the damaged region from healthy neural tissue. While the reconstructed glia limitans prevents further secondary injury, it also acts as an impediment to the regeneration of damaged axons and prevents the restructuring of synaptic connections within the scarred tissue (Kimura-Kuroda *et al.*, 2010). Additionally, factors secreted into the injury microenvironment inhibit neurite outgrowth and axon regeneration (Cafferty *et al.*, 2010).

The severe damage TBI and SCI impart to adult CNS circuitry ultimately results from the inability of non-neurogenic tissues to induce neurogenesis for active replacement of irreversibly damaged neurons. Although neural progenitors migrating from proliferating neurogenic zones to non-neurogenic lesion sites can generate neurons, these new neurons survive, mature, and integrate with limited frequency (Ming and Song, 2005; Lagace, 2012). Therefore, the repair processes following a traumatic insult often facilitate damage control but promote only minimal functional recovery. This has inspired a search for therapeutic techniques that enhance functional recovery post injury. Recent advances in cell identity reprogramming enable the induction of neurons from non-neuronal precursors and might offer an elegant solution for the replacement of trauma-damaged neurons. At present, two approaches predominate: (1) *in vitro* cell identity reprogramming followed by transplantation and (2) *in vivo* reprogramming of resident cells.

Neurogenesis-Inspired Cell Fate Reprogramming

The discovery that terminally differentiated somatic cells can be induced to pluripotency and a variety of distinct neural identities redefined the landscape of regenerative therapeutics. This concept enables us to apply the biological factors, mechanisms, and signaling pathways inherent to early NSC differentiation to the specification of subtype-specific neurons and glia for therapeutic applications. Two paradigms have emerged in the pursuit of TBI and SCI therapies. First, *in vitro* reprogramming utilizes an easily accessible source of somatic cells for transdifferentiation and transplantation. More recently, endogenous cells of the glial scar or surrounding non-neurogenic tissue have been reprogrammed *in vivo* to bypass the requirement for transplantation. Here, we briefly summarize recent advances in cell identity reprogramming and the ongoing challenges that face the clinical application of this technology.

In vitro reprogramming methodologies

Induced neural cells can be generated either directly from precursor cells or indirectly differentiated after passing through a pluripotent progenitor state. These pluripotent and neural fates have been achieved through a multitude of techniques, including transcription factor overexpression (Takahashi *et al.*, 2007; Zeng *et al.*, 2010; Shimada *et al.*, 2012; Karumbayaram *et al.*, 2009; Krencik *et al.*, 2011; Ring *et al.*, 2012; Lujan *et al.*, 2012; Yang *et al.*, 2013; Najm *et al.*, 2013; Vierbuchen *et al.*, 2010; Son *et al.*, 2011; Liu *et al.*, 2013; Kim *et al.*, 2011; Caiazzo *et al.*, 2011; Pfisterer *et al.*, 2011; Karow *et al.*, 2012; Berninger *et al.*, 2007; Heinrich *et al.*, 2010; Heinrich *et al.*, 2011; Takahashi and Yamanaka, 2006; Rais *et al.*, 2013), protein knock-down (Xue *et al.*, 2013; Sun *et al.*, 2014), chemical treatment (Hou *et al.*, 2013), and microRNA overexpression (Anokye-Danso *et al.*, 2011; Yoo *et al.*, 2011). Readily accessible somatic cells like skin fibroblasts are often the precursor cell of choice for translational research, while cultured neural cells are often used to screen, optimize, and evaluate the feasibility of *in vivo* reprogramming protocols (Figure 1).

The seminal discovery that human and mouse fibroblasts could be induced to pluripotency catalyzed a revolution in our under-standing of the mechanisms that govern the specification of cellular identity and terminal differentiation (Takahashi and Yamanaka, 2006). Rapid advances in the high-efficiency generation of induced pluripotent stem cells (IPSC) from fibroblasts quickly followed (Rais *et al.*, 2013). Astonishingly, a plethora of new techniques for somatic cell-IPSC reprogramming began to emerge. Numerous studies have demonstrated that the canonical set of four transcription factors is replaceable with small molecules (Hou *et al.*, 2013) or microRNAs (Anokye-Danso *et al.*, 2011; Yoo *et al.*, 2011). With these pluripotent progenitors in hand, much interest shifted to the specification of distinct cell types, particularly neural lineages. This pursuit led not only to the induction of neuronal cells from IPSCs (Takahashi *et al.*, 2007), but the defined production of glutamatergic forebrain neurons (Zeng *et al.*, 2010), dopaminergic midbrain neurons (Zeng *et al.*, 2010), serotonergic neurons (Shimada *et al.*, 2012), cholinergic motor neurons (Zeng *et al.*, 2010; Karumbayaram *et al.*, 2009), and astrocytes (Krencik *et al.*, 2011).

Although transformative for biological research, these ground-breaking advances in cell fate regulation and pluripotency are not without clinical drawbacks. The potential for engrafted IPSCs to

In vitro direct cell fate reprogramming

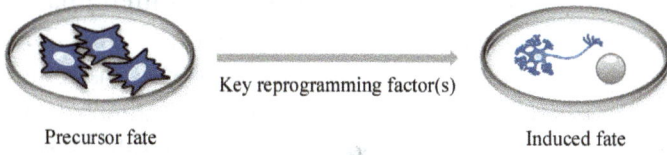

Key reprogramming factor(s)

Precursor fate		Induced fate
Fibroblast		
ME, HF	SOX2	Neural stem cell (Ring et al. 2012)
ME	SOX2, BRN2, FOXG1	Neural stem cell (Lujan et al. 2012)
RE	SOX10, OLIG2, ZFP536	NG2-OPC (Yang et al. 2013)
ME	OLIG1, OLIG2, NKX2.2, ST18, NKX6.3, SOX10, GM98, MYT1	NG2-OPC (Najm et al. 2013)
ME, MP	ASCL1, BRN2, MYT1L	Neuron (Vierbuchen et al. 2010)
ME	miR-124	Neuron (Xue et al. 2013)
HF, HA	P16 and/or P19 depletion	Neuron (Sun et al. 2014)
HF	NGN2, forskolin, dorsomorphin	Cholinergic neuron (Liu et al. 2013)
ME, HF, HA	ASCL1, NURR1, LMX1A	Dopaminergic neuron (Caiazzo et al. 2011)
MP	ASCL1, PITX3, NURR1, LMX1A, FOXA2, EN1	Dopaminergic neuron (Kim et al. 2011)
HE, HP	ASCL1, BRN2, MYT1L, LMX1A, FOXA2	Dopaminergic neuron (Pfisterer et al. 2011)
ME, HE	ASCL1, BRN2, MYT1L, NGN2, LHX3, ISL1, HB9	Motor neuron (Son et al. 2011)
Cortical astrocyte		
MP	NGN2 or ASCL1	Neuron (Breninger et al. 2007)
MP	NGN2	Glutamatergic neuron (Heinrich et al. 2010)
MP	DLC1	GABAergic neuron (Heinrich et al. 2010)
Cortical pericyte		
HA	SOX2 and ASCL1	GABAergic interneuron-like cell (Karow et al. 2012)

Figure 1.   A selection of *in vitro* direct cell fate reprogramming methodologies. In addition to the key factors described, induction media containing growth factors and small molecules is often required for survival and maturation of the induced fate. Defined abbreviations: A, adult; E, embryonic; F, fetal; H, human; M, mouse; NG2-OPC, NG2-oligodendrocyte precursor cell; P, postnatal; R, rat.

develop into a teratoma is of particular concern (Gutierrez-Aranda *et al.*, 2010). Therefore, many have looked to the principles of neurogenesis and induced NSCs for a solution. Induced NSCs retain the potential to differentiate into neurons, astrocytes, and oligodendrocytes but exhibit a significantly reduced tumorigenicity (Ring *et al.*, 2012). NSCs have been induced and differentiated *in vitro* using the combination of transcription factors SOX2, BRN2, and FOXG1 (Lujan *et al.*, 2012). Remarkably, only SOX2 is required for the induction of tripotent NSCs, which differentiate upon transplantation (Ring *et al.*, 2012). Induced NG2-OPCs have also garnered attention as multipotent progenitors (Yang *et al.*, 2013; Najm *et al.*, 2013). While this plasticity is highly desirable for some TBI and SCI applications, the indirect generation of subtype-specific neurons from intermediate progenitors is a relatively time-consuming, low-yield process. Therefore, the ability to directly differentiate a somatic or glial precursor cell into a lineage-specific neuron offers multiple advantages, such as a reduced time-scale of generation, reduced tumorigenic potential, and enhanced reprogramming efficiency.

Neurons have been directly induced from a variety of somatic and glial cell types via neurogenesis-inspired mechanisms (Vierbuchen *et al.*, 2010; Son *et al.*, 2011; Liu *et al.*, 2013; Kim *et al.*, 2011; Caiazzo *et al.*, 2011; Pfisterer *et al.*, 2011; Karow *et al.*, 2012; Berninger *et al.*, 2007; Heinrich *et al.*, 2010; Heinrich *et al.*, 2011; Xue *et al.*, 2013). Heterogeneous pools of excitatory glutamatergic and inhibitory GABAergic neurons have been generated from fibroblasts by either the overexpression of three proneural transcription factors or the modulation of endogenous microRNA expression profiles (Vierbuchen *et al.*, 2010; Xue *et al.*, 2013). Building on this core set of neuron-inducing transcription factors, cholinergic spinal motor neurons were specified from fibroblasts with the inclusion of NGN2, LHX3, ISL1, and HB9 (Son *et al.*, 2011). Interestingly, NGN2 itself is sufficient to induce homogeneous populations of cholinergic neurons from human fibroblasts when combined with two small molecules (Liu *et al.*, 2013). In addition to cholinergic neurons, fibroblasts have been specifically reprogrammed into dopaminergic neurons with various combinations of transcription factors (Kim *et al.*, 2011; Caiazzo *et al.*, 2011; Pfisterer *et al.*, 2011). Further, transplantation studies have demonstrated that induced midbrain dopaminergic neurons injected into mouse striatal tissue lesioned by 6-hydroxydopamine ameliorate the Parkinson's disease-associated symptoms typically observed in this model (Kim *et al.*, 2011). Similarly, induced spinal motor neurons engrafted into the developing chick spinal cord functionally integrate and project axons toward musculature suggesting these cells might have the potential to repair trauma-damaged circuits following SCI (Son *et al.*, 2011).

Alternative approaches to *in vitro* fibroblast reprogramming have targeted the pericyte lineage for neuronal conversion (Karow *et al.*, 2012). Present in brain and spinal cord injury sites, these cells are strong candidates for *in vivo* reprogramming therapies following TBI or SCI. Likewise, cultured astrocytes have been functionally reprogrammed into both glutamatergic and GABAergic neurons (Berninger *et al.*, 2007; Heinrich *et al.*, 2010; Heinrich *et al.*, 2011). While these *in vitro* reprogramming studies have shed light on the mechanisms governing cell identity and offer new models for drug screening, the clinical adoption of reprogramming and transplantation techniques must overcome several hurdles. Immune rejection, tumor formation, limited survival of neurons post transplantation, and aberrant synaptic integration are among the challenges facing this technology (Zhao *et al.*, 2011; Wernig *et al.*, 2008; Okano *et al.*, 2003; Emborg *et al.*, 2013). For these reasons, the clinical relevance of this technology might be best appreciated through the *in vivo* reprogramming of resident brain and spinal cord cells.

In vivo reprogramming methodologies

The multilineage applications of *in vivo* cell identity reprogramming have been broadly demonstrated by the transient expression of pluripotency factors in mice (Abad *et al.*, 2013). The ability to induce IPSCs in numerous specialized organ tissues underscores the vast regenerative potential for *in vivo* reprogramming in terminally differentiated systems (Abad *et al.*, 2013). Therefore, state-of-the-art strategies have begun to explore both the indirect and direct induction of functional neurons from neuroglia resident to non-neurogenic CNS regions (Figure 2; Niu *et al.*, 2013; Su *et al.*, 2014; Guo *et al.*, 2014; Torper *et al.*, 2013; Rouaux and Arlotta, 2010; Rouaux and Arlotta, 2013; Rossa *et al.*, 2013).

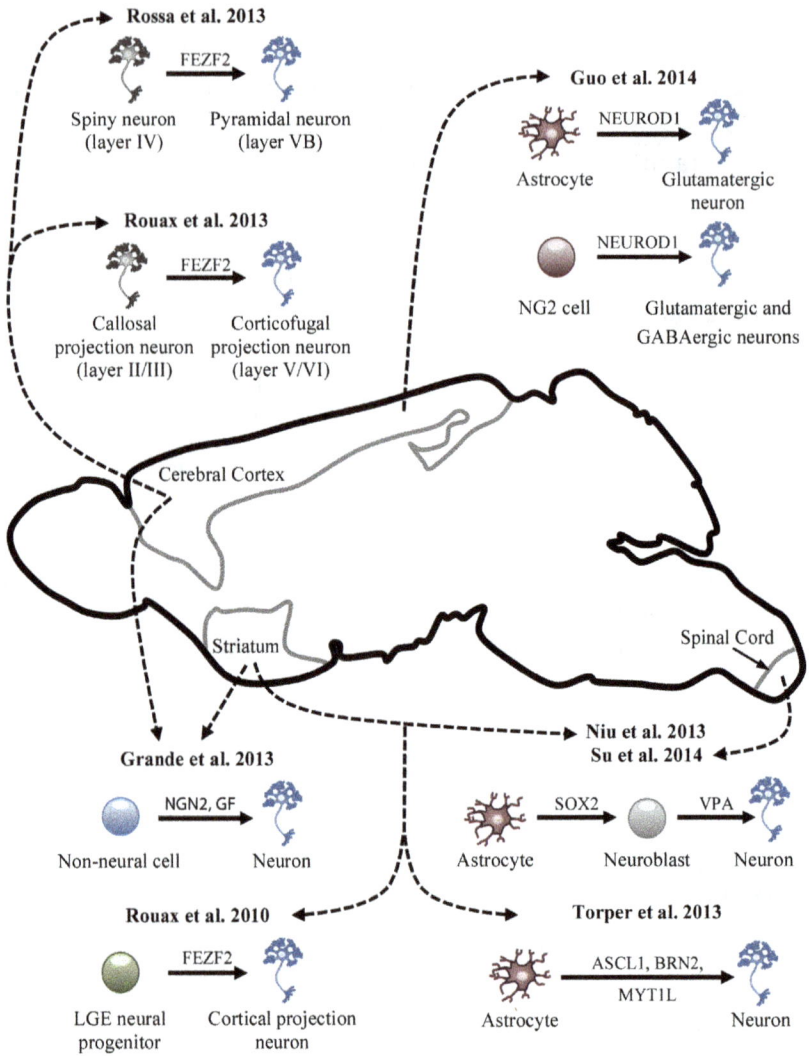

Figure 2. A selection of *in vivo* reprogramming methodologies. These approaches fall under two distinct developmental stages: embryonic or early postnatal (Rossa *et al.*, 2013; Rouax *et al.*, 2010; Rouax *et al.*, 2013) and adult (Grande *et al.*, 2013; Guo *et al.*, 2014; Niu *et al.*, 2013; Su *et al.*, 2014; Torper *et al.*, 2013). Defined abbreviations: GF, growth factor; LGE, lateral ganglionic eminence; VPA, valproic acid.

Drawing from the mechanisms of adult neurogenesis and NSC multipotency, lentiviral-mediated SOX2 expression was used to transform striatal astrocytes into neuroblasts in the adult mouse brain (Niu *et al.*, 2013). The targeted conversion of resident striatal astrocytes was achieved by lentivirus-mediated *GFAP* promoter-driven *Sox2* expression and confirmed by linage tracing in *GFAP-Cre; Rosa-YFP* mice. Induced neuroblasts traced with bromodeoxyuridine were observed to pass through a proliferative state and were coaxed to adopt neuronal fate by treatment with valproic acid (VPA), a histone-deacetylase inhibitor with established roles in the neuronal differentiation of NSCs (Hsieh *et al.*, 2004), or a combination of brain-derived neurotrophic factor and noggin. Remarkably, these indirectly induced neurons matured and functionally integrated into local neuronal circuitry. In parallel with this finding, SOX2 overexpression in astrocytes of the injured spinal cord induces a neuroblast identity that differentiates into mature synapse-forming interneuron-like cells (Su *et al.*, 2014). This single factor *in vivo* conversion of cellular identity highlights a surprising plasticity in glial cells of the adult CNS.

Reminiscent of the striking role for SOX2 in neuroblast induction, the retroviral expression of NEUROD1 in the mouse cortex following TBI is sufficient to promote neurogenesis in reactive astrocytes and NG2-glia (Guo *et al.*, 2014). Interestingly, reactive astrocytes directly transition to an excitatory glutamatergic identity, while NG2-glia reprogram into a heterogeneous population of glutamatergic and GABAergic neurons. In addition to reprogramming reactive glia triggered by stab-wound injury, NEUROD1 overexpression induces resident cortical astrocytes in a transgenic mouse model of Alzheimer's disease to convert into neurons with robust synaptic activity within 14–16 days. The functional integration of these induced neurons into local brain circuitry suggests the *in vivo* reprogramming of reactive glia might offer a mechanism for the reconstruction of synapses destroyed by focal injury and neurodegenerative disease.

To investigate the feasibility and clinical potential of this approach, human astrocytes and human fibroblasts transplanted into striatal and hippocampal regions of the adult rat brain were successfully *in vivo* reprogrammed to neuronal identity by doxycycline-regulated transgene expression (Torper *et al.*, 2013). This finding indicates that the brain microenvironment might be conductive to the *in vivo* reprogramming and survival of induced human neurons.

The specification of subtype-specific human neuron populations is a central focus of *in vitro* reprogramming research and remains a barrier to the development of clinically-relevant *in vivo* translational models. Therefore, it will be crucial to define the intricate transcriptional mechanisms that instruct region- and subtype-specific neuron development. The transcription factor FEZF2 has played an integral role in the dissection of these mechanisms in the mouse cortex. In the developing mouse embryo, neural progenitors of the lateral ganglionic eminence normally differentiate into GABAergic medium spiny neurons and interneurons; however, the electroporation of these cells with FEZF2 is sufficient to instruct a new genetic program that results in the generation of glutamatergic corticofugal projection neuron-like cells (Rouaux and Arlotta, 2010). Further, this factor is sufficient to reprogram post-mitotic layer II/III excitatory callosal projection neurons and layer IV interneurons to a similar corticofugal fate (Rouaux and Arlotta, 2013; Rossa *et al.*, 2013). Importantly, these induced cells not only acquire the morphological and molecular properties of corticofugal projection neurons, but self-direct the rearrangement of axonal connections to mimic the architecture of *in vivo* neuronal circuitry in a functionally meaningful manner (Rouaux and Arlotta, 2013; Rossa *et al.*, 2013). These *in vivo* reprogramming studies have offered insight into the molecular underpinnings that regulate neural fate specification and provide a blueprint for engineering protocols that will enable the production of new neurons in postmitotic, non-neurogenic CNS tissues.

Therapeutic Applications and Challenges

As the point of origin for all endogenous human neurons, the multipotent NSC is an ideal candidate for the therapeutic regeneration of damaged CNS neuronal circuitry. Problematically, reservoirs of these cells in the adult CNS are narrowly localized and often promote only minimal functional recovery after trauma (Ming and Song, 2005; Lagace, 2012). Cell fate reprogramming technologies aim to harness the neurogenic potential of these cells by inducing neurogenesis in non-neurogenic regions of the adult brain and spinal cord. The *de novo* generation of neurons from induced neural progenitors and directly converted glial cells provides patient-specific methods for repairing the currently irreversible damage imparted by TBI, SCI, neurodegenerative disease, and aging.

One of the primary obstacles to functional recovery following focal TBI or SCI is the inhibition of axon regrowth by glial and fibrotic scarring (Wanner *et al.*, 2013; Soderblom *et al.*, 2013; Kimura-Kuroda *et al.*, 2010). Therefore, current reprogramming strategies have targeted reactive astrocytes and pericytes in an attempt to curtail secondary injury and emphasize axon regenera-tion (Karow *et al.*, 2012; Berninger *et al.*, 2007; Heinrich *et al.*, 2010; Heinrich *et al.*, 2011; Su *et al.*, 2014; Guo *et al.*, 2014). The direct induction of functional neurons in mouse cortical tissue following injury (Guo *et al.*, 2014) and the self-reorganization of outgoing synaptic connections from induced corticofugal projection neu-rons (Rouaux and Arlotta, 2013; Rossa *et al.*, 2013) lends a promis-ing outlook to the development of effective *in vivo* reprogramming therapies.

As an alternative to direct one-to-one neuronal conversion, the induction of proliferative neural progenitor cells with the capacity to yield multiple neurons would be an asset in cases of both acute injury and diffuse neurodegenerative disease resulting in substantial neuron loss (Niu *et al.*, 2013; Su *et al.*, 2014). Induced neuroblasts differentiable to a variety of neuron subtypes could prove to be an invaluable source of replacement neurons in patients affected by Parkinson's disease, Alzheimer's disease, Huntington's disease, and amyotrophic lateral sclerosis. The ability to induce neuroblasts in aged mouse brains suggests these cells may even find application in the treatment of age-related neurodegeneration (Niu *et al.*, 2013).

Although noteworthy strides have been made in neurogene-sis-inspired cell fate reprogramming in recent years, the enthusiasm behind this relatively new technology must be tempered with an understanding of the barriers to clinical relevance. One of the most intractable problems facing this technology is the development of a safe delivery system for reprogramming factors. The prevalent method for introducing exogenous factors to neural tissue is the stereotaxic injection of retrovirus or lentivirus (Niu *et al.*, 2013; Su *et al.*, 2014; Guo *et al.*, 2014; Rouaux and Arlotta, 2010; Rouaux and Arlotta, 2013; Rossa *et al.*, 2013). In addition to secondary tissue damage created at the injection site, the random integration of viral DNA into the human genome could disrupt transcriptional regulation resulting in cell death or cancer. To circumvent these issues, small molecules have been utilized to dedifferentiate somatic cells *in vitro* (Hou *et al.*, 2013); however, BBB permeability remains an untested challenge. Further, medically-relevant systems must target site- and identity-specific cell populations with controlled activity and limited off-target effects. To overcome these diverse challenges, new fate conversion methodologies will likely focus on integration-free reprogramming without the use of viral vectors, recombinant DNA, and factors that induce permanent genetic modification (Heng and Fussenegger, 2014).

Recent innovations in somatic and glial cell reprogramming have enabled the directed production of multiple neuron subtypes *in vitro* (Zeng *et al.*, 2010; Shimada *et al.*, 2012; Karumbayaram *et al.*, 2009; Krencik *et al.*, 2011; Son *et al.*, 2011; Liu *et al.*, 2013; Kim *et al.*, 2011; Caiazzo *et al.*, 2011; Pfisterer *et al.*, 2011). Transcriptional, proteomic, and epigenetic analyses will be instrumental in defining the relationship between these induced neurons and their endogenous counterparts. Moreover, the insights garnered during these investigations will bolster methods focused on the controlled specification of a variety of nuanced neuronal identities. While transplantation models indicate human neurons can be induced in the CNS, the long-term survival of these cells is largely dependent on the injury or disease microenvironment (Torper *et al.*, 2013; Grande *et al.*, 2013). Therefore, reprogramming modalities that enhance the *in vivo* survival and maturation of induced neurons and NSC-like intermediates must be developed. Further, the directed and meaningful integration of surviving neurons, including both synaptic targeting and dendritic branching, must be achieved to restore lost function in damaged circuits.

Finally, the immense potential for pluripotent IPSCs in regenerative medicine is stifled by their propensity to form cancerous tumors

(Gutierrez-Aranda *et al.*, 2010; Knoepfler, 2009). Induced multipotent NSCs, on the other hand, exhibit a significantly reduced tumorigenicity (Ring *et al.*, 2012). For example, the SOX2-mediated induction of neuroblasts in the mouse brain and spinal cord did not result in any tumor formation when examined 50 weeks post reprogramming (Niu *et al.*, 2013; Su *et al.*, 2014). Furthermore, the direct reprogramming of tumorigenic glioblastoma stem-like cells to post-mitotic fates is being actively investigated as a method to curb the progression of this aggressive brain cancer (Guichet *et al.*, 2013; Hide *et al.*, 2009).

Although numerous obstacles must be cleared before these neurogenesis-inspired reprogramming methods find therapeutic application, the rapid evolution and refinement of this technology has laid the groundwork for an extremely promising future.

Conclusion

Neurogenesis-inspired cell identity reprogramming has enabled researchers to investigate the mechanisms of cell fate specification, commitment, and plasticity from a novel perspective that has yielded remarkable insights into the biological mechanisms that govern neural identity. As a new and rapidly evolving technology, reprogramming still faces numerous practical limitations that challenge its clinical utility. In the coming years, as these limitations are overcome through refinement and innovation, we believe a multitude of novel reprogramming methodologies will emerge to establish a new milestone in patient-specific regenerative medicine.

References

Abad M, Mosteiro L, Pantoja C, Cañamero M, Rayon T, Ors I, Graña O, Megías D, Domínguez O, Martínez D, Manzanares M, Ortega S, Serrano M (2013) Reprogramming *in vivo* produces teratomas and iPS cells with totipotency features. *Nature* 502:340–345.

Abbott NJ, Rönnbäck L, Hansson E (2006) Astrocyte-endothelial interactions at the blood-brain barrier. *Nat Rev Neurosci* 7:41–53.

Alvarez-Buylla A, García-Verdugo JM (2002) Neurogenesis in adult subventricular zone. *J Neurosci* 22:629–634.

Anokye-Danso F, Trivedi CM, Juhr D, Gupta M, Cui Z, Tian Y, Zhang Y, Yang W, Gruber PJ, Epstein JA, Morrisey EE (2011) Highly efficient miRNA-mediated reprogramming of mouse and human somatic cells to pluripotency. *Cell Stem Cell* 8:376–388.

Berninger B, Costa MR, Koch U, Schroeder T, Sutor B, Grothe B, Götz M (2007) Functional properties of neurons derived from *in vitro* reprogrammed postnatal astroglia. *J Neurosci* 27:8654–8664.

Burda JE, Sofroniew MV (2014) Reactive gliosis and the multicellular response to CNS damage and disease. *Neuron* 81:229–248.

Cafferty WBJ, Duffy P, Huebner E, Strittmatter SM (2010) MAG and OMgp synergize with Nogo-A to restrict axonal growth and neurological recovery after spinal cord trauma. *J Neurosci* 30:6825–6837.

Caiazzo M, Dell'Anno MT, Dvoretskova E, Lazarevic D, Taverna S, Leo D, Sotnikova TD, Menegon A, Roncaglia P, Colciago G, Russo G, Carninci P, Pezzoli G, Gainetdinov RR, Gustincich S, Dityatev A, Broccoli V (2011) Direct generation of functional dopaminergic neurons from mouse and human fibroblasts. *Nature* 476:224–227.

Emborg ME, Liu Y, Xi J, Zhang X, Yin Y, Lu J, Joers V, Swanson C, Holden JE, Zhang S-C (2013) Induced pluripotent stem cell-derived neural cells survive and mature in the nonhuman primate brain. *Cell Rep* 3:646–650.

Eriksson PS, Perfilieva E, Björk-Eriksson T, Alborn A-M, Nordborg C, Peterson DA, Gage FH (1998) Neurogenesis in the adult human hippocampus. *Nature* 4:1313–1317.

Gadea A, Schinelli S, Gallo V (2008) Endothelin-1 regulates astrocyte proliferation and reactive gliosis via a JNK/c-Jun signaling pathway. *J Neurosci* 28:2394–2408.

Göritz C, Dias DO, Tomilin N, Barbacid M, Shupliakov O, Frisén J (2011) A pericyte origin of spinal cord scar tissue. *Science* 333:238–242.

Götz M, Huttner, WB (2005) The cell biology of neurogenesis. *Nat Rev Mol Cell Biol* 6:777–788.

Grande A, Sumiyoshi K, López-Juárez A, Howard J, Sakthivel B, Aronow B, Campbell K, Nakafuku M (2013) Environmental impact on direct neuronal reprogramming *in vivo* in the adult brain. *Nat Commun* 4:2373.

Guichet P-O, Bieche I, Teigell M, Serguera C, Rothhut B, Rigau V, Scamps F, Ripoll C, Vacher S, Taviaux S, Chevassus H, Duffau H, Mallet J, Susini A, Joubert D, Bauchet L, Hugnot J-P (2013) Cell death and neuronal differentiation of glioblastoma stem-like cells induced by neurogenic transcription factors. *Glia* 61:225–239.

Guo Z, Zhang L, Zheng W, Chen Y, Wang F, Chen G (2014) *In vivo* direct reprogramming of reactive glial cells into functional neurons after brain injury and in an Alzheimer's disease model. *Cell Stem Cell* 14:188–202.

Gutierrez-Aranda I, Ramos-Mejia V, Bueno C, Munoz-Lopez M, Real PJ, Mácia A, Sanchez L, Ligero G, Garcia-Parez JL, Menendez P (2010) Human induced pluripotent stem cells develop teratoma more efficiently and faster than human embryonic stem cells regardless the site of injection. *Stem Cells* 28:1568–1570.

Heinrich C, Blum R, Gascón S, Masserdotti G, Tripathi P, Sánchez R, Tiedt S, Schroeder T, Götz M, Berninger B (2010) Directing astroglia from the cerebral cortex into subtype specific functional neurons. *PLoS Biol* 8:e1000373.

Heinrich C, Gascón S, Masserdotti G, Lepier A, Sanchez R, Simon-Ebert T, Schroeder T, Götz M, Berninger B (2011) Generation of subtype-specific neurons from postnatal astroglia of the mouse cerebral cortex. *Nat Protoc* 6:214–228.

Heng BC and Fussenegger M (2014) Chapter 6: Integration-free reprogramming of human somatic cells to induced pluripotent stem cells (iPSCs) without viral vectors, recombinant DNA, and genetic modification. *Methods Mol Biol* 1151:75–94.

Hevner RF (2006) From radial glia to pyramidal-projection neuron. *Mol Neurobiol* 33:33–50.

Hide T, Takezaki T, Nakatani Y, Nakamura H, Kuratsu J-i, Kondo T (2009) Sox11 prevents tumorigenesis of glioma-initiating cells by inducing neuronal differentiation. *Cancer Res* 69:7953–7959.

Hsieh J (2012) Orchestrating transcriptional control of adult neurogenesis. *Genes Dev* 26:1010–1021.

Hsieh J, Nakashima K, Kuwabara T, Mejia E, Gage FH (2004) Histone deacetylase inhibition-medicated neuronal differentiation of multipotent adult neural progenitor cells. *Proc Natl Acad Sci U S A* 101:16659–16664.

Hou P, Li Y, Zhang X, Liu C, Guan J, Li H, Zhao T, Ye J, Yang W, Liu K, Ge J, Xu J, Zhang Q, Zhao Y, Deng H (2013) Pluripotent stem cells induced from mouse somatic cells by small-molecule compounds. *Science* 341:651–654.

Hughes EG, Kang SH, Fukaya M, Bergles DE (2013) Oligodendrocyte progenitors balance growth with self-repulsion to achieve homeostasis in the adult brain. *Nat Neurosci* 16:668–676.

Karow M, Sánchez R, Schichor C, Masserdotti G, Felipe O, Heinrich C, Gascón S, Khan MA, Lie DC, Dellavalle A, Cossu G, Goldbrunner R, Götz M, Berninger B (2012) Reprogramming of pericyte-derived cells of the adult human brain into induced neuronal cells. *Cell Stem Cell* 11:471–476.

Karumbayaram S, Novitch BG, Patterson M, Umbach JA, Richter L, Lindgren A, Conway AE, Clark AT, Goldman SA, Plath K, Wiedau-Pazos M, Kornblum HI, Lowry WE (2009) Directed differentiation of human-induced pluripotent stem cells generates active motor neurons. *Stem Cells* 27:806–811.

Kim J, Su SC, Wang H, Cheng AW, Cassady JP, Lodato MA, Lengner CJ, Chung C-Y, Dawlaty MM, Tsai L-H, Jaenich R (2011) Functional integration of dopaminergic neurons directly converted from mouse fibroblasts. *Cell Stem Cell* 9:413–419.

Kimura-Kuroda J, Teng X, Komuta Y, Yoshioka N, Sango K, Kawamura K, Raisman G, Kawano H (2010) An in vitro model of the inhibition of axon growth in the lesion scar formed after central nervous system injury. *Mol Cell Neurosci* 43:177–187.

Knoepfler PS (2009) Deconstructing stem cell tumorigenicty: a roadmap to safe regenerative medicine. *Stem Cells* 27:1050–1105.

Krencik R, Weick JP, Liu Y, Zhang Z-J, Zhang S-C (2011) Specification of transplantable astroglial subtypes from human pluripotent stem cells. *Nat Biotechnol* 29:528–534.

Lagace DC (2012) Does the endogenous neurogenic response alter behavioral recovery following stroke? *Behav Brain Res* 227:426–432.

Liu M-L, Zang T, Zou Y, Chang JC, Gibson JR, Huber KM, Zhang C-L (2013) Small molecules enable neurogenin 2 to efficiently convert human fibroblasts into cholinergic neurons. *Nat Commun* 4:2183.

Lujan E, Chanda S, Ahlenius H, Südhof TC, Wernig M (2012) Direct conversion of mouse fibroblasts to self-renewing, tripotent neural precursor cells. *Proc Natl Acad Sci U S A* 109:2527–2532.

Ming G-L, Song H (2005) Adult neurogenesis in the mammalian central nervous system. *Annu Rev Neurosci* 28:223–250.

Najm FJ, Lager AM, Zaremba A, Wyatt K, Caprariello AV, Factor DC, Karl RT, Maeda T, Miller RH, Tesar PJ (2013) Transcription factor-mediated reprogramming of fibroblasts to expandable, myelinogenic oligodendrocyte progenitor cells. *Nat Biotechnol* 31:426–433.

Nishiyama A, Komitova M, Suzuki R, Zhu X (2009) Polydendrocytes (NG2 cells): multifunctional cells with lineage plasticity. *Nat Rev Neurosci* 10:9–22.

Niu W, Zang T, Zou Y, Fang S, Smith DK, Bachoo R, Zhang C-L (2013) *In vivo* reprogramming of astrocytes to neuroblasts in the adult brain. *Nat Cell Biol* 15:1164–1175.

Okano H, Ogawa Y, Nakamura M, Kaneko S, Iwanami A, Toyama Y (2003) Transplantation of neural stem cells into the spinal cord after injury. *Semin Cell Dev Biol* 14:191–198.

Panayiotou E, Malas, S (2013) Adult spinal cord ependymal layer: a promising pool of quiescent stem cells to treat spinal cord injury. *Front Physiol* 4:430.

Pfisterer U, Kirkeby A, Torper O, Wood J, Nelander J, Dufour A, Björklund A, Lindvall O, Jakobsson J, Parmar M (2011) Direct conversion of human fibroblasts to dopaminergic neurons. *Proc Natl Acad Sci U S A* 108: 10343–10348.

Rais Y, *et al.* (2013) Deterministic direct reprogramming of somatic cells to pluripotency. *Nature* 502:65–70.

Raivich G, Bohatschek M, Kloss CUA, Werner A, Jones LL, Kreutzberg GW (1999) Neuroglial activation repertoire in the injured brain: graded response, molecular mechanisms and cues to physiological function. *Brain Res Rev* 30:77–105.

Ring KL, Tong LM, Balestra ME, Javier R, Andrews-Zwilling Y, Li G, Walker D, Zhang WR, Kreitzer AC, Huang Y (2012) Direct reprogramming of mouse and human fibroblasts into multipotent neural stem cells with a single factor. *Cell Stem Cell* 11:100–109.

Rossa AD, Bellone C, Golding B, Vitali I, Moss J, Toni N, Lüscher C, Jabaudon D (2013) *In vivo* reprogramming of circuit connectivity in postmitotic neocortical neurons. *Nat Neurosci* 16:193–200.

Rouaux C, Arlotta P (2010) Fezf2 directs the differentiation of corticofugal neurons from striatal progenitors *in vivo*. *Nat Neurosci* 13:1345–1347.

Rouaux C, Arlotta P (2013) Direct lineage reprogramming of post-mitotic callosal neurons into corticofugal neurons *in vivo*. *Nat Cell Biol* 15: 214–221.

Shimada T, Takai Y, Shinohara K, Yamasaki A, Tominaga-Yoshino K, Ogura A, Toi A, Asano K, Shintani N, Hayata-Takano A, Baba A, Hashimoto H (2012) A simplified method to generate serotonergic neurons from mouse embryonic stem and induced pluripotent stem cells. *J Neurochem* 122:81–93.

Sirko S, *et al.* (2013) Reactive glia in the injured brain acquire stem cell properties in response to sonic hedgehog (corrected). *Cell Stem Cell* 12:426–439.

Soderblom C, Luo X, Blumenthal E, Bray E, Lyapichev K, Ramos J, Krishnan V, Lai-Hsu C, Park KK, Tsoulfas P, Lee JK (2013) Perivascular fibroblasts form the fibrotic scar after contusive spinal cord injury. *J Neurosci* 33:13882–13887.

Sofroniew MV (2009) Molecular dissection of reactive astrogliosis and glial scar formation. *Trends Neurosci* 32:638–647.

Sofroniew MV, Vinters HV (2010) Astrocytes: biology and pathology. *Acta Neuropathol* 119:7–35.

Son EY, Ichida JK, Wainger BJ, Toma JS, Rafuse VF, Woolf CJ, Eggan K (2011) Conversion of mouse and human fibroblasts into functional spinal motor neurons. *Cell Stem Cell* 9:205–218.

Streit WJ, Walter SA, Pennell NA (1999) Reactive microgliosis. *Prog Neurobiol* 57:563–581.

Su Z, Niu W, Liu M-L, Zou Y, Zhang C-L (2014) *In vivo* conversion of astrocytes to neurons in the injured adult spinal cord. *Nat Commun* 5:3338.

Sun C-K, Zhou D, Zhang Z, He L, Zhang F, Wang X, Yuan J, Chen Q, Wu L-G, Yang Q (2014) Senescence impairs direct conversion of human somatic cells to neurons. *Nat Commun* 5:4112.

Takahashi K, Tanabe K, Ohnuki M, Narita M, Ichisaka T, Tomoda K, Yamanaka S (2007) Induction of pluripotent stem cells from adult human fibroblasts by defined factors. *Cell* 131:861–872.

Takahashi K, Yamanaka S (2006) Induction of pluripotent stem cells from mouse embryonic and adult fibroblast cultures by defined factors. *Cell* 126:663–676.

Torper O, Pfisterer U, Wolf DA, Pereira M, Lau S, Jakobsson J, Björklund A, Grealish S, Parmar M (2013) Generation of induced neurons via direct conversion *in vivo*. *Proc Natl Acad Sci U S A* 110:7038–7043.

Vierbuchen T, Ostermeier A, Pang ZP, Kokubu Y, Südhof TC, Wernig M (2010) Direct conversion of fibroblasts to functional neurons by defined factors. *Nature* 463:1035–1041.

Wanner IB, Anderson MA, Song B, Levine J, Fernandez A, Gray-Thompson Z, Ao Y, Sofroniew MV (2013) Glial scar borders are formed by newly proliferated, elongated astrocytes that interact to corral inflammatory and fibrotic cells via STAT3-dependent mechanisms after spinal cord injury. *J Neurosci* 33:12870–12886.

Weiss S, Dunne C, Hewson J, Wohl C, Wheatley M, Peterson AC, Reynolds BA (1996) Multipotent CNS stem cells are present in the adult mammalian spinal cord and ventricular neuroaxis. *J Neurosci* 16:7599–7609.

Wernig M, Zhao J-P, Pruszak J, Hedlund E, Fu D, Soldner F, Broccoli V, Constantine-Paton M, Isacson O, Jaenisch R (2008) Neurons derived from reprogrammed fibroblasts functionally integrate into the fetal brain and improve symptoms of rats with Parkinson's disease. *Proc Natl Acad Sci U S A* 105:5856–5861.

Xue Y, Ouyang K, Huang J, Zhou Y, Ouyang H, Li H, Wang G, Qijia W, Wei C, Bi Y, Jiang L, Cai Z, Sun H, Zhang K, Zhang Y, Chen J, Fu X-D (2013) Direct conversion of fibroblasts to neurons by reprogramming PTB-regulated microRNA circuits. *Cell* 152:82–96.

Yang N, Zuchero JB, Ahlenius H, Marro S, Ng YH, Vierbuchen T, Hawkins JS, Geissler R, Barres BA, Wernig M (2013) Generation of oligodendroglial cells by direct lineage conversion. *Nat Biotechnol* 31:434–439.

Yoo AS, Sun AX, Li L, Shcheglovitov A, Portmann T, Li Y, Lee-Messer C, Dolmetsch RE, Tsien RW, Crabtree GR (2011) MicroRNA-mediated conversion of human fibroblasts to neurons. *Nature* 476:228–231.

Zeng H, Guo M, Martins-Taylor K, Wang X, Zhang Z, Park JW, Zhan S, Kronenberg MS, Lichtler A, Liu H-X, Chen F-P, Yue L, Li X-J, Xu R-H (2010) Specification of region-specific neurons including forebrain glutamatergic neurons from human induced pluripotent stem cells. *PloS One* 7:e11853.

Zhang D, Hu X, Qian L, O'Callaghan JP, Hong J-S (2010) Astrogliosis in CNS pathologies: is there a role for microglia? *Mol Neurobiol* 41: 232–241.

Zhao T, Zhang Z-N, Rong Z, Xu Y (2011) Immunogenicity of induced pluripotent stem cells. *Nature* 474:212–215.

Chapter 13

Neural Stem Cell Therapy for Parkinson's Disease

Marcel M. Daadi

Dopaminergic (DA) neurons are involved in many critical functions within the central nervous system (CNS) and dopamine neurotransmission impairment underlies a wide range of disorders from motor control deficiencies, such as Parkinson's disease (PD) to psychiatric disorders, such as alcoholism, drug addictions, bipolar disorders and depression. The ability to consistently grow purified and well-characterized populations of DA neurons from pluripotent stem cells or other cell sources is invaluable for disease modeling and drug discovery and for cell therapy approaches to diseased or injured brain. Approximately one million people in the US suffer from PD with an economic burden of $6 billion annually. Cell transplantation of differentiated neural stem cells (NSCs) into a functionally compromised nervous system has shown promising results as a treatment for PD. However, in order for cell-based therapy and regenerative medicine to become a viable option in the future, commercially feasible biological products need to be developed and proven to be consistent, predictable and efficacious. This requires meeting and overcoming numerous challenges in process development and manufacturing to enable product commercialization. Some of the critical steps are defining the optimal process for cell production and cryopreservation that will not compromise the safety or efficacy of cellular product. Here, we briefly summarize recent advances in NSCs derivation from various sources and their differentiation methods into dopaminergic lineage. We also highlight the current challenges to bring these cells into the clinical stage.

Introduction

Over the past 20 years, there has been growing interest in the potential of regenerative therapy for neuronal disease and brain injuries. The use of self-renewable multipotent neural stem cells (NSCs) to repair cellular defects or injured brain represents promising technology with significant humanitarian, societal and economic impact. The favorable characteristic that is disposing NSCs towards clinical use is their ability to generate, under controlled conditions, a large number of progeny with the potential to differentiate into functionally specialized groups of neural cells.

Parkinson's disease (PD) is a neurodegenerative disorder characterized by the loss of dopamine (DA) neurons in the substantia nigra pars compacta (SN), resulting in decreased dopaminergic input to the striatum. PD is the second most common chronic neurodegenerative disease after Alzheimer's and symptoms include tremor, rigidity, bradykinesia and instability. In the United States, over a million persons suffer from PD and 60,000 new cases are diagnosed every year with an estimated annual cost of $27 billion (Obeso *et al.*, 2000). Neural cell transplantation is a promising strategy for improving dopaminergic dysfunction and restoring dopaminergic neurotransmission in PD. Over three decades of research on fetal mesencephalic (MS) tissue as a source of DA neurons has demonstrated the therapeutic potential of cell therapy in rodents, non-human primate (NHP) animal models and human patients (Barker and Dunnett; 1999; Olanow *et al.*, 1997; Sortwell *et al.*, 1998; Brundin *et al*; 1988; Burdin *et al.*, 2000; Perlow *et al.*, 1979; Bjorklund and Stenevi, 1979; Lindvall *et al.*, 1992; Sladek *et al.*, 1993; Kordower *et al.*, 1998; Remy *et al.*, 1995; Mendez *et al.*, 2002; Mendez *et al.*, 2008; Freeman *et al.*, 1995; Peschanski *et al.*, 1994; Barker *et al.*, 2013; Freed *et al.*, 1992). Clinical trials have reported that the grafted neural cells survive, densely reinnervate the host putamen with new dopamine fibers and improve motor function in patients. Although fetal MS tissue demonstrated proof of principal that transplantation of DA neurons into the putamen of PD patients restores dopaminergic neurotransmission and improves L-DOPA pharmacotherapy, the enthusiasm for this source is diminished by the unpractical logistical and safety concerns, ethical issues and the lack of commercial viability. Nevertheless, the clinical research with the fetal MS tissue has been extremely insightful and is paving the way for developing NSC-based cell replacement therapy for PD.

Neural Stem Cell Sources of Dopaminergic Neurons

A promising source of DA neurons may be the multipotent and self-renewable human (h)NSCs because under controlled conditions, large numbers of specific neurons can be generated. Previous studies have demonstrated that instructive cues, known as floor plate-secreted Shh and FGF8, are required for the generation and specification of the midbrain DA neurons (Hynes *et al.*, 1995; Hynes *et al.*, 1995; Ye *et al.*, 1998) and the transcription factors Nurr1 and FoxA2 are also essential (Kittappa *et al.*, 2007; Zetterstrom *et al.*, 1997; Saucedo-Cardenas *et al.*, 1998). Then, the question was: do these developmental cues and transcription factors control DA phenotype in NSC-derived progeny, similarly to the developing floor plate in the midbrain?

NSC progeny are clusters of cells derived from multipotent neural precursors in response to EGF with or without FGF2 and LIF treatment (Reynolds and Weiss, 1992; Carpenter *et al.*, 1999; Uchida *et al.*, 2000). We reported that SHH was inefficient in inducing the DA phenotype in self-renewable NSCs, while glial-secreted dopamine-inducing factors (GSDF) were instructive in generating dopaminergic neurons (Daadi and Weiss, 1999; Daadi, 2008). DA neurons may provide therapeutic benefits through either reinnervation of the putamen, non-synaptic release of DA or neurotrophic support for the remaining host residual DA terminals. So far it has been challenging to maintain the hNSC-derived DA neurons *in vivo* after grafting.

There has also been a great effort to generate DA neurons from self-renewable CNS-derived stem cell lines. The potency of the instructive cues to induce TH varies with the properties of the stem cell line. These properties may be influenced by the origin and method of derivation. Early studies have demonstrated rare TH-positive neurons derived from the EGF-responsive hNSCs grown for 10, 14 or 28 days *in vitro* and transplanted into 6-OHDA denner-vated rat striatum (Svendsen *et al.*, 1997; Burnstein *et al.*, 2004). In early reports, hNSCs isolated by using EGF, FGF2 and LIF used a combination of cytokines and neurotrophic factors consisting of IL-1, IL-11 and GDNF to induce the TH expression (Carpenter *et al.*, 1997). The engraftment, midbrain identity and stability of the DA phenotype of these cells in animal models have not been reported.

Another approach taken to induce dopaminergic phenotype in non-midbrain-derived NSCs has been to insert critical genes involved in the development of mesencepahalon (VM)-DA neurons, specifi-cally *Nurr1* (Zetterstrom *et al.*, 1997; Saucedo-Cardenas *et al.*, 1998; Wagner *et al.*, 1999), via *ex vivo* genetic modification and co-culture with astrocytes (Daadi and Weiss, 1999; Wagner *et al.*, 1999). In con-trast, Sakurada and colleagues reported that *Nurr1* did not appear to influence the neuronal fate of the NSCs while in the presence of either forskolin or retinoic acid, although *Nurr-1* directly activated the TH gene expression in NSCs derived from adult hippocampus (Sakurada *et al.*, 1999). Recent studies have taken this genetic engi-neering approach to the extreme by demonstrating that the over-expression of a set of transcription factors including *Ascl1*, *Nurr1* and *Lmx1a* (Caiazzo *et al.*, 2011) or *Ascl1*, *Brn2* and *Myt1l* followed by *Lmx1a* and *FoxA2* (Pfisterer *et al.*, 2011) are sufficient to induce the conversion of fibroblasts to functional DA neurons. The effi-cacy of these cells to innervate and provide functional dopamine replacement in animal models of PD remains to be determined.

The requirement of these key-DA-specific transcription factors is inciting to isolate normal hNSCs from the VM. However, to this end, attempts to isolate such a normal ventral VM hNSCs have shown encouraging but limited success without immortalization (Villa *et al.*, 2009). Precursors isolated from the E12 rat VM and grown in

FGF for 1 week, then induced to differentiate in absence of FGF2 and presence of fetal bovine serum for 7 more days yielded an increase of TH-expressing from 6% to 18% of neurons. The increase in TH-immunorective (IR) neurons was due to a 10-fold increase in cell proliferation. In these cultures, ascorbic acid and low oxygen concentration potentiated the cell proliferation and led to more DA neurons (56% of neurons) (Studer *et al.*, 2000; Yan *et al.*, 2001). The effect of low O_2 levels (3 ± 2%) was partially mimicked by erythropoietin. Interestingly, interleukin-1 (IL-1) induced the TH gene expression in the midbrain-derived progenitors and VM-derived DA clone (Potter *et al.*, 1999). Although it has been shown that DA-inducing conditions up-regulate the expression of *Nurr1* and *Pitx3*, a key transcription factor of the midbrain DA neurons, *FoxA2*, does not appear to be expressed either before or after the DA-induction treatment. This suggests that the DA neurons generated from these hNSCs may not express all transcription factors that identify midbrain DA neurons. Further *in vitro* and *in vivo* characterization of these cells and correlation with the behavioral outcome, will be insightful on the therapeutic properties of these hNSCs.

Tremendous progress has been made in deriving DA neurons from pluripotent stem cells including human ESCs (hESCs) and human induced pluripotent stem cells (hiPSCs). Recent studies have reported the induction of the floor plate and DA neurons in the pluripotent stem cells using small molecules (Sundberg *et al.*, 2013; Kriks *et al.*, 2011; Lindvall, 2012; Kirkeby *et al.*, 2012; Xi *et al.*, 2012). The technique consists of first generating neural lineage from hESCs or iPSCs then inducing DA neurons. The successive exposure of iPSCs or hESCs to SMAD dual inhibitors LDN193189 and SB431542 and sonic hedgehog (SHH), FGF8 and to small molecule, CHIR99021 (CHIR), a potent GSK3B inhibitor that strongly activates WNT signaling, leads to the selective enrichment for midbrain DA precursor markers. Further maturation of the DA neurons is carried out in Neurobasal/B27 medium supplemented with ascorbic acid, BDNF, GDNF, TGFb3 and dibutyryl (db) cyclic AMP (Kriks *et al.*, 2011; Lindvall, 2012). Transplantation of 250,000 cells into rat-6OHDA model led to an average of 15,000 TH+/FOXA2+ cells and to behavioral recovery demonstrated by the amphetamine-induced rotational test, stepping test and the forepaw exploratory cylinder test (Kriks *et al.*, 2011). This approach has been improved upon recently by adding a cell sorting step for the neural lineage (NCAM+/CD29^{low}) that eliminates non-neural lineage in the cell preparation (Sundberg *et al.*, 2013). This protocol generates DA neurons that express midbrain transcription factors, differentiate into DA neurons *in vivo* and alleviate PD symptoms in rat-6OHDA model.

A more targeted purification approach of the midbrain DA from iPSCs was reported and utilized the cell surface marker Corin (Chung *et al.*, 2011; Ono *et al.*, 2007; Jonsson *et al.*, 2009; Doi *et al.*, 2014), a serine protease expressed in the developing brain specifically in the floor plate where DA neurons are born. Using hiPSCs, sorted Corin+ cells differentiated for 28 days were more efficacious in improving amphetamine-induced rotational behavior in the 6-OHDA lesioned rats than those differentiated for 42 days (Doi *e al.*, 2014).

We previously reported a purification method of self-renewable NSCs from hESC (Daadi *et al.*, 2008) (Figure 1). When treated with GSDF, these NSCs differentiate into DA neurons in a dose-dependent manner while control cultures show very low to no DA expression (Daadi *et al.*, 2012). This DA differentiation process leads to approximately 27% of neurons becoming TH+ and co-expressing transcription factors that characterize them as midbrain DA neurons including, Nurr1, Pitx3, FoaxA2, En1, Lmx1b and ALDH2 (Daadi *et al.*, 2012). To test the engraftability and the stability of the phenotype, the DA-induced neurons were transplanted into the caudate of an MPTP lesioned NHP (Daadi *et al.*, 2012). Two months post-transplantation, the grafted DA neurons were detected with human-specific nuclei and cytoplasmic markers. Approximately 10% of the hNSCs expressed the dopaminergic phenotype (10,000 to 15,000 TH+ cells/graft). These dopaminergic neurons extended neurite outgrowths that co-localized the synaptic marker synaptophysin, suggesting connectivity with the host cells (Daadi *et al.*, 2012). Transplantation of the GSDF-induced DA neurons into the 6-OHDA-lesioned rat model of PD led to functional recovery in the

Partial Cell Dissociation with Collagenase
DMEM/F12+EGF+bFGF+LIF   Single Cell Dissociation

3 DIV	7 DIV	15 +4×7 DIV

| hESCs Pluripotent | → | 1° Spheres Replate - I | → | 2° Spheres Replate - II | → | NSCs Multipotent |

Oct4+
SSEA4+
Nanog+

Primitive NSC
Oct4-, SSEA- Nanog-
SOX2+, Nest+

Definitive NSC
Nest+, NCAM+, Notch1+
NF-M+, GFAP+, MBP+

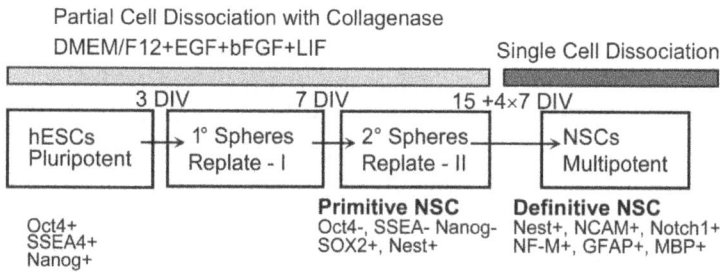

Figure 1. Schematic representation of the isolation of self-renewable definitive NSCs. Neural stem cells were derived from hESCs and propagated using defined media supplemented with EGF, FGF and LIF. The developmental progression of the *in vitro* neural specification and patterning was monitored by the expression of lineage markers as indicated at each neuralization stage [Adapted from (Daadi *et al.*, 2008)].

apomorphin test and the forepaw exploratory cylinder test at a dose of 300,000 cells with a TH+ neurons survival rate of $12 \pm 3\%$ (~9,000 TH+/graft). However, head-to-head comparison of these purification and differentiation approaches of DA neurons from PSCs in the cellular composition and in the efficacy of reinnervating the striatum in animal models of PD remain to be determined.

With the current preclinical and clinical data on fetal cells, stem cell-based therapy for Parkinson's disease is progressing cautiously toward the clinical arena. Some of the critical remaining questions and challenges are, for instance, the degree of innervation by dopaminergic neurons derived from CNS, iPSCs or hESCs sources of NSCs. The ideal stem cell-based cellular products will strike an optimal balance between the safety of the cells and the purity and scalability of derivation method of the midbrain DA neurons with a proven therapeutic innervation capacity.

References

Barker RA, Dunnett SB. (1999) Functional integration of neural grafts in Parkinson's disease. *Nat Neurosci* 2:1047–1048.

Barker RA, Barrett J, Mason SL, Bjorklund A (2013) Fetal dopaminergic transplantation trials and the future of neural grafting in Parkinson's disease. *Lancet Neurol* 12:84–91.

Bjorklund A, Stenevi U (1979) Reconstruction of the nigrostriatal dopamine pathway by intracerebral nigral transplants. *Brain Res* 177: 555–560.

Brundin P *et al.* (1988) Human fetal dopamine neurons grafted in a rat model of Parkinson's disease: immunological aspects, spontaneous and drug-induced behaviour, and dopamine release. *Exp Brain Res* 70: 192–208.

Brundin P *et al.* (2000) Bilateral caudate and putamen grafts of embryonic mesencephalic tissue treated with lazaroids in Parkinson's disease. *Brain* 123 (Pt 7):1380–1390.

Burnstein RM *et al.* (2004) Differentiation and migration of long term expanded human neural progenitors in a partial lesion model of Parkinson's disease. *Int J Biochem Cell Biol* 36:702–713.

Caiazzo M *et al.* (2011) Direct generation of functional dopaminergic neurons from mouse and human fibroblasts. *Nature* 476:224–227.

Carpenter MK *et al.* (1999) *In vitro* expansion of a multipotent population of human neural progenitor cells. *Experimental Neurology* 158:265–278.

Chung S *et al.* (2011) ES cell-derived renewable and functional midbrain dopaminergic progenitors. *Proc Natl Acad Sci U S A* 108:9703–9708.

Daadi MM, Weiss S (1999) Generation of tyrosine hydroxylase-producing neurons from precursors of the embryonic and adult forebrain. *J Neurosci* 19:4484–4497.

Daadi MM (2008) *In vitro* assays for neural stem cell differentiation: Induction of Dopaminergic phenotype. *Methods in Molecular Biology* 438:205–212.

Daadi MM, Grueter BA, Malenka RC, Redmond DE, Jr, Steinberg GK (2012) Dopaminergic neurons from midbrain-specified human embryonic stem cell-derived neural stem cells engrafted in a monkey model of Parkinson's disease. *PLoS ONE* 7:e41120.

Daadi MM, Maag AL, Steinberg GK (2008) Adherent self-renewable human embryonic stem cell-derived neural stem cell line: functional engraftment in experimental stroke model. *PLoS ONE* 3:e1644.

Doi D *et al.* (2014) Isolation of human induced pluripotent stem cell-derived dopaminergic progenitors by cell sorting for successful transplantation. *Stem Cell Reports* 2:337–350.

Freed CR *et al.* (1992) Survival of implanted fetal dopamine cells and neurologic improvement 12 to 46 months after transplantation for Parkinson's disease. *NE J Med* 327:1549–1555.

Freeman TB *et al.* (1995) Bilateral fetal nigral transplantation into the post-commissural putamen in Parkinson's disease. *Ann Neurol* 38:379–388.

Hynes M *et al.* (1995) Induction of midbrain dopaminergic neurons by Sonic hedgehog. *Neuron* 15:35–44.

Hynes M, Poulsen K, Tessier-Lavigne M, Rosenthal A (1995) Control of neuronal diversity by the floor plate: contact-mediated induction of midbrain dopaminergic neurons. *Cell* 80:95–101.

Jonsson ME, Ono Y, Bjorklund A, Thompson LH (2009) Identification of transplantable dopamine neuron precursors at different stages of midbrain neurogenesis. *Exp Neurol* 219:341–354.

Kirkeby A *et al.* (2012) Generation of regionally specified neural progenitors and functional neurons from human embryonic stem cells under defined conditions. *Cell Rep* 1:703–714.

Kittappa R, Chang WW, Awatramani RB, McKay RD (2007) The foxa2 gene controls the birth and spontaneous degeneration of dopamine neurons in old age. *PLoS Biol* 5:e325.

Kordower JH *et al.* (1998) Fetal nigral grafts survive and mediate clinical benefit in a patient with Parkinson's disease. *Mov Disord* 13:383–393.

Kriks S *et al.* (2011) Dopamine neurons derived from human ES cells efficiently engraft in animal models of Parkinson's disease. *Nature* 480: 547–551.

Lindvall O (2012) Dopaminergic neurons for Parkinson's therapy. *Nat Biotechnol* 30:56–58.

Lindvall O *et al.* (1992) Transplantation of fetal dopamine neurons in Parkinson's disease: One-year clinical and neurophysiological observations in two patients with putamminal implants. *Annals of Neurology* 31: 155–165.

Mendez I *et al.* (2002) Simultaneous intrastriatal and intranigral fetal dopaminergic grafts in patients with Parkinson disease: a pilot study. Report of three cases. *J Neurosurg* 96:589–596.

Mendez I *et al.* (2008) Dopamine neurons implanted into people with Parkinson's disease survive without pathology for 14 years. *Nat Med* 14: 507–509.

Obeso JA, Olanow CW, Nutt JG (2000) Levodopa motor complications in Parkinson's disease. *Trends Neurosci* 23:S2–7.

Olanow CW, Freeman TB, Kordower JH (1997) Neural transplantation as a therapy for Parkinson's disease. *Adv Neurol* 74:249–269.

Ono Y *et al.* (2007) Differences in neurogenic potential in floor plate cells along an anteroposterior location: midbrain dopaminergic neurons originate from mesencephalic floor plate cells. *Development* 134:3213–3225.

Perlow MJ *et al.* (1979) Brain grafts reduce motor abnormalities produced by destruction of nigrostriatal dopamine system. *Science* 204:643–647.

Peschanski M *et al.* (1994) Bilateral motor improvement and alteration of L-dopa effect in two patients with Parkinson's disease following intra-striatal transplantation of foetal ventral mesencephalon. *Brain* 117 (Pt 3):487–499.

Pfisterer U *et al.* (2011) Direct conversion of human fibroblasts to dopaminergic neurons. *Proc Natl Acad Sci U S A* 108:10343–10348.

Potter ED, Ling ZD, Carvey PM (1999) Cytokine-induced conversion of mesencephalic-derived progenitor cells into dopamine neurons. *Cell Tissue Res* 296:235–246.

Remy P *et al.* (1995) Clinical correlates of [18F]fluorodopa uptake in five grafted parkinsonian patients. *Ann Neurol* 38:580–588.

Reynolds BA, Weiss S (1992) Generation of neurons and astrocytes from isolated cells of the adult mammalian central nervous system. *Science* 255:1707–1710.

Sakurada K, Ohshima-Sakurada M, Palmer TD, Gage FH (1999) Nurr1, an orphan nuclear receptor, is a transcriptional activator of endogenous tyrosine hydroxylase in neural progenitor cells derived from the adult brain. *Development* 126:4017–4026.

Saucedo-Cardenas O *et al.* (1998) Nurr1 is essential for the induction of the dopaminergic phenotype and the survival of ventral mesence-phalic late dopaminergic precursor neurons. *Proc Natl Acad Sci U S A* 95:4013–4018.

Sladek JR, Jr *et al.* (1993) Fetal dopamine cell survival after transplantation is dramatically improved at a critical donor gestational age in nonhuman primates. *Exp Neurol* 122:16–27.

Sortwell CE *et al.* (1998) Pattern of synaptophysin immunoreactivity within mesencephalic grafts following transplantation in a parkinsonian primate model. *Brain Res* 791:117–124.

Studer L *et al.* (2000) Enhanced proliferation, survival, and dopaminergic differentiation of CNS precursors in lowered oxygen. *J Neurosci* 20: 7377–7383.

Sundberg M *et al.* (2013) Improved cell therapy protocols for Parkinson's disease based on differentiation efficiency and safety of hESC-, hiPSC-, and non-human primate iPSC-derived dopaminergic neurons. *Stem Cells* 31:1548–1562.

Svendsen CN *et al.* (1997) Long-term survival of human central nervous system progenitor cells transplanted into a rat model of Parkinson's disease. *Exp Neurol* 148:135–146.

Uchida N *et al.* (2000) Direct isolation of human central nervous system stem cells. *Proc Natl Acad Sci U S A* 97:14720–14725.

Villa A *et al.* (2009) Generation and properties of a new human ventral mesencephalic neural stem cell line. *Exp Cell Res* 315:1860–1874.

Wagner J *et al.* (1999) Induction of a midbrain dopaminergic phenotype in Nurr1-overexpressing neural stem cells by type 1 astrocytes. *Nat Biotechnol* 17:653–659.

Xi J *et al.* (2012) Specification of midbrain dopamine neurons from primate pluripotent stem cells. *Stem Cells* 30:1655–1663.

Yan J, Studer L, McKay RD (2001) Ascorbic acid increases the yield of dopaminergic neurons derived from basic fibroblast growth factor expanded mesencephalic precursors. *J Neurochem* 76:307–311.

Ye W, Shimamura K, Rubenstein JL, Hynes MA, Rosenthal A (1998) FGF and Shh signals control dopaminergic and serotonergic cell fate in the anterior neural plate. *Cell* 93:755–766.

Zetterstrom RH *et al.* (1997) Dopamine neuron agenesis in *Nurr1*-deficient mice. *Science* 276:248–250.

Chapter 14

Stem Cell-Based Neuroprotective Strategies in Stroke

*Ike dela Peña, Alesia Antoine, Stephanny Reyes,
Diana Hernandez, Sandra Acosta, Mibel Pabon,
Naoki Tajiri, Yuji Kaneko, and Cesar V. Borlongan*

The ability to produce and harvest sufficient amount of stem cells from diverse sources fueled significant progress in stem cell-based therapies for stroke. Nevertheless, what deserves further research is determining optimal conditions of stem cell transplantation. Stem cell derivations not only provide promise but also present a number of challenges when employed as stroke therapies. Here, we review the advantages and limitations of various stem cell-based therapies for neuroprotection in stroke.

Stem Cell Therapy for Stroke: An Overview

Stroke remains to be one of the top killers of Americans and poses a significant threat to millions of others worldwide (Koton *et al.*, 2014). It is a highly prevalent disease with scarce therapeutic options, and most of the currently used stroke therapies show limited efficacy in restoring lost neurological functions. Furthermore, the only FDA-approved drug for stroke, namely tissue plasminogen activator (tPA) presents serious limitations and complications, which include a limited therapeutic window (4.5 hr from stroke onset to tPA administration) and detrimental side effects associated with delayed treatment (e.g. hemorrhagic transformation), resulting in a mere 3% of ischemic stroke patients actually benefiting from tPA therapy (Graham, 2003; Yip and Demaerschalk, 2007). The lack of effective therapies and other significant unmet clinical needs for stroke prompted both preclinical and clinical research for novel stroke interventions. A promising approach to stroke therapy is the use of exogenous stem cells. Stem cell-based therapies, as opposed to pharmacologic agents/compounds, show efficacy when initiated in acute and sub-acute phases, as well as at later time-points following stroke onset and have been demonstrated to address the complex pathophysiology of stroke, providing neurological improvement. Furthermore, a number of preclinical studies have documented the ability of transplanted stem cells to improve stroke-induced brain and behavioral pathology robustly early on and stably over long-term post-insult than any available stroke treatments (e.g. Xiao *et al.*, 2005; Cui *et al.*, 2012; Rowe *et al.*, 2012).

Adult stem cells derived from different tissues may serve as donor cells for transplantation therapy in stroke. In stem cell therapy, it is imperative to consider mode of stem cell treatment, i.e., autologous or allogeneic, the latter entails receiving cells from an unrelated donor, while the former involves obtaining cells from the same individual receiving them. However, an issue or limitation associated with the use of allogeneic stem cell grafts is that they may elicit immunogenic complication with the host such as graft rejection. Nevertheless, different stem cell sources have their own strengths and inherent limitations (e.g. low cell yield, limited proliferation capacity of stem cells and immunogenicity). In particular, when utilizing stem cell-based therapies for stroke, it is important to consider cell yield, proliferation capacity, and optimal time for delivery of these stem cells, as demonstrated by previous research with umbilical cord blood transplantation. Ideally, stem cells should be delivered within 48 hours post-stroke (Newcomb *et al.*, 2006), which is rather a short time period to generate enough amount of stem cells from freshly harvested autologous tissue sources.

Meanwhile, an issue associated with using neural stem cell for stroke is harvesting these cells, which may require highly invasive surgical procedures. Indeed, ease of harvesting may have greater influence over the practicality of therapeutic potential of stem cells.

Immunological reactions, such as graft vs. host, and secondary complications that arise from adjunctive immunosuppression also present additional challenges in stem cell treatment for stroke. Accordingly, Cyclosporine A, an immunosuppressant, induces endogenous neural stem cell activity and migration aiding in the recovery of cortical injury following stroke (Erlandsson *et al.*, 2011). Studies in immune-compromised stroked animals demonstrated elevated endogenous neurogenesis via a CD4+ T cell-, but not a CD25+ T cell-dependent mechanism (Saino *et al.*, 2010). Nevertheless, despite the possibility for stem cells to produce an immunogenic response, it is widely believed that cell immunogenicity is influenced by differentiation state of these cells, i.e., the more naïve or less lineage-specific a cell is, the less likely it is to induce an immune response. As an example, due to immunological immaturity of umbilical cord blood, transplantation of these cells is less likely to require immunosuppression. Therefore, human leukocyte antigen (HLA) matching may be less strict before transplantation of umbilical cord blood while cell viability remains high compared to the requirements for bone marrow transplants (Willing *et al.*, 2007). On the other hand, some cells may be more immunosuppressive than bone marrow-derived cells, such as chorionic plate-derived mesenchymal stem cells which display higher expression of HLA-G (Hunt *et al.*, 2005), a contributing factor in the induction of stronger immunosuppression and indicator of graft tolerance (Menier *et al.*, 2010), compared with bone marrow-derived and adipose tissue-derived mesenchymal stem cells (Lee *et al.*, 2012). Conversely, placenta derived-mesenchymal stem cells demonstrate less inhibition of stimulation of CD4+ T cells compared with bone marrow-derived stem cells (Fazekasova *et al.*, 2011).

The purpose of this review is to provide insights on the different tissues used to harvest stem cells and to discuss advantages and limitations of these tissue-derived stem cells for neuroprotection in stroke. This review is limited to utilizing stem cells for neuroprotection, in lieu of neurorestoration, of which goals include remodeling of the damaged brain tissue rather than preserving the tissue at risk (neuroprotection), treatment is usually initiated at several days, months or even years after stroke onset (i.e., when the infarct area and penumbra have already stabilized), and therapeutic benefit is not immediate, evolving progressively over several weeks, accompanied by neurological recovery processes which are also presented in a delayed manner (Herman, 2010) (Figure 1). In this regard, we posit that early initiation of therapeutic intervention post-stroke will result in increased likelihood of a better clinical outcome. Nevertheless, considering the harsh local microenvironment which may not allow survival of transplanted stem cells, and the limitations of neuroprotective treatments which benefit only a few eligible

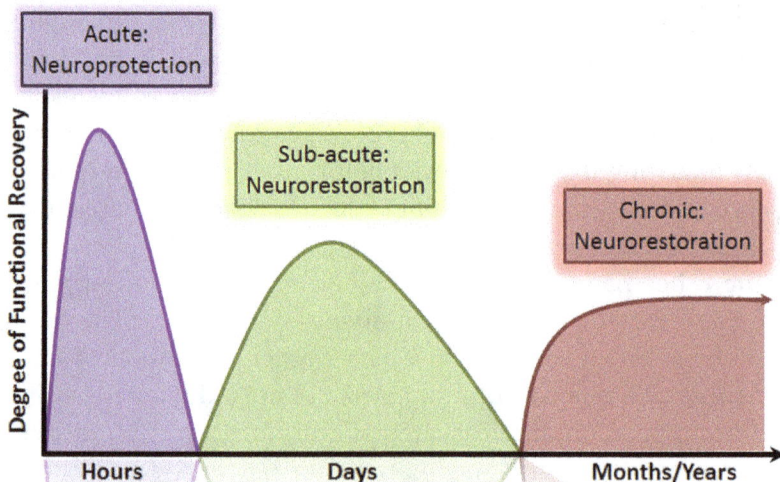

Figure 1. Diagram depicting the "time windows of opportunity" for stroke therapy. The neuroprotective window, is short, lasting hours, and treatments are usually initiated after stroke onset in order to preserve the tissue at risk. In contrast, the neurorestoration window, an area of opportunity for remodeling the damaged brain tissue, is usually initiated at several days, months or even years after stroke onset.

stroke patients, the benefits of tailoring stem cells for neurorestoration may outweigh the neuroprotective promise of stem cells (Huang *et al.*, 2010). A review on various stem cells currently being investigated for neurorestoration can be found elsewhere (Huang *et al.*, 2010).

Embryonic Stem Cells

Embryonic stem (ES) cells provide access to an indefinite supply of stem cells that populate the three germ layers. Hence, they are considered as the yardstick of "stemness" properties of stem cells. ES cell transplantation in stroke animals ameliorated stroke-induced neuronal (Hayashi *et al.*, 2006) and vascular deficits (Oyamada *et al.*, 2008) in these subjects resulting in functional recovery (Wei *et al.*, 2005; Yanagisawa *et al.*, 2006; Pignataro *et al.*, 2007; Theus *et al.*, 2008; Yang *et al.*, 2009). The neurotrophic, angiogenic, and anti-apoptotic effects of transplanted ES cells have also been documented in many previous studies (Wei *et al.*, 2005; Pignataro *et al.*, 2007; Li *et al.*, 2008; Theus *et al.*, 2008; Yang *et al.*, 2009). Moreover, ES cells deposition in both the brain and the periphery following transplantation has also been revealed using various imaging techniques (Hoehn *et al.*, 2002; Lappalainen *et al.*, 2008). However, some caveats associated with ES cell transplants, such as ethical concerns and high risk of tumorigenesis, limit their use for stroke therapy.

Adult Stem Cells

Due to the diverse nature of stroke and the complex mode of action of stem cells, it is necessary to use specific stem cell derivatives to treat distinct stroke conditions. In this regard, it may be challenging to use stem cells derived from adult tissues in stroke as obviously, they contain non-stem cells which have differentiated into specific lineages. Thus, adult tissue-derived stem cells may have to be purified in order to obtain homogeneous stem cell populations for transplantation.

Neural stem cells

Neural stem cells (NSCs) appear to be an obvious solution to repair brain damage caused by stroke. Endogenous stem cells are located in the subgranular zone (SGZ) of the dentate gyrus and subventricular zone (SVZ), as well as in the subependymal zone (SEZ) of the spinal cord. In light of upregulated cellular activity in these zones, it can be assumed that cell replacement and eventually, full functional repair may be accomplished following a stroke-like event. However, despite the presence of NSCs at the site of ischemic lesions as soon as day 1 after stroke in human patients (Nakayama *et al.*, 2010), these effects have not been observed.

Although NSCs in the SVZ migrate into ischemic lesions after stroke, very few or even possibly none of the newborn cells develop into mature neurons (Arvidsson *et al.*, 2002; Nygren *et al.*, 2006; Deierborg *et al.*, 2009). It has been assumed that NSCs from the SVZ may be redirected from their normal route through the rostral stream into a redefined direction to reach ischemic regions along blood vessels providing a scaffold for migration (Jin *et al.*, 2003; Thored *et al.*, 2007; Kojima *et al.*, 2010). Furthermore, the course of SVZ NSC migration to the ischemic area via blood vessels is influenced by chemokine signals such as stromal-derived factor-1 (SDF-1), vascular endothelial growth factor (VEGF), and angiopoietin, which are released from the ischemic tissue (Barkho *et al.*, 2008; Liu *et al.*, 2009; Zhang *et al.*, 2009; Carbajal *et al.*, 2010). Microglia are also believed to play a crucial role in differentiation of neural progenitor cells (NPCs). This phenomenon has been observed in *ex vivo* cultures of rat brain cells, which showed that microglia from the ischemic, but not the intact brain have the ability to promote differentiation of SVZ NSCs into neurons (Deierborg *et al.*, 2010).

Although endogenous NPCs in the SVZ migrate and differentiate into mature neurons, this process may not be sufficient for self-repair of the ischemic brain. Therefore, recent research has explored the possibility of exogenous stem cell transplantation to boost endogenous stem cell production at the site of injury (Bachstetter *et al.*, 2008; Park *et al.*, 2010; van Velthoven *et al.*, 2010; Jin *et al.*, 2011). Of note, intravenous infusion of neural progenitor cells resulted in increased dendritic length and increased number of branch points in host neurons but also decreased neurogenesis (Minnerup *et al.*, 2011).

Despite the benefits of NSC transplantation on endogenous stem cell proliferation, NSCs are not without limitations. A major challenge involves acquiring sufficient amount of NSCs, which in the case of autologous treatment may require invasive surgery prior to therapy. Moreover, allogenic grafts would likely require a fetal source or derivation from an alternative cell type. To address this, one may consider harvesting cells during other surgical procedures although this may not be very advantageous (Chaichana *et al.*, 2009).

The tumorigenic potential of stem cells has been one of the foremost concerns with stem cell transplantation. Typically, cells that are less differentiated exhibit higher risk for tumorigenicity, somewhat contrary to immunogenicity of stem cells. Therefore, adult stem cells may be less likely tumorigenic than their embryonic counterparts due to the progressive differentiation of these cells. Nevertheless, it is important to transplant a purified cell population when utilizing stem cells (Jandial and Snyder, 2009; Amariglio and Renchavi, 2010) as previous studies reported formation of glioneuronal neoplasm in a patient with ataxia telangiectasia transplanted with a heterogeneous mixture of fetally-derived neural stem cells (Amariglio *et al.*, 2009).

The decreased tumorigenic potential of adult-derived stem cells has been attributed to their reduced capacity to proliferate relative to embryonic stem cells. Accordingly, while circumventing the issue of neoplasticity associated with embryonic stem cells, a problem may arise when attempting to produce ample amount of adult-derived stem cells for transplantation. A number of methods have been suggested to address this propagation limitation of adult-derived stem cells, including long-term culturing, immortalization, insertion of oncogenes and even deriving neural stem cells from more immature tissues (e.g., placenta, amnion fluid, cord blood) or pluripotent stem cells (i.e., iPS), and closely monitoring safety outcomes to prevent tumorigenesis. These methods, however, have their own inherent limitations. For instance, long-term culturing presents the risk of spontaneous conversion to a non-neural cell type like a tumor precursor cell (Wu *et al.*, 2011). Although teratocarcinoma-derived hNT neuron cell lines have advanced into a phase II clinical trial in stroke (Newman *et al.*, 2005), transplantation of these cells did not improve conditions of stroke patients (Kondziolka *et al.*, 2005). Insertion of oncogenes may also be a promising method. ReNeuron LTD, a stem cell therapeutics company based in England has reported generation of an immortalized neural cell line via incorporation of c-MYc regulator gene and mutated estrogen receptor transgene (Pollock *et al.*, 2006), a method currently investigated in clinical trials as a potential stroke therapy in the United Kingdom (Mack, 2011).

Bone marrow-derived stem cells

Recent research suggests feasibility of bone marrow-derived stem cells (BMDCs) for stroke therapy. Emerging data demonstrate mobilization of BMDCs from the bone marrow to the peripheral blood in response to injury, and the ability of these cells to migrate to the central nervous system (CNS) to influence neuronal injury (Borlongan *et al.*, 2011). As the bone marrow consists of a diverse population of cells (i.e. BMDCs), it is important to purify these cells in order to harvest a specific cell type, although they can also be used as a mixture. The bone marrow is composed of various types of cells, including hematopoietic stem cells (HSCs), mesenchymal stem cells (MSCs), endothelial progenitor cells (EPCs), and very small embryonic-like stem cells (VSELs) (Herzog *et al.*, 2003). The therapeutic potentials of these bone marrow derived stem cell lines are discussed in the following sections.

Hematopoietic stem cells

A cerebrovascular injury such as stroke induces migration of HSCs via cytokines produced by the CNS (Lapidot *et al.*, 2005; Nervi *et al.*, 2006; Papayannopoulou and Scadden, 2008; Lapidot and Kollet, 2010). Neurotransmitters, most notably, catecholamines, can induce mobilization of HSCs via a nerve ending paracrine signal directly into the bone marrow or through sympathetic release into blood circulation (Kalinkovich *et al.*, 2006). The cytokine-mediated concept of stem cell recruitment has been employed by current treatment protocols such as administration of granulocyte-colony stimulating factor (G-CSF) (Nervi *et al.*, 2006; Papayannopoulou and Scadden, 2008). Clinical studies reported migration by peripheral blood immature hematopoietic CD34+ cells, colony-forming cells, and long-term culture-initiating cells (LTC-IC), and correlation of magnitude of mobilization of these cells with functional recovery in acute stroke patients (Hennemann *et al.*, 2008, Dunac *et al.*, 2007). Infusion of autologous bone marrow mononuclear cells into patients with acute, subacute, and chronic stroke also revealed promising results without reports of adverse effects of transplantation (Battistela *et al.*, 2011; Savitz *et al.*, 2011; Friedrich *et al.*, 2012; Monich *et al.*, 2012). Transplantation of bone marrow mononuclear cells have also been shown to increase plasma B-nerve growth factor (Moniche *et al.*, 2012). The amount of CD34+ cells in transplanted mononuclear cells somewhat correlated with functional recovery (Moniche *et al.*, 2012). Due to these positive findings, bone marrow-derived HSCs have also been considered for other medical conditions such cardiovascular system, bone and cartilage disorders.

Mesenchymal stromal cells

Mesenchymal stromal cells can be found in almost all tissues of the body. We discuss in this section two types of MSCs namely, bone marrow-derived and non-bone marrow-derived MSCs.

Functional recovery of neurological deficits following cerebral ischemia has been reported with transplantation of bone marrow-derived MSCs in animal models of stroke (Chopp and Li, 2002; Rempe and Kent, 2002; Song *et al.*, 2004). However, a limitation with regard to mesenchymal stromal cell therapy is mode of delivery due to very low graft survival rates of cells when transplanted using intravenous, intracarotid, and intracerebral delivery techniques (Shen *et al.*, 2007). However, the benefits of MSCs may be enhanced by introducing neurotrophic factors such as hepatocyte growth factor (HGF) (Chopp and Li, 2002; Chop *et al.*, 2002), vascular endothelial growth factor (VEGF) (Chen *et al.*, 2003), nerve growth factor (NGF) (Li *et al.*, 2001), brain-derived neurotrophic factor (BDNF) (Li *et al.*, 2001), basic fibroblast growth factor [bFGF, FGF-2 (Chen *et al.*, 2003)], and insulin growth factor-1 (IGF-1) (Zhang *et al.*, 2004), which can activate endogenous brain tissue. In addition to secreting neurotrophic factors, MSCs may also promote migration of primary stem cells from the rostral subventricular zone (SVZ) and hippocampal subgranular zone (SGZ) to the site of injury, and reduction of apoptosis in the penumbral zone of the lesion (Li *et al.*, 2001; Chen *et al.*, 2003). It has also been demonstrated that intravenous infusion of autologous bone marrow-derived mesenchymal stromal cells in stroke patients resulted in a significant functional improvement without adverse effects (Bang *et al.*, 2005). MSC-infused patients also showed higher survival rate and functional improvement than non-infused patients according to long-term, i.e. five years after MSC transplantation, follow-up studies (Lee *et al.*, 2010).

Arguably, MSCs are the most commonly studied stem cells derived from the extraembryonic tissue. Unlike neural stem cells from ectoderm-derived tissues of the nervous system, mesoderm-derived mesenchymal stromal cells can be obtained from almost all mesenchymal tissues in the body, including: bone marrow, placenta, teeth, and adipose tissues. Because there are multiple sources of MSCs, these cells are a favorable line for autologous transplantation. However, there have been discrepancies with defining and classifying mesenchymal stromal cells, which prompted the International Society for Cellular Therapy (ISCT) to suggest these criteria: plastic adherence, cluster differentiation (CD) expression, and differentiation ability (Dominici *et al.*, 2006).

Some evidence suggest that origin of mesenchymal stromal cells and the method by which these cells are harvested, isolated and proliferated may influence functional activity of these cells although they may be harvested from mesenchyme-derived tissues (Barlow *et al.*, 2008; Jansen *et al.*, 2010; Kim *et al.*, 2011; Dmitrieva *et al.*, 2012; Strioga *et al.*, 2012). Therefore, MSCs extracted from a specific tissue site may be more qualified as a specific therapy than cells derived from another source. There are also disparities in characteristics between mesenchyme-derived stromal cells and other stem cell types. For instance, bone marrow-derived stem cells in horses are known to reach senescence at earlier passages than adipose and umbilical cord-derived cells in mesenchymal tissues (Vidal *et al.*, 2012).

It has also been demonstrated that MSCs induce neurogenesis after a stroke, although transplanted MSCs do not survive long enough after transplantation, and it is still unclear whether they also differentiate into functional neurons (Chen *et al.*, 2003). Similar to NSCs, the benefits of MSCs may be attributed to the production of neurotrophic factors such as BDNF and β-NGF (Crigler *et al.*, 2006), and the modulation of vasculature as demonstrated by MSCs derived from bone marrow, adipose tissue, skeletal muscle, and myocardium (Lin *et al.*, 2012). However, like NSCs, MSCs also have the propensity to develop into tumors. An important study demonstrated formation of a sarcoma in the lungs of mice infused with MSCs (Tolar *et al.*, 2007). Moreover, MSC secretions also affect tumor formation as exemplified by the interleukin-6 (IL-6) and vascular endothelial growth factor (VEGF)-A secreted from MSCs which increased the migration of breast cancer cell lines (De Luca *et al.*, 2012). Breast cancer cells stimulate *de novo* secretion of the chemokine CCL5 from MCSs, which acts in a paracrine fashion on cancer cells enhancing their motility and invasiveness, and also metastasis (Karnoub *et al.*, 2007). It has also been shown that MSCs of specific derivations may have greater likelihood for tumorigenesis and in inducing metastasis, although this may not be possible with mesenchyme-derived stromal cells. Previous research has also shown that unlike bone-marrow-derived MSCs, umbilical cord mesenchymal stem cells do not appear to develop into tumor progenitor cells in the presence of tumor cells (Subramanian *et al.*, 2012).

Endothelial progenitor cells

An important stroke etiology is disruption in the integrity of the vasculature, causing vessel vulnerability that predisposes the region to a stroke-like event. The endothelium, a monolayer of endothelial cells that line the interior surface of blood vessels and lymphatic vessels, modulates blood brain barrier permeability and therefore, stroke recovery. Endothelial progenitor cells (EPCs) are precursors of mature endothelium that line the vascular system. Previous studies have shown deposition of transplanted EPCs in the newly vascularized epithelium of surgically induced ischemic limb injury in rabbits (Asahara *et al.*, 1997). Moreover, recent studies reported mobilization of bone marrow-derived EPCs that differentiate into endothelial cells in sites of neovascularization (Masuda and Asahara, 2003; Kawamoto and Losordo, 2008). Tail vein injection of EPCs in diabetic mice subjected to middle cerebral artery occlusion (MCAO) has been shown to reduce infarct induction (Chen *et al.*, 2011). Furthermore, intravenous injection of autologous EPCs produced functional improvement, reduced infarct area and the number of apoptotic cells, and increased microvessel density in the ischemic boundary area of rabbits subjected to MCAO (Chen *et al.*, 2008; Chen *et al.*, 2011). A correlational study in human stroke patients showed positive relationship between levels of circulating EPCs and improvement on the National Institute of Health Stroke Scale (Yip *et al.*, 2008). Research on EPCs and stroke-related vascularization is still sparse. However, accumulating evidence suggest constitutional role of EPCs in the prevention of stroke and treatment after an injury.

Very small embryonic-like stem cells

Very small embryonic-like stem cells (VSELs) are believed to be epiblast-derived pluripotent stem cells that are deposited during early embryonic development (Ratajczak *et al.*, 2007; Kucia *et al.*, 2008), which function as reserves within the tissue that can be used for rejuvenation. Accordingly, the brain is one important location for a large number of cells that display VSEL characteristics (Kucia *et al.*, 2005; Zuba-Surma *et al.*, 2008). Microglia VSELs are a strong candidate for stroke therapy as they have been shown to differentiate into neurons, oligodendrocytes, and astrocytes and to repair damage to the CNS (Borlongan *et al.*, 2011). Interestingly, similar to hematopoetic stem cells, VSELs are also mobilized from adult tissues into peripheral blood following a stroke event (Kucia *et al.*, 2008; Paczkowska *et al.*, 2009; Ratajczak *et al.*, 2010). However, a major drawback of VSELs for stroke therapy includes difficulty in harvesting enough cells for transplantation. Furthermore, levels of VSELs have been shown to decrease with age exacerbating the difficulty to harvest adequate amount of cells, particularly in elderly individuals (Ratajczak *et al.*, 2011). This concern may be addressed via *in vitro* VSEL proliferation prior to transplantation (Borlongan *et al.*, 2011).

Extraembryonic stem cells

Umbilical cord, placenta, amnion, and Wharton's jelly are rich sources of extraembryonic stem cells. Aside from mesenchymal stem cells, amniotic epithelial cells, amnion-derived stem cells, placental-derived stem cells, and umbilical cord matrix stem cells found in extraembryonic tissues are potential stem cell sources (Marcus and Woodbury, 2008). Much like NSCs and mesenchymal stromal cells, extraembryonic stem cells pertain to different germ layers. Accordingly, the ectoderm gives rise to amniotic epithelium while the amnion-derived mesenchymal stromal cells constitute the mesodermal layer (Yu *et al.*, 2009). As a result, amnion-derived stem cells may exhibit higher capacity for mesodermal cell lineages than the ectoderm (Diaz-Prado *et al.*, 2010). Moreover, amnion mesenchymal stromal cells display less endothelial capabilities providing further evidence for potential embryonic specificity (Konig *et al.*, 2012).

The effects of placental-derived mesenchymal stromal cell transplantation have been investigated in animal models of stroke. As expected, these cells not only replaced damaged cells but also provided a microenvironment conducive for endogenous neurogenesis (Yarygin *et al.*, 2009; Kranz *et al.*, 2010; Chen *et al.*, 2012). Research has also been made to determine effects of umbilical cord lining mesenchymal stromal cells in rat stroke models, which reported functional recovery accompanied by increased vascular density, increased expression of VEGF and basic fibroblast growth factor (Liao *et al.*, 2009). Moreover, umbilical cord lining mesenchymal stromal cells also exhibited an immunosuppressive effect on the immune cascade, and greater immune immaturity compared with aged-bone marrow mesenchymal stromal cells (Deuse *et al.*, 2011), which has been attributed to increased leukemia inhibitory factor (LIF) in umbilical cord lining mesenchymal stromal cells (Najar *et al.*, 2010). Meanwhile, Wharton's jelly-derived mesenchymal stromal cells also differentiated into glial, neuronal, doublecortin[+], CXCR4[+], and vascular endothelial cells and enhanced neuroplasticity in the ischemic brain (Ding *et al.*, 2007).

Other sources of adult stem cells

Adipose tissue

Adipose tissue contains adipose-derived stem cells which have more than 90% homologous phenotype as compared to bone-marrow-derived mesenchymal stromal cells (Gimble *et al.*, 2007). These cells are plastic adherent cell populations that can differentiate into neural, glial, and vascular endothelial cells and exhibit higher proliferative activity with a greater production of VEGF and hepatocyte growth factor compared to bone marrow-derived stromal cells (Ikegame *et al.*, 2011). Treatment with adipose-derived stem cells reduced infarct size, cerebral improved neurological function, and attenuated cerebral inflammation and chronic degeneration in an intracerebral model of hemorrhage (Kim *et al.*, 2007; Leu *et al.*, 2010). Adipose-derived stem cells also improved ischemic damage in ischemic stroke model of mice (Ikegame *et al.*, 2011).

A caveat with the use of adipose-derived stem cells, however, is that extensive passaging of these cells may cause spontaneous mutations within the cell line leading to a cancerous state (Rubio *et al.*, 2005). This observation, however, has not been replicated in other studies (de la Fuente *et al.*, 2010) and recent findings indicate that adipose-derived stem cells per se, do not cause tumors, but they do promote pre-existing cancer cells to produce tumors (Ra *et al.*,

2011). Indeed, a stringent analysis on the risk-to-benefit ratio of stem cells is required in order to advance safe and effective cell therapy for stroke.

Breast milk

Breast milk has long been known to confer both immunologic and nutritive benefits. Emerging research has attempted to elucidate the potential for vertical transmission of stem cells from mother to off-spring (Meng *et al.*, 2007). The mammary tissue includes stem cells and differentiated stem cells that enter breast milk via cellular migration and turnover, and/or as a result of the mechanical shear forces of breastfeeding (Cregan *et al.*, 2007; Hassiotou *et al.*, 2012). Breast milk stem cells exhibit stem cell-like morphology and pheno-type and can be differentiated *in vitro* to form all three germ layers (Hassiotou *et al.*, 2012). Stem cells in breast milk provide a great advantage for harvesting cells without the need for invasive methods (McGregor and Rogo, 2006). Aside from ease of harvesting, breast milk stem cells also present a potential opportunity for autologous transplantation.

Dental tissue

Dental tissue-derived stem cells such as post-natal dental pulp stem cells (DPSCs) (Gronthos *et al.*, 2000), stem cells from exfoliated deciduous teeth (SHED) (Seo *et al.*, 2004), periodontal ligament stem cells (PDLSCs) (Seo *et al.*, 2004), stem cells from apical papilla (SCAP) (Sonoyama *et al.*, 2006; Sonoyama *et al.*, 2008), and dental follicle precursor cells (DFPCs) (Morsczeck *et al.*, 2005) which show mesenchymal stromal cell-like abilities, have been identified [for review, see (Huang *et al.*, 2009)] and suggested to be important future resources for stem cell. Dental tissue-derived stem cells can differentiate into variable cell types including neural cells, adipo-cytes, and odontoblasts (Miura *et al.*, 2003). Transplantation of these cells into an intact mouse brain indicated cell survival coupled with expression of neuronal markers (Miura *et al.*, 2003). MCAO rats showed improvement in motor function post-transplantation of dental tissue-derived stem cells into the dorsolateral striatum (Yang *et al.*, 2009). More potent neurogenicity has been observed with transplantation of dental tissue-derived stem cells compared to bone marrow-derived stem cells (Karaoz *et al.*, 2011), probably due to the neural crest origin of dental tissue-derived stem cells (Huang *et al.*, 2009).

Menstrual blood

The endometrium or uterine lining, is another source of adult stem cells. These cells generate uterine tissue each month as part of the menstrual cycle. Two laboratories have independently isolated stem cells from menstrual blood, although it is uncertain if they have obtained similar cell lines due to differences in culturing methods (Meng *et al*, 2007; Patel *et al.*, 2008). Stem cells from menstrual blood exhibit multipotency. In an oxygen-glucose deprivation (OGD) *in vitro* model of stroke, menstrual blood-derived stem cells have been shown to secrete essential trophic factors such as VEGF, BDNF, and neurotrophin-3. Menstrual blood-derived stem cells or its conditioned medium co-cultured with rat primary neurons improved cell survival rate after exposure to OGD. Moreover, intracerebral and intravenous transplantation of menstrual blood-derived cells enhanced host cell survival and behavioral functions in animal models of stroke (Borlongan *et al.*, 2010). In addition, these cells have been implemented for *in vivo* surgical MCAO rat studies without immunosuppression (Borlongan *et al.*, 2010; Allickson *et al.*, 2011; Rodrigues *et al.*, 2012).

Umbilical cord blood

The increasing popularity of umbilical cord banking has raised enthusiasm for umbilical cord blood transplantation in stroke. Umbilical cord blood (UCB) has broad therapeutic potential considering the possibility for both allogenic and autologous use. UCB refers to the mononuclear fraction which includes: hematopoetic progenitors, lymphocytes, monocytes, and mesenchymal stromal cells. These heterogeous cells are considered as immunologically immature, therefore, they show capacity to modulate the immune response and reduce levels of pro-inflammatory cytokines (Vendrame *et al.*, 2005). The early investigations on effects of umbilical cord blood transplantation in experimental models of stroke have shown promising results. Accordingly, functional recovery, reduction of infarct size and increased expression of neuroprotective factors such as BDNF and VEGF have been observed in stroke rats, which benefit from umbilical cord blood transplants (Willing *et al.*, 2003, Vendrame *et al.*, 2004; Xiao *et al.*, 2005; Chung *et al.*, 2009). Current research suggests a combination of intravenous administration, 48 hr post-stroke, and a therapeutic dose of 1 million cells to achieve optimal results (Newcomb *et al.*, 2006; Willing *et al.*, 2003; Vendrame *et al.*, 2004).

Induced pluripotent stem cells

The advent of induced pluripotent stem cells (iPSCs) dispelled the widely-held belief that differentiation of stem cells is unidrectional. Moreover, via retrograde manipulation, it has been possible to regenerate embryonic-like stem cells regenerated from fibroblasts via transfection of specific transcription factors (Takahashi and Yamanaka, 2006). This technique has also been applied to increase the potency of umbilical cord, placental mesenchymal stromal cells, NSCs, and adipose-derived precursor cells (Cai *et al.*, 2010; Tat *et al.*, 2010). Indeed, a primary advantage with retrograde conversion is enhanced proliferation capacity of precursor cells. Transplantation of iPSCs in animal models of stroke showed improvement in sensorimotor functions (Chen *et al.*, 2010; Jiang *et al.*, 2011), reduced infarct size, reduction of pro-inflammatory cytokines, and increased number of anti-inflammatory cytokines (Chen *et al.*, 2010). Some studies, however, revealed tumorigenesis and immunogenicity as drawbacks of IPSCs. iPSCs are generated using transcription factors of known oncogenicity. Indeed, a higher rate of tumorigenesis after transplantation of undifferentiated iPSCs has been reported (Kawai *et al.*, 2010; Yamashita *et al.*, 2011). Furthermore, even when autologous, these cells provoke an immune response leading to rejection (Zhao *et al.*, 2011). Recent reports also demonstrated that relative to embryonic stem cells, iPSCs exhibited lower efficacy and higher likelihood to differentiate into neuroepithelial cells in culture (Hu *et al.*, 2010).

Regulatory Control of Transplanted Stem Cells

Several fundamental biological and engineering challenges need to be overcome before stem cell-based interventions could be successfully transferred from the bench to the clinic. These include improving the survival and controlling self-renewal of stem cells, directing the lineage/tissue-specific stem cell differentiation, *in vivo* delivery, and integration to the host milieu [for review see (Hwang *et al.*, 2008)] (Figure 2). In particular, a number of factors may influence cell survival in the acute phase of cerebral ischemia such as limited blood supply, hypoxia, trophic factor deficiency, oxidative stress, inflammatory response, and others (White *et al.*, 2000). Several approaches have been designed to enhance survival of transplanted stem cells such as injection of neurotrophic factors e.g., FGF, EGF and BDNF, overexpression of growth factor genes including VEGF, GDNF, BDNF, and Akt1 which have been shown to promote the survival of NSCs in stroke animal model [(Kelly *et al.* 2004; Lee *et al.*, 2007; 2008; 2009); for review, see (Hao *et al.* 2014)]. Gene modifications with various factors such as Bcl-2 and placental growth factor (PlGF), have also been reported to promote the survival of ESCs and MSCs (Liu *et al.*, 2006; Wei *et al.*, 2005). Furthermore, preconditioning with IL-6 protected the grafted NSCs from ischemic reperfusion injury in a mouse model of ischemic stroke (Sakata *et al.*, 2006). Minocycline preconditioning also enhanced the survival, proliferative capacity, and paracrine effects of NSCs, and also accounted for improved neurological recovery post-stroke (Rueger *et al.*, 2012). The use of biomaterial scaffolding has also been documented to facilitate survival of NSCs after intracerebral transplantation in the ischemic brain (Jin *et al.*, 2010). Recent studies also showed that

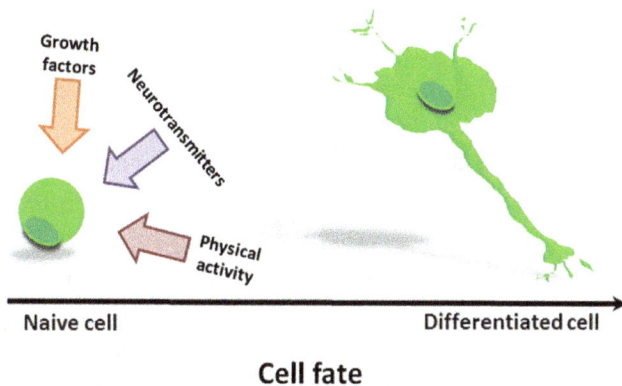

Cell fate

Figure 2. Strategies to improve survival and differentiation of transplanted stem cells. Injection or overexpression of growth or neurotrophic factors (e.g., FGF, EGF and BDNF, VEGF), has been shown to enhance the survival of transplanted stem cells. Other methods such as preconditioning with pro-inflammatory cytokines (e.g. IL-6) or antibiotics, or providing a biomaterial scaffolding have also showed promise in controlling massive grafted-cell death after transplantation thereby enhancing the efficacy of transplanted stem cells. To aid stem cell differentiation, different strategies have been explored which include application of neurotransmitters (e.g. glutamate, GABA and ACh), that can influence stem cell fate, and physical activity (e.g. exercise) that reportedly aided the differentiation and synaptic integration of stem cells.

transduction of TAT-heat shock protein 70 (Hsp70) *in vitro*, which reduces apoptosis and inflammation after hypoxic-ischemic injury, significantly boosted the survival of NSCs intracerebrally transplanted in post-stroke mice brain (Doeppner *et al.*, 2012). Moreover, some evidence revealed greater survival and enhanced homing of hypoxia-treated BMSCs to ischemic region, and superior property of promoting angiogenesis and neurogenesis after administration into rat subjected to MCAO (Wei *et al.*, 2012).

Application of neurotransmitters such as GABA, glutamate and acetylcholine has also been shown to affect stem cell fate corresponding to the roles of these neurotransmitters in the differentiation of neuronal cells and during brain development [for review, see (Berg *et al.*, 2013)]. Accordingly, GABA released spontaneously by adult-generated neuroblasts activated adult neural stem cells and inhibited their proliferation [for review, see (Kriegstein, 2005)].

The downstream mechanisms of glutamate-mediated regulation of progenitor cell proliferation is not yet fully understood, although glutamate signaling has been thought to induce expression of neurotrophic factors such as BDNF, NGF and FGF (Uchida *et al.*, 1998; Zafra *et al.*, 1991; Mackowiak *et al.*, 2002). Moreover, long-term treatment with the ionotropic acetylcholine receptor agonist nicotine decreased cell proliferation in the DG (Abrous *et al.*, 2002; Jang *et al.*, 2002), while activation of muscarinic M1 receptors improved cell proliferation in the SGZ (Van Kampen and Eckman, 2010). Some studies have also reported influence of physical activity on differentiation and synaptic integration of stem cells. For instance, exercise has been shown to improve functional recovery via enhancement of NSCs proliferation, and migration potentially through activation of the SDF-1α/CXCR4 axis after ischemic stroke (Lou *et al.*, 2014; Zheng *et al.*, 2014).

Co-Transplantation of Stem Cells and Combination Treatment with Therapeutic Molecules: A New Approach in Stem Cell Therapy

Different stem cell types confer discrete therapeutic benefits. It is, therefore, worth investigating the beneficial effects of simultaneous therapy or combination treatment of multiple stem cell lines. Some studies reported synergistic effects of co-transplantation of neural stem cells and adipose-derived stem cells in neural cell survival (Oh *et al.*, 2011). Decreased tumorigenesis has also been observed when bone marrow-derived stromal cells were co-transplanted with embryonic stem cells (Matsuda *et al.*, 2009). Neural stem cells combined with epithelial cells also increased cell survival and differentiation (Nakagomi *et al.*, 2009). Furthermore, combination therapy, in the same fashion as co-transplantation of two cell lines, can incorporate a non-stem cell substrate increasing the efficacy of transplantation. For example, the combination of bone marrow-derived stromal cells with trophic factors has been shown to enhance survival and potentiation (Zhang *et al.*, 2010), and provide a scaffold for stem cell adherence (Jin *et al.*, 2010). While the techniques of co-transplantation and combination therapy are still novel, methods to enhance stem cell survival while simultaneously decreasing adverse events is an emerging field of research.

Concluding Remarks

The increased capacity to harvest stem cells from various sources necessitates better understanding of the advantages and limitations of stem cell-based therapies for stroke. Several factors need to be considered prior to utilization of stem cell transplantation for stroke therapy, some of which have been addressed in this review (e.g. immunogenicity, tumorigenicity, harvesting techniques, survival, proliferation capacity, differentiation and overall feasibility of stem cells) and elsewhere (Sanberg *et al.*, 2012). We previously investigated the influence of these factors with umbilical cord blood transplantation for various conditions such as amyotrophic lateral sclerosis, Alzheimer's disease, and Sanfilippo syndrome (Sanberg *et al.*, 2012). However, data in stroke are still missing. Despite the limitations identified and the considerations still needing concrete exploration, there is optimism with regard to future utilization of cell therapy for stroke as evidenced by successful entry of stem cell-based therapies in clinical studies. Nevertheless, it is still crucial to optimize the safety and efficacy of stem cells for clinical applications, which could be achieved by conducting more rigorous, and comprehensive laboratory investigations. Of note, we and other members of the consortium created the Stem Cell Therapies as an Emerging Paradigm in Stroke (STEPS) in order to promote standardized procedures in interpreting results from stroke studies (Borlongan *et al.*, 2008; Borlongan, 2009; Chopp *et al.*, 2009; Borlongan and Weiss, 2011).

References

Abrous DN, Adriani W, Montaron MF, Aurousseau C, Rougon G, Le Moal M, Piazza PV (2002) Nicotine self-administration impairs hippocampal plasticity. *J Neurosci* 22(9):3656–3662.

Allickson JG, Sanchez A, Yefimenko N, Borlongan CV, Sanberg PR (2011) Recent studies assessing the proliferative capability of a novel adult stem cell identified in menstrual blood. *Open Stem Cell J* 3:4–10.

Amariglio N, Cohen Y, Constantini S, Hirshberg A, Koren-Michowitz M, Leider-Trejo L, Loewenthal R, Paz N, Rechavi G, Scheithauer BW, Toren A, Trakhtenbrot L, Waldman D (2009) Donor-derived brain tumor following neural stem cell transplantation in an ataxia telangiectasia patient. *PLoS Med* 6:e1000029.

Amariglio N, Rechavi G (2010) On the origin of glioneural neoplasms after neural cell transplantation. *Nat Med* 16:157–158.

Arvidsson A, Collin T, Kirik D, Kokaia Z, Lindvall O (2002) Neuronal replacement from endogenous precursors in the adult brain after stroke. *Nat Med* 8:963–970.

Asahara T, Murohara T, Sullivan A, Silver M, van der Zee R, Li T, Witzenbichler B, Schatteman G, Isner JM (1997) Isolation of putative progenitor endothelial cells for angiogenesis. *Science* 275:964–967.

Bachstetter AD, Pabon MM, Cole MJ, Hudson CE, Sanberg PR, Willing AE, Bickford PC, Gemma C (2008) Peripheral injection of human umbilical cord blood stimulates neurogenesis in the aged rat brain. *BMC Neurosci* 9:22.

Bang OY, Lee JS, Lee PH, Lee G (2005) Autologous mesenchymal stem cell transplantation in stroke patients. *Ann Neurol* 57:874–882.

Barkho BZ, Munoz AE, Li X, Li L, Cunningham LA, Zhao X (2008) Endogenous matrix metalloproteinase (MMP)-3 and MMP-9 promote the differentiation and migration of adult neural progenitor cells in response to chemokines. *Stem Cells* 26:3139–3149.

Barkho BZ, Munoz AE, Li X, Li L, Cunningham LA, Zhao X (2008) Endogenous matrix metalloproteinase (MMP)-3 and MMP-9 promote the differentiation and migration of adult neural progenitor cells in response to chemokines. *Stem Cells* 26:3139–3149.

Barlow S, Brooke G, Chatterjee K, Price G, Pelekanos R, Rossetti T, Doody M, Venter D, Pain S, Gilshenan K, Atkinson K (2008) Comparison of human placenta- and bone marrow-derived multipotent mesenchymal stem cells. *Stem Cells Dev* 17:1095–1107.

Battistella V, de Freitas GR, da Fonseca LMB, Mercante D, Gutfilen B, Goldenberg RCS, Dias JV, Kasai-Brunswick TH, Wajnberg E, Rosado-de-Castro PH, Alves-Leon SV, Mendez-Otero R, Andre C (2011) Safety of autologous bone marrow mononuclear cell transplantation in patients with nonacute ischemic stroke. *Regen Med* 6:45–52.

Berg DA, Belnoue L, Song H, Simon A (2013) Neurotransmitter-mediated control of neurogenesis in the adult vertebrate brain. *Development* 140(12):2548–2561.

Borlongan CV (2009) Cell therapy for stroke: remaining issues to address before embarking on clinical trials. *Stroke* 40: S146–148.

Borlongan CV, Weiss MD (2011) Baby STEPS: a giant leap for cell therapy in neonatal brain injury. *Pediatr Res* 70:3–9.

Borlongan CV, Chopp M, Steinberg GK, Bliss TM, Li Y, Lu M, Hess DC, Kondziolka D (2008) Potential of stem/progenitor cells in treating stroke: the missing steps in translating cell therapy from laboratory to clinic. *Regen Med* 3:249–250.

Borlongan CV, Kaneko Y, Maki M, Yu SJ, Ali M, Allickson JG, Sanberg CD, Kuzmin-Nichols N, Sanberg PR (2010) Menstrual blood cells display stem cell-like phenotypic markers and exert neuroprotection following transplantation in experimental stroke. *Stem Cells Dev* 19:439–452.

Borlongan CV, Glover LE, Tajiri N, Kaneko Y, Freeman TB (2011) The great migration of bone marrow-derived stem cells toward the ischemic brain: therapeutic implications for stroke and other neurological disorders. *Prog Neurobiol* 95:213–228.

Cai J, Li W, Su H, Qin D, Yang J, Zhu F, Xu J, He W, Guo X, Labuda K, Peterbauer A, Wolbank S, Zhong M, Li Z, Wu W, So KF, Redl H, Zeng L, Esteban MA, Pei D (2010) Generation of human induced pluripotent stem cells from umbilical cord matrix and amniotic membrane mesenchymal cells. *J Biol Chem* 285:11227–11234.

Carbajal KS, Schaumburg C, Strieter R, Kane J, Lane TE (2010) Migration of engrafted neural stem cells is mediated by CXCL12 signaling through CXCR4 in a viral model of multiple sclerosis. *Proc Natl Acad Sci U S A* 107:11068–11073.

Chaichana KL, Guerrero-Cazares H, Capilla-Gonzalez V, Zamora-Berridi G, Achanta P, Gonzalez-Perez O, Jallo GI, Garcia-Verdugo JM, Quinones-Hinojosa A (2009) Intra-operatively obtained human tissue: protocols and techniques for the study of neural stem cells. *J Neurosci Methods* 180:116–125.

Chang AE, Ge R, He Q, Li Q, Li X, Lu A, Shen L, Wu W, Zhang X, Zhen H (2011) Long-term cultured human neural stem cells undergo spontaneous transformation to tumor-initiating cells. *Int J Biol Sci* 7: 892–901.

Chen J, Shehadah A, Pal A, Zacharek A, Cui X, Cui Y, Roberts C, Lu M, Zeitlin A, Hariri R, Chopp M (2013) Neuroprotective effect of human placenta-derived cell treatment of stroke in rats. *Cell Transplant* 22(5):871–879.

Chen SJ, Chang CM, Tsai SK, Chang YL, Chou SJ, Huang SS, Tai LK, Chen YC, Ku HH, Li HY, Chiou SH (2010) Functional improvement of focal cerebral ischemia injury by subdural transplantation of induced pluripotent stem cells with fibrin glue. *Stem Cells Dev* 19:1757–1767.

Chen J, Chen SZ, Chen YS, Zhang C, Wang JJ, Zhang WF, Liu G, Zhao B, Chen YF (2011) Circulating endothelial progenitor cells and cellular membrane microparticles in db/db diabetic mouse: possible implications in cerebral ischemic damage. *Am J Physiol Endocrinol Metab* 301: E62–E71.

Chen J, Li Y, Katakowski M, Chen X, Wang L, Lu D, Lu M, Gautam SC, Chopp M (2003) Intravenous bone marrow stromal cell therapy reduces apoptosis and promotes endogenous cell proliferation after stroke in female rat. *J Neurosci Res* 73:778–786.

Chen J, Li Y, Wang L, Lu M, Chopp M (2002) Caspase inhibition by Z-VAD increases the survival of grafted bone marrow cells and improves functional outcome after MCAo in rats. *J Neurol Sci* 199:17–24.

Chen ZZ, Jiang XD, Zhang LL, Shang JH, Du MX, Xu G, Xu RX (2008) Beneficial effect of autologous transplantation of bone marrow stromal cells and endothelial progenitor cells on cerebral ischemia in rabbits. *Neurosci Lett* 445:36–41.

Chopp M, Steinberg GK, Kondziolka D, Lu M, Bliss TM, Li Y, Hess DC, Borlongan CV (2009) Who's in favor of translational cell therapy for stroke: STEPS forward please? *Cell Transplant* 18:691–693.

Chopp M, Li Y (2002) Treatment of neural injury with marrow stromal cells. *Lancet Neurol* 1:92–100.

Chung DJ, Choi CB, Lee SH, Kang EH, Lee JH, Hwang SH, Han H, Lee JH, Choe BY, Lee SY, Kim HY (2009) Intraarterially delivered human umbilical cord blood-derived mesenchymal stem cells in canine cerebral ischemia. *J Neurosci Res* 87:3554–3567.

Cregan MD, Fan YP, Appelbee A, Brown ML, Klopcic B, Koppen J, Mitoulas LR, Piper KME, Choolani MA, Chong YS, Hartmann PE (2007) Identification of nestin-positive putative mammary stem cells in human breastmilk. *Cell Tissue Res* 329:129–136.

Crigler L, Robey RC, Asawachaicharn A, Gaupp D, Phinney DG (2006) Human mesenchymal stem cell subpopulations express a variety of neuro-regulatory molecules and promote neuronal cell survival and neuritogenesis. *Exp Neurol* 198:54–64.

Cui X, Chopp M, Shehadah A, Zacharek A, Kuzmin-Nichols N, Sanberg D, Dai J, Zhang C, Ueno Y, Roberts C, Chen J (2012) Therapeutic benefit of treatment of stroke with simvastin and human umbilical cord blood cells: Neurogenesis, synaptic plasticity, and axon growth. *Cell Transplant* 21:845–856.

de la Fuente R, Bernad A, Garcia-Castro J, Martin MC, Cigudosa JC (2010) Retraction: Spontaneous human adult stem cell transformation. *Cancer Res* 70:6682.

De Luca A, Lamura L, Gallo M, Maffia V, Normanno N (2012) Mesenchymal stem cell-derived interleukin-6 and vascular endothelial growth factor promote breast cancer cell migration. *J Cell Biochem* 113:3363–3370.

Deierborg T, Roybon L, Inacio AR, Pesic J, Brundin P (2010) Brain injury activates microglia that induce neural stem cell proliferation ex vivo and promote differentiation of neurosphere-derived cells into neurons and oligodendrocytes. *Neuroscience* 171:1386–1396.

Deierborg T, Staflin K, Pesic J, Roybon L, Brundin P, Lundberg C (2009) Absence of striatal newborn neurons with mature phenotype following defined striatal and cortical excitotoxic brain injuries. *Exp Neurol* 219:363–367.

Deuse T, Stubbendorff M, Tang-Quan K, Phillips N, Kay M.A, Eiermann T, Phan TT, Volk HD, Reichenspurner H, Robbins RC, Schrepfer S (2011) Immunogenicity and immunomodulatory properties of umbilical cord lining mesenchymal stem cells. *Cell Transplant* 20:655–667.

Diaz-Prado S, Muinos-Lopez E, Hermida-Gomez T, Rendal-Vazquez ME, Fuentes-Boquete I, de Toro FJ, Blanco FJ (2010) Multilineage differentiation potential of cells isolated from the human amniotic membrane. *J Cell Biochem* 111:846–857.

Ding DC, Shyu WC, Chiang MF, Lin SZ, Chang YC, Wang HJ, Su CY, Li H (2007) Enhancement of neuroplasticity through upregulation of beta 1-integrin in human umbilical cord-derived stromal cell implanted stroke model. *Neurobiol Dis* 27:339–353.

Dmitrieva RI, Minullina IR, Bilibina AA, Tarasova OV, Anisimov SV, Zaritskey AY (2012) Bone marrow- and subcutaneous adipose tissue-derived mesenchymal stem cells: differences and similarities. *Cell Cycle* 11:377–383.

Doeppner TR, Ewert TA, Tönges L, Herz J, Zechariah A, ElAli A, Ludwig AK, Giebel B, Nagel F, Dietz GP, Weise J, Hermann DM, Bähr M (2012) Transduction of neural precursor cells with TAT-heat shock protein

70 chaperone: therapeutic potential against ischemic stroke after intra-striatal and systemic transplantation. *Stem Cells* 30(6):1297–1310.

Dominici M, Le Blanc K, Mueller I, Slaper-Cortenbach I, Marini F, Krause D, Deans R, Keating A, Prockop D, Horwitz E (2006) Minimal criteria for defining multipotent mesenchymal stromal cells. The International Society for Cellular Therapy position statement. *Cytotherapy* 8:315–317.

Dunac A, Frelin C, Popolo-Blondeau M, Chatel M, Mahagne MH, Philip PJ (2007) Neurological and functional recovery in human stroke are associated with peripheral blood CD34+ cell mobilization. *J Neurol* 254:327–332.

Erlandsson A, Lin CH, Yu F, Morshead CM (2011) Immunosuppression promotes endogenous neural stem and progenitor cell migration and tissue regeneration after ischemic injury. *Exp Neurol* 230:48–57.

Fazekasova H, Lechler R, Langford K, Lombardi G (2011) Placenta-derived MSCs are partially immunogenic and less immunomodulatory than bone marrow-derived MSCs. *J Tissue Eng Regen Med* 5:684–694.

Friedrich MAG, Martins MP, Araujo MD, Klamt C, Vedolin L, Garicochea B, Raupp EF, El Ammar JS, Machado DC, da Costa JC, Nogueira RG, Rosado-de Castro PH, Mendez-Otero R, de Freitas GR (2012) Intra-arterial infusion of autologous bone marrow mononuclear cells in patients with moderate to severe middle cerebral artery acute ischemic stroke. *Cell Transplant* 21:S13–S21.

Gimble JM, Katz AJ, Bunnell BA (2007) Adipose-derived stem cells for regenerative medicine. *Circ Res* 100:1249–1260.

Graham, GD (2003) Tissue plasminogen activator for acute ischemic stroke in clinical practice: a meta-analysis of safety data. *Stroke* 34: 2847–2850.

Gronthos S, Mankani M, Brahim J, Robey PG, Shi S (2000) Postnatal human dental pulp stem cells (DPSCs) *in vitro* and *in vivo*. *Proc Natl Acad Sci U S A* 97:13625–13630.

Hao L, Zou Z, Tian H, Zhang Y, Zhou H, Liu L (2014) Stem cell-based therapies for ischemic stroke. *Biomed Res Int* 2014:468748.

Hassiotou F, Beltran A, Chetwynd E, Stuebe AM, Twigger AJ, Metzger P, Trengove N, Lai CT, Filgueira L, Blancafort P, Hartmann PE (2012) Breastmilk is a novel source of stem cells with multilineage differentiation potential. *Stem Cells* 30:2164–2174.

Hayashi J, Takagi Y, Fukuda H, Imazato T, Nishimura M, Fujimoto M, Takahashi J, Hashimoto N, Nozaki K (2006) Primate embryonic stem cell-derived neuronal progenitors transplanted into ischemic brain. *J Cereb Blood Flow Metab* 26:906–914.

Hennemann B, Ickenstein G, Sauerbruch S, Luecke K, Haas S, Horn M, Andreesen R, Bogdahn U, Winkler J (2008) Mobilization of CD34+ hematopoietic cells, colony-forming cells and long-term culture-initiating cells into the peripheral blood of patients with an acute cerebral ischemic insult. *Cytotherapy* 10:303–311.

Herman DM (2010) Neuroprotection and neurorestoration: ready for translation to clinics? *Swiss Arch Neurol Psychiatry* 161:274–275.

Herzog EL, Chai L, Krause DS (2003) Plasticity of marrow-derived stem cells. *Blood* 102:3483–3493.

Hoehn M, Kustermann E, Blunk J, Wiedermann D, Trapp T, Wecker S, Focking M, Arnold H, Hescheler J, Fleischmann BK, Schwindt W, Buhrle C (2002) Monitoring of implanted stem cell migration *in vivo*: A highly resolved *in vivo* magnetic resonance imaging investigation of experimental stroke in rat. *Proc Natl Acad Sci U S A* 99:16267–16272.

Hu BY, Weick JP, Yu J, Ma LX, Zhang XQ, Thomson JA, Zhang SC (2010) Neural differentiation of human induced pluripotent stem cells follows developmental principles but with variable potency. *Proc Natl Acad Sci U S A* 107:4335–4340.

Huang GTJ, Gronthos S, Shi S (2009) Mesenchymal stem cells derived from dental tissues vs. those from other sources: their biology and role in regenerative medicine. *J Dent Res* 88:792–806.

Huang H, Chen L, Sanberg P (2010) Cell therapy from bench to bedside translation in CNS neurorestoratology era. *Cell Med* 1:15–46.

Hunt JS, Petroff MG, McIntire RH, Ober C (2005) HLA-G and immune tolerance in pregnancy. *FASEB J* 19:681–693.

Hwang NS, Varghese S, Elisseeff J (2008) Controlled differentiation of stem cells. *Adv Drug Deliv Rev* 60(2):199–214.

Ikegame Y, Yamashita K, Hayashi SI, Mizuno H, Tawada M, You F, Yamada K, Tanaka Y, Egashira Y, Nakashima S, Yoshimura SI, Iwama T (2011) Comparison of mesenchymal stem cells from adipose tissue and bone marrow for ischemic stroke therapy. *Cytotherapy* 13:675–685.

Jandial R, Snyder EY (2009) A safer stem cell: on guard against cancer. *Nat Med* 15:999–1001.

Jang MH, Shin MC, Jung SB, Lee TH, Bahn GH, Kwon YK, Kim EH, Kim CJ (2002) Alcohol and nicotine reduce cell proliferation and enhance apoptosis in dentate gyrus. *Neuroreport* 13(12):1509–13.

Jansen BJ, Gilissen C, Roelofs H, Schaap-Oziemlak A, Veltman JA, Raymakers RA, Jansen JH, Kogler G, Figdor CG, Torensma R, Adema GJ (2010) Functional differences between mesenchymal stem cell populations are reflected by their transcriptome. *Stem Cells Dev* 19:481–490.

Jiang M, Lv L, Ji H, Yang X, Zhu W, Cai L, Gu X, Chai C, Huang S, Sun J, Dong Q (2011) Induction of pluripotent stem cells transplantation therapy for ischemic stroke. *Mol Cell Biochem* 354:67–75.

Jin K, Mao X, Xie L, Galvan V, Lai B, Wang Y, Gorostiza O, Wang X, Greenberg DA (2010) Transplantation of human neural precursor cells in Matrigel scaffolding improves outcome from focal cerebral ischemia after delayed postischemic treatment in rats. *J Cereb Blood Flow Metab* 30:534–544.

Jin K, Sun YJ, Xie L, Peel A, Mao XO, Batteur S, Greenberg DA (2003) Directed migration of neuronal precursors into the ischemic cerebral cortex and striatum. *Mol Cell Neurosci* 24:171–189.

Jin K, Xie L, Mao X, Greenberg MB, Moore A, Peng B, Greenberg RB, Greenberg DA (2011) Effect of human neural precursor cell transplantation on endogenous neurogenesis after focal cerebral ischemia in the rat. *Brain Res* 1374:56–62.

Kalinkovich A, Spiegel A, Shivtiel S, Kollet O, Jordaney N, Piacibello W, Lapidot T (2009) Blood-forming stem cells are nervous: direct and indirect regulation of immature human CD34+ cells by the nervous system. *Brain Behav Immun* 23:1059–1065.

Karaoz E, Demircan PC, Saglam O, Aksoy A, Kaymaz F, Duruksu G (2011) Human dental pulp stem cells demonstrate better neural and epithelial stem cell properties than bone marrow-derived mesenchymal stem cells. *Histochem Cell Biol* 136:455–473.

Karnoub AE, Dash AB, Vo AP, Sullivan A, Brooks MW, Bell GW, Richardson AL, Polyak K, Tubo R, Weinberg RA (2007) Mesenchymal stem cells within tumour stroma promote breast cancer metastasis. *Nature* 449:557–U554.

Kawai H, Yamashita T, Ohta Y, Deguchi K, Nagotani S, Zhang XM, Ikeda Y, Matsuura T, Abe K (2010) Tridermal tumorigenesis of induced pluripotent stem cells transplanted in ischemic brain. *J Cereb Blood Flow Metab* 30:1487–1493.

Kawamoto A, Losordo DW (2008) Endothelial progenitor cells for cardiovascular regeneration. *Trends Cardiovasc Med* 18:33–37.

Kelly S, Bliss TM, Shah AK, Sun GH, Ma M, Foo WC, Masel J, Yenari MA, Weissman IL, Uchida N, Palmer T, Steinberg GK (2004) Transplanted human fetal neural stem cells survive, migrate, and differentiate in ischemic rat cerebral cortex. *Proc Natl Acad Sci U S A* 101(32):11839–11844.

Kim JM, Lee ST, Chu K, Jung KH, Song EC, Kim SJ, Sinn DI, Kim JH, Park DK, Kang KM, Hyung Hong N, Park HK, Won CH, Kim KH, Kim M,

Kun Lee S, Roh JK (2007) Systemic transplantation of human adipose stem cells attenuated cerebral inflammation and degeneration in a hemorrhagic stroke model. *Brain Res* 1183:43–50.

Kim SH, Kim YS, Lee SY, Kim KH, Lee YM, Kim WK, Lee YK (2011) Gene expression profile in mesenchymal stem cells derived from dental tissues and bone marrow. *J Periodontal Implant Sci* 41:192–200.

Kojima T, Hirota Y, Ema M, Takahashi S, Miyoshi I, Okano H, Sawamoto K (2010) Subventricular zone-derived neural progenitor cells migrate along a blood vessel scaffold toward the post-stroke striatum. *Stem Cells* 28:545–554.

Kondziolka D, Steinberg GK, Wechsler L, Meltzer CC, Elder E, Gebel J, Decesare S, Jovin T, Zafonte R, Lebowitz J, Flickinger JC, Tong D, Marks MP, Jamieson C, Luu D, Bell-Stephens T, Teraoka J (2005) Neurotransplantation for patients with subcortical motor stroke: a phase 2 randomized trial. *J Neurosurg* 103:38–45.

Konig J, Huppertz B, Desoye G, Parolini O, Frohlich JD, Weiss G, Dohr G, Sedlmayr P, Lang I (2012) Amnion-derived mesenchymal stromal cells show angiogenic properties but resist differentiation into mature endothelial cells. *Stem Cells Dev* 21:1309–1320.

Koton S, Schneider AL, Rosamond WD, Shahar E, Sang Y, Gottesman RF, Coresh J (2014) Stroke incidence and mortality trends in US communities, 1987 to 2011. *JAMA* 312(3):259–268.

Kranz A, Wagner DC, Kamprad M, Scholz M, Schmidt UR, Nitzsche F, Aberman Z, Emmrich F, Riegelsberger UM, Boltze J (2010) Transplantation of placenta-derived mesenchymal stromal cells upon experimental stroke in rats. *Brain Res* 1315:128–136.

Kriegstein AR (2005) GABA puts the brake on stem cells. *Nat Neurosci* 8(9):1132–1133.

Kucia M, Ratajczak J, Ratajczak MZ (2005) Are bone marrow stem cells plastic or heterogenous–that is the question. *Exp Hematol* 33: 613–623.

Kucia M, Wysoczynski M, Ratajczak J, Ratajczak MZ (2008) Identification of very small embryonic like (VSEL) stem cells in bone marrow. *Cell Tissue Res* 331:125–134.

Kucia M, Zhang YP, Reca R, Wysoczynski M, Machalinski B, Majka M, Ildstad ST, Ratajczak J, Shields CB, Ratajczak MZ (2006) Cells enriched in markers of neural tissue-committed stem cells reside in the bone marrow and are mobilized into the peripheral blood following stroke. *Leukemia* 20:18–28.

Lapidot T, Dar A, Kollet O (2005) How do stem cells find their way home? *Blood* 106:1901–1910.

Lapidot T and Kollet O (2010) The brain-bone-blood triad: traffic lights for stem-cell homing and mobilization. *Hematology Am Soc Hematol Educ Program* 2010:1–6.

Lappalainen RS, Narkilahti S, Huhtala T, Liimatainenn T, Suuronen T, Narvanen A, Suuronen R, Hovatta O, Jolkkonen J (2008) The SPECT imaging shows the accumulation of neural progenitor cells into internal organs after systemic administration in middle cerebral artery occlusion rats. *Neurosci Lett* 440:246–250.

Lee HJ, Kim KS, Park IH, Kim SU (2007) Human neural stem cells overexpressing VEGF provide neuroprotection, angiogenesis and functional recovery in mouse stroke model. *PLoS ONE* 2(1):e156.

Lee HJ, Kim MK, Kim HJ, Kim SU (2009) Human neural stem cells genetically modified to overexpress Akt1 provide neuroprotection and functional improvement in mouse stroke model," *PLoS ONE* 4(4):e5586.

Lee JM, Jung J, Lee HJ, Jeong SJ, Cho KJ, Hwang SG, Kim GJ (2012) Comparison of immunomodulatory effects of placenta mesenchymal stem cells with bone marrow and adipose mesenchymal stem cells. *Int Immunopharmacol* 13:219–224.

Lee JS, Hong JM, Moon GJ, Lee PH, Ahn YH, Bang OY, STARTING Collaborators (2010) A long-term follow-up study of intravenous autologous mesenchymal stem cell transplantation in patients with ischemic stroke. *Stem Cells* 28:1099–1106.

Lee ST, Chu K, Jung KH, Kim SJ, Kim DH, Kang KM, Hong NH, Kim JH, Ban JJ, Park HK, Kim SU, Park CG, Lee SK, Kim M, Roh JK (2008) Anti-inflammatory mechanism of intravascular neural stem cell transplantation in haemorrhagic stroke. *Brain* 131(3):616–629.

Leu S, Lin YC, Yuen CM, Yen CH, Kao YH, Sun CK, Yip HK (2010) Adipose-derived mesenchymal stem cells markedly attenuate brain infarct size and improve neurological function in rats. *J Transl Med* 8:63.

Li Y, Chen J, Wang L, Lu M, Chopp M (2001) Treatment of stroke in rat with intracarotid administration of marrow stromal cells. *Neurology* 56:1666–1672.

Li Z, McKercher SR, Cui J, Nie ZG, Soussou W, Roberts AJ, Sallmen T, Lipton JH, Talantova M, Okamoto SI, Lipton SA (2008) Myocyte enhancer factor 2C as a neurogenic and antiapoptotic transcription factor in murine embryonic stem cells. *J Neurosci* 28:6557–6568.

Liao WB, Xie J, Zhong J, Liu YJ, Du L, Zhou B, Xu J, Liu PX, Yang SG, Wang JM, Han ZB, Han ZC (2009) Therapeutic effect of human umbilical cord multipotent mesenchymal stromal cells in a rat model of stroke. *Transplantation* 87:350–359.

Lin RZ, Moreno-Luna R, Zhou B, Pu WT, Melero-Martin JM (2012) Equal modulation of endothelial cell function by four distinct tissue-specific mesenchymal stem cells. *Angiogenesis* 15(3):443–455.

Liu H, Honmou O, Harada K, Nakamura K, Houkin K, Hamada H, Kocsis JD (2006) Neuroprotection by PlGF gene-modified human mesenchymal stem cells after cerebral ischaemia. *Brain* 129(10):2734–2745.

Liu XS, Chopp M, Zhang RL, Hozeska-Solgot A, Gregg SC, Buller B, Lu M, Zhang ZG (2009) Angiopoietin 2 mediates the differentiation and migration of neural progenitor cells in the subventricular zone after stroke. *J Biol Chem* 284:22680–22689.

Luo J, Hu X, Zhang L, Li L, Zheng H, Li M, Zhang Q (2014) Physical exercise regulates neural stem cells proliferation and migration via SDF-1α/CXCR4 pathway in rats after ischemic stroke. *Neurosci Lett* 22(578):203–208.

Mack GS (2011) ReNeuron and StemCells get green light for neural stem cell trials. *Nat Biotechnol* 29:95–97.

Mackowiak M, O'Neill MJ, Hicks CA, Bleakman D, Skolnick P (2002) An AMPA receptor potentiator modulates hippocampal expression of BDNF: an *in vivo* study. *Neuropharmacology* 43(1):1–10.

Marcus AJ, Woodbury D (2008) Fetal stem cells from extra-embryonic tissues: do not discard. *J Cell Mol Med* 12:730–742.

Masuda H, Asahara T (2003) Post-natal endothelial progenitor cells for neovascularization in tissue regeneration. *Cardiovasc Res* 58: 390–398.

Matsuda R, Yoshikawa M, Kimura H, Ouji Y, Nakase H, Nishimura F, Nonaka J, Toriumi H, Yamada S, Nishiofuku M, Moriya K, Ishizaka S, Nakamura M, Sakaki T (2009) Cotransplantation of mouse embryonic stem cells and bone marrow stromal cells following spinal cord injury suppresses tumor development. *Cell Transplant* 18:39–54.

McGregor JA and Rogo LJ (2006) Breast milk: an unappreciated source of stem cells. *J Hum Lact* 22:270–271.

Meng X, Ichim TE, Zhong J, Rogers A, Yin Z, Jackson J, Wang H, Ge W, Bogin V, Chan KW, Thebaud B, Riordan NH (2007) Endometrial regenerative cells: a novel stem cell population. *J Transl Med* 5:57.

Menier C, Rouas-Freiss N, Favier B, LeMaoult J, Moreau P, Carosella ED (2010) Recent advances on the non-classical major histocompatibility complex class I HLA-G molecule. *Tissue Antigens* 75:201–206.

Minnerup J, Kim JB, Schmidt A, Diederich K, Bauer H, Schilling M, Strecker JK, Ringelstein EB, Sommer C, Scholer HR, Schabitz WR (2011) Effects of neural progenitor cells on sensorimotor recovery and endogenous repair mechanisms after photothrombotic stroke. *Stroke* 42:1757–1763.

Miura M, Gronthos S, Zhao M, Lu B, Fisher LW, Robey PG, Shi S (2003) SHED: stem cells from human exfoliated deciduous teeth. *Proc Natl Acad Sci U S A* 100:5807–5812.

Moniche F, Gonzalez A, Gonzalez-Marcos JR, Carmona M, Pinero P, Espigado I, Garcia-Solis D, Cayuela A, Montaner J, Boada C, Rosell A, Jimenez MD, Mayol A, Gil-Peralta A (2012) Intra-arterial bone marrow mononuclear cells in ischemic stroke a pilot clinical trial. *Stroke* 43(8):2242–2244.

Morsczeck C, Gotz W, Schierholz J, Zellhofer F, Kuhn U, Mohl C, Sippel C, Hoffmann KH (2005) Isolation of precursor cells (PCs) from human dental follicle of wisdom teeth. *Matrix Biol* 24:155–165.

Najar M, Raicevic G, Boufker HI, Fayyad-Kazan H, De Bruyn C, Meuleman N, Bron D, Toungouz M, Lagneaux L (2010) Adipose-tissue-derived and Wharton's jelly-derived mesenchymal stromal cells suppress lymphocyte responses by secreting leukemia inhibitory factor. *Tissue Eng Part A* 16:3537–3546.

Nakagomi N, Nakagomi T, Kubo S, Nakano-Doi A, Saino O, Takata M, Yoshikawa H. Stern DM, Matsuyama T, Taguchi A (2009) Endothelial cells support survival, proliferation, and neuronal differentiation of transplanted adult ischemia-induced neural stem/progenitor cells after cerebral infarction. *Stem Cells* 27(9):2185–2195.

Nakayama D, Matsuyama T, Ishibashi-Ueda H, Nakagomi T, Kasahara Y, Hirose H, Kikuchi-Taura A, Stern DM, Mori H, Taguchi A (2010) Injury-induced neural stem/progenitor cells in post-stroke human cerebral cortex. *Eur J Neurosci* 31:90–98.

Nervi B, Link DC, DiPersio JF (2006) Cytokines and hematopoietic stem cell mobilization. *J Cell Biochem* 99:690–705.

Newcomb JD, Ajmo CT Jr., Sanberg CD, Sanberg PR, Pennypacker KR, Willing AE (2006) Timing of cord blood treatment after experimental stroke determines therapeutic efficacy. *Cell Transplant* 15:213–223.

Newman MB, Misiuta I, Willing AE, Zigova T, Karl RC, Borlongan CV, Sanberg PR (2005) Tumorigenicity issues of embryonic carcinoma-derived stem cells: relevance to surgical trials using NT2 and hNT neural cells. *Stem Cells Dev* 14:29–43.

Nygren J, Wieloch T, Pesic J, Brundin P, Deierborg T (2006) Enriched environment attenuates cell genesis in subventricular zone after focal ischemia in mice and decreases migration of newborn cells to the striatum. *Stroke* 37:2824–2829.

Oh JS, Kim KN, An SS, Pennant WA, Kim HJ, Gwak SJ, Yoon do H, Lim MH, Choi BH, Ha Y (2011) Cotransplantation of mouse neural stem cells (mNSCs) with adipose tissue-derived mesenchymal stem cells improves mNSC survival in a rat spinal cord injury model. *Cell Transplant* 20: 837–849.

Oyamada N, Itoh H, Sone M, Yamahara K, Miyashita K, Park K, Taura D, Inuzuka, Sonoyama T, Tsujimoto H, Fukunaga Y, Tamura N, Nakao K (2008) Transplantation of vascular cells derived from human embryonic stem cells contributes to vascular regeneration after stroke in mice. *J Transl Med* 30(6):54.

Paczkowska E, Kucia M, Koziarska D, Halasa M, Safranow K, Masiuk M, Karbicka A, Nowik M, Nowacki P, Ratajczak MZ, Machalinski B (2009) Clinical evidence that very small embryonic-like stem cells are mobilized into peripheral blood in patients after stroke. *Stroke* 40: 1237–1244.

Papayannopoulou T, Scadden DT (2008) Stem-cell ecology and stem cells in motion. *Blood* 111:3923–3930.

Park DH, Eve DJ, Sanberg PR, Musso J 3rd, Bachstetter AD, Wolfson A, Schlunk A, Baradez MO, Sinden JD, Gemma C (2010) Increased neuronal proliferation in the dentate gyrus of aged rats following neural stem cell implantation. *Stem Cells Dev* 19:175–180.

Patel AN, Park E, Kuzman M, Benetti F, Silva FJ, Allickson JG (2008) Multipotent menstrual blood stromal stem cells: isolation, characterization, and differentiation. *Cell Transplant* 17:303–311.

Pignataro G, Studer FE, Wilz A, Simon RP, Boison D (2007) Neuroprotection in ischemic mouse brain induced by stem cell-derived brain implants. *J Cereb Blood Flow Metab* 27:919–927.

Pollock K, Stroemer P, Patel S, Stevanato L, Hope A, Miljan E, Dong Z, Hodges H, Price J, Sinden JD (2006) A conditionally immortal clonal stem cell line from human cortical neuroepithelium for the treatment of ischemic stroke. *Exp Neurol* 199:143–155.

Ra JC, Shin IS, Kim SH, Kang SK, Kang BC, Lee HY, Kim YJ, Jo JY, Yoon EJ, Choi HJ, Kwon E (2011) Safety of intravenous infusion of human adipose tissue-derived mesenchymal stem cells in animals and humans. *Stem Cells Dev* 20:1297–1308.

Ratajczak J, Shin DM, Wan W, Liu R, Masternak MM, Piotrowska K, Wiszniewska B, Kucia M, Bartke A, Ratajczak MZ (2011) Higher number of stem cells in the bone marrow of circulating low Igf-1 level Laron dwarf mice–novel view on Igf-1, stem cells and aging. *Leukemia* 25:729–733.

Ratajczak MZ, Kim CH, Wojakowski W, Janowska-Wieczorek A, Kucia M, Ratajczak J (2010) Innate immunity as orchestrator of stem cell mobilization. *Leukemia* 24:1667–1675.

Ratajczak MZ, Machalinski B, Wojakowski W, Ratajczak J, Kucia M (2007) A hypothesis for an embryonic origin of pluripotent Oct-4(+) stem cells in adult bone marrow and other tissues. *Leukemia* 21:860–867.

Rempe DA and Kent TA (2002) Using bone marrow stromal cells for treatment of stroke. *Neurology* 59:486–487.

Rodrigues MC, Voltarelli J, Sanberg PR, Allickson JG, Kuzmin-Nichols N, Garbuzova-Davis S, Borlongan CV (2012) Recent progress in cell therapy for basal ganglia disorders with emphasis on menstrual blood transplantation in stroke. *Neurosci Biobehav Rev* 36:177–190.

Rowe D, Leonardo C, Recio J, Collier L, Willing A, Pennypacker K (2012) Human umbilical cord blood cells protect oligodendrocytes from brain ischemia through Akt signal transduction. *J Biol Chem* 287:4177–4187.

Rubio D, Garcia-Castro J, Martin MC, de la Fuente R, Cigudosa JC, Lloyd AC, Bernad A (2005) Spontaneous human adult stem cell transformation. *Cancer Res* 65:3035–3039.

Rueger MA, Muesken S, Walberer M, Jantzen SU, Schnakenburg K, Backes H, Graf R, Neumaier B, Hoehn M, Fink GR, Schroeter M (2012) Effects of minocycline on endogenous neural stem cells after experimental stroke. *Neuroscience* 215:174–183.

Saino O, Taguchi A, Nakagomi T, Nakano-Doi A, Kashiwamura S, Doe N, Nakagomi N, Soma T, Yoshikawa H, Stern DM, Okamura H, Matsuyama T (2010) Immunodeficiency reduces neural stem/progenitor cell apoptosis and enhances neurogenesis in the cerebral cortex after stroke. *J Neurosci Res* 88:2385–2397.

Sakata H, Narasimhan P, Niizuma K, Maier CM, Wakai T, Chan PH (2012) Interleukin 6-preconditioned neural stem cells reduce ischaemic injury in stroke mice. *Brain* 135:3298–3310.

Sanberg PR, Eve DJ, Cruz LE, Borlongan CV (2012) Neurological disorders and the potential role for stem cells as a therapy. *Br Med Bull* 101: 163–181.

Savitz SI, Misra V, Kasam M, Juneja H, Cox CS, Alderman S, Aisiku I, Kar S, Gee A, Grotta JC (2011) Intravenous autologous bone marrow mono-nuclear cells for ischemic stroke. *Ann Neurol* 70:59–69.

Seo BM, Miura M, Gronthos S (2004) Investigation of multipotent postna-tal stem cells from human periodontal ligament. *Lancet* 364:1756.

Shen LH, Li Y, Chen J, Zacharek A, Gao Q, Kapke A, Lu M, Raginski K, Vanguri P, Smith A, Chopp M (2007) Therapeutic benefit of bone mar-row stromal cells administered 1 month after stroke. *J Cereb Blood Flow Metab* 27: 6–13.

Song S, Kamath S, Mosquera D, Zigova T, Sanberg P, Vesely DL, Sanchez-Ramos J (2004) Expression of brain natriuretic peptide by human bone marrow stromal cells. *Exp Neurol* 185:191–197.

Sonoyama W, Liu Y, Fang DAJ, Yamaza T, Seo BM, Zhang CM, Liu H, Gronthos S, Wang CY, Shi ST, Wang SL (2006) Mesenchymal stem cell-mediated functional tooth regeneration in swine. *Plos One* 1:e79.

Sonoyama W, Liu Y, Yamaza T, Tuan RS, Wang S, Shi S, Huang GTJ (2008) Characterization of the apical papilla and its residing stem cells from human immature permanent teeth: a pilot study. *J Endod* 34:166–171.

Strioga M, Viswanathan S, Darinskas A, Slaby O, Michalek J (2012) Same or not the same? comparison of adipose tissue-derived versus bone marrow-derived mesenchymal stem and stromal cells. *Stem Cells Dev* 21(14):2724–2752.

Subramanian A, Shu-Uin G, Kae-Siang N, Gauthaman K, Biswas A, Choolani M, Bongso A, Chui-Yee F (2012) Human umbilical cord Wharton's jelly mesenchymal stem cells do not transform to tumor-associated fibroblasts in the presence of breast and ovarian cancer cells unlike bone marrow mesenchymal stem cells. *J Cell Biochem* 113:1886–1895.

Takahashi K, Yamanaka S (2006) Induction of pluripotent stem cells from mouse embryonic and adult fibroblast cultures by defined factors. *Cell* 126: 663–676.

Tat PA, Sumer H, Jones KL, Upton K, Verma PJ (2010) The efficient gen-eration of induced pluripotent stem (iPS) cells from adult mouse adipose tissue-derived and neural stem cells. *Cell Transplant* 19:525–536.

Theus MH, Wei L, Cui L, Francis K, Hu XY, Keogh C, Yu SP (2008) *In vitro* hypoxic preconditioning of embryonic stem cells as a strategy of promoting cell survival and functional benefits after transplantation into the ischemic rat brain. *Exp Neurol* 210:656–670.

Thored P, Wood J, Arvidsson A, Cammenga J, Kokaia Z, Lindvall O (2007) Long-term neuroblast migration along blood vessels in an area with transient angiogenesis and increased vascularization after stroke. *Stroke* 38:3032–3039.

Tolar J, Nauta AJ, Osborn MJ, Panoskaltsis Mortari A, McElmurry RT, Bell S, Xia L, Zhou N, Riddle M, Schroeder TM, Westendorf JJ, McIvor RS, Hogendoorn PC, Szuhai K, Oseth L, Hirsch B, Yant SR, Kay MA, Peister A, Prockop DJ, Fibbe WE, Blazar BR (2007) Sarcoma derived from cultured mesenchymal stem cells. *Stem Cells* 25:371–379.

Uchida N, Kiuchi Y, Miyamoto K, Uchida J, Tobe T, Tomita M, Shioda S, Nakai Y, Koide R, Oguchi K (1998) Glutamate-stimulated proliferation of rat retinal pigment epithelial cells. *Eur J Pharmacol* 343(2–3): 265–273.

Van Kampen JM and Eckman CB (2010) Agonist-induced restoration of hippocampal neurogenesis and cognitive improvement in a model of cholinergic denervation. *Neuropharmacology* 58(6):921–929.

van Velthoven CT, Kavelaars A, van Bel F, Heijnen CJ (2010) Mesenchymal stem cell treatment after neonatal hypoxic-ischemic brain injury improves behavioral outcome and induces neuronal and oligodendrocyte regeneration. *Brain Behav Immun* 24:387–393.

Vendrame M, Cassady J, Newcomb J, Butler T, Pennypacker KR, Zigova T, Sanberg CD, Sanberg PR, Willing AE (2004) Infusion of human umbilical cord blood cells in a rat model of stroke dose-dependently rescues behavioral deficits and reduces infarct volume. *Stroke* 35:2390–2395.

Vendrame M, Gemma C, de Mesquita D, Collier L, Bickford PC, Sanberg CD, Sanberg PR, Pennypacker KR, Willing AE (2005) Anti-inflammatory effects of human cord blood cells in a rat model of stroke. *Stem Cells Dev* 14:595–604.

Vidal MA, Walker NJ, Napoli E, Borjesson DL (2012) Evaluation of senescence in mesenchymal stem cells isolated from equine bone marrow, adipose tissue, and umbilical cord tissue. *Stem Cells Dev* 21:273–283.

Wei L, Cui L, Snider BJ, Rivkin M, Yu SS, Lee CS, Adams LD, Gottlieb DI, Johnson EM, Yu SP, Choi DW (2005) Transplantation of embryonic stem cells overexpressing Bcl-2 promotes functional recovery after transient cerebral ischemia. *Neurobiol Dis* 19:183–193.

Wei L, Fraser JL, Lu ZY, Hu X, Yu SP (2012) Transplantation of hypoxia preconditioned bone marrow mesenchymal stem cells enhances angiogenesis and neurogenesis after cerebral ischemia in rats. *Neurobiol Dis* 46(3):635.

White BC, Sullivan JM, DeGracia DJ, O'Neil BJ, Neumar RW, Grossman LI, Rafols JA, Krause GS (2000) Brain ischemia and reperfusion: molecular mechanisms of neuronal injury. *J Neurol Sci* 179(S 1–2):1–33.

Willing AE, Eve DJ, Sanberg PR (2007) Umbilical cord blood transfusions for prevention of progressive brain injury and induction of neural recovery: an immunological perspective. *Regen Med* 2:457–464.

Willing AE, Lixian J, Milliken M, Poulos S, Zigova T, Song S, Hart C, Sanchez-Ramos J, Sanberg PR (2003) Intravenous versus intrastriatal cord blood administration in a rodent model of stroke. *J Neurosci Res* 73:296–307.

Xiao J, Nan Z, Motooka Y, Low WC (2005) Transplantation of a novel cell line population of umbilical cord blood stem cells ameliorates neurological deficits associated with ischemic brain injury. *Stem Cells Dev* 14:722–733.

Yamashita T, Kawai H, Tian FF, Ohta Y, Abe K (2011) Tumorigenic development of induced pluripotent stem cells in ischemic mouse brain. *Cell Transplant* 20:883–891.

Yanagisawa D, Qi M, Kim DH, Kitamura Y, Inden M, Tsuchiya D, Takata K, Taniguchi T, Yoshimoto K, Shimoama S, Akaike A, Sumi S, Inoue K (2006) Improvement of focal ischemia-induced rat dopaminergic dysfunction by striatal transplantation of mouse embryonic stem cells. *Neurosci Lett* 407:74–79.

Yang KL, Chen MF, Liao CH, Pang CY, Lin PY (2009) A simple and efficient method for generating Nurr1-positive neuronal stem cells from human wisdom teeth (tNSC) and the potential of tNSC for stroke therapy. *Cytotherapy* 11:606–617.

Yang T, Tsang KS, Poon WS, Ng HK (2009) Neurotrophism of bone marrow stromal cells to embryonic stem cells: Noncontact induction and transplantation to a mouse ischemic stroke model. *Cell Transplant* 18:391–404.

Yarygin KN, Kholodenko IV, Konieva AA, Burunova VV, Tairova RT, Gubsky LV, Cheglakov IB, Pirogov YA, Yarygin VN, Skvortsova VI (2009) Mechanisms of positive effects of transplantation of human placental mesenchymal stem cells on recovery of rats after experimental ischemic stroke. *Bull Exp Biol Med* 148:862–868.

Yip HK, Chang LT, Chang WN, Lu CH, Liou CW, Lan MY, Liu JS, Youssef AA, Chang HW (2008) Level and value of circulating endothelial progenitor cells in patients after acute ischemic stroke. *Stroke* 39:69–74.

Yip TR and Demaerschalk BM (2007) Estimated cost savings of increased use of intravenous tissue plasminogen activator for acute ischemic stroke in Canada. *Stroke* 38:1952–1955.

Yu SJ, Soncini M, Kaneko Y, Hess DC, Parolini O, Borlongan CV (2009) Amnion: a potent graft source for cell therapy in stroke. *Cell Transplant* 18:111–118.

Zafra F, Castrén E, Thoenen H, Lindholm D (1991) Interplay between glutamate and gamma-aminobutyric acid transmitter systems in the physiological regulation of brain-derived neurotrophic factor and nerve growth factor synthesis in hippocampal neurons. *Proc Natl Acad Sci U S A* 88(22):10037–10041.

Zhang J, Li Y, Chen J, Yang M, Katakowski M, Lu M, Chopp M (2004) Expression of insulin-like growth factor 1 and receptor in ischemic rats treated with human marrow stromal cells. *Brain Res* 1030:19–27.

Zhang RL, Chopp M, Gregg SR, Toh Y, Roberts C, Letourneau Y, Buller B, Jia L, S PND, Zhang ZG (2009) Patterns and dynamics of subventricular zone neuroblast migration in the ischemic striatum of the adult mouse. *J Cereb Blood Flow Metab* 29:1240–1250.

Zhang W, Yan Q, Zeng YS, Zhang XB, Xiong Y, Wang JM, Chen SJ, Li Y, Bruce IC, Wu W (2010) Implantation of adult bone marrow-derived mesenchymal stem cells transfected with the neurotrophin-3 gene and pretreated with retinoic acid in completely transected spinal cord. *Brain Res* 1359:256–271.

Zhao T, Zhang ZN, Rong Z, Xu Y (2011) Immunogenicity of induced pluripotent stem cells. *Nature* 2474(7350):212–215.

Zheng HQ, Zhang LY, Luo J, Li LL, Li M, Zhang Q, Hu XQ (2014) Physical exercise promotes recovery of neurological function after ischemic stroke in rats. *Int J Mol Sci* 15(6):10974–10988.

Zuba-Surma EK, Kucia M, Wu W, Klich I, Lillard JW Jr., Ratajczak J, Ratajczak MZ (2008) Very small embryonic-like stem cells are present in adult murine organs: ImageStream-based morphological analysis and distribution studies. *Cytometry A* 73A:1116–1127.

Chapter 15

Neural Stem Cell Therapy for Easing Status Epilepticus Induced Hippocampus Dysfunction and Chronic Temporal Lobe Epilepsy

Ashok K. Shetty and Bharathi Hattiangady

Neural stem cell (NSC) transplantation has potential for inhibiting status epilepticus (SE)-induced epileptogenesis as well as controlling spontaneous recurrent seizures in chronic temporal lobe epilepsy (TLE). The reasoning behind the use of NSCs for treating SE and chronic TLE stems from their competence to spontaneously generate sizable numbers of interneurons synthesizing the inhibitory neurotransmitter gamma-amino butyric acid and large numbers of astrocytes secreting a multitude of neurotrophic factors, including some anticonvulsant proteins, after their transplantation into an injured or epileptic brain region. Furthermore, NSC transplantation strategy can be beneficial for recovering cognitive and mood function after SE and TLE. This is because these cells can secrete as well as stimulate the production of multiple pro-cognitive and anti-inflammatory factors, which in turn may enhance hippocampus neurogenesis, a substrate contributing to the maintenance of hippocampus-dependent cognitive and mood function. The objective of this chapter is to confer the current perception and provide insights on NSC-based therapies for SE-induced injury and chronic TLE. The initial section of this review discusses the efficacy of early NSC grafting after hippocampus injury or SE for restraining the evolution of initial precipitating injury into chronic TLE and related co-morbidities. The subsequent segment confers the usefulness of NSC grafting intervention performed in the chronic phase of TLE for restricting spontaneous seizures and improving cognitive and mood function.

Introduction

Epilepsy, characterized by recurrent seizures, is among the world's most common serious neurological disorders. It afflicts over 50 million people worldwide and over 2.2 million Americans. A seizure is exemplified by a short-lived incident of unintentional quivering that may comprise only a portion of the body (a partial seizure) or the whole body (a generalized seizure) and loss of consciousness. Seizures are due to extreme electrical discharges in a group or groups of neurons in the brain. Temporal lobe epilepsy (TLE), one of the most common types of partial epilepsy, typified by various structural and functional aberrations in the hippocampus, a region of brain important for functions such as learning, memory and mood (Engel, 2001, Devinsky, 2004). It typically commences at the end of a first or second decade of life in most instances, ensuing either a seizure with fever (febrile seizures) or an initial precipitating injury (IPI) to the brain in the form of status epilepticus (SE), traumatic brain injury (TBI), stroke or brain tumors. A significant loss of neurons in the hippocampus is one of the conspicuous features of TLE. This involves both excitatory neurons (mossy cells, and CA1 and CA3 pyramidal neurons) as well as several subclasses of inhibitory gamma-amino butyric acid positive (GABA-ergic) interneurons (de Lanerolle *et al.*, 1989; Shetty and Turner, 2000, 2009). An IPI usually also modifies the extent of generation of new neural cells from endogenous neural stem cells (NSCs), migration, and neuronal differentiation of newly born cells in the hippocampus leading to an increased and abnormal neurogenesis in the early phase after injury and greatly decreased neurogenesis in the chronic phase (Shetty and Hattiangady, 2007; Parent and Murphy, 2008; Kuruba *et al.*, 2009a). Abnormally migrated newly born neurons in the dentate hilus develop aberrant connectivity with afferent axons coming from the entorhinal cortex and the efferent CA3 pyramidal neurons (Scharfman and Pierce, 2012). Furthermore, the newly born neurons that incorporate into the granule cell layer develop increased connectivity with other granule cells through sprouting of their axons into the dentate molecular layer, also referred to as aberrant mossy fiber sprouting (Hester and Danzer, 2013). Additionally, neurodegeneration also triggers inflammation that persists for prolonged periods after an IPI. This involves astrocyte hypertrophy and hyperplasia and increased occurrence of activated microglia with increased levels of pro-inflammatory cytokines (Vezzani *et al.*, 2011). Astrocytes also show other multiple abnormalities, which deplete endogenous anticonvulsant proteins such as adenosine as a result of increased adenosine kinase synthesis by astrocytes (Boison, 2012) and the glial cell line-derived neurotrophic factor due to altered synthesis by astrocytes (Waldau *et al.*, 2010). All of these changes initially contribute to hippocampal hyperexcitability due to an increase in the overall excitatory tone vis-à-vis the inhibitory function (Kobayashi and Buckmaster, 2003). This eventually evolves into a chronic epileptic state typified by spontaneous recurrent seizures and co-morbidities such as cognitive impairments and depression.

Antiepileptic drug (AED) therapy is the major treatment offered for patients afflicted with SE or chronic TLE. While this strategy is efficacious for controlling seizures in most patients, over 35% of patients afflicted with chronic TLE display seizures that are pharmacoresistant in nature (Engel, 2001; Litt *et al.*, 2001; Spencer, 2002). Besides, long-term AED therapy can lead to several side effects and does not alleviate memory and mood impairments associated with TLE (Devinsky, 2004; Strine *et al.*, 2005; Maino *et al.*, 2007). Hence, alternative therapies that are efficacious not only for restraining the frequency and intensity of spontaneous recurrent seizures (SRS) but also for alleviating memory and mood impairments on a long-term basis are urgently needed. Multiple pre-clinical studies have shown great interest in testing the efficacy of neural cell grafting approaches as an alternative therapy for excitotoxin- or SE-induced hippocampus injury and TLE (Shetty, 2011, 2014). The working hypothesis is that an early neural cell grafting intervention after an IPI such as SE or TBI would restrain multiple epileptogenic changes through neuroprotective, antiepileptogenic, antiinflammatory, and circuitry altering effects. This may prevent or delay the onset of TLE or at least reduce the severity of TLE and related co-morbidities (Shetty, 2011, 2014). On the other hand, neural cell grafting intervention performed after the onset of chronic epilepsy is hypothesized to restrain the frequency and intensity of SRS and improve cognitive and mood function through disease modification effects, which may include suppression of aberrant mossy fiber sprouting, insertion of new GABA-ergic interneurons to the hippocampus circuitry, and addition of new astrocytes releasing anticonvulsant and pro-cognitive factors (Shetty *et al.*, 2005; Waldau *et al.*, 2010; Hunt *et al.*, 2013; Cunningham *et al.*, 2014).

The principal goal of this chapter is to evaluate the present perception and to put forward viewpoints about NSC transplantation strategy for TLE. Considering the focus of this book on NSCs and NSC-based therapies for neurological disorders, this chapter is consciously restricted to discussion of investigations that examined the usefulness of NSC transplants in SE and TLE models. The first segment of this chapter confers different donor cell types that are being considered for grafting in epilepsy and advantages of using NSCs over other neural cell types for treating TLE. The subsequent section deliberates the prospects for averting or curtailing SRS using NSC transplantation strategies that are executed soon after an IPI, such as a direct excitotoxic lesion or SE. The final segment discusses the potential of NSC transplantation for controlling SRS and improving learning and memory function when intervened shortly or at a protracted time-point after the onset of TLE. Additionally, major issues that are critical to be addressed before the clinical translation of NSC grafting therapy for TLE are also conferred.

Ideal Donor Cell Types for Grafting after Hippocampus Injury, SE or the Onset of TLE

The efficacy of grafting of multiple donor cell types has been and are being examined in animal models of SE and chronic TLE. These include fetal hippocampal cells, GABA-ergic cells from medial and lateral ganglionic eminences of the fetal brain, genetically engineered GABA-producing cells, and GABA-ergic precursors generated from human embryonic stem cells (hESCs) and human induced pluripotent stem cells (hiPSCs). Many of these studies have reported encouraging results for alleviating seizures and/or improving cognitive function in a variety of hippocampus injury and epilepsy models (Shetty and Turner, 2000; Shetty *et al.*, 2005; Rao *et al.*, 2007; Hattiangady *et al.*, 2008; Waldau *et al.*, 2010; Shetty, 2011; Hattiangady and Shetty, 2012; Hunt *et al.*, 2013; Henderson *et al.*, 2014; Cunningham *et al.*, 2014). However, the suitability of these cell types for clinical application in conditions such as TLE is still unclear. Transplantation of hippocampal or GABA-ergic cells derived from the fetal brain will be hard to translate due to difficulty in obtaining the required amount of fetal tissues from aborted fetuses. While it is possible to generate such specific neural cells in large quantifies from hESCs in culture (Cunningham *et al.*, 2014), the use of hESCs is still ethically controversial. On the other hand, generating specific neural cells from hiPSCs seems ideal, as their use not only avoids ethical issues but also facilitates grafting of patient-specific cells. Nonetheless, the protocols for generating large amounts of specific cell types (e.g. GABA-ergic cells) from iPSCs in a reasonable period of time without contamination of PSCs are still in the process of evolving and refinement (Liu *et al.*, 2013). Furthermore, issues such as an increased propensity for teratoma and potential genetic abnormalities after multiple passaging are delaying the clinical use of iPSC-derived cells for treating neurological as well as other diseases (Huo *et al.*, 2014). From these perspectives, the use of NSCs as donor cells seems attractive. This is because multipotent NSCs can be expanded in culture for extended periods from diverse sources such as the fetal, postnatal and adult brain

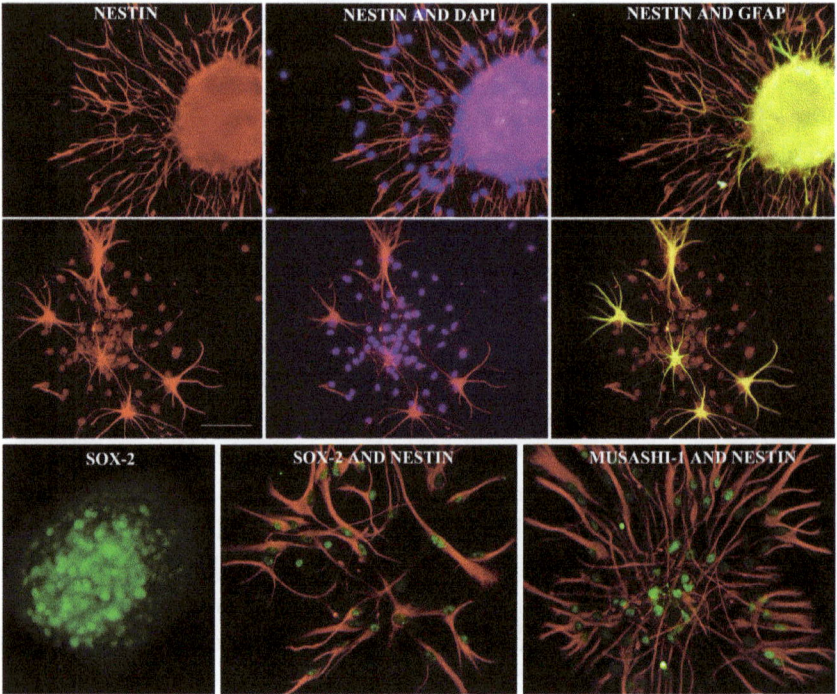

Figure 1.   Expression of neural stem cell specific markers in cells expanded as neurospheres from the postnatal hippocampus. The upper two rows show the expression of nestin and glial fibrillary acidic protein (GFAP) whereas the lower row demonstrates the expression of Sox-2, nestin and musashi-1.   Scale bar, 50 µm. *(Figure reproduced from Shetty and Hattiangady, Int J Dev Neuro Sci, 31: 646–656, 2013).*

(Reynolds and Weiss, 1992; Shetty and Turner, 1998; Palmer *et al.*, 1999; Barkho and Zhao, 2011). Such cells typically display the expression of NSC-specific markers (Figure 1). Moreover, newly developed technologies allow direct conversion of somatic cells (such as fibroblasts, lymphocytes or glia) into multipotent NSCs (Han *et al.*, 2012; Ring *et al.*, 2012; Cassady *et al.*, 2014), which may facilitate grafting of patient-specific NSCs in the future. These cells are believed to have much lesser propensity for developing teratoma or tumors than iPSCs (Ring *et al.*, 2012).

The potential of NSC transplantation approach for restraining SRS after SE or in TLE principally stems from their ability to:

(1) spread expansively into various layers of the hippocampus; (2) generate a sizable population of interneurons synthesizing the inhibitory neurotransmitter GABA;   (3) give rise to astrocytes synthesizing the anticonvulsant factor GDNF (Waldau *et al.*, 2010); and (4) induce neuroprotective and antiinflammatory effects (Cusimano *et al.*, 2012; Hattiangady and Shetty, 2012; Butti *et al.*, 2012; Huang *et al.*, 2014). NSC grafting is also believed to improve cognitive and mood function through several pro-cognitive effects, which include secretion of a multitude of beneficial neurotrophic factors by NSCs (Figure 2) and addition of new NSCs to the neurogenic region of the epileptic hippocampus (Hattiangady and Shetty, 2012). Both of

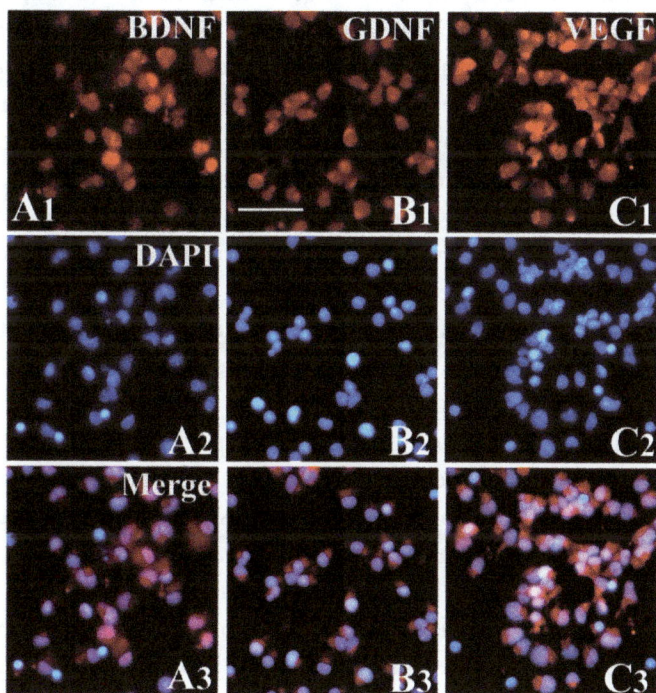

Figure 2. Expression of neurotrophic factors, the brain-derived neurotrophic factor (BDNF), the glial cell-line derived neurotrophic factor (GDNF) and the vascular endothelial growth factor (VEGF) in neural stem/progenitor cells expanded from the anterior subventricular zone of the postnatal rat brain. Scale bar, 50 µm *(Figure reproduced from Hattiangady and Shetty, Stem Cells Transl Med, 1:696–708, 2012).*

these changes can lead to enhanced NSC proliferation and improved net hippocampal neurogenesis (Hattiangady *et al.*, 2007), one of the substrates vital for sustaining the hippocampus-dependent cognitive function and mood (Sahay and Hen, 2007; Dupret *et al.*, 2008; Deng *et al.*, 2010).

Early NSC Grafting Intervention into the Hippocampus after Injury Prevents Impairments in Memory, Mood and Neurogenesis

The potential of early NSC transplantation strategy for reducing hippocampus dysfunction after injury has been demonstrated in several studies. A study by Hattiangady and Shetty (2012) showed that transplantation of NSCs expanded from the subventricular zone (SVZ) of the postnatal brain into the hippocampus of adult rats early after an intracerebroventricular kainic acid (KA) induced injury can prevent memory and mood dysfunction typically found in the chronic phase after injury. Preservation of normal memory and mood function in these animals was associated with excellent survival and widespread migration of graft-derived cells and differentiation of significant percentages of NSC graft-derived cells into different subtypes of GABA-ergic interneurons expressing the calcium binding proteins calbindin and parvalbumin (PV) and a large number of astrocytes (Figure 3).

In addition, transplantation of NSCs prevented several pathological features that ensue after injury, which are believed to contribute to cognitive and mood impairments, as well as the development of chronic epilepsy. These include aberrant neurogenesis in the early phase after injury and greatly declined neurogenesis in the chronic phase. Transplantation of NSCs normalized both the extent and pattern of neurogenesis in the injured hippocampus with proliferation of NSCs in the neurogenic SGZ maintained to levels seen in the age-matched intact hippocampus (Figure 4). Interestingly, normalization of neurogenesis was associated with the protection of a subclass of GABA-ergic neurons expressing reelin in the DG that are believed to be important for guiding newly-born neurons generated

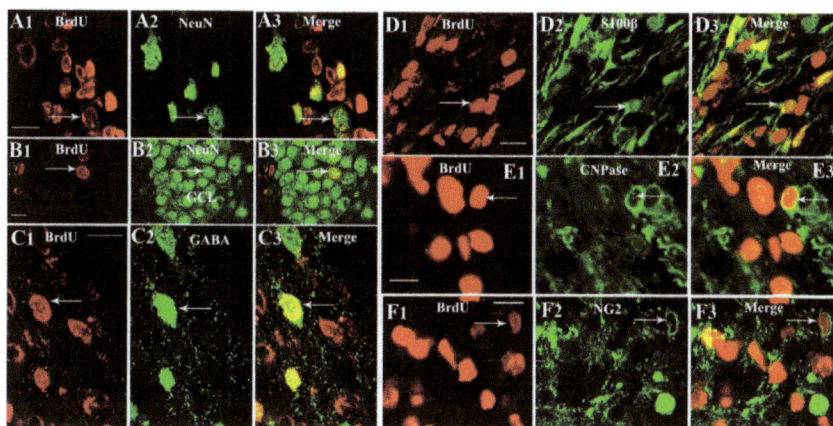

Figure 3. Differentiation of 5′-bromodeoxyuridine positive (red) cells derived from a neural stem cell graft into: (1) neuron-specific nuclear antigen (NeuN) positive neurons near the graft core (A1–A3) and the granule cell layer (GCL; B1–B3); (2) gamma-amino butyric acid (GABA) positive neurons (C1–C3), S100β+ astrocytes (D1–D3), 2′,3′-Cyclic-nucleotide 3′-phosphodiesterase (CNPase) positive oligodendrocytes (E1–E3) and NG2+ oligodendrocyte progenitors (F1–F3). Scale bar, A1–A3: 200 µm; B1–B3, C1–C3, D1–D3, E1–E3: 10 µm; F1–F3 = 20 µm. (*Figure reproduced from Hattiangady and Shetty, Stem Cells Transl Med, 1:696–708, 2012*).

from NSCs into the granule cell layer (Gong *et al.*, 2007). Because a close association between hippocampal neurogenesis and cognitive and mood function has been established in several models (Deng *et al.*, 2010; Koehl and Abrous, 2011; Snyder *et al.*, 2011; Aimone *et al.*, 2011; Sahay *et al.*, 2011), preservation of normal memory and mood function in this study is at least partially due to NSC grafting-mediated stabilization of the extent and pattern of neurogenesis in the injured hippocampus. Enhanced levels of neurotrophic factors GDNF, BDNF, FGF-2, and VEGF in the hippocampus may have also played a role, as significant fractions of graft-derived cells expressed them and these factors are known to have beneficial effects on cognitive and mood function (Schmidt and Duman, 2010; Perez *et al.*, 2009; Pertusa *et al.*, 2008; Graham and Richardson, 2009; Kiyota *et al.*, 2011).

Furthermore, GDNF being an endogenous anticonvulsant compound can suppress the occurrence of seizures (Kanter-Schlifke

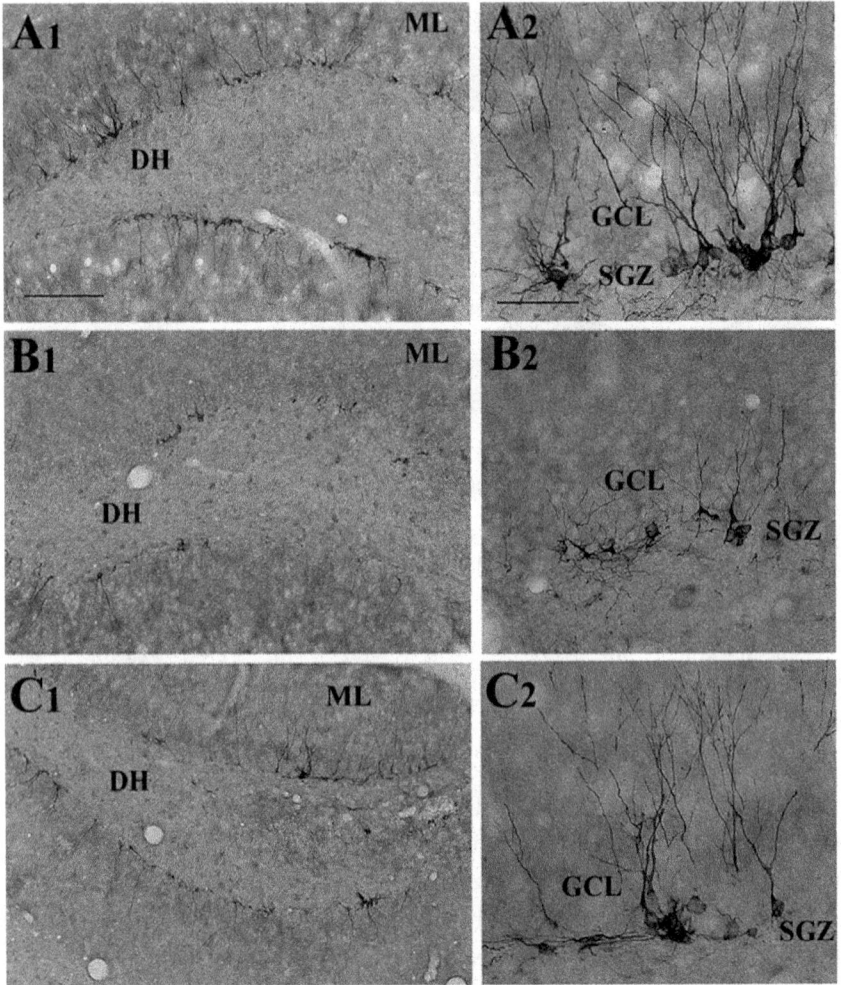

Figure 4. Grafting of subventricular zone-neural stem cells (SVZ-NSCs) into the injured hippocampus maintains neurogenesis at levels comparable to the intact control hippocampus. A1–C2: Extent of neurogenesis measured through double-cortin immunostaining. Note that, in comparison to naïve control rats (A1–A2), rats receiving sham-grafting surgery after hippocampal injury exhibit: (1) decreased neurogenesis (B1–B2). In contrast, rats receiving SVZ-NSC grafts after hippocampal injury display neurogenesis (C1–C2) to levels observed in naïve control rats. *(Figure reproduced from Hattiangady and Shetty, Stem Cells Transl Med, 1:696–708, 2012).*

et al., 2007) whereas BDNF and FGF-2 are known to reduce epileptogenesis and hyperexcitability that ensue after hippocampus injury (Paradiso *et al.*, 2011). Additionally, the influence of increased levels of GABA cannot be ruled out because NSC grafting added considerable numbers of new GABA-ergic interneurons to the injured hippocampus and GABA has the ability to reduce hippocampus hyperexcitability and positively influence neurogenesis, cognition and mood (Luscher *et al.*, 2011; Damgaard *et al.*, 2011; Koh *et al.*, 2010). Another study in a mouse model of bilateral hippocampal injury also reported similar findings (Miltiadous *et al.*, 2013). In summary, these studies demonstrated that early NSC grafting intervention after hippocampal injury is efficacious for ameliorating mood and memory dysfunction as well as reduced and abnormal neurogenesis.

NSC Transplantation into the Injured Hippocampus Early after SE Restrains Chronic Epilepsy Development and Cognitive Dysfunction

Quite a few investigations have examined the usefulness of administration/grafting of NSCs for containing seizures in various prototypes of hippocampal injury and SE via measurement of SRS or spike activity, through frequent behavioral surveillances or electroencephalographic (EEG) recordings over variable periods after NSC transplantation. Some studies have also examined the effects of this approach for preventing cognitive impairments. In these studies, NSCs were administered or grafted within 10 days after an excitotoxic lesion or SE-induced injury to examine their effects on the evolution of an IPI into chronic epilepsy and/or cognitive impairments.

Chu and colleagues investigated the usefulness of intravenous administration of beta-galactosidase (β-gal)-encoded human NSCs a day after the induction of SE on SRS at 28–35 days post-SE, using a rat pilocarpine prototype of TLE (Chu *et al.*, 2004). This investigation reported that only 13% of SE-rats that received NSCs displayed SRS whereas 87% of SE-rats that did not receive NSCs exhibited SRS. Furthermore, SE-rats receiving NSCs displayed diminished severity of SRS as well as smaller field excitatory postsynaptic potentials (fEPSP), in comparison to SE-rats receiving no NSCs. Additionally, SE-rats receiving NSCs exhibited the presence of β-gal positive cells in multiple regions of the brain, including the hippocampal CA1 and CA3 subfields and the dentate hilus. A smaller fraction of NSC-derived cells also differentiated into PV-positive GABA-ergic interneurons and glial fibrillary acidic protein (GFAP) positive astrocytes. Considering these, it is plausible that addition of new GABA-synthesizing cells into the inhibitory circuitry of the injured hippocampus has contributed to decreased neuronal excitability and reduced SRS observed in this study. However, the precise mechanism underlying the beneficial effect in this study remains unknown.

Jing and associates examined the effects of grafts of NSCs expanded in culture as neurospheres from the adult subventricular zone (SVZ) in a rat model of unilateral hippocampal injury inflicted through an intracerebroventricular administration of an excitotoxin kainic acid (KA) (Jing *et al.*, 2009). They placed NSC grafts into the rat hippocampus a week after hippocampus injury and examined the effects of grafts on spontaneous spike activity for three weeks post-grafting. The SVZ is one of the principal neurogenic niches that persist in the adult brain where NSCs continuously generate neuroblasts, which typically migrate into the olfactory bulb (OB) where they differentiate into interneurons (Alvarez-Buylla *et al.*, 2008). The use of SVZ-NSCs is attractive because these cells can be isolated from the brain of any age and are amenable for expansion in culture for extended periods without exhausting their self-renewal and multipotent characteristics (Leonard *et al.*, 2009; Ayuso-Sacido *et al.*, 2008). Furthermore, these NSCs display competence for giving rise to sizable numbers of GABA-ergic interneurons, astrocytes and oligodendrocytes *in vitro* as well as *in vivo* after grafting (Hattiangady and Shetty, 2012). The study by Jing *et al.* (2009) did not find differences in the abnormal spike frequencies from the injured hippocampus in the first week after grafting between KA-treated rats that were grafted with NSCs and KA-treated rats that received non-specific cell grafts. Interestingly, at subsequent time-points (i.e. at 2–3 weeks post-grafting), the injured hippocampus receiving NSC grafts displayed reduced occurrences of deviant spikes in contrast to the injured hippocampus grafted with non-specific cells, implying that NSC grafts restrained the progression of epileptogenesis. This study did not determine the effects of NSC grafts on SRS however. Characterization of the hippocampus revealed survival of graft-derived cells and their differentiation into GFAP+ astrocytes and NeuN+ neurons. Although precise mechanisms underlying the beneficial effect mediated by NSC grafts could not be ascertained, analysis of the injured host hippocampus demonstrated improved survival of subclasses of host GABA-ergic interneurons and diminished abnormal sprouting of mossy fibers into the dentate molecular layer. Because both loss of interneurons and aberrant mossy fiber sprouting are considered major epileptogenic changes that contribute to the development of chronic epilepsy after a hippocampus injury or SE, the above results imply anti-epileptogenic effects of NSC grafts.

Additional studies have examined the efficacy of grafting of NSCs expanded from the hippocampus or the SVZ in SE models (Kuruba *et al.*, 2009b; Hattiangady *et al.*, 2010). In one of these studies, NSCs from the embryonic day 19 hippocampus were expanded *in vitro* as neurospheres in chlorodeoxyuridine (CldU; a thymidine analog and cell birth-dating marker) containing proliferation medium. This facilitated labeling of virtually all neurosphere cells with CldU. Neurospheres were triturated and suspensions of neurosphere cells were grafted into the hippocampus of adult rats that underwent SE induction seven days prior through graded intraperitoneal injections of KA (Rao *et al.*, 2006). Analyses of SRS at 4–6 months post-grafting revealed greatly reduced frequency and intensity of SRS in SE-rats receiving NSC grafts, in comparison to SE-rats receiving sham-grafting surgery (Kuruba *et al.*, 2009b). Additional analyses through EEG recordings also confirmed that SE-rats receiving NSC grafts displayed diminished frequency and intensity of SRS in the chronic phase after SE than SE-rats receiving no grafts or SE-rats receiving sham-grafting surgery (Hattiangady *et al.*, 2010). These results suggested that the beneficial effects observed after NSC grafting were specific to the presence of NSC-derived cells. Characterization of the grafted hippocampus using immunohistochemical and dual immunofluorescence methods revealed widespread migration of NSC graft-derived cells as well as differentiation into GABA-ergic neurons and mature astrocytes (Hattiangady *et al.*, 2010). NSC grafting also had a protective effect on the survival of host interneurons expressing the neuropeptide Y (NPY) and PV. Hence, addition of new GABA-ergic neurons and preservation of host GABA-ergic interneurons are likely among mechanisms underlying the suppression of SRS in this study.

Another study by Hattiangady and colleagues examined the effects of grafting of NSCs from the postnatal SVZ (SVZ-NSCs) into the hippocampus in the same model of SE as described above (Hattiangady *et al.*, 2012). This study grafted SVZ-NSCs into the hippocampus seven days after the induction of SE and analyzed behavioral SRS at 3–5 months post-grafting via behavioral observations as well as EEG recordings. The results revealed substantially reduced frequency and intensity of SRS in SE-rats receiving NSC grafts, in comparison to those receiving none, demonstrated by considerable reductions in the frequency of all SRS, frequency of stage-V SRS, duration of individual SRS and the percentage of recorded time spent in SRS. Furthermore, in sharp contrast to SE-rats receiving no grafts, SE-rats receiving NSC grafts displayed preserved memory function in a novel object recognition test and greatly reduced depressive-like behavior in a forced swim test (Hattiangady *et al.*, 2012). Immunohistochemical and dual immunofluorescence analyses of hippocampal tissues from SE-rats receiving NSC grafts demonstrated excellent yield of graft-derived cells (equaling ~89% of injected cells) and differentiation of graft-derived cells into neurons expressing NeuN (~24% of graft-derived cells). Considerable percentages of graft-derived cells also migrated into the neurogenic SGZ-granule cell layer of the DG where ~75% of them integrated as neurons. Moreover, graft-derived cells differentiated into GABA-ergic interneurons (~22%) and astrocytes secreting neurotrophic factors (~60%). Furthermore, NSC transplantation greatly preserved subclasses of host GABA-ergic interneurons synthesizing the NPY and PV in the dentate gyrus. Considerable protection of these interneurons by NSC grafting has functional relevance. With regard to NPY, it is clear from previous studies that this neuropeptide can inhibit the activity of excitatory neurons in the dentate gyrus via hyperpolarization and inhibition of glutamate release and act as a robust anticonvulsant protein (Redrobe *et al.*, 1999; Fu and van den Pol, 2007) as well as a potent stimulator of NSC proliferation in the hippocampus (Rodrigo *et al.*, 2010; Howell *et al.*, 2005). On the other hand, PV (a calcium-binding protein expressed conspicuously in fast-spiking GABA-ergic hippocampal interneurons) plays an important role in the synchronization of excitatory neurons during network oscillations and maintenance of cognitive function (Klausberger *et al.*, 2005; Korotkova *et al.*, 2010). Taken together, the above studies demonstrate that early intervention with NSC grafting following an injury to the hippocampus or an insult such as SE is beneficial as a prophylactic treatment. Such approaches have the promise to prevent or considerably delay the occurrence of chronic epilepsy after a hippocampus injury or at least reduce the overall severity of spontaneous seizures and cognitive impairments in chronic epilepsy.

NSC Grafting into the Chronically Epileptic Hippocampus can Diminish the Frequency and Intensity of Spontaneous Seizures

The most likely candidates for cell grafting therapy among TLE patients are those suffering from pharmacoresistant TLE. In conditions where seizures can be controlled with AED or other non-invasive therapies, invasive intracerebral cell transplantation may not be the best approach. Hence, studies on NSCs grafts in chronic TLE prototypes where animals exhibit robust SRS at the time of grafting have immense value. Because SRS in TLE predominantly originate from the hippocampus and are associated with memory problems, it is also vital to investigate the effects of NSC grafts in animals that exhibit SRS as well as memory impairments at the time of grafting.

However, only a few studies have examined the efficacy of NSC grafts in chronic epilepsy models so far. A study by Waldau and colleagues rigorously examined whether grafting of NSCs that are capable of adding new GABA-ergic interneurons and the GDNF-expressing astrocytes into the epileptic hippocampus can restrain SRS in animals exhibiting chronic TLE (Waldau *et al.*, 2010). In order to ascertain the efficacy of NSC grafts for treating chronic TLE, this study grafted NSCs bilaterally into the hippocampus (four grafts/hippocampus, 80,000 live cells/graft) of adult rats displaying chronic TLE with cognitive impairments for prolonged periods. Rats with chronic epilepsy were generated through kainate-induced SE (Rao *et al.*, 2006). Because the frequency and severity of SRS can vary considerably between animals, a group of age-matched rats with chronic epilepsy displaying similar frequency and severity of SRS were picked from a larger pool of rats that were chronically epileptic for ~12 months. Chronically epileptic rats selected for NSC grafting were also surveyed with a water maze test to verify the spatial learning and memory dysfunction prior to grafting. The donor NSCs were expanded from the embryonic medial ganglionic eminence (MGE) in this study (Figure 5).

The rationale for choosing MGE-NSCS is based on facts that embryonic MGE is the source of GABA-ergic interneurons for the hippocampus during development, and GABA-ergic interneurons derived from the MGE display ability for both functional integration and increasing the extent of inhibition when grafted into the normal postnatal brain (Alvarez-Dolado *et al.*, 2006). The results showed reduced frequency and severity of SRS in chronically epileptic rats receiving NSC grafts but not in rats receiving sham-grafting surgery. The reductions in NSC-treated rats were 43% for the frequency of SRS, 51% for the duration of individual SRS, and 90% for the frequency of stage V seizures (the most severe form of SRS). In addition, the total time spent in seizures was reduced by 74% in the third month after grafting. Analyses of grafted hippocampi revealed considerable dispersion of graft-derived cells into different layers of the hippocampus and a graft yield that was equivalent to 28% of injected cells.

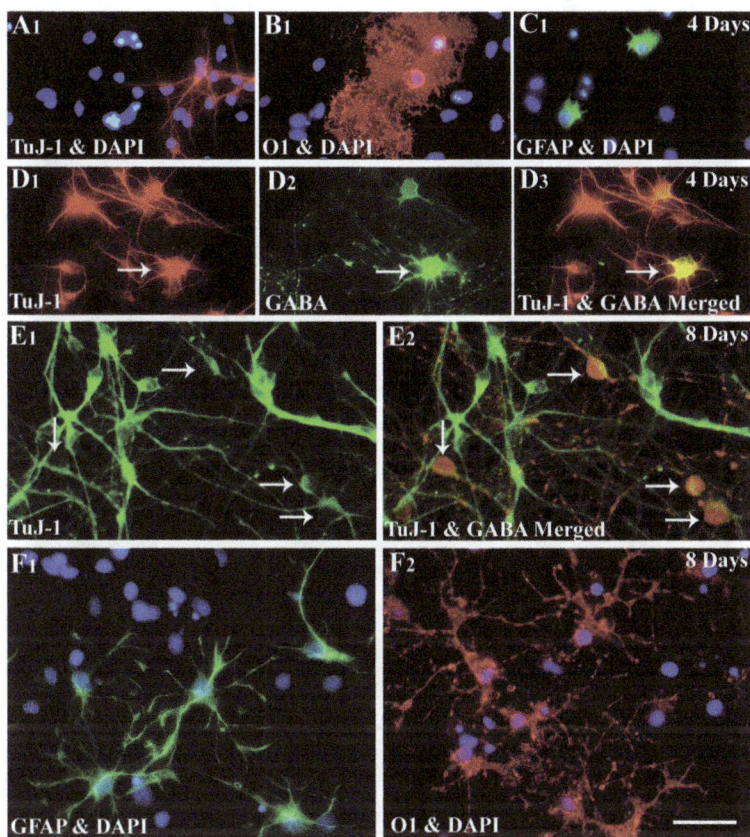

Figure 5. Differentiation of medial ganglionic eminence-neural stem cells (MGE-NSCs) after their dissociation from CldU-labeled neurospheres and incubation in the differentiation medium for four days (A1–D3) or eight days (E1–F2). Differentiation of fractions of MGE-NSCs into TuJ-1+ neurons (A1, E1), O1+ oligo-dendrocytes (B1, F2), and GFAP+ astrocytes (C1, F1) could be seen at both time-points. Furthermore, fractions of MGE-NSCs also differentiate into GABA-ergic neurons (arrows in D1–D3 and E1–E2). Scale bar: 50 μm. *(Figure reproduced from Waldau et al, Stem Cells, 28:1153–1164, 2010).*

Dual immunofluorescence and confocal microscopic analyses revealed that MGE-NSC grafting resulted in addition of ~10,000 new neurons, ~46,000 new astrocytes, ~2,000 new oligodendrocyte pro-genitors, ~8,000 new GABA-ergic neurons, and ~40,000 new GDNF+ astrocytes (Figure 6) into each hippocampus of chronically epileptic

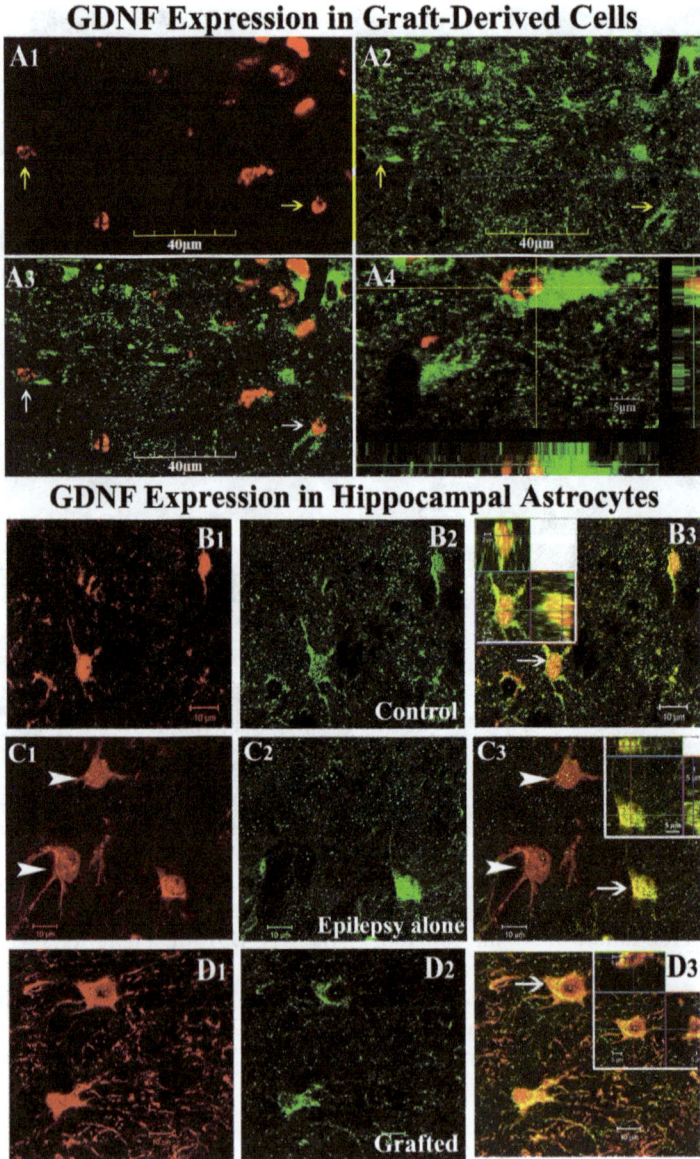

Figure 6. Expression of glial cell-line derived neurotrophic factor (GDNF) in cells derived from medial ganglionic eminence-neural stem cell (MGE-NSC) grafts (A1–A4), and MGE-NSC grafting mediated changes in GDNF expression of host hippocampal astrocytes (B1–D3). Arrows in figures A1–A3 show examples of graft-derived CldU+ cells (red) that express GDNF (green). A4 shows orthogonal

◄

Figure 6. (*Continued*)   views of a GDNF+ graft derived cell (with CldU+ red nucleus and GDNF+ green cytoplasm). Scale bar, A1–A3 = 40 µm; A4 = 5 µm. Figures B1–D3 show confocal microscopic images of S-100β+ hippocampal astrocytes (red) that exhibit GDNF expression (green) in an age-matched control rat (B1–B3), a rat with chronic epilepsy alone (C1–C3) and a chronically epileptic rat that received MGE-NSC grafts (D1–D3). The insets in B3, C3, and D3 show orthogonal views of cells indicated by arrows. Note that these cells are positive for both S-100β and GDNF. Arrowheads in C1 and C3 denote S-100β+ astrocytes that lack GDNF expression in the epilepsy alone group. Scale bar, B1–D3 = 10 µm. (*Figure reproduced from Waldau et al, Stem Cells, 28:1153–1164, 2010*).

rats. Moreover, this study demonstrated that chronic epilepsy is associated with loss of GDNF (an anticonvulsant protein) in a vast majority of astrocytes in the hippocampus, while NSC grafting restores GDNF synthesis in host astrocytes (Figure 6). The mechanisms underlying the suppression of SRS in this study likely include addition of new GABA-ergic neurons and new astrocytes expressing GDNF along with normalization of GDNF expression in the host hippocampal astrocytes. Addition of ~8,000 new GABA-ergic neurons is considered significant because GABA-ergic interneuron loss and loss of the functional inhibition are some of the conspicuous features of chronic TLE (de Lanerolle *et al.*, 1989; Turner and Wheal, 1991; Shetty and Turner, 2000; Shetty *et al.*, 2009). In addition, the grafting of cells that release GABA can also facilitate transient anti-seizure effects (Castillo *et al.*, 2008; Loscher *et al.*, 2008; Thompson, 2009). However, grafting of NSCs in this chronic TLE model neither improved spatial learning and memory function nor hippocampus neurogenesis. Since neurogenesis is one of the vital substrates contributing to the maintenance of hippocampus-dependent learning and memory function (Deng *et al.*, 2010), it is likely that the inability of NSC grafts to enhance the greatly waned neurogenesis in the chronically epileptic hippocampus (Hattiangady *et al.*, 2004; Hattiangady and Shetty, 2010) contributed to their failure to induce better cognitive outcome. Another reason for lack of improved cognitive function may be that NSC grafts did not give rise to CA1 or CA3 pyramidal neurons to restore the neuron loss in their respective cell layers. It is plausible that restoration of cognitive pathways may require grafting of cells that have the ability to differentiate into hippocampal pyramidal neurons and restore the damaged CA1–CA3 circuitry (Shetty and Turner, 2000; Shetty *et al.*, 2005; Rao *et al.*, 2007).

A study by Shindo and colleagues examined the effects of grafts of NSCs derived from mouse ESCs in the hippocampus of kindled rats exhibiting stage V seizures (Shindo *et al.*, 2010). Measurement of SRS at six weeks post-grafting via behavioral surveillances uncovered some recovery from SRS in animals receiving NSC grafts in the form of decreases in the intensity of SRS (i.e. occurrence of stage III/IV seizures instead of stage V seizures). However, the recovery was significant in comparison to the sham-operated rats displaying predominantly stage V seizures during the same time period. Histological analyses showed some differentiation of graft-derived cells into neurons those positive for the GABA synthesizing enzyme, glutamic acid decaroboxylase-67. Thus, NSCs derived from the ES cells are also efficient for controlling SRS in a TLE model. However, this study has some limitations, which include intermittent analyses of SRS for brief periods, lack of SRS measurements via EEG recordings and lack of correlative analyses between the phenotype of the NSC-graft derived cells and SRS.

Another recent study evaluated the therapeutic potential of human NSCs in animal models of TLE. In this study, NSCs derived from aborted fetuses expanded as neurospheres in culture were grafted into animals that were either kindled or treated with pilocarpine (Lee *et al.*, 2014). The results showed that NSC grafting reduced the duration of behavioral seizures and after discharges in kindled animals, and the frequency and the duration of SRS in pilocarpine-treated animals. Histological characterization revealed differentiation of ~24% of cells into GABA-ergic neurons and restoration of GDNF expression in host astrocytes. Nonetheless, NSC grafting did not improve spatial learning or memory function, consistent with the results of Waldau *et al.* (2010) described above.

Conclusions and Required Future Studies

Studies conducted so far in animal models have demonstrated that grafting of NSCs into the hippocampus early after an IPI such as hippocampus injury or SE is beneficial for easing injury-induced epileptogenesis, SRS development and cognitive and mood impairments. Such a prophylactic strategy has the promise for preventing or considerably delaying the occurrence of chronic epilepsy or, at least, reducing the overall severity of spontaneous seizures and cognitive impairments when chronic epilepsy develops. Clinical application of NSC grafting as a prophylactic treatment may be feasible in the future for patients suffering head injury or severe SE with considerable damage to the hippocampus. Nevertheless, because antiepileptic drug (AED) therapy controls seizures in most patients, the ostensible candidates for grafting therapy among epilepsy patients are those suffering from pharmacoresistant epilepsy. In such patients, the grafting approach is ideal as an alternative to hippocampus resection surgery, if found efficacious in animal models of chronic TLE. Therefore, long-term studies on NSC grafts in chronic TLE prototypes where animals exhibit robust SRS at the time of grafting have immense value. Indeed, transplantation of NSCs into the hippocampus shortly or at prolonged periods after the onset of TLE has also shown significant efficacy for reducing the frequency and intensity of SRS (Waldau *et al.*, 2010; Shindo *et al.*, 2010). While the specific mechanisms that underlie the control of seizures by NSC grafting are yet to be ascertained, correlative analyses point to several potential mechanisms behind this beneficial effect. These include the addition of significant numbers of new GABA-ergic neurons and GDNF secreting new astrocytes into the epileptic host hippocampus and restoration of the GDNF in the host hippocampal astrocytes by NSC grafts.

Nonetheless, prior to the clinical application of NSC grafts for treating chronic TLE, studies on the following aspects are critically needed. First of all, it is imperative to examine the long-term behavior of multiple types of human NSCs in rodent models of chronic TLE. The donor NSCs may include those derived from the fetal, postnatal and adult brain tissues, a direct conversion of somatic cells, ESCs, and iPSCs. Moreover, grafting outcome measurements should include rigorous analyses of their efficiency for long-term survival, long-lasting seizure suppression, improving cognitive and mood function, and generating substantial numbers of GABA-ergic interneurons (including subclasses that undergo substantial decline in TLE) and GDNF secreting astrocytes. Furthermore, it will be important to assess whether or not an appropriate synaptic integration of NSC graft-derived GABA-ergic interneurons is critical or just bystander effects of cells derived from NSC grafts (such as the release of neurotrophic factors and anticonvulsant proteins, neurogenesis-promoting and antiinflammatory effects) are sufficient for seizure suppression and improved cognitive and mood function in chronically epileptic prototypes. Besides, it is important to note that approaches which are efficacious for reducing the frequency and intensity of SRS (e.g. increased inhibition) may not necessarily improve the cognitive and mood function in chronic TLE (Waldau *et al.*, 2010). Hence, it will be important to examine the efficacy of combination therapies, which may include transplantation of NSCs into the hippocampus followed by systemic administration of neurogenesis enhancing compounds such as NSC mitogenic and neuronal differentiation factors or antioxidant and antiinflammatory drugs that ease the ongoing oxidative stress and inflammation in chronic TLE. Such approaches may control SRS as well as improve cognitive and mood function in chronic TLE through increased neurogenesis. In addition, novel approaches that are efficacious for not only enhancing the overall yield of NSC graft-derived GABA-ergic neurons and the GDNF secreting astrocytes but also promote the functional engraftment of graft-derived NSCs into neurogenic niches of the hippocampus will be needed to restore the greatly waned hippocampal neurogenesis observed in chronic TLE.

Acknowledgements

The studies described in this chapter from the author's laboratory were supported by grants from the National Institute of Neurological Disorders and Stroke (RO1 NS054780 to A.K.S.), the Department of Veterans Affairs (VA Merit Award to A.K.S.) and the State of Texas (Emerging Technology Funds to A.K.S.). The authors thank Drs. B. Waldau, R. Kuruba and B. Shuai for their excellent contributions to the NSC grafting studies performed in Dr. Shetty's laboratory at the Duke University Medical Center, the Durham Veterans Affairs Medical Center and the Institute for Regenerative Medicine at the Texas A&M Health Science Center.

References

Aimone JB, Deng W, Gage FH (2011) Resolving new memories: A critical look at the dentate gyrus, adult neurogenesis, and pattern separation. *Neuron* 70:589–596.

Alvarez-Buylla A, Kohwi M, Nguyen TM, Merkle FT (2008) The heterogeneity of adult neural stem cells and the emerging complexity of their niche. *Cold Spring Harb Symp Quant Biol* 73:357–365.

Alvarez-Dolado M, Calcagnotto ME, Karkar KM, Southwell DG, Jones-Davis DM, Estrada RC, Rubenstein JL, Alvarez-Buylla A, Baraban SC (2006) Cortical inhibition modified by embryonic neural precursors grafted into the postnatal brain. *J Neurosci* 26:7380-7389.

Ayuso-Sacido A, Roy NS, Schwartz TH, Greenfield JP, Boockvar JA (2008) Long-term expansion of adult human brain subventricular zone precursors. *Neurosurgery* 62:223–229; discussion 229–231.

Barkho BZ, Zhao X (2011) Adult neural stem cells: Response to stroke injury and potential for therapeutic applications. *Curr Stem Cell Res Ther* 6:327–338.

Boison D (2012) Adenosine dysfunction in epilepsy. *Glia* 60(8):1234–43.

Butti E, Bacigaluppi M, Rossi S, Cambiaghi M, Bari M, Cebrian Silla A, Brambilla E, Musella A, De Ceglia R, Teneud L, De Chiara V, D'Adamo P, Garcia-Verdugo JM, Comi G, Muzio L, Quattrini A, Leocani L, Maccarrone M, Centonze D, Martino G (2012) Subventricular zone neural progenitors protect striatal neurons from glutamatergic excitotoxicity. *Brain* 135:3320–3335.

Cassady JP, D'Alessio AC, Sarkar S, Dani VS, Fan ZP, Ganz K, Roessler R, Sur M, Young RA, Jaenisch R (2014) Direct lineage conversion of adult mouse liver cells and B lymphocytes to neural stem cells. *Stem Cell Reports* 3:948–956.

Castillo CG, Mendoza-Trejo S, Aguilar MB, Freed WJ, Giordano M (2008) Intranigral transplants of a GABAergic cell line produce long-term alleviation of established motor seizures. *Behav Brain Res* 193:17–27.

Chu K, Kim M, Jung KH, Jeon D, Lee ST, Kim J, Jeong SW, Kim SU, Lee SK, Shin HS, Roh JK (2004) Human neural stem cell transplantation reduces spontaneous recurrent seizures following pilocarpine-induced status epilepticus in adult rats. *Brain Res* 1023:213–221.

Cunningham M, Cho JH, Leung A, Savvidis G, Ahn S, Moon M, Lee PK, Han JJ, Azimi N, Kim KS, Bolshakov VY, Chung S (2014) hPSC-derived maturing GABAergic interneurons ameliorate seizures and abnormal behavior in epileptic mice. *Cell Stem Cell* 15:559–573.

Cusimano M, Biziato D, Brambilla E, Donega M, Alfaro-Cervello C, Snider S, Salani G, Pucci F, Comi G, Garcia-Verdugo JM, De Palma M, Martino G, Pluchino S (2012) Transplanted neural stem/precursor cells instruct phagocytes and reduce secondary tissue damage in the injured spinal cord. *Brain* 135:447–460.

Damgaard T, Plath N, Neill JC, Hansen SL (2011) Extrasynaptic GABAA receptor activation reverses recognition memory deficits in an animal model of schizophrenia. *Psychopharmacology* 214:403–413.

de Lanerolle NC, Kim JH, Robbins RJ, Spencer DD (1989) Hippocampal interneuron loss and plasticity in human temporal lobe epilepsy. *Brain Res* 495:387–395.

Deng W, Aimone JB, Gage FH (2010) New neurons and new memories: How does adult hippocampal neurogenesis affect learning and memory? *Nat Rev Neurosci* 11:339–350.

Devinsky O (2004) Therapy for neurobehavioral disorders in epilepsy. *Epilepsia* 45 Suppl 2:34–40.

Dupret D, Revest JM, Koehl M, Ichas F, De Giorgi F, Costet P, Abrous DN, Piazza PV (2008) Spatial relational memory requires hippocampal adult neurogenesis. *PLoS One* 3:e1959.

Engel J, Jr (2001) Mesial temporal lobe epilepsy: What have we learned? *Neuroscientist* 7:340–352.

Fu LY, van den Pol AN (2007) GABA excitation in mouse hilar neuropeptide Y neurons. *J Physiol* 579:445–464.

Gong C, Wang TW, Huang HS, Parent JM (2007) Reelin regulates neuronal progenitor migration in intact and epileptic hippocampus. *J Neurosci* 27:1803–1811.

Graham BM, Richardson R (2009) Acute systemic fibroblast growth factor-2 enhances long-term extinction of fear and reduces reinstatement in rats. *Neuropsychopharmacology* 34:1875–1882.

Han DW, Tapia N, Hermann A, Hemmer K, Hoing S, Arauzo-Bravo MJ, Zaehres H, Wu G, Frank S, Moritz S, Greber B, Yang JH, Lee HT, Schwamborn JC, Storch A, Scholer HR (2012) Direct reprogramming of fibroblasts into neural stem cells by defined factors. *Cell Stem Cell* 10:465–472.

Hattiangady B, Shetty AK (2010) Decreased neuronal differentiation of newly generated cells underlies reduced hippocampal neurogenesis in chronic temporal lobe epilepsy. *Hippocampus* 20:97–112.

Hattiangady B, Shetty AK (2012) Neural stem cell grafting counteracts hippocampal injury-mediated impairments in mood, memory, and neurogenesis. *Stem Cells Transl Med* 1:696–708.

Hattiangady B, Rao MS, Shetty AK (2004) Chronic temporal lobe epilepsy is associated with severely declined dentate neurogenesis in the adult hippocampus. *Neurobiol Dis* 17:473–490.

Hattiangady B, Shuai B, Cai J, Coksaygan T, Rao MS, Shetty AK (2007) Increased dentate neurogenesis after grafting of glial restricted progenitors or neural stem cells in the aging hippocampus. *Stem Cells* 25:2104–2117.

Hattiangady B, Rao MS, Shetty AK (2008) Grafting of striatal precursor cells into hippocampus shortly after status epilepticus restrains chronic temporal lobe epilepsy. *Exp Neurol* 212:468–481.

Hattiangady B, Kuruba R, Parihar VK, Shetty AK (2010) Intrahippocampal grafting of NSCs after status epilepticus eases both spontaneous seizures & cognitive dysfunction in a rat model of temporal lobe epilepsy. *Soc Neurosci Abstr*, 29.30.

Hattiangady B, Kuruba R, Shuai B, Waldau B, Shetty AK (2012) Neural stem cell grafting after status epilepticus restrains spontaneous recurrent seizures and preserves cognitive and mood function. *Soc Neurosci Abstr*, 35.07.

Henderson KW, Gupta J, Tagliatela S, Litvina E, Zheng X, Van Zandt MA, Woods N, Grund E, Lin D, Royston S, Yanagawa Y, Aaron GB, Naegele JR (2014) Long-term seizure suppression and optogenetic analyses of synaptic connectivity in epileptic mice with hippocampal grafts of GABAergic interneurons. *J Neurosci* 34:13492–13504.

Hester MS, Danzer SC (2013) Accumulation of abnormal adult-generated hippocampal granule cells predicts seizure frequency and severity. *J Neurosci* 33:8926–8936.

Howell OW, Doyle K, Goodman JH, Scharfman HE, Herzog H, Pringle A, Beck-Sickinger AG, Gray WP (2005) Neuropeptide Y stimulates neuronal precursor proliferation in the post-natal and adult dentate gyrus. *J Neurochem* 93:560–570.

Huang L, Wong S, Snyder EY, Hamblin MH, Lee JP (2014) Human neural stem cells rapidly ameliorate symptomatic inflammation in early-stage ischemic-reperfusion cerebral injury. *Stem Cell Res Ther* 5:129.

Hunt RF, Girskis KM, Rubenstein JL, Alvarez-Buylla A, Baraban SC (2013) GABA progenitors grafted into the adult epileptic brain control seizures and abnormal behavior. *Nat Neurosci* 16:692–697.

Huo JS, Zambidis ET (2013) Pivots of pluripotency: The roles of non-coding RNA in regulating embryonic and induced pluripotent stem cells. *Biochim Biophys Acta* 1830:2385–2394.

Jing M, Shingo T, Yasuhara T, Kondo A, Morimoto T, Wang F, Baba T, Yuan WJ, Tajiri N, Uozumi T, Murakami M, Tanabe M, Miyoshi Y, Zhao S, Date I (2009) The combined therapy of intrahippocampal transplantation of adult neural stem cells and intraventricular erythropoietin-infusion ameliorates spontaneous recurrent seizures by suppression of abnormal mossy fiber sprouting. *Brain Res* 1295:203–217.

Kanter-Schlifke I, Georgievska B, Kirik D, Kokaia M (2007) Seizure suppression by GDNF gene therapy in animal models of epilepsy. *Mol Ther* 15:1106–1113.

Kiyota T, Ingraham KL, Jacobsen MT, Xiong H, Ikezu T (2011) FGF2 gene transfer restores hippocampal functions in mouse models of Alzheimer's disease and has therapeutic implications for neurocognitive disorders. *Proc Natl Acad Sci U S A* 108:E1339–48.

Klausberger T, Marton LF, O'Neill J, Huck JH, Dalezios Y, Fuentealba P, Suen WY, Papp E, Kaneko T, Watanabe M, Csicsvari J, Somogyi P (2005) Complementary roles of cholecystokinin- and parvalbumin-expressing GABAergic neurons in hippocampal network oscillations. *J Neurosci* 25:9782–9793.

Kobayashi M, Buckmaster PS (2003) Reduced inhibition of dentate granule cells in a model of temporal lobe epilepsy. *J Neurosci* 23: 2440–2452.

Koehl M, Abrous DN (2011) A new chapter in the field of memory: Adult hippocampal neurogenesis. *Eur J Neurosci* 33:1101–1114.

Koh MT, Haberman RP, Foti S, McCown TJ, Gallagher M (2010) Treatment strategies targeting excess hippocampal activity benefit aged rats with cognitive impairment. *Neuropsychopharmacology* 35:1016–1025.

Korotkova T, Fuchs EC, Ponomarenko A, von Engelhardt J, Monyer H (2010) NMDA receptor ablation on parvalbumin-positive interneurons impairs hippocampal synchrony, spatial representations, and working memory. *Neuron* 68:557–569.

Kuruba R, Hattiangady B, Shetty AK (2009a) Hippocampal neurogenesis and neural stem cells in temporal lobe epilepsy. *Epilepsy Behav* 14 Suppl 1:65–73.

Kuruba R, Hattiangady B, Shuai B, Shetty AK (2009b) Effects of grafting of hippocampal stem/progenitor cells shortly after status epilepticus on the development of chronic epilepsy. *Cell Transplant* 18:221–221.

Lee R, Kim IS, Han N, Yun S, Park KI, Yoo KH (2014) Real-time discrimination between proliferation and neuronal and astroglial differentiation of human neural stem cells. *Sci Rep* 4:6319.

Leonard BW, Mastroeni D, Grover A, Liu Q, Yang K, Gao M, Wu J, Pootrakul D, van den Berge SA, Hol EM, Rogers J (2009) Subventricular zone neural progenitors from rapid brain autopsies of elderly subjects with and without neurodegenerative disease. *J Comp Neurol* 515: 269–294.

Litt B, Esteller R, Echauz J, D'Alessandro M, Shor R, Henry T, Pennell P, Epstein C, Bakay R, Dichter M, Vachtsevanos G (2001) Epileptic seizures may begin hours in advance of clinical onset: A report of five patients. *Neuron* 30:51–64.

Liu Y, Liu H, Sauvey C, Yao L, Zarnowska ED, Zhang SC (2013) Directed differentiation of forebrain GABA interneurons from human pluripotent stem cells. *Nat Protoc* 8:1670–1679.

Loscher W, Gernert M, Heinemann U (2008) Cell and gene therapies in epilepsy — promising avenues or blind alleys? *Trends Neurosci* 31:62–73.

Luscher B, Shen Q, Sahir N (2011) The GABAergic deficit hypothesis of major depressive disorder. *Mol Psychiatry* 16:383–406.

Mainio A, Alamaki K, Karvonen K, Hakko H, Sarkioja T, Rasanen P (2007) Depression and suicide in epileptic victims: A population-based study of suicide victims during the years 1988–2002 in northern Finland. *Epilepsy Behav* 11:389–393.

Miltiadous P, Kouroupi G, Stamatakis A, Koutsoudaki PN, Matsas R, Stylianopoulou F (2013) Subventricular zone-derived neural stem cell grafts protect against hippocampal degeneration and restore cognitive function in the mouse following intrahippocampal kainic acid administration. *Stem Cells Transl Med* 2:185–198.

Palmer TD, Markakis EA, Willhoite AR, Safar F, Gage FH (1999) Fibroblast growth factor-2 activates a latent neurogenic program in neural stem cells from diverse regions of the adult CNS. *J Neurosci* 19:8487–8497.

Paradiso B, Zucchini S, Su T, Bovolenta R, Berto E, Marconi P, Marzola A, Navarro Mora G, Fabene PF, Simonato M (2011) Localized overexpression of FGF–2 and BDNF in hippocampus reduces mossy fiber sprouting and spontaneous seizures up to 4 weeks after pilocarpine–induced status epilepticus. *Epilepsia* 52:572–578.

Parent JM, Murphy GG (2008) Mechanisms and functional significance of aberrant seizure-induced hippocampal neurogenesis. *Epilepsia* 49 Suppl 5:19–25.

Perez JA, Clinton SM, Turner CA, Watson SJ, Akil H (2009) A new role for FGF2 as an endogenous inhibitor of anxiety. *J Neurosci* 29:6379–6387.

Pertusa M, Garcia-Matas S, Mammeri H, Adell A, Rodrigo T, Mallet J, Cristofol R, Sarkis C, Sanfeliu C (2008) Expression of GDNF transgene in astrocytes improves cognitive deficits in aged rats. *Neurobiol Aging* 29:1366–1379.

Rao MS, Hattiangady B, Reddy DS, Shetty AK (2006) Hippocampal neuro-degeneration, spontaneous seizures, and mossy fiber sprouting in the F344 rat model of temporal lobe epilepsy. *J Neurosci Res* 83:1088–1105.

Rao MS, Hattiangady B, Rai KS, Shetty AK (2007) Strategies for promoting anti-seizure effects of hippocampal fetal cells grafted into the hippo-campus of rats exhibiting chronic temporal lobe epilepsy. *Neurobiol Dis* 27:117–132.

Redrobe JP, Dumont Y, St-Pierre JA, Quirion R (1999) Multiple receptors for neuropeptide Y in the hippocampus: Putative roles in seizures and cognition. *Brain Res* 848:153–166.

Reynolds BA, Weiss S (1992) Generation of neurons and astrocytes from isolated cells of the adult mammalian central nervous system. *Science* 255:1707–1710.

Ring KL, Tong LM, Balestra ME, Javier R, Andrews-Zwilling Y, Li G, Walker D, Zhang WR, Kreitzer AC, Huang Y (2012) Direct reprogramming of mouse and human fibroblasts into multipotent neural stem cells with a single factor. *Cell Stem Cell* 11:100–109.

Rodrigo C, Zaben M, Lawrence T, Laskowski A, Howell OW, Gray WP (2010) NPY augments the proliferative effect of FGF2 and increases the expression of FGFR1 on nestin positive postnatal hippocampal precursor cells, via the Y1 receptor. *J Neurochem* 113:615–627.

Sahay A, Hen R (2007) Adult hippocampal neurogenesis in depression. *Nat Neurosci* 10:1110–1115.

Sahay A, Scobie KN, Hill AS, O'Carroll CM, Kheirbek MA, Burghardt NS, Fenton AA, Dranovsky A, Hen R (2011) Increasing adult hippocampal neurogenesis is sufficient to improve pattern separation. *Nature* 472:466–470.

Scharfman HE, Pierce JP (2012) New insights into the role of hilar ectopic granule cells in the dentate gyrus based on quantitative anatomic analysis and three-dimensional reconstruction. *Epilepsia* 53 Suppl 1:109–115.

Schmidt HD, Duman RS (2010) Peripheral BDNF produces antidepressant-like effects in cellular and behavioral models. *Neuropsychopharmacology* 35:2378–2391.

Shetty AK (2011) Progress in cell grafting therapy for temporal lobe epilepsy. *Neurotherapeutics* 8:721–735.

Shetty AK (2014) Hippocampal injury-induced cognitive and mood dysfunction, altered neurogenesis, and epilepsy: Can early neural stem cell grafting intervention provide protection? *Epilepsy Behav* 38: 117–124.

Shetty AK, Hattiangady B (2007) Concise review: Prospects of stem cell therapy for temporal lobe epilepsy. *Stem Cells* 25:2396–2407.

Shetty AK, Turner DA (1998) *In vitro* survival and differentiation of neurons derived from epidermal growth factor-responsive postnatal hippocampal stem cells: Inducing effects of brain-derived neurotrophic factor. *J Neurobiol* 35:395–425.

Shetty AK, Turner DA (2000) Fetal hippocampal grafts containing CA3 cells restore host hippocampal glutamate decarboxylase-positive interneuron numbers in a rat model of temporal lobe epilepsy. *J Neurosci* 20:8788–8801.

Shetty AK, Zaman V, Hattiangady B (2005) Repair of the injured adult hippocampus through graft-mediated modulation of the plasticity of the dentate gyrus in a rat model of temporal lobe epilepsy. *J Neurosci* 25:8391–8401.

Shetty AK, Hattiangady B, Rao MS (2009) Vulnerability of hippocampal GABA-ergic interneurons to kainate-induced excitotoxic injury during old age. *J Cell Mol Med* 13:2408–2423.

Shindo A, Nakamura T, Matsumoto Y, Kawai N, Okano H, Nagao S, Itano T, Tamiya T (2010) Seizure suppression in amygdala-kindled mice by transplantation of neural stem/progenitor cells derived from mouse embryonic stem cells. *Neurol Med Chir* 50:98–105; discussion 105–106.

Snyder JS, Soumier A, Brewer M, Pickel J, Cameron HA (2011) Adult hippocampal neurogenesis buffers stress responses and depressive behaviour. *Nature* 476:458–461.

Spencer SS (2002) When should temporal-lobe epilepsy be treated surgically? *Lancet Neurol* 1:375–382.

Strine TW, Kobau R, Chapman DP, Thurman DJ, Price P, Balluz LS (2005) Psychological distress, comorbidities, and health behaviors among U.S. adults with seizures: Results from the 2002 national health interview survey. *Epilepsia* 46:1133–1139.

Thompson K (2009) Transplantation of GABA-producing cells for seizure control in models of temporal lobe epilepsy. *Neurotherapeutics* 6:284–294.

Turner DA, Wheal HV (1991) Excitatory synaptic potentials in kainic acid-denervated rat CA1 pyramidal neurons. *J Neurosci* 11:2786–2794.

Vezzani A, French J, Bartfai T, Baram TZ (2011) The role of inflammation in epilepsy. *Nat Rev Neurol* 7:31–40.

Waldau B, Hattiangady B, Kuruba R, Shetty AK (2010) Medial ganglionic eminence-derived neural stem cell grafts ease spontaneous seizures and restore GDNF expression in a rat model of chronic temporal lobe epilepsy. *Stem Cells* 28:1153–1164.

Chapter 16

Prospects of Neural Stem Cell Therapy for Alzheimer's Disease

Samuel E. Marsh and Mathew Blurton-Jones

Alzheimer's disease (AD) is the most common cause of age-related neurodegeneration, affecting over 5 million people in the United States alone. Unfortunately, all of the currently approved therapies for AD provide only transient palliative benefit and recent Phase III clinical trials have failed to meet their primary endpoints of slowing cognitive decline. It is therefore critical to develop novel therapeutic approaches to slow the progression of this prevalent and debilitating disease. Researchers had previously speculated that AD was too diffuse a brain disorder to benefit from a stem cell-based therapy, yet new evidence suggests this may not be the case. In this chapter, we will review recent work demonstrating the preclinical feasibility of using neural stem cell transplantation to treat and slow the progression of AD. We will also provide a critical overview of some of the mechanisms of action by which NSCs appear to mediate their effects and discuss some of the remaining hurdles to translation of NSC transplantation toward human clinical trials. Lastly, we will consider the importance of new technologies, such as induced pluripotent stem cells and direct reprogramming, that are beginning to offer new ways to enhance our knowledge and understanding of NSC transplantation and offer a glimpse of the potential for personalized medicine approaches to treat AD.

Introduction

Alzheimer's disease (AD) is the most prevalent age-related neurodegenerative disorder in the world. Today, over 5 million people living in the United States alone have a diagnosis of AD, and this number is expected to nearly triple by 2050 (Alzheimer's Association, 2013). Unfortunately, currently approved therapies target only symptomatic aspects of the disease, having no effect on the underlying pathology or long-term progression of AD. There is therefore a critical need to identify and develop innovative new therapies to treat the rapidly growing population of patients suffering from AD. One novel approach that has gained considerable attention in the last few years aims to harness the regenerative potential of neural stem cells (NSCs). Initial studies are indeed suggesting that NSC transplantation may offer a promising new alternative to traditional pharmaceutical-based treatments for AD.

Alzheimer's disease

Alzheimer's disease is characterized by a progressive loss of memory and cognitive function that eventually robs patients of their ability to care for themselves and carry out basic daily activities (Alzheimer's Association, 2013). Pathologically, AD is characterized by two hallmark protein aggregates, amyloid plaques and neurofibrillary tangles (NFTs), which accumulate in the brain and are composed of beta-amyloid (Aβ) and hyperphosphorylated tau proteins, respectively (Selkoe, 2001). In addition to these characteristic aggregates, AD patients also exhibit widespread synaptic and neuronal loss (Terry *et al.*, 1991). Importantly, synaptic loss begins early in the disease course and, interestingly, correlates far better with cognitive decline than either plaques or tangles (Terry *et al.*, 1991; Masliah *et al.*, 2001).

The prevailing theory in AD research, the amyloid hypothesis, postulates that overproduction and/or impaired clearance of Aβ results in the accumulation and aggregation of this peptide which in turn initiates a pathological cascade including hyperphosphorylation of tau, inflammation, synaptic loss, neuronal death, and progressive cognitive dysfunction (Hardy and Selkoe, 2002). The view that amyloid is the trigger of the pathological cascade of AD is supported by strong genetic evidence from rare dominantly inherited familial forms of AD. In some of these families early-onset AD is associated with mutations or triplication within the gene coding for amyloid precursor protein (APP), which as the name implies can be cleaved to produce beta-amyloid. Other families with early-onset AD carry mutations in either presenilin-1 or presenilin-2, genes which produce the catalytic component of the enzyme complex that liberates beta-amyloid from APP (Selkoe, 2001; Tanzi, 2012). This convincing genetic evidence has led many researchers and the pharmaceutical industry to focus almost exclusively on developing therapies that could either reduce the production of Aβ or enhance its clearance from the brain. However, to date none of these drugs has succeeded in preventing or slowing cognitive decline in late stage clinical trials (Golde *et al.*, 2011). While some have criticized the amyloid hypothesis itself for the failure of these trials, recent research demonstrates that amyloid begins to accumulate up to 15 years prior to the first signs of cognitive dysfunction and by that time, levels of amyloid within the brain may have even begun to plateau (Jack *et al.*, 2013). This has led to a reformulation of anti-amyloid therapies with new trials now underway to test whether Aβ-targeting drugs can be used to prevent, rather than treat AD. While such approaches may eventually prove useful in slowing or preventing the development of AD, our current diagnostic abilities limit the application of such therapies. The past failures of anti-amyloid therapies also suggest that is critical for the field to diversify its efforts and expand the examination of alternative drug targets and innovative therapeutic approaches. One such approach that is gaining considerable attention is the potential use of stem cell transplantation for AD. Given the unique regenerative capacity of stem cells, they may be just what is required to combat this devastating degenerative condition.

Are NSCs a viable therapy for AD?

The idea of harnessing the regenerative potential of NSCs for a neurodegenerative disorders is not revolutionary. Researchers have been exploring the use of fetal tissue transplantation and more recently, stem cell therapy for Parkinson's disease (PD) for over 20 years (Lindvall *et al.*, 1988). However, unlike AD, PD patients suffer from a more focal degeneration that primarily affects the dopamine producing cells within the substantia nigra. In contrast, AD involves far more widespread neuronal and synaptic loss in addition to the accumulation of the two hallmark proteinopathies. Consequently, AD researchers have often suggested that stem cell-based therapies could not provide a viable therapeutic option for a diffuse disorder such as AD. However, recent results have shown this may not be the case and that NSCs could be developed as a potential therapy for Alzheimer's disease. In this chapter we will provide an overview of the current state of research involving NSC transplantation for AD, discuss the potential mechanisms of action behind NSC-mediated benefits, review some of the hurdles that remain, and consider what the future of NSC therapies for AD may hold.

Investigating the Potential of NSCs as Therapy for AD

The number of studies examining NSC transplantation in AD animal models has expanded rapidly in the past decade. Studies have been conducted in a wide variety of animal models with a number of proposed mechanisms of action underlying the therapeutic benefit of NSC transplantation. However, the majority of studies have pointed toward four primary mechanisms of action that, either alone or in concert, allow NSCs to improve function in AD models. These proposed mechanisms include: cell replacement, neurotrophic support, therapeutic peptide delivery, and immune modulation (Figure 1).

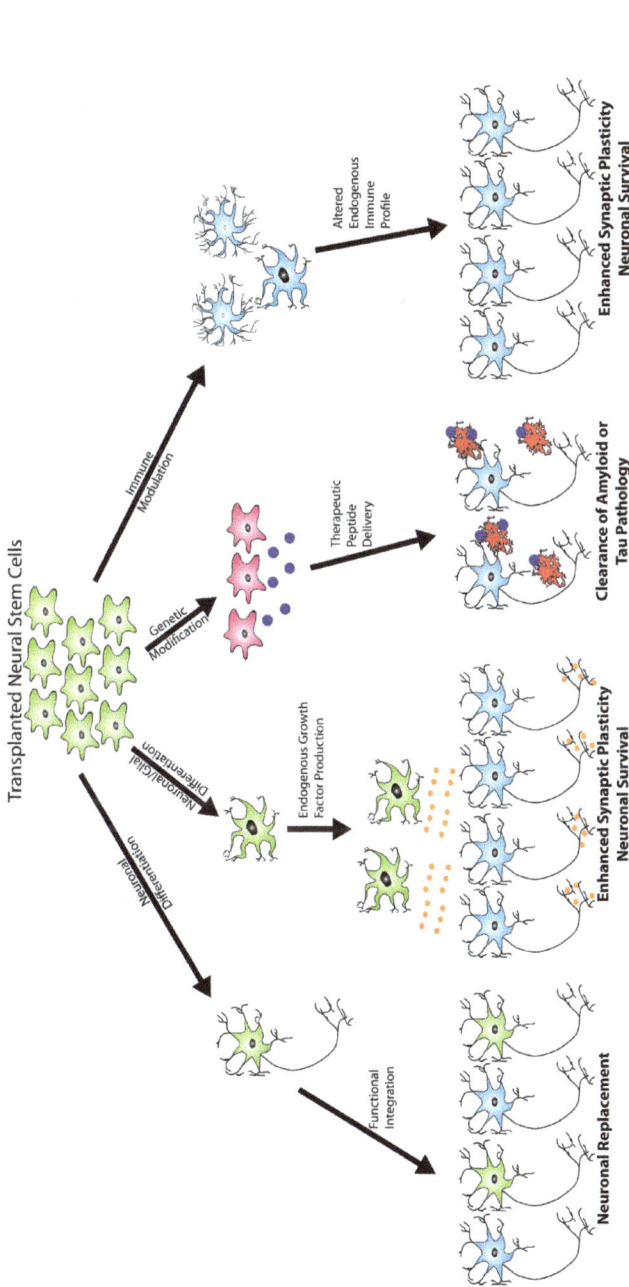

Figure 1. Mechanisms of action of transplanted neural stem cells (NSCs). Transplanted NSCs (green) may exert benefits via multiple mechanisms. **Neuronal Replacement** (far left): Following neuronal differentiation (neuron; green) cells could potentially integrate with host neuronal circuitry (blue) to replace neurons that have died during the course of AD. **Neurotrophic support** (2nd from the left): following differentiation (i.e. astrocyte; green) transplanted cells can produce growth factors (i.e. BDNF, GDNF; orange) which may enhance synaptic plasticity and neuronal survival. **Therapeutic peptide delivery** (2nd from right): NSCs can be genetically modified (purple) to generate and secrete therapeutic peptides (i.e. Aβ-degrading enzymes; blue) that reduce amyloid (red) or tau pathology. **Immune Modulation** (far right): Transplantation of NSCs may also induce alterations in host immune profiles (i.e. microglia and astrocytes; blue) that could enhance neuronal survival and/or synaptic plasticity and potentially decrease AD-associated pathology.

Neuronal replacement

Many neurological disorders are characterized by dysfunction and loss of neurons within specific brain regions. Replacement of these dead or dying cells is one mechanism by which neural stem cells could potentially exert therapeutic benefit (Figure 1; far left). However, unlike diseases such as Parkinson's where the degeneration is more focal, the neurodegeneration that occurs in AD is widespread, making a cell replacement strategy extremely daunting. Even in the case of PD, double-blind placebo-controlled fetal cell transplantation trials found that cell transplantation had no significant effect on disease progression (Morizane *et al.*, 2008).

Despite the incredible challenges of a neuronal replacement paradigm, some researchers have attempted to use neural stem cells to replace a specific population of neurons lost in AD, the cholinergic neurons of the basal forebrain (Auld *et al.*, 2002). Researchers have likely focused on these neurons as significant loss of function and death of the cholinergic forebrain neurons occurs in AD and correlates well with cognitive impairment (Perry *et al.*, 1978; DeKosky *et al.*, 1992). It has also been well established that cholinergic basal forebrain neurons, which connect strongly with both the cortex and hippocampus, play an important role in learning and memory. In order to model the loss of cholinergic neurons, researchers typically employ neurotoxic lesion models to create focal cholinergic cell loss. There are several types of lesions but the basic procedure involves the stereotactic delivery of the lesioning agent, such as ibotenic acid, to the nucleus basalis of Meynert (NBM), thereby depleting cholinergic innervation of the cerebral cortex and hippocampus and leading to cognitive dysfunction (Toledano and Alvarez, 2011).

One study used this model to examine the ability of NSCs to improve cognition and replace lost cholinergic innervation within mice. Following the lesion, the researchers transplanted green fluorescent protein (GFP)-labeled mouse embryonic stem cell-derived NSCs or undifferentiated mouse embryonic stem cells (ESCs) at four sites within the cortex (Wang *et al.*, 2006). Two months after transplantation, mice that received NSCs performed similarly to control non-lesioned animals in an eight-arm radial maze, a task that measures working and reference memory, whereas animals that just received the lesion were significantly impaired. Examination of the animals that received undifferentiated ESCs revealed significantly impaired performance compared to both lesion animals and controls. Subsequent analysis revealed that the impairment was due to tumors that had formed in all animals that received ESC grafts. When the researchers examined the fate of the transplanted NSCs *in vivo*, no glial differentiation was observed. However, many cells expressing markers indicating the production of acetylcholine and serotonin were identified. The group suggested that NSCs had differentiated into functional cholinergic and serotonergic neurons, which in turn led to the observed improvements in cognition.

However, there are several questions that remain. For example, the neurons were transplanted into one of the target regions, the cortex, rather than the basal forebrain. This approach would therefore not be expected to fully recapitulate the endogenous normal circuitry but perhaps instead provide a more tonic release of acetylcholine to the target neurons. It also remains unclear whether the transplanted cells formed active synapses with host neurons and integrated into the local cortical circuitry. This approach may therefore not necessarily have been an example of neuronal replacement so much as an example of targeted neurotransmitter supplementation.

While neuronal replacement may seem like a reasonable theory, the reality is much more complicated than simply replacing dead cells. In order for such a therapy to be truly viable, the transplanted cells must accomplish several difficult tasks. First, NSCs must differentiate into the appropriate phenotype of the lost cells, which has proven to be a very difficult task to accomplish *in vivo*. A recent study utilizing the same ibotenic lesion mouse model attempted to prime neuronal precursors towards cholinergic fate *in vitro* prior to transplantation, in order to more effectively replace the cholinergic neurons lost following the lesion (Moghadam *et al.*, 2009). The authors reported that priming of neuronal precursors resulted in twice as many cholinergic neurons generated *in vitro* compared to unprimed neuronal precursors. Despite the increase seen *in vitro,* no difference was found in the number of engrafted cholinergic neurons between primed and unprimed cells following transplantation. A second issue with attempting cell replacement in AD is that basal forebrain cholinergic neurons are not the only cells or region of the brain that degenerates in AD. In order for cell replacement to truly be a viable therapy, NSCs would need to become multiple different cell types in different regions of the brain, requiring either extensive migration or multiple invasive surgeries. Third, to truly replace lost neurons transplanted NSCs would be required to establish appropriate dendritic and axonal projections, and form appropriate synaptic connections with target neurons, a difficult feat that is normally only accomplished during neural development *in utero.* The ability of transplanted cells to correctly integrate into the existing adult neuronal circuitry, in a brain with 100 billion neurons and 100 trillion synapses (Kandel *et al.,* 2000), is likely the most difficult aspect of cell replacement therapy. However, even if this could be achieved, neuronal replacement would be unlikely to alter the underlying pathology of AD and therefore transplanted neurons would likely be just as susceptible to death and dysfunction as the host neurons they are intended to replace.

Neurotrophic support

Recently numerous studies have shown the ability of stem cells to provide therapeutic benefits without directly replacing dead or dying neurons. One mechanism behind this beneficial effect is hypothesized to be through the neurotrophic support of endogenous circuitry (Figure 1; 2nd from the left). Neurotrophic growth factors are key regulators of survival, plasticity, and activity in neurons within the adult brain (Tuszynski and Gage, 1995). For example, brain-derived neurotrophic factor (BDNF) is known to be a critical factor in the regulation of synaptic plasticity associated with hippocampal-dependent learning and memory, such that reduction of BDNF leads to profound cognitive deficits (Heldt *et al.,* 2007). This is particularly relevant to AD as the hippocampus is one of the brain regions critical for the formation and storage of memory and consequently, one of the areas most affected in the course of the disease (Geula, 1998). Deficits in the expression and transport of neurotrophic factors, including BDNF, have also been found to occur in AD and MCI patients as well as animal and cell models and these impairments likely play a role in synaptic loss (Salehi *et al.*, 2006; Arancio and Chao, 2007; Poon *et al.*, 2011). Finally, several lines of NSCs have been found to express and secrete high levels of several different neurotrophic factors including BDNF, glial-derived neurotrophic factor (GDNF), and nerve growth factor (NGF) (Lu *et al.*, 2003; Kamei *et al.*, 2007; Blurton-Jones *et al.*, 2009). Therefore, researchers have begun to examine whether transplanted NSCs could help support the endogenous neural circuitry through the secretion of neurotrophins.

Assessing the role of specific neuronal populations in learning and memory is a difficult task. Lesion models, like ibotenic acid lesions of the NBM, are not an ideal, because while they result in the death of cholinergic neurons, they can lack specificity and induce the death of other neuronal cell types and the activation of glia (Toledano and Alvarez, 2011). To circumvent this problem, we and others have utilized an inducible genetic model of neuronal loss (referred to as CaM/Tet mice) that allows for selective and regulatable ablation of hippocampal CA1 neurons (Yamasaki *et al.*, 2007). Cognitive testing of CaM/Tet mice illustrates the specificity of the model as mice display deficits in hippocampal- but not cortical-dependent cognitive tasks. This model is therefore ideal to study the effect of NSC transplantation on neuronal loss similar to the loss that occurs in the AD brain.

In one study, we examined the effect of GFP-mouse-NSC (mNSC) transplantation following the ablation of CA1 neurons in CaM/Tet mice (Yamasaki *et al.*, 2007). When cognition was examined one month after intrahippocampal mNSC transplantation, there was a non-significant trend towards behavioral improvement. However, by three months post-transplantation, mice that received mNSCs displayed significant improvements in memory compared to vehicle-injected lesioned mice. Immunohistochemical analysis following cognitive testing revealed that mice which received NSCs had increased synaptic density as well as robust increases in the number of CA1 neurons. On the basis of this result alone, it would be tempting to speculate that transplanted NSCs differentiated into new neurons and formed functional synapses with the surrounding tissue and therefore neuronal replacement mediated the cognitive effects. However, we found that less than 2% of transplanted cells expressed neuronal markers, while the majority of cells differentiated toward glial lineages. Therefore the increase in CA1 neurons was likely due to the ability of transplanted NSCs to provide support to vulnerable endogenous hippocampal neurons, enhancing their survival and promoting increased connectivity of the host neurons. While this study provides intriguing results for the ability of stem cells to promote functional recovery after severe neuronal loss, an important caveat which remains is that despite selective neuronal loss, this model suffers from one of the same limitations as other lesion models, a lack of underlying AD pathology. Though NSCs rescued cognition after the termination of neuronal loss, an argument could be made that the functional gains might not occur in a mouse where synaptotoxic pathology was also present.

In order to address this concern and further examine the potential efficacy of NSC transplantation for AD, we undertook an additional study with a widely utilized transgenic AD model, the triple transgenic mouse (3xTg-AD). The 3xTg-AD mouse recapitulates both of the primary proteinopathies of AD, amyloid plaques and neurofibrillary tangles (NFT), and develops cognitive deficits (Oddo *et al.*, 2003). Another critical factor of AD pathogenesis better replicated by this model is the impact of aging on the pathogenesis of AD and the general microenvironment of the aged brain. Together these represent distinct advantages of the 3xTg-AD model compared to cholinergic lesion models which lack pathology and often fail to account for the impact of aging (Toledano and Alvarez, 2011).

Utilizing the same NSCs as in the CaM/Tet study, 18-month-old 3xTg-AD and wild-type (WT) mice received bilateral stereotactic intrahippocampal injections of mNSCs or equivalent volume of vehicle. One month later, 3xTg-AD mice that received NSCs

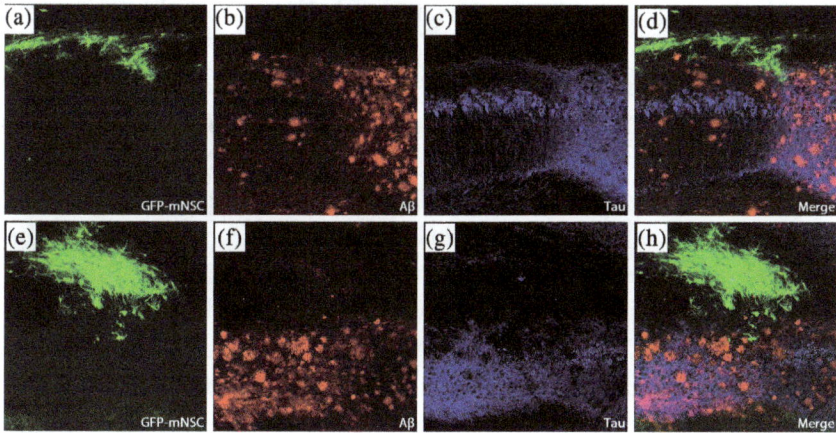

Figure 2. Neural stem cells (NSCs) survive and engraft well despite the presence of both amyloid and tau pathology. The 3xTg-AD mouse model recapitulates both of the major AD proteinopathies: amyloid plaques labeled by OC antibody (**b, f**) and neurofibrillary tangles labeled with AT8 antibody (**c, g**) and thus is an excellent model in which to study the therapeutic potential of NSC (**a, e**) transplantation. Several studies in our lab (Blurton-Jones *et al.*, 2009; Blurton-Jones *et al.*, 2014) have shown that GFP-mouse NSCs (**a, e**) are capable of engraftment and survival even in the presence of these established pathologies (D, H).

exhibited cognitive improvements in two cognitive tasks examining hippocampal-dependent memory whereas 3xTg-AD mice that received vehicle displayed impaired cognition. Given the presence of amyloid and tau pathology in this model, it was possible that a reduction in either or both of these pathologies might underlie the observed behavioral improvement. However, analysis of several measures of amyloid and tau pathology revealed that NSC transplantation has no impact on either pathology (Figure 2).

While amyloid and tau were unchanged, analysis of synaptic density in animals receiving NSC transplants revealed significant increases within the hippocampus, mirroring the prior results observed with the Cam/Tet lesion model. Neuronal differentiation of NSCs was also low in 3xTg-AD mice, indicating neuronal replacement was unlikely to be responsible for the observed synaptic plasticity. To further elucidate the mechanism of action behind the changes in synaptic density, we examined whether NSCs might be providing neurotrophic support to the endogenous hippocampal circuitry. Examination of the neurotrophin BDNF found that not only did NSCs produce high levels of BDNF *in vitro,* transplanted animals also exhibited increased BDNF via both biochemical and histological measures. In order to confirm that BDNF was necessary for the improved cognition and increased synaptic density, the experiment was repeated after knocking down BDNF in the mNSCs. Animals transplanted with knockdown cells displayed impaired cognition at similar levels to vehicle injected 3xTg-AD mice, while NSC transplanted animals again displayed improved cognition. Interestingly, the knockdown cells still increased synaptic plasticity compared to vehicle-injected animals although the increase was not as great as the increase seen with unmodified NSCs. This increase in synaptic plasticity even when BDNF was knocked down indicates that while the majority of the effect on cognition is BDNF-dependent, there are likely multiple neurotrophins or mechanisms involved in the enhancement of synaptic density mediated by NSC transplantation.

Another study that found similar benefits of NSC transplantation examined the effects of mouse NSCs in a mouse model of tauopathy (Hampton *et al.,* 2010). This tau model utilized exhibits robust cortical neuronal loss and accumulation of hyperphosphorylated tau. Researchers utilized a unilateral surgery protocol where animals received NSCs, derived from GFP-mice, on one side of the cortex and received a control surgery on the other side. Examination of neuron loss revealed that the NSC-treated side of cortex had a greater number of neurons compared to the side that received the control injection. Similar to results from our own studies, most of the NSC differentiation that was observed was glial, predominantly astrocytes, and again ruling out neuronal replacement as the mechanism responsible for the observed results. To further elucidate the mechanism by which NSCs influenced neuronal survival, Hampton and colleagues quantified mRNA levels of several neurotrophins within the transplanted tissue. Levels of BDNF and NGF mRNA were unchanged between NSC and control treated tissue but levels of GDNF mRNA were increased over 4-fold on the NSC transplanted side. Immunohistochemical analysis also confirmed high levels of GDNF protein expression in engrafted NSCs. Finally, owing to the predominantly astrocytic differentiation, the research- ers decided to examine whether transplanted astrocytes were just as neuroprotective as NSCs. The initial experiment was repeated with *ex vivo*-differentiated astrocytes instead of NSCs. Neuronal survival was again increased in the transplanted cortex, demonstrating that astrocytes alone were capable of mediating the neuroprotective effects, likely through secretion of GDNF.

Taken together the results of these studies, as well as research in other disease models, demonstrate that a large proportion of the beneficial effect of NSC transplantation may stem from secretion of neurotrophic factors. While the results of these studies were due to endogenous production of neurotrophins by NSCs, several research- ers have also begun to genetically modify NSCs to secrete high levels of certain neurotrophic factors in the hopes that this will further enhance their regenerative abilities. Successes have been reported using this technique in models of Parkinson's and amyotrophic lat- eral sclerosis (ALS) (Suzuki *et al.*, 2007; Ebert *et al.*, 2008). It will be intriguing to determine whether similar overexpression approaches can provide additional benefit in models of AD. While delivery of neurotrophic factors could also be achieved through gene therapy techniques, stem cells offer the unique ability to migrate throughout the brain, theoretically achieving a far greater distribution of thera- peutic proteins than viral approaches (Muller *et al.*, 2006; de Backer *et al.*, 2010). Another interesting aspect of the results in AD models is that rescue was achieved without impacting the underlying amy- loid or tau pathology. While none of the engrafted cells in these studies showed any accumulation of AD pathology, they also failed to moderate the progression of existing pathology. Evidence from long-term stem cells grafts in human Parkinson's disease patients have shown the presence of α-synuclein pathology accompanied by an apparent decrease in their functional potential (Chu and Kordower, 2010). While instances of host-to-graft transmission were rare, these data suggest that engrafted cells might be vulnerable to existing pathology. Despite many remaining questions, these initial studies demonstrate a tremendous potential for neurotrophic-based NSC therapy for AD.

Therapeutic peptide delivery

The use of NSCs as delivery vehicles for therapeutic peptides is not limited to endogenous or overexpressed neurotrophic factors; it can potentially be applied to a wide range of proteins and enzymes (Figure 1; 2nd from the right). Recent evidence has shown that rather than increased production of Aβ, it is impaired clearance that results in the accumulation of amyloid in the majority of AD cases [For review, see (Wildsmith *et al.*, 2013)]. Studies have also revealed that levels of Aβ degrading enzymes are decreased with normal aging and this decrease may be exacerbated in AD patients and transgenic mouse models (Caccamo *et al.*, 2005; Wang *et al.*, 2010). Therefore, engineering NSCs to express and secrete enzymes capable of degrading Aβ are of particular interest.

One such study, genetically engineered mouse GFP-NSCs to express Metalloproteinase 9 (MMP9), an enzyme known to degrade Aβ both *in vitro* and *in vivo* (Njie *et al.*, 2012). Using a unilateral study design researchers performed NSC, MMP9-NSC, or control transplantations into one hippocampus of the animals and a mock surgery on the contralateral hippocampus. Interestingly, both the NSCs and the MMP9-NSCs appeared to reduce plaque load in the hippocampus on the transplanted-side although no difference was observed in Aβ clearance between the two cell types. The authors speculated that since MMP9 is already being endogenously produced, then the MMP9-NSCs might not have secreted enough additional MMP9 to be therapeutically relevant. The authors also suggest that the local reduction in Aβ observed in response to NSC transplantation is due to a secondary effect of transplantation and not necessarily the cells themselves as graft size did not correlate at all with Aβ clearance. Curiously, the authors report the presence of microglia in their NSC cultures *in vitro*, yet the effects of transplanted microglia were not directly examined. If microglia persisted following transplantation, it is possible that they play a key role in the increased degradation of Aβ with both NSC transplanted groups.

While MMP9 modified cells failed to show efficacy, it is possible that other Aβ degrading enzymes may have more of an effect.

Another Aβ degrading enzyme that has garnered particular interest in the field is neprilysin. However, since neprilysin is normally membrane bound, simply overexpressing neprilysin may not be sufficient. Recently, we have shown that NSCs engineered to express a secreted form of neprilysin can reduce plaque load following transplantation into the hippocampus of two independent transgenic AD models (Blurton-Jones *et al.*, 2014). Interestingly, plaque loads were also reduced in the amygdala and medial septum, regions which receive direct projections from the hippocampus. This study provides just one example of how NSCs might be used as a delivery vehicle for anti-Aβ or anti-tau therapeutics. It will no doubt be important to determine whether this combinatorial approach provides additional functional benefits.

Immune modulation

Another mechanism by which NSCs may exert beneficial effects that has garnered considerable attention is through the potential modulation of endogenous immune activity (Figure 1; far right). It is well known that chronic inflammation plays an important role in many neurodegenerative disorders including Alzheimer's (Akiyama *et al.*, 2000). Therefore, enhancement of endogenous anti-inflammatory activity may yield beneficial effects on pathology and cognition. Much of this recent work has focused on the ability of mesenchymal stem cells to modulate neuroinflammation, but discussion of those results is beyond the scope of this chapter. However, one study by Ryu *et al.* (2009) has examined the ability of NSCs to modulate inflammation in an Aβ injection mouse model.

This AD model is created by injecting aggregated Aβ42, thought to be the most toxic Aβ species (Selkoe, 2001), directly into the hippocampus of rats. This injection induces localized neuroinflammatory changes and neuronal damage. Three days after the injection of Aβ, researchers transplanted mouse NSCs into the hippocampus and then examined their effect one week later. Examination of NSC differentiation revealed, not surprisingly given the very brief engraftment period, that cells were still nestin and GFAP positive, suggesting the cells were still largely in an undifferentiated NSC state. Examination of inflammatory makers found that Aβ42 injected animals exhibited increases in expression of the microglial marker Iba1, astrocytic GFAP, and tumor necrosis factor alpha (TNF-α), a proinflammatory cytokine. After only one week of engraftment, NSC-injected animals displayed decreases in Iba1 and TNF-α, while GFAP expression remained unchanged. Examination of neuronal damage in this model revealed that rats which received NSCs in addition to Aβ42 had significant increases in neuronal viability within the dentate gyrus of the hippocampus compared to Aβ42-injected rats. The concomitant reduction of TNF-α and Iba1 is logical as microglia are a major source of TNF-α in the CNS (Wyss-Coray and Rogers, 2012). Furthermore, increased neuronal viability found by Ryu *et al.* (2006) is also in agreement with research demonstrating that Aβ-induced activation of microglia *in vitro* leads to production of TNF-α which is required for Aβ's neurotoxic effect on neuronal cultures (Combs *et al.*, 2001).

There are some caveats to the study worth addressing in regards to anti-inflammatory capability of NSCs, perhaps the most prevalent is the model utilized in this study. By definition, injection of Aβ induces a number of non-physiological responses that could have dramatic effects on the inflammation observed including breaking the blood brain barrier and using non-physiological solvent to solubilize Aβ. The short time window between Aβ injection, stem cell delivery, and animal sacrifice also increases the likelihood that a robust acute immune response would be present that may not accurately mimic the more chronic inflammation that occurs in AD. While Aβ injection clearly leads to a localized acute inflammatory change, how closely those changes mimic the chronic global inflammation that occurs in AD is unclear (Van Dam and De Deyn, 2011). Further research in transgenic animal models which combine the presence of pathology, age, and chronic inflammation are needed to truly examine the potential immune-modulatory effects of NSCs.

Remaining Challenges in the Potential Translation of NSC Therapy for AD

The studies discussed support the potential of NSC-based therapies for AD but considerable research is clearly needed before these preclinical studies can be translated into a potential human clinical trial. Some of those limitations have already been discussed but other challenges clearly remain. Continued investigation and identification of the mechanisms involved is critical. Such studies will not only aid in the identification of optimal human NSC lines and refinement of therapeutic design, but may also uncover additional therapeutic targets and approaches. One limitation is that preclinical studies often focus on uncovering a single mechanistic explanation for the observed results. Yet, NSCs likely exert beneficial effects through modulation of multiple systems (Redmond *et al.*, 2007) making experimental manipulations and interpretation of results much more complex and challenging.

Another major challenge in the translation of these findings toward the clinic is the wide variety of methodology employed by different research groups, which complicates the ability to compare across and between studies. While this can be said of most fields of research, it is particularly true in studies of stem cell transplantation. For example, a wide variety of negative controls have been used including phosphate buffered saline (PBS), PBS+growth factors, culture medium, and dead cells (Tang *et al.*, 2008; Wu *et al.*, 2008; Blurton-Jones *et al.*, 2009; Hampton *et al.*, 2010). Differential reaction of the host tissue to these various controls could partially underlie why similar studies sometimes arrive at conflicting results. Another critical methodological consideration is the need for more complete disclosure of methods in publications. For instance, all of the studies discussed in the chapter thus far detailed how many cells were injected at each injection site, but none of the studies clearly state the viability of the cell suspension at the time of transplantation. It stands to reason that comparison of transplantation of 100,000 cells with a viability of 90% and 100,000 cells with 50%

viability may exhibit highly discrepant results. Finally, use of consistent and reliable cell labeling of NSCs prior to transplant is essential. Some studies examining NSC transplantation have utilized BrdU or fluorescent dyes in order to label cells prior to transplant. However, studies have shown that both BrdU and fluorescent dyes can spread from transplanted cells to host tissue (Coyne *et al.*, 2006; Li *et al.*, 2013). Thus accurate identification of graft vs. host cells is compromised and can lead to errors in analysis of survival and differentiation. In order for NSC-based therapies for AD to move closer to clinical translation, greater continuity of results is required and more standardized and detailed methodology should help in that regard.

Investigation of the safety and efficacy of human NSCs (hNSCs) in animal models of AD is also a critical requirement for translation to clinical trials. It is especially important to identify stem cell lines that have been grown under good manufacturing processes (GMP) that are capable of improving function as the FDA will only allow cells prepared under these kind of stringent conditions to be used in clinical trials. One major challenge to these evaluations is how to achieve stable engraftment of human cells following xenotransplantation into rodent models [For review see (Anderson *et al.*, 2011)]. Many studies utilize common pharmaceutical immunosuppressant paradigms, such as the calcineurin inhibitors FK506 or Cyclosporine-A. These chronic pharmacologic immune suppression paradigms are less than ideal as grafts survive initially but are eventually fully rejected (Anderson *et al.*, 2011) and long-term use of the drugs can be highly toxic in rodents (Mollison *et al.*, 1998). Use of immune suppression drugs in AD models has also been shown to modulate amyloid and tau pathology, potentially obscuring and complicating interpretation of results (Yoshiyama *et al.*, 2007; Hong *et al.*, 2010). One alternative to traditional immune suppression approach is the use of immune-deficient mouse models. These models allow for xenotransplantation without rejection of grafted tissue. However, currently no immune-incompetent mouse that also exhibits AD pathology exists. A final aspect complicating the use of hNSCs is a lack of data on the functional differences between fetal-derived NSCs and embryonic-derived NSCs. Our own unpublished data suggest that these cells differentiate and migrate in very different ways. For example, while fetal-derived hNSCs can migrate extensively in the adult mouse brain, ESC and iPSC-derived hNSCs show very little migration. Studies are therefore needed to better understand the effects of cell source and maturation on their functional capacity. Methods of derivation, cell culture, and cell sorting also likely lead to further differences between lines, even when derived from same type of source tissue. Much more work is needed in order to gain a better understanding of the different properties of different lines and what characteristics are optimal for a particular application.

Finally, before human clinical trials can begin, rigorous well-powered preclinical efficacy and safety studies must, of course, be performed. Most basic research studies, including those reviewed in this chapter, are often performed with relatively few animals. Unfortunately, many animal studies of AD and other neurodegenerative conditions have thus far failed to translate into effective therapies. It is therefore critical that rigorous, well-controlled, and appropriately blinded, pre-clinical studies are conducted and independently replicated prior to the initiation of any human trials.

The Future of NSC Transplantation in Alzheimer's Disease

Despite several important challenges, the future of NSC transplantation remains bright. The studies discussed in this chapter have provided a foundation for future work that will no doubt expand and enhance our understanding of NSC transplantation and its potential application to AD. Additionally, several recent advances in the field of stem cell biology may provide valuable tools to further drive the potential clinical application of stem cell therapies for AD.

The creation of induced pluripotent stem cells (iPSCs) from adult human tissue provided a transformative new technology that is accelerating our understanding of human development and disease (Takahashi *et al.*, 2007). This technology is also providing a novel approach to generate renewable sources of patient-derived NSCs. Not only does this circumvent the potential ethical concerns surrounding embryonic- or fetal-based NSC therapy, but it also opens up the possibility of a personalized medicine approach to NSC transplantation. By reprogramming a person's own cells, one can in principle generate autologous NSCs that can be transplanted without the need for immune suppression. Furthermore, utilizing gene correction techniques, it is also possible to potentially correct disease-associated mutations in iPSC lines prior to transplantation (Fong *et al.*, 2013).

NSCs, as well as differentiated neurons, astrocytes, etc., derived from iPSCs, are also proving to be invaluable tools to allow researchers to study the causes of AD and to test potential pharmacological interventions in human primary cells. For instance, several clinical trials in the past decade have tested gamma-secretase-modulators (GSMs) which aim to decrease generation of the more toxic Aβ42 peptide. Many studies have shown that these drugs can be efficacious in animal models as well as non-neuronal cell lines. However, all clinical trials with GSMs have failed in human patients. Recently, scientists created iPSCs from AD patients and healthy controls, differentiated them into neurons, and treated them with several GSMs to examine the efficacy of the drugs (Mertens *et al.*, 2013). Interestingly, it was found that while GSMs showed efficacy in non-neuronal cell lines, they had no effect when they were tested on patient-derived human neurons. Thus, studies in AD iPSCs may improve our ability to predict the clinical effects of a given treatment and inform the development of better pharmacologic-based treatments. Although more work is needed to better understand the characteristics of iPSC-derived NSCs and to examine the capability of these cells to improve cognition or alter pathology, they represent an exciting avenue of research for the future of cell therapy in AD.

Another exciting new stem cell technology that may lead to the development of additional therapeutic approaches is the direct *in vivo* reprogramming of cells within the CNS. Two recent studies using different techniques have shown the ability to reprogram mouse astrocytes within the brain into either neuroblasts or directly into neurons (Niu *et al.*, 2013; Guo *et al.*, 2014). These studies have demonstrated that the reprogrammed cells are electrophysiologically functional and are capable of becoming both glutamatergic and GABAergic neurons. Furthermore, one of the studies demonstrated that not only was reprogramming possible in normal mouse brain but also within a transgenic AD model. This innovative technology potentially offers a way to replace dead or dying neurons after injury or neurodegeneration without the need for direct NSC transplantation. There are several questions that still need to be addressed regarding this innovative technology. Similar to iPSCs, analysis of the ability of *in vivo* reprogramed cells to moderate pathology or recuse cognition in models of injury or neurodegeneration will be needed. Additionally, examination of the long-term survival, migration, and functionality of the reprogrammed cells will be important.

Conclusions

As we have discussed in this chapter, neural stem cell-based treatments for AD offer an innovative therapeutic approach for an otherwise untreatable disease. The studies examined in this chapter have laid the groundwork for stem cell-based therapies for AD by demonstrating the feasibility of this approach and defining several mechanisms through which NSCs likely exert their effects. While initial stem cell studies in related neurodegenerative conditions aimed to replace degenerating neurons, it now appears that this strategy is extremely challenging and complex. For a widespread disease such as AD, neuronal replacement represents an extremely daunting challenge that will likely take many decades of intense research to develop. Neurotrophic support, immune modulation, and use of NSCs as a peptide delivery vehicle in contrast are avenues which currently offer the most promise in regards to translation of a stem cell therapy toward human clinical trials. Our understanding of the mechanisms involved in NSC transplantation for AD has clearly progressed, but additional research will be needed to elucidate the cellular and molecular pathways by which NSCs exert their beneficial effects. While a number of challenges still remain, recent results and new technologies offer great hope that NSCs may one day provide a viable therapy for AD.

References

Akiyama H, Barger S, Barnum S, Bradt B, Bauer J, Cole GM, Cooper NR, Eikelenboom P, Emmerling M, Fiebich BL, Finch CE, Frautschy S, Griffin WS, Hampel H, Hull M, Landreth G, Lue L, Mrak R, Mackenzie IR, McGeer PL, O'Banion MK, Pachter J, Pasinetti G, Plata-Salaman C, Rogers J, Rydel R, Shen Y, Streit W, Strohmeyer R, Tooyoma I, Van Muiswinkel FL, Veerhuis R, Walker D, Webster S, Wegrzyniak B, Wenk G, Wyss-Coray T (2000) Inflammation and Alzheimer's disease. *Neurobiol Aging* 21:383–421.

Alzheimer's Association (2013) 2013 Alzheimer's disease facts and figures. *Alzheimers Dement* 9:208–245.

Anderson AJ, Haus DL, Hooshmand MJ, Perez H, Sontag CJ, Cummings BJ (2011) Achieving stable human stem cell engraftment and survival in the CNS: is the future of regenerative medicine immunodeficient? *Regen Med* 6:367–406.

Arancio O, Chao MV (2007) Neurotrophins, synaptic plasticity and dementia. *Curr Opin Neurobiol* 17:325–330.

Auld DS, Kornecook TJ, Bastianetto S, Quirion R (2002) Alzheimer's disease and the basal forebrain cholinergic system: relations to beta-amyloid peptides, cognition, and treatment strategies. *Prog Neurobiol* 68:209–245.

Blurton-Jones M, Kitazawa M, Martinez-Coria H, Castello NA, Muller FJ, Loring JF, Yamasaki TR, Poon WW, Green KN, LaFerla FM (2009) Neural stem cells improve cognition via BDNF in a transgenic model of Alzheimer disease. *Proc Natl Acad Sci U S A* 106:13594–13599.

Blurton-Jones M, Spencer B, Michel S, Castello NA, Agazaryan AA, Davis JL, Müller F-J, Loring JF, Masliah E, LaFerla FM (2014) Neural stem cells genetically-modified to express neprilysin reduce pathology in Alzheimer transgenic models. *Stem Cells Res Ther* 5:46–59.

Caccamo A, Oddo S, Sugarman MC, Akbari Y, LaFerla FM (2005) Age- and region-dependent alterations in Abeta-degrading enzymes: implications for Abeta-induced disorders. *Neurobiol Aging* 26:645–654.

Chu Y, Kordower JH (2010) Lewy body pathology in fetal grafts. *Ann N Y Acad Sci* 1184:55–67.

Combs CK, Karlo JC, Kao SC, Landreth GE (2001) beta-Amyloid stimulation of microglia and monocytes results in TNFalpha-dependent expression of inducible nitric oxide synthase and neuronal apoptosis. *J Neurosci* 21:1179–1188.

Coyne TM, Marcus AJ, Woodbury D, Black IB (2006) Marrow stromal cells transplanted to the adult brain are rejected by an inflammatory response and transfer donor labels to host neurons and glia. *Stem Cells* 24:2483–2492.

de Backer MW, Brans MA, Luijendijk MC, Garner KM, Adan RA (2010) Optimization of adeno-associated viral vector-mediated gene delivery to the hypothalamus. *Hum Gene Ther* 21:673–682.

DeKosky ST, Harbaugh RE, Schmitt FA, Bakay RA, Chui HC, Knopman DS, Reeder TM, Shetter AG, Senter HJ, Markesbery WR (1992) Cortical biopsy in Alzheimer's disease: diagnostic accuracy and neurochemical, neuropathological, and cognitive correlations. Intraventricular Bethanecol Study Group. *Ann Neurol* 32:625–632.

Ebert AD, Beres AJ, Barber AE, Svendsen CN (2008) Human neural progenitor cells over-expressing IGF-1 protect dopamine neurons and restore function in a rat model of Parkinson's disease. *Exp Neurol* 209:213–223.

Fong H, Wang C, Knoferle J, Walker D, Balestra ME, Tong LM, Leung L, Ring KL, Seeley WW, Karydas A, Kshirsagar MA, Boxer AL, Kosik KS, Miller BL, Huang Y (2013) Genetic correction of tauopathy phenotypes in neurons derived from human induced pluripotent stem cells. *Stem Cell Reports* 1:226–234.

Geula C (1998) Abnormalities of neural circuitry in Alzheimer's disease: hippocampus and cortical cholinergic innervation. *Neurology* 51: S18–29; discussion S65.

Golde TE, Schneider LS, Koo EH (2011) Anti-abeta therapeutics in Alzheimer's disease: the need for a paradigm shift. *Neuron* 69:203–213.

Guo Z, Zhang L, Wu Z, Chen Y, Wang F, Chen G (2014) *In vivo* direct reprogramming of reactive glial cells into functional neurons after brain injury and in an Alzheimer's disease model. *Cell Stem Cell* 14: 188–202.

Hampton DW, Webber DJ, Bilican B, Goedert M, Spillantini MG, Chandran S (2010) Cell-mediated neuroprotection in a mouse model of human tauopathy. *J Neurosci* 30:9973–9983.

Hardy J, Selkoe DJ (2002) The amyloid hypothesis of Alzheimer's disease: progress and problems on the road to therapeutics. *Science* 297: 353–356.

Heldt SA, Stanek L, Chhatwal JP, Ressler KJ (2007) Hippocampus-specific deletion of BDNF in adult mice impairs spatial memory and extinction of aversive memories. *Mol Psychiatry* 12:656–670.

Hong HS, Hwang JY, Son SM, Kim YH, Moon M, Inhee MJ (2010) FK506 reduces amyloid plaque burden and induces MMP-9 in AbetaPP/PS1 double transgenic mice. *J Alzheimers Dis* 22:97–105.

Jack CRJ, Knopman DS, Jagust WJ, Petersen RC, Weiner MW, Aisen PS, Shaw LM, Vemuri P, Wiste HJ, Weigand SD, Lesnick TG, Pankratz VS, Donohue MC, Trojanowski JQ (2013) Tracking pathophysiological processes in Alzheimer's disease: an updated hypothetical model of dynamic biomarkers. *Lancet Neurol* 12:207–216.

Kamei N, Tanaka N, Oishi Y, Hamasaki T, Nakanishi K, Sakai N, Ochi M (2007) BDNF, NT-3, and NGF released from transplanted neural progenitor cells promote corticospinal axon growth in organotypic cocultures. *Spine (Phila Pa 1976)*, 32:1272–1278.

Kandel ER, Schwartz JH, Jessell TM (2000) *Principles of Neural Science.* McGraw-Hill Health Professions Division: New York.

Li P, Zhang R, Sun H, Chen L, Liu F, Yao C, Du M, Jiang X (2013) PKH26 can transfer to host cells *in vitro* and *vivo*. *Stem Cells Dev* 22:340–344.

Lindvall O, Rehncrona S, Gustavii B, Brundin P, Astedt B, Widner H, Lindholm T, Bjorklund A, Leenders KL, Rothwell JC, Frackowiak R, Marsden CD, Johnels B, Steg G, Freedman R, Hoffer BJ, Seiger L, Stromberg I, Bygdeman M, Olson L (1988) Fetal dopamine-rich mesencephalic grafts in Parkinson's disease. *Lancet* 2(8626–8627): 1483–1484.

Lu P, Jones LL, Snyder EY, Tuszynski MH (2003) Neural stem cells constitutively secrete neurotrophic factors and promote extensive host axonal growth after spinal cord injury. *Exp Neurol* 181:115–129.

Masliah E, Mallory M, Alford M, DeTeresa R, Hansen LA, McKeel DW, Morris JC (2001) Altered expression of synaptic proteins occurs early during progression of Alzheimer's disease. *Neurology* 56:127–129.

Mertens J, Stuber K, Wunderlich P, Ladewig J, Kesavan JC, Vandenberghe R, Vandenbulcke M, van Damme P, Walter J, Brustle O, Koch P (2013) APP Processing in Human Pluripotent Stem Cell-Derived Neurons Is Resistant to NSAID-Based gamma-Secretase Modulation. *Stem Cell Rep* 1:491–498.

Moghadam FH, Alaie H, Karbalaie K, Tanhaei S, Nasr Esfahani MH, Baharvand H (2009) Transplantation of primed or unprimed mouse embryonic stem cell-derived neural precursor cells improves cognitive function in Alzheimerian rats. *Differentiation* 78:59–68.

Mollison KW, Fey TA, Krause RA, Andrews JM, Bretheim PT, Cusick PK, Hsieh GC, Luly JR (1998) Nephrotoxicity studies of the immunosuppressants tacrolimus (FK506) and ascomycin in rat models. *Toxicology* 125:169–181.

Morizane A, Li JY, Brundin P (2008) From bench to bed: the potential of stem cells for the treatment of Parkinson's disease. *Cell Tissue Res* 331:323–336.

Muller FJ, Snyder EY, Loring JF (2006) Gene therapy: can neural stem cells deliver? *Nat Rev Neurosci* 7:75–84.

Niu W, Zang T, Zou Y, Fang S, Smith DK, Bachoo R, Zhang CL (2013) *In vivo* reprogramming of astrocytes to neuroblasts in the adult brain. *Nat Cell Biol* 15:1164–1175.

Njie EG, Kantorovich S, Astary GW, Green C, Zheng T, Semple-Rowland SL, Steindler DA, Sarntinoranont M, Streit WJ, Borchelt DR (2012) A preclinical assessment of neural stem cells as delivery vehicles for anti-amyloid therapeutics. *PLoS One* 7:e34097.

Oddo S, Caccamo A, Shepherd JD, Murphy MP, Golde TE, Kayed R, Metherate R, Mattson MP, Akbari Y, LaFerla FM (2003) Triple-transgenic model of Alzheimer's disease with plaques and tangles: intracellular Abeta and synaptic dysfunction. *Neuron* 39:409–421.

Perry EK, Tomlinson BE, Blessed G, Bergmann K, Gibson PH, Perry RH (1978) Correlation of cholinergic abnormalities with senile plaques and mental test scores in senile dementia. *Br Med J* 2:1457–1459.

Poon WW, Blurton-Jones M, Tu CH, Feinberg LM, Chabrier MA, Harris JW, Jeon NL, Cotman CW (2011) beta-Amyloid impairs axonal BDNF retrograde trafficking. *Neurobiol Aging* 32:821–833.

Redmond DEJ, Bjugstad KB, Teng YD, Ourednik V, Ourednik J, Wakeman DR, Parsons XH, Gonzalez R, Blanchard BC, Kim SU, Gu Z, Lipton SA, Markakis EA, Roth RH, Elsworth JD, Sladek JRJ, Sidman RL, Snyder EY (2007) Behavioral improvement in a primate Parkinson's model is associated with multiple homeostatic effects of human neural stem cells. *Proc Natl Acad Sci U S A* 104:12175–12180.

Salehi A, Delcroix JD, Belichenko PV, Zhan K, Wu C, Valletta JS, Takimoto-Kimura R, Kleschevnikov AM, Sambamurti K, Chung PP, Xia W, Villar A, Campbell WA, Kulnane LS, Nixon RA, Lamb BT, Epstein CJ,

Stokin GB, Goldstein LS, Mobley WC (2006) Increased App expression in a mouse model of Down's syndrome disrupts NGF transport and causes cholinergic neuron degeneration. *Neuron*, 51:29–42.

Selkoe DJ (2001) Alzheimer's disease: genes, proteins, and therapy. *Physiol Rev*, 81:741–766.

Suzuki M, McHugh J, Tork C, Shelley B, Klein SM, Aebischer P, Svendsen CN (2007) GDNF secreting human neural progenitor cells protect dying motor neurons, but not their projection to muscle, in a rat model of familial ALS. *PLoS One* 2:e689.

Takahashi K, Tanabe K, Ohnuki M, Narita M, Ichisaka T, Tomoda K, Yamanaka S (2007) Induction of pluripotent stem cells from adult human fibroblasts by defined factors. *Cell* 131:861–872.

Tang J, Xu H, Fan X, Li D, Rancourt D, Zhou G, Li Z, Yang L (2008) Embryonic stem cell-derived neural precursor cells improve memory dysfunction in Abeta(1-40) injured rats. *Neurosci Res* 62:86–96.

Tanzi RE (2012) *The genetics of Alzheimer disease. Cold Spring Harb Perspect Med* 2.

Terry RD, Masliah E, Salmon DP, Butters N, DeTeresa R, Hill R, Hansen LA, Katzman R (1991) Physical basis of cognitive alterations in Alzheimer's disease: synapse loss is the major correlate of cognitive impairment. *Ann Neurol* 30:572–580.

Toledano A, Álvarez MI (2011) *Lesion-Induced Vertebrate Models of Alzheimer Dementia.* (De D, Peter Paul, Van D, Debby, eds), pp 295–345. Totowa, NJ: Humana Press.

Tuszynski MH, Gage FH (1995) Maintaining the neuronal phenotype after injury in the adult CNS. Neurotrophic factors, axonal growth substrates, and gene therapy. *Mol Neurobiol* 10:151–167.

Van Dam D, De Deyn PP (2011) Animal models in the drug discovery pipeline for Alzheimer's disease. *Br J Pharmacol* 164:1285–1300.

Wang Q, Matsumoto Y, Shindo T, Miyake K, Shindo A, Kawanishi M, Kawai N, Tamiya T, Nagao S (2006) Neural stem cells transplantation in cortex in a mouse model of Alzheimer's disease. *J Med Invest* 53:61–69.

Wang S, Wang R, Chen L, Bennett DA, Dickson DW, Wang DS (2010) Expression and functional profiling of neprilysin, insulin-degrading enzyme, and endothelin-converting enzyme in prospectively studied elderly and Alzheimer's brain. *J Neurochem* 115:47–57.

Wildsmith KR, Holley M, Savage JC, Skerrett R, Landreth GE (2013) Evidence for impaired amyloid beta clearance in Alzheimer's disease. *Alzheimers Res Ther* 5:33.

Wu S, Sasaki A, Yoshimoto R, Kawahara Y, Manabe T, Kataoka K, Asashima M, Yuge L (2008) Neural stem cells improve learning and memory in rats with Alzheimer's disease. *Pathobiology* 75:186–194.

Wyss-Coray T, Rogers J (2012) Inflammation in Alzheimer disease-a brief review of the basic science and clinical literature. *Cold Spring Harb Perspect Med* 2:a006346.

Yamasaki TR, Blurton-Jones M, Morrissette DA, Kitazawa M, Oddo S, LaFerla FM (2007) Neural stem cells improve memory in an inducible mouse model of neuronal loss. *Neurosci* 27:11925–11933.

Yoshiyama Y, Higuchi M, Zhang B, Huang SM, Iwata N, Saido TC, Maeda J, Suhara T, Trojanowski JQ, Lee VM (2007) Synapse loss and microglial activation precede tangles in a P301S tauopathy mouse model. *Neuron* 53:337–351.

Chapter 17

Neural Stem Cell Therapy for Spinal Cord Injury

Christopher J. Haas, Joseph F. Bonner, George Ghobrial,
and Itzhak Fischer

Introduction to Spinal Cord Injury

Spinal cord injury (SCI) is a complex disorder that manifests as varying degrees of motor, sensory, and autonomic dysfunction depending upon the location and severity of the lesion. Early clinical assessment, prompt surgical intervention, and a continued multidisciplinary approach to patient care are critical not only for immediate patient stabilization and limiting further primary and secondary injury, but also for stratification of patients for clinical trials of promising experimental therapies. Cellular transplantation utilizing neural stem cells (NSC) and neural progenitors has been demonstrated to be a promising therapeutic tool for SCI in animal models, holding the potential to improve the injured environment, replace lost cells, and promote functional recovery. Promising preclinical studies have ushered in a wave of clinical trials, directed at modulating various aspects of SCI pathology. This review will briefly discuss the pathophysiology and clinical presentation of SCI, including acute standard of care patient management, examine the potential therapeutic targets of SCI, and explore the various cellular

467

therapies, focusing on transplantation of NSC and progenitors that have shown therapeutic potential and those that are currently progressing to clinical trials.

Clinical presentation of SCI

The common definition of SCI is an insult to the spinal cord tissues, resulting in either a temporary or permanent deficit in motor, sensory, or autonomic function. SCI is a devastating condition that profoundly affects the quality of life of the injured individuals with respect to psychological, social, and financial burdens. It is estimated that 12,000 new cases of SCI occur annually in the United States with a total population of up to 332,000 affected individuals. Young males are disproportionately affected, and are estimated to incur lifetime costs as high as $4,633,137 for an individual with a high cervical lesion (C1–C4) suffered at age 25 (NSCISC, 2013). Furthermore, new data from the Christopher and Dana Reeve Foundation suggests that the number of individuals currently with paralysis could be as high as 1.2 million. SCI in human populations vary widely in the etiology, level of injury, severity and comorbidity. Traumatic SCI occurs mostly as a result of motor vehicle accidents with additional cases coming from sport accidents and violence (e.g., gun shots); however, over the past 20 years, increasing life expectancy has led to higher rates of new-onset SCI in the elderly, whom are prone to falls. SCI patients are often transferred to regional SCI specialty centers by 24 hours post-injury for specialized treatment (and potentially for entry into clinical trials). Clinical severity of SCI is categorized using the American Spinal Injury Association (ASIA) scale of impairment (where A is complete injury, B is motor complete, C and D are incomplete, and E is no impairment). Most patients affected by SCI have incomplete contusion/compression injuries that are classified as AIS B or C (Marino *et al.*, 2003). Although advances in patient care have brought life expectancy for patients with incomplete injuries (ASIA C/D) to near that of the general population, sequelae associated with SCI, including pressure ulcers, autonomic dysreflexia and neuropathic pain, contribute to an increased morbidity and mortality, resulting in costs to the United States healthcare system of billions of dollars per year (Albin *et al.*, 1980). As we may have reached the limits of SCI symptom management, a treatment that restores or protects sensory, autonomic and/or motor control is needed more than ever. Progress in the understanding of the pathophysiology of SCI, the development of promising strategies that utilize cell-based therapy to limit secondary injury and promote axonal regeneration to promote recovery, and the remarkable advances in neurorehabilitation and imaging techniques have resulted in the initiation of several clinical trials for SCI. In this chapter, we will focus on the state of stem cell therapy in SCI beginning with a discussion on the pathophysiology of SCI and the corresponding therapeutic targets, summarize the sources and properties of NSC, review the research on transplantation of these cells, and finally discuss ongoing clinical trials.

Pathophysiology of SCI

Primary injury

The mechanical force associated with the primary phase of the injury disrupts spinal tissue and in most cases results in a contusion, which continues as a compression injury caused by fractured bones (Norenberg *et al.*, 2004). The injury can also be associated with laceration, rotation, and stretching of the cord. Taken together these primary insults result in cell death, traumatic axonal injury of ascending and descending tracts, interruption of the blood brain barrier, invasion of immune cells and disruption of ionic balance. These events are characterized in the clinic by acute hemorrhage, swelling, spinal cord ischemia as well as irregularities of autonomic system. They are therefore treated at the acute stage with decompression strategies and stabilization of vital functions.

Secondary injury

Following primary insult, the injury undergoes a process of expansion, with an increase in cellular damage and death, axonal dysfunction, and the formation of an injury site that inhibits endogenous repair. Secondary injury is characterized by: (1) a sequence of inflammatory and immune responses (initially involving endogenous microglia and astrocytes followed by the recruitment and invasion of peripheral macrophages and lymphocytes); (2) excitotoxicity (e.g., glutamate, free radicals) leading to oxidative stress and further cell death of neurons, astrocytes, and oligodendrocytes; (3) demyelination leading to axonal dysfunction; and (4) the production of a physical and chemical glial scar. The glial scar, a potent inhibitor of repair, contains reactive astrocytes and inhibitory molecules such as chondroitin sulfated proteoglycans (CSPGs), which when combined with myelin-associated inhibitory molecules, such as myelin associated glycoprotein (MAG) and NoGo, further limits axonal regeneration and sprouting.

The cascade of events in secondary injury presents multiple neuroprotective therapeutic targets in the time shortly after SCI. These include strategies to reduce excitotoxicity (e.g., antioxidants), modulate inflammation (e.g., anti-inflammatory cytokines), inhibit cell death (anti-apoptotic reagents), and minimize the inhibitory environment (e.g., digest the CSPG components of the scar). These therapeutic targets share one critical component: timing. The timing of administration is critical to the success of any therapy aimed at neuroprotection.

Chronic stage

At the chronic stage (months and years post-injury) the lesion develops into a fluid-filled, cystic cavity surrounded by a glial scar, which serves to isolate the injury site, but also blocks axonal regeneration, precluding functional recovery. Besides the sensorimotor deficits, the chronic stage of the injury is also associated with neuropathic pain, autonomic dysreflexia and problems in bladder, sexual and digestive functions. Treatments of chronic SCI currently include symptom management, but hope remains that regenerative and/or cell-mediated therapies could restore lost function long after SCI.

Neural Stem Cells and Progenitors

SCI is defined by a cascade of complex pathological processes that show temporal and spatial specificity, and therefore present multiple therapeutic targets specific to the stage of the injury process. In general, therapeutic strategies can be divided into approaches that: (1) provide neuroprotection designed to limit the effects of secondary injury and (2) promote repair by promoting regeneration and plasticity. Neuroprotective strategies must be applied before the neuropathology of SCI has completely developed. Although this time is not well defined, neuroprotective strategies in animal models are generally applied within hours to days after SCI. Proof of principle studies may even be applied before injury or at the same time of injury. Strategies that promote regeneration or plasticity are not tied directly to the development of the injury but may work best when applied prior to the development of the glial scar or the death of surrounding cells. In short, although regenerative strategies do not *require* neuroprotective strategies, a combination of strategies that protects as well as regenerates would be ideal. NSC therapies are an attractive SCI therapy because they have the potential to be neuroprotective while also supporting regeneration and contributing to plasticity. We will now discuss types of stem cells and the characteristics that make different types of NSC desirable for SCI therapy.

Neural stem cell sources and properties

Stem cells are defined by the capacity to both self-renew and differentiate, but these properties vary dramatically among the different types of stem cells. Several terms may be used to describe NSC. We will use the term NSC to refer only to multipotent cells capable of producing neurons, astrocytes, and oligodendrocytes. We will use the terms progenitors and precursor cells to denote cells with restrictive proliferative abilities and differentiation potential. The origins of a stem cell population determine the potential and ability for self-renewal. Thus, when reviewing the options of NSC therapy it is important to consider the origin of these cells.

Pluripotent cells

Pluripotent embryonic stem (ES) cells derived from the inner cell mass of a blastocyst have (1) unlimited ability for self-renewal and (2) a multi-lineage differentiation potential that includes all three embryonic layers (endoderm, mesoderm and ectoderm). ES cells have been generated from different species including mice, rats, and humans allowing the banking and sharing of ES lines and allowing derivation of multipotent stem cells with restricted fate, including a variety of NSC. Pluripotent cells can also be induced by reprogramming mature cells, such as fibroblasts, into an ES cell-like state (termed induced pluripotent, iPS cells) using a process that initially required the induced expression of four master genes (c-myc, Oct4, Sox2 and Klf4) (Takahashi and Yamanaka, 2006). This method has been continually improved to avoid the use of viral vectors and oncogenes (Stadtfeld *et al.*, 2008; Kim *et al.*, 2009), increasing the safety of these cells. Nevertheless, significant hurdles remain to be addressed relative to the efficiency of reprogramming (see Chapter 11). The discovery and refinement of the iPS cell process have important implications for the future of stem cell research and their clinical application due to the possibility of autologous cell transplantation, avoiding the need for immune suppression (see Chapter 11).

Pluripotent ESC and iPSC offer significant advantages compared to other cells. Due to their replicative capacity, these cells provide a nearly unlimited stock of source material that can be banked. Furthermore, these cells possess the ability, given the proper environmental cues, to differentiate into a range of neural phenotypes, including NSC, more committed progenitors, or mature neurons, astrocytes, or oligodendrocytes. However, use of these cell populations mandates that careful preparation, derivation, and sorting quality control measures be followed prior to transplantation, as undifferentiated pluripotent ESC and iPSC have the potential to form teratomas after transplantation *in vivo*. While the use of hESC poses significant ethical concerns, the fact that current stocks of hESC do not reflect the genetic diversity of the population also represent a significant obstacle that requires the use of long-term immunosuppressive therapy. iPSC, in contrast, circumvent ethical concerns and the need for immunosuppression, offering the potential for autologous therapy, but are limited by varied reprogramming efficiency to the pluripotent state, a lack of understanding of differences between different iPSC-derived neural populations with respect to their ability to support recovery, and the need for FDA approval of each individual iPSC-derived line to be used in the clinic. Further obstacles to the routine use of hESCs in addition to the lengthy culturing time, are the procurement of a cell stock and the need for immunosuppression.

Multipotent cells

Multipotent NSC and progenitors can be prepared directly from the embryonic and adult nervous system, from which distinct populations of cells can be isolated using cell surface markers, or induced from ES and iPS cells using specific differentiation factors. The preparation of multipotent NSC from the embryonic spinal cord is closely related to the developmental events that begin in rats at E10.5 with the proliferation of neural epithelial cells lining the ventricular cavity of the caudal neural tube. Multipotent NSC cells can be isolated from rat E10.5 spinal cord and cultured either as neurospheres in suspension or grown as adherent cultures on a fibronectin substrate in the presence of mitogens such as fibroblast growth factor and epidermal growth factor. These cells can produce neuronal and glial progenitors, as well as mature neurons, astrocytes and oligodendrocytes *in vitro* and *in vivo*, consistent with their multipotent properties. Multipotent cells can also be found in the adult central nervous system (CNS) where they continue to proliferate and generate neurons in the subventricular zone (SVZ) and the subgranular zone (SGZ) of the hippocampal dentate gyrus. These highly specialized niches are the only regions of the adult CNS where neurogenesis occurs. Multipotent cells can be isolated from other regions of the CNS, including the cells lining the central canal of the spinal cord. Although the spinal cord niche does not support neurogenesis, spinal cord NSC can be prepared as multipotent neurospheres capable of generating neurons *in vitro*, demonstrating the importance of the environment.

Progenitor cells

In contrast to the multipotent NSC, fate-restricted progenitors are present in the embryonic rat spinal cord at later stages of development. Neuronal restricted progenitors (NRP) will only generate neurons and can be isolated from E13.5 or E14 rat spinal cord by immunopanning or sorting with antibodies against the embryonic neural cell adhesion molecule (E-NCAM) or the polysialic form (PSA-NCAM). Spinal cord derived-NRP are committed to the generation of neurons *in vitro* and *in vivo*, capable of producing multiple neurotransmitter phenotypes and can integrate with brain and spinal cord neural circuits (Yang *et al.*, 2000). GRP represent multiple classes of progenitors ranging from the tripotential GRP, which can generate two types of astrocytes and oligodendrocyte, to a variety of other progenitors such as oligodendrocyte-type 2 astrocyte (O2A) cells, oligodendrocyte progenitor cells (OPC), and astrocyte progenitor cells (APC). These progenitors can be selected based on the surface expression of antigens such as A2B5 and characterized by their potential to generate specific astrocyte phenotypes and oligodendrocyte *in vitro* and *in vivo*. Oligodendrocyte progenitors have been of particular interest to the field, due to their potential to restore myelination after SCI. The precise lineage of OPC in relation to other glial progenitors is complex and may depend on the developmental stage and specific region of the CNS from which these progenitors are isolated. In general, the two factors that regulate oligodendrocyte specification during development are Sonic Hedgehog (SHH), which promotes the oligogenic fate, and Bone Morphogenetic Protein (BMP), which drives differentiation into an astrocyte fate. Importantly, these cells can also be prepared from ES cells by various differentiation protocols.

NSC have also been identified and characterized in humans. In parallel, there are new differentiation protocols for preparation of NSC and progenitors from human ES and human iPS cells, exploiting the availability of well-defined lines and taking advantage of their potential application as autologous cells. As an example, the FDA has recently approved clinical trials for human ES-derived OPC by Geron, human stem cells derived from the CNS by StemCells Inc. and human fetal NSC prepared by Neuralstem Inc. (see discussion on clinical trials below). Similarly, a production process for human GRP from the embryonic CNS, which is consistent with FDA protocols (Q-Therapeutics), has facilitated a series of preclinical studies designed to initiate clinical trials.

Other cell types

Other cell types that cannot be used for canonical cell replacement in the injured spinal cord are attractive for cell-mediated therapies. Adult bone marrow stromal cells (MSCs), for example, have permissive properties that promote neuroprotection and regeneration of injured axons and can be used as autologous grafts, which circumvent the need for immunosuppressive agents. This makes them attractive candidates for cellular therapies, as is shown by the relatively large number of ongoing clinical trials. However, they are not suitable for replacement of neural cells (e.g., neurons) (Neuhuber *et al.*, 2004) despite claims of their neurogenic differentiation (Sanchez-Ramos 2002; Sanchez-Ramos 2000; Song 2007). Other promising candidates for cell transplantation include non-neural cells such as adipocytes, cells derived from the umbilical cord and placenta, and neural cells such as olfactory ensheathing cells (OEC) and Schwann cells, some of which have already been implemented in clinical trials.

Therapeutic Strategies

Therapeutic strategies can be applied by a variety of methods including pharmacological approaches by drug delivery, genetic approaches by *in vivo* and *ex vivo* gene therapy, cellular transplantation with a focus on cell replacement, and rehabilitation using specific protocols of physical therapy designed to promote neural plasticity and the retraining of spared neural circuits for maximum efficiency. In reality, most of these strategies have the potential to provide multiple therapeutic effects. While these therapies may give therapeutic benefit, the potential for adverse effects, such as neuropathic pain, spasticity, or tumorigenicity, must be considered in the preclinical application of these treatments, prior to proceeding to clinical trials. For example, transplantation of oligodendrocyte precursor cells (OPC), like those used in the Geron Stem Cell Trial, designed to replace oligodendrocytes and improve myelination are also capable of providing neuroprotection and limiting the expansion of the injury. These cells, however, may pose a risk of tumorigenicity upon transplantation if the methods of derivation from ESC fail to remove all pluripotent ESCs that failed to successfully differentiate (see section on Oligodendrocyte replacement). It has also become clear that an effective treatment plan may require combinatorial strategies designed to address the different phases of the injury or multiple components at a particular injury stage. For example, a strategy that is designed to promote regeneration will likely benefit from an early intervention that reduces cell death and axonal damage, thus maximizing the population of neurons available for regeneration. At the chronic injury state, alternative combinatorial strategies, such as those designed to enhance the intrinsic regenerative capacity of CNS neurons (e.g., by activating specific signaling pathway such a mTOR) when coupled with the reduction of local inhibitors of axon growth (e.g., glial scar digestion using Chondroitinase) may also be necessary for axonal regeneration. Ongoing combinatorial therapies have also focused on the inclusion of rehabilitation, as an activity-dependent strategy that can facilitate the effects of regeneration, plasticity, and motor learning (Liu *et al.*, 2012; Houle and Cote, 2013). For example, in forming a relay across a dorsal column lesion to reconnect the disrupted sensory axons with their target at the brainstem (Bonner *et al.*, 2011), it is important to consider connectivity not only at the anatomical and synaptic level, but also at the functional level. It is reasonable to assume that such connectivity, even when optimized, will not recreate the exact circuit nor form the precise sensory maps relative to the uninjured CNS. It may therefore be necessary to include an activity-dependent step that will not only facilitate such connectivity by strengthening active synapses, but also interpreting the new sensory data in a way that is functionally relevant. Studies that have shown the reorganization of the cortex after injury and following repair (Aguilar *et al.*, 2010; Kao *et al.*, 2011; Graziano *et al.*, 2013) support this hypothesis and bring the concepts of neural plasticity and activity to the forefront of the therapeutic stage.

Cell Transplantation with Neural Stem Cells and Progenitors

Although a variety of cells are available for transplantation in models of SCI (Fehlings and Vawda, 2011), this review is focused on the therapeutic potential of NSC and progenitor transplantation. The advantages of cell therapy include the potential to address the multifactorial nature of injury and repair, the ability to deliver permissive factors by genetic modification of transplantable cells, using transplants that can promote both neuroprotection and repair, and the possibility for cell replacement. The disadvantages of cellular therapy depend on the specific type of cells used for transplantation and include: the cost of isolation, expansion, and storage of cells, potential tumorigenicity and immune rejection (see Table 1).

In recent years there have been important advances in the field of cell therapy for SCI, with significant progress in understanding the properties of NSC, identifying different sources for the preparation of these cells and developing transplantation protocols that target the distinct phases of injury and recovery, including replacement therapy (Tetzlaff *et al.*, 2011; Garbossa *et al.*, 2012; Mothe and Tator, 2013). NSC and progenitors represent one class of the growing candidates for cellular therapy in SCI. Utilizing this specific class of cells for clinical application depends on a multitude of factors that include: (1) understanding the basic biology of NSC and their mechanism of their action; (2) developing effective methods for the isolation, preparation, expansion, and cryopreservation by a clinically-compatible, good laboratory manufacturing process that can get FDA approval; (3) defining the specific target of therapy (e.g.,

Table 1. Sources of neural stem cells and progenitors.

Cells	Source	Properties	Advantages	Problems
ES Cells	Blastocyst	Pluripotent	Self-renewal Multiple Phenotypes	Tumorigenicity Differentiation Protocols
iPS Cells	Reprogrammed Somatic Cells	Pluripotent	Self Renewal Multiple Phenotypes Autologous Transplantation	Reprogramming Tumorigenicity Differentiation Protocols
Embryonic NSCs	Embryonic CNS	Multipotent	Large Numbers (by expansion) Differentiation to all neural phenotypes (neurons, astrocytes, oligodendrocytes)	Environmental Dependence
Embryonic Progenitors	Embryonic CNS — lineage restricted	Phenotypically Committed	Control over phenotype	Limited Numbers Limited Self-renewal Capacity Limited Differentiation Capacity
Adult NSC	Adult CNS —	Multipotent or lineage restricted	No need for embryonic tissue	Limited Numbers

neuronal cell replacement); (4) assessing risk factors relative to benefits (e.g., potential tumor formation when using ESC and iPSC); and finally, (5) preparing transplantation protocols that can be easily and effectively applied (e.g., noninvasive delivery of cells).

Fetal tissue transplants

Transplants of fetal spinal cord (FSC) tissue into the injured spinal cord, which started 30 years ago, have been the predecessor for the therapeutic use of NSC and progenitors. These pioneering studies tested the efficacy of segmental and dissociated FSC from rats, and discovered that transplants derived from E11–14 integrated with host tissue and generated differentiated neural cells including neurons (Reier *et al.*, 1992). Interestingly, the FSC grafts initially experienced extensive cell death, followed by subsequent proliferation and expansion, likely from a population of NSC and progenitors present in the FSC at corresponding developmental stage (Kalyani *et al.*, 1998). Indeed, a direct comparison of transplants from E14 FSC tissue to transplants of neuronal and glial restricted progenitors (NRP/GRP) derived from the same developmental stage showed remarkable similarities (Lepore and Fischer, 2005). The presence of both neuronal and glial progenitors creates a supportive microenvironment for the survival and differentiation of neurons likely through the generation of permissive astrocytes. This is a lesson learned from the development of the embryonic spinal cord, reproduced with FSC transplants, and then applied to the grafting of neural progenitors. Despite encouraging results that demonstrated that FSC transplants promote modest improvement of function and axonal growth into and out of the graft (Bregman and Reier, 1986; Houle and Reier, 1988; Bernstein-Goral and Bregman, 1997), there was no evidence of bridging across the graft/injury site or generation of functional relays. This approach was limited by the inability to detect graft-derived cells (with these experimental studies lacking transgenic animals or viral vectors for reliable analysis of transplanted tissue) and by the complexities of preparing sufficient fetal tissue for transplantation experiments.

However, renewed interest in FSC has been sparked by the availability of transgenic rats [expressing Alkaline Phosphatase (AP) or Green Fluorescent Protein (GFP)], which have afforded researchers to undertake a more detailed analysis of the grafts with respect to their phenotype and growth. Furthermore, this technology demonstrated the formation of graft-derived neurons, axon growth from grafted cells out of the graft (Lepore and Fischer, 2005), as well as support of respiratory function following upper cervical injury (White *et al.*, 2010). More recent experiments demonstrated that grafting of E14 spinal cord (which have been dissociated and trypsinized) subacutely into a complete transection together with a complex mixture of 10 growth factors and matrix molecules resulted in extensive and long distance growth of graft axons and connectivity associated with improved locomotion (Lu *et al.*, 2012). However, some of the conclusions regarding connectivity and improved function of this study have now been challenged in a replication study (Sharp *et al.*, 2014). Additional lessons pertaining to effective strategies for stem cell transplantation can be learned from our own recent studies comparing the survival of FSC transplants with neural progenitors in a complete transection injury. In this study (Medalha *et al.*, 2014), we demonstrated poor survival of NRP/GRP grafts compared to those of FSC in the complete transection model. These results were surprising as the mix of NRP/GRP was very effective in a hemisection injury, not only in terms of survival and generation of neurons, but also in forming a functional relay (Bonner *et al.*, 2011). When rats that underwent a complete transection were acutely grafted with E14 FSC, without the addition of any exogenous factors, as opposed to the use of NRP/GRP grafts, the grafted cells survived, integrated with host tissue, and generated neurons. These results indicate that in a severe injury (or scaling any injury to large animals), there is a need for additional measures to generate an appropriate microenvironment that achieves effective transplantation. The comparison of E14 FSC to the corresponding progenitors (NRP/GRP) suggests that the presence of other cells (e.g., endothelial cell to improve vascularization), matrix molecules, and survival and growth factors may play an integral role in the survival, differentiation, and integration of grafted cells in complex injury models.

Neuronal cell replacement

Following injury, the spinal cord fails to generate neurons from endogenous NSC. Although these cells have multipotent properties *in vitro*, the adult spinal cord — unlike the SVZ and hippocampus — lacks the neurogenic niche necessary for neuronal differentiation and they are directed towards a glial fate. Thus, neuronal cell replacement using NSC transplants remains challenging due to gliogenic environment of the injured spinal cord. Furthermore, neuronal replacement requires integration of newborn neurons into a functional circuit without aberrant connections that can induce undesired effects, such as neuropathic pain. A classical neuronal replacement approach in the context of SCI could target either motor neurons or interneurons that are damaged following the primary and secondary stages of injury, particularly when they occur in the cervical and lumbar regions. Alternatively, it is possible to transplant NSC and progenitors that will generate neurons *in vivo* and form functional relays to reconnect disrupted tracts. The concept of connectivity by relays is also related to spontaneous and induced plasticity and reorganization of the CNS, in which ascending or descending tracts can reconnect through local circuits of interneurons and circumvent the need for long distance regeneration (Bareyre *et al.*, 2004).

Motor neuron replacement

Replacement of motor neurons in the spinal cord requires the generation of not only of the correct neuronal phenotype, but also the recapitulation of afferent connectivity at the level of the ventral horn with descending control from the cortex (in a spatially organized manner)and axonal projections through the ventral roots to innervate muscle targets. Such a replacement therapy could be applicable for SCI and a variety of degenerative spinal disorders like ALS (Koliatsos *et al.*, 2008). Consequently, there has been impressive progress in the development of differentiation protocols that generate motor neurons from ES cells (Hester *et al.*, 2011). There has also been a breakthrough in the development of reprogramming methods that allow the conversion of mouse and human fibroblasts into functional spinal motor neurons, termed induced motor neurons by the Eggan laboratory (Son *et al.*, 2011). Several studies have recently shown a proof-of-concept for the ability to generate graft-derived motor neurons from a preparation of ES cells that survived and integrated with the host spinal cord (Lee *et al.*, 2007; Soundararajan *et al.*, 2007; Chipman *et al.*, 2012; Takazawa *et al.*, 2012). When combined with treatments that promote directional axon growth, these motor neurons were able to innervate distal musculature and form functional synapses (Yohn *et al.*, 2008; Umbach *et al.*, 2012). Nevertheless, this approach is still at the very early stages of research and most of the therapeutic efforts have been directed to improve neuroprotection and slow the degenerative process, particularly in the field of ALS, with potential for translation to SCI. In fact, studies that have used transplants of human NSCs, isolated from fetal tissue, showed that these cells integrate and form functional synapses with the motor circuitry (Xu *et al.*, 2009; Hefferan *et al.*, 2012), which could provide trophic support to injured or degenerating motor neurons. Similarly, transplantation of embryonic motor neurons into the peripheral nerve re-innervated the muscle and thus reduced motor neuron atrophy (Grumbles *et al.*, 2012).

Interneurons

In the lumbar cord, a replacement strategy directed to the interneuronal circuit that composes the central pattern generator (CPG) (Butt and Kiehn, 2003) could be utilized for functional reconnectivity. Although the anatomy of the CPG locomotor circuitry is poorly understood, the physiological and functional properties with respect to rhythmicity have been extensively studied. Based on cellular and molecular studies that elucidated the developmental program of the spinal cord, it was discovered that the ventral region of the cord is formed along a SHH gradient to generate domains known as p3, pMN, p2, p1 and p0, which express a unique set of transcription factors that define the profile of the corresponding progenitor cells in each region. Utilizing these transcription factors, it was therefore possible to prepare effective protocols that could "prime" multipotent NSC towards distinct progenitors of the ventral spinal cord. Such protocols include the addition of retinoic acid as a caudalizing factor to pattern development of the spinal cord with subsequent application of SHH as a ventralizing factor (Li *et al.*, 2008; Hu and Zhang, 2010) to pattern the ventral spinal cord. There are also specific markers to identify the specific subpopulation of ventral interneurons (e.g., V0, V1, V2 and V3), relying on an array of transcription factors that define the corresponding domains. Preliminary studies directed at replacement of ventral interneurons began with the development of a gray matter kainic acid lesion in the spinal cord, which specifically targeted the ventral interneuron population (Hadi *et al.*, 2000; Magnuson *et al.*, 2001) and the grafting of neural progenitors that were primed to become ventral interneurons (See J, 2008, See J, 2009).

Relay

In contrast to the classical cellular replacement strategies, the spinal cord also offers an opportunity to test the formation of functional neuronal relays, where the impetus for long distance growth is removed from the injured axon and placed on NSC-derived neurons. The relay strategy requires that graft-derived neurons bridge the injured spinal cord by: (1) making a local synapse at the injury site with the disrupted axons (necessitating the short distance regeneration of injured host axons into the graft); (2) graft-derived neurons extend axons to a target beyond the injury; and (3) the formation of a second synaptic connection between the graft-derived neurons and the target, thus allowing the transmission of signals and restoration of connectivity. We have studied the formation of a functional relay in a cervical dorsal column injury model that disrupts sensory tracts, which connect the DRG with the dorsal column

nucleus (DCN) in the brainstem. In a series of studies, we first demonstrated that a mixed population of neuronal and glial restricted
progenitors (NRP and GRP) is needed to produce neurons within
the injury site (Lepore and Fischer, 2005), including excitatory glutamatergic neurons that are critical for a relay (Bonner *et al.*, 2010).
Astrocytes generated by the grafted GRP provide a supportive environment for the survival and differentiation of graft-derived neurons. In fact, the NRP/GRP mix allowed the axotomized sensory
axons to regenerate into the graft and form synaptic connection
with graft-derived neurons without additional intervention (Bonner
et al., 2011). In subsequent studies, we confirmed the permissive
properties of GRP, demonstrating that GRP alone (or astrocytes
derived from these GRP) promote the same level of regeneration of
sensory axons into the graft (Haas *et al.*, 2012; Haas and Fischer,
2013); see section on astrocyte replacement. To connect graft-
derived neurons with the brain stem target, we generated a neurotrophin gradient that served as an axonal guidance cue for
graft-derived neurons, by injection of a BDNF-expressing lentivirus
into the DCN target (see Figure 1). The anatomical analysis of graft
phenotype, axonal growth, and synapse formation was facilitated by
the use of cells derived from alkaline phosphatase (AP) transgenic
rats and verified by tracing experiments and immunoelectron
microscopy that revealed excitatory synaptic connections (Bonner
et al., 2011). Functional analyses were carried out first by stimulus-
evoked c-Fos expression and subsequently confirmed by electrophysiological recording, demonstrating not only that host axons
formed active synapses with graft-derived neurons at the injury site,
but also that graft-derived neurons sent axons which formed active
synapses with the DCN target. Importantly, by electrophysiological
recording, the signal propagating to the DCN had a temporal delay
consistent with a bi-synaptic relay (rather than the original mono-
synaptic connection). These results highlight the potential for
NRP/GRP grafts to form functional relays in other injury models,
such as lesions of the descending corticospinal tract (CST). Indeed,
GRP grafts differentiated into permissive astrocytes and supported
the modest growth of severed CST axons into the graft (Haas,

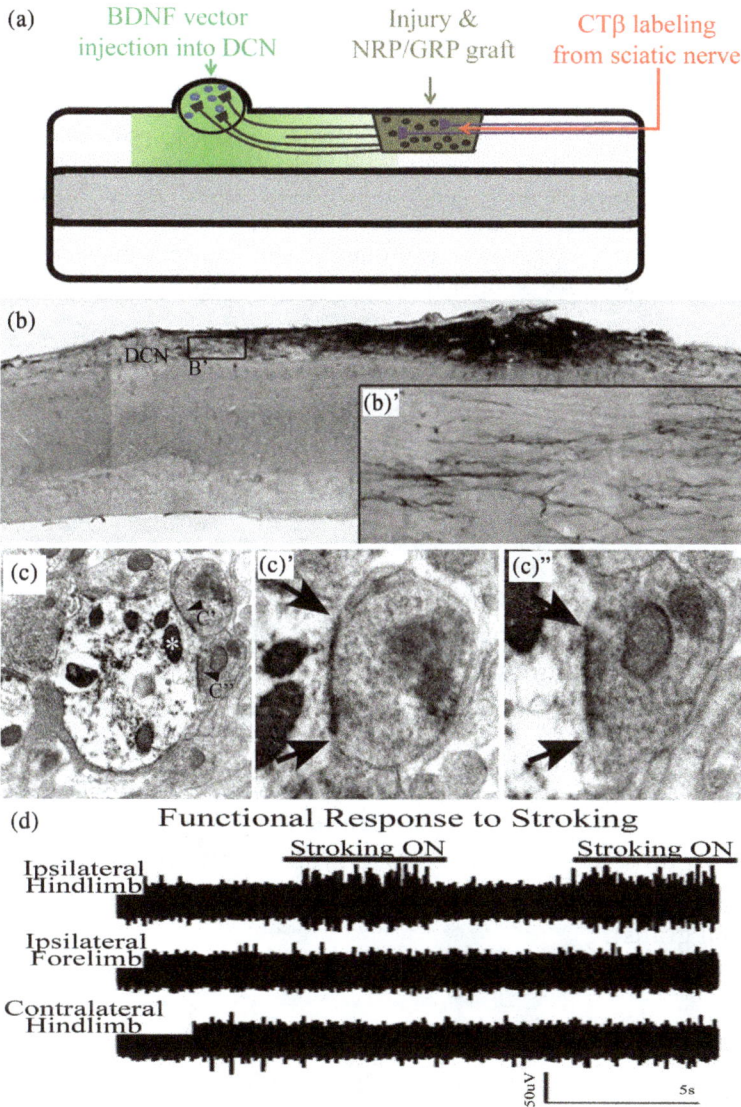

Figure 1. Forming a functional relay in the dorsal column sensory system. Diagram of the components necessary for the formation of a functional relay in the lesioned dorsal column sensory system (a). Grafts of NRP/GRP survive acute transplantation into the injured spinal cord, support the regeneration of lesioned dorsal column sensory axons traced from the ipsilateral sciatic nerve with Cholera toxin b (CTB) into the graft, and graft-derived neurons extend axons under lentivrial-mediated expression of BDNF to the normal target of sensory axons, the

◄──

Figure 1. (*Continued*)   DCN (b). b' represents area of high magnification in B showing AP+ axons extending to the DCN. Regenerating CTB-traced axons formed structural synaptic connections with graft-derived neurons [indicated by white asterisk (*)], as demonstrated by Immunoelectron microscopy (c). c' and c" represent high magnification of areas in c, while arrowheads depict post-synaptic densities. Graft-derived neurons formed synaptic relays between regenerating axons derived from the sciatic nerve and with neurons located in the DCN as demonstrated by recorded electrophysiological activity in response to tactile stimulation (e.g., stroking hindlimb ipsilateral to the graft) to the ipsilateral hindlimb, but not the ipsilateral forelimb or contralateral forelimb (d). Adapted from (Bonner *et al.*, 2011).

unpublished studies), compatible with previous reports that demonstrated permissive astrocyte bridges are integral in supporting regeneration of CST axons (Zukor *et al.*, 2013). Taken together, this data represents an important initial step in promoting relay formation with NRP/GRP grafts.

Similar attempts to form a relay with neural progenitors using a severe injury model of transection failed due of the poor survival of the graft. However, these experiments allowed survival and connectivity when using E14 spinal cord tissue that contains the same populations of neural progenitors (Lu *et al.*, 2012; Medalha *et al.*, 2014). These experiments indicate that additional components, such as growth factors, extracellular matrix molecules, and possibly endothelial cells, present in the fetal tissue preparation are needed to support the survival and differentiation of progenitor cells (see section on fetal grafts).

Oligodendrocyte cell replacement — myelination

Remyelination is an important therapeutic target for SCI and a promising application for NSC in general and OPC in particular (Mekhail *et al.*, 2012). The focus on promoting remyelination by oligodendrocyte replacement originates with the vulnerability of these cells to the processes of ischemia and secondary injury that occur after SCI. The resulting oligodendrocyte death causes loss of conduction and demyelinated axons are exposed to further damage and dysfunction. Endogenous OPC present at the injury proliferate, but fail to fully myelinate axons underscoring the complexities of endogenous cell composition and fate determination in the micro-environment of the injured spinal cord (McDonald and Belegu, 2006). Efforts have continued to identify and characterize glial precursors that generate oligodendrocytes and effective methods for the preparation of cells that can be grafted to promote myelination [reviewed by (Faulkner and Keirstead, 2005; Franklin and Ffrench-Constant, 2008; Almad *et al.*, 2011)]. Proof-of-principle experiments designed to test the ability of grafted cells to myelinate axons utilized an ethidium bromide demyelination lesion (Oka *et al.*, 2004) and the congenitally demyelinated shiverer mouse (Warrington *et al.*, 1993; Yandava *et al.*, 1999; Windrem *et al.*, 2004), demonstrated the potential of transplanted cells to myelinate axons. One of the most promising approaches has been the use of OPC, alone, or in combination with growth factors that enhance oligodendrocyte differentiation and survival and ultimately contributing to restoration of function. For example, transplantation of OPC derived from human ES cells (Keirstead *et al.*, 2005) have shown increased myelination associated with improved function in subacute, but not chronic, SCI. However, transplantation of OPCs may also confer other benefits by providing neurotrophic support to surrounding tissue (Zhang *et al.*, 2006) that provides neuroprotection and sparing of damaged tissue (Sharp *et al.*, 2010). Similar transplantation experiments with rodent progenitors derived from the embryonic spinal cord (Cao *et al.*, 2005b; Cao *et al.*, 2010) or adult CNS (Windrem *et al.*, 2004) promoted remyelination, conduction through the spinal cord, and recovery of function. These transplantation experiments have been combined with delivery of growth factors by either *ex vivo* gene therapy where the cells were modified to express neurotrophins (Cao *et al.*, 2005b) or CNTF (Cao *et al.*, 2010), or by inclusion of a battery of growth factors that promote survival, including platelet-derived growth factor, basic fibroblast growth factor, and epidermal growth factor (Karimi-Abdolrezaee *et al.*, 2006). Some progress has also been demonstrated in chronic SCI where a combination therapy utilizing adult progenitors, together with growth factor and Chondroitinase supplementation, generated oli-godendrocytes, but also enhanced the growth of descending axons (Karimi-Abdolrezaee *et al.*, 2010). Alternative myelination strategies can be provided by Schwann cell transplantation (Oudega and Xu, 2006).

It is important to note that it is very difficult to separate the effects of neuroprotection by the grafted cells from the effects on remyelination and recovery of function. Theoretically, selective ablation of the grafted cells that reverses functional recovery will support the latter interpretation (Cummings *et al.*, 2005). Caution should be used when interpreting results in strategies utilizing ablation techniques, as the ablation process itself can generate inflammation and local damage that will confound an unequivocal conclusion. In any case, the challenge for effective remyelination is the need for long-term survival and integration of the replacement oligodendrocytes. This goal likely necessitates the development of effective strategies for the isolation or pre-differentiation of oligodendrocyte precursors from the fetal or adult CNS or from pluripotent stem cells, the inclusion of factors to support survival and differentiation of trans-planted cells, and caution with respect to formation of tumors by ES/iPS-derived cells and unwanted side effects such as allodynia (Hofstetter *et al.*, 2005).

Astrocyte replacement

Astrocytes play an important role in the maintenance and function of the nervous system by providing a scaffold for neuronal architecture, modulating the blood-brain barrier, regulating metabolic and trophic activity, and supporting the formation and function of synapses (Pekny and Nilsson, 2005; Freeman, 2010; Sofroniew and Vinters, 2010; Zhang and Barres, 2010; Nag, 2011; Haas *et al.*, 2012). Astrocytes respond to SCI by undergoing a spectrum of morphological, biochemical, and functional alterations that are triggered by local cues and are dependent on the location, severity, and time course of the injury (White and Jakeman, 2008). Traditionally this response has been thought of as detrimental, as these reactive astrocytes produce an inhibitory glial scar and secrete factors that limit axonal growth (Fitch and Silver, 2008); however, there is growing evidence that the changes in host astrocytes following injury include a wide spectrum of dynamic properties — both toxic and protective (Sofroniew, 2009; Sofroniew and Vinters, 2010; Lepore and Maragakis, 2011; Lepore *et al.*, 2011). For example, astrocytes are capable of providing support for axonal growth and neuroprotection in a process that limits secondary injury (Bush *et al.*, 1999; Faulkner *et al.*, 2004; Fitch and Silver, 2008; Rolls *et al.*, 2009; Sofroniew and Vinters, 2010).

Early transplantation studies explored astrocyte replacement for SCI using astrocytes derived from the developing CNS. Transplantation of primary astrocytes, derived from the embryonic (Kliot *et al.*, 1990) or neonatal (Smith *et al.*, 1986; Smith and Silver, 1988; Smith *et al.*, 1990; Smith and Miller, 1991; Wang *et al.*, 1995; Olby and Blakemore, 1996; Joosten *et al.*, 2004) CNS into a variety of injury models, confirmed the beneficial properties of immature astrocyte transplantation, demonstrating a variety of beneficial outcomes including decreased glial scar formation, decreased lesion area and necrosis of host tissue, axonal sprouting and regeneration, and modest recovery of function.

During CNS development astrocytes may originate from a variety of progenitor cells including GRP, which have the potential to give rise to both astrocytes and oligodendrocytes. GRP can be isolated from the embryonic spinal cord by cell surface expression of the A2B5 marker (Rao and Mayer-Proschel, 1997; Rao *et al.*, 1998; Wu *et al.*, 2002), often accompanied by negative selection of NRP using the cell surface expression of E-NCAM. These cells are capable of extensive proliferation in the presence of basic fibroblast growth factor (Rao *et al.*, 1998; Haas *et al.*, 2012), allowing for the expansion and cryopreservation of large cell stocks, as well as differentiation into astrocytes *in vitro* (Rao *et al.*, 1998; Gregori *et al.*, 2002; Haas *et al.*, 2012) and *in vivo* (Herrera *et al.*, 2001; Han *et al.*, 2004). The established procedures for the isolation, and expansion of GRP and their ability to differentiate into astrocyte stand in contrast to the more tedious and limiting methods for preparation of primary cultures of astrocytes from the post-natal CNS. These properties make GRP attractive candidates for translational research and therefore, recent studies sought to examine the therapeutic potential of GRP following transplantation into the injured spinal cord. Acute transplantation of GRP into a thoracic contusion injury model demonstrated a variety of beneficial effects on the environment of the injured spinal cord, including decreased glial scarring and growth of injured host sensory and motor axons (Hill *et al.*, 2004), without adverse effects, such as allodynia or hyperalgesia. Similarly, transplantation of human GRP and human BMP4-derived astrocytes into a contusion model of SCI promoted anatomical and functional recovery in the absence of neuropathic pain (Jin *et al.*, 2011; Haas and Fischer, 2013). Other studies utilized GRP in combinatorial strategies involving rolipram delivery (Nout *et al.*, 2011) or multi-neurotrophin (D15A) expression (Cao *et al.*, 2005a; Fan *et al.*, 2013) and observed benefits in clinically important outcomes such as bladder and sexual function, or locomotion, respectively. Furthermore, GRP grafts supported the modest growth of CST axons into the graft following cervical dorsal hemisection (Haas, unpublished studies), compatible with previous reports (Zukor *et al.*, 2013). Taken together, this data on sensory and motor axons suggests that GRP are capable of promoting modest axonal regeneration into the graft, but that combinatorial strategies utilizing GRP as a therapeutic platform, which combine GRP with either NRP for relay formation or enhancing the intrinsic growth capacity of injured axons for long distance regeneration, may be necessary for reconnectivity across the injured spinal cord.

In contrast, a series of studies by Davies and colleagues demonstrated that rodent and human GRP-derived astrocytes, predifferentiated utilizing Bone Morphogenetic Protein-4 (BMP4), promoted extensive axonal growth and partial functional recovery when acutely grafted into a cervical dorsal column hemisection model of SCI (Davies *et al.*, 2006; Davies *et al.*, 2008; Davies *et al.*, 2011). Surprisingly, transplantation of GRP or GRP pre-differentiated into astrocytes utilizing ciliary neurotrophic factor (CNTF) failed to promote axonal growth and functional recovery, and had

adverse effects, including thermal hyperalgesia and mechanical allodynia. We did not observe any differences between transplants of
GRP or astrocytes pre-differentiated from GRP utilizing BMP-4 or
CNTF when utilizing GRP isolated from E13.5 rodent spinal cord,
or prepared by a clinically-compatible protocol from human CNS
tissue. Transplants of either GRP or GRP-derived astrocytes supported the growth of axons into, but not out of the graft, following
a cervical SCI (Haas *et al.*, 2012; Haas and Fischer, 2013), with no
differences amongst the groups. These results are consistent with
previous studies that demonstrated the beneficial effects of GRP
transplants in a contusion model of SCI (Hill *et al.*, 2004; Jin *et al.*,
2011; Nout *et al.*, 2011; Fan *et al.*, 2013).

The generation of different types of astrocytes with distinct
properties during development or following injury is determined by
the interaction of an intrinsic expression program with external
signals that depend on the state of the environment (White and
Jakeman, 2008; Freeman, 2010). Similarly, the differentiation of
glial precursors into various astrocyte subtypes depends on the specific population of precursors and the factors present in the culture.
Indeed, GRP treatment with BMP4 or CNTF *in vitro* produced distinct astrocyte phenotypes (Davies *et al.*, 2006; Davies *et al.*, 2008;
Davies *et al.*, 2011) that nevertheless remained heterogeneous (Haas
et al., 2012; Haas and Fischer, 2013). Specifically, GRP treated with
BMP4 produced predominantly stellate GFAP+ astrocytes, whereas
CNTF treatment produced predominantly long-process GFAP+
astrocytes that retained markers characteristic of immature GRP,
such as A2B5 and Ki67. Importantly, though the directed differentiation of GRP *in vitro* can give rise to clearly identifiable subpopulations of astrocytes, such cultures retain significant heterogeneity,
reflecting the complexity of astrocyte biology. Evidence suggests that
GRP have multiple and divergent fate potentials depending upon
their rostrocaudal location in the CNS, as well as their dorsoventral
positioning (Gregori *et al.*, 2002; Hochstim *et al.*, 2008; Hewett,
2009). The challenges of obtaining uniform populations are further
underscored by the divergent effects of morphogens, such as BMP
signaling through BMPR1a and BMPR1b (Sahni *et al.*, 2010).

Furthermore, several reports have noted that time in culture, combined with the use of mitogens, can affect not only the capacity for cellular differentiation but also the functional properties of GRP and astrocytes *in vitro* and *in vivo* [(Haas unpublished studies) (*in vitro* and *in vivo*) (Smith *et al.*, 1990; Rao *et al.*, 1998; Noble, 2006; Bithell *et al.*, 2008)].

Advances in the field of stem cell biology have now allowed the opportunity to prepare and test GRP and astrocytes derived from human ESC and iPSC. A number of recent studies have examined diverse protocols for astrocyte differentiation from pluripotent stem cells. Krenick and colleagues were able to direct astrocyte differentiation through a process that transitioned through a NSC/neural progenitor stage prior to treatment with CNTF to generate astrocytes. Following developmental principles, these immature astrocytes transitioned sequentially through an A2B5+ GRP and CD44+ astrocyte precursor stage, prior to expressing GFAP, the characteristic astrocyte marker. The transition to the progenitor and astrocyte stages required extensive differentiation *in vitro*, with approximately 90 and 180 days to reach the CD44+ and GFAP+ stage, respectively (Krencik *et al.*, 2011; Krencik and Zhang, 2011). Emdad and colleagues used a similar approach involving pluripotent stem cell growth on irradiated mouse fibroblasts, prior to differentiation with CNTF, in combination with Matrigel, to achieve significant astrocyte differentiation in as little as 35 days (Emdad *et al.*, 2012). Using a novel, chemically-defined, xeno-free culture system, Shaltouki and colleagues were also able to rapidly prepare cryopreservable astrocyte restricted precursors and astrocytes from NSC derived from hESC and iPSC in 21 and 35 days, respectively (Shaltouki *et al.*, 2013). Importantly, the astrocytes derived from these studies were capable of exerting functional effects, such as increasing synapsin-1 expression in neurons when co-culture was performed, glutamate transport, and calcium wave propagation (Krencik *et al.*, 2011; Krencik and Zhang, 2011; Shaltouki *et al.*, 2013). Furthermore, transplantation into the uninjured rodent CNS demonstrated that transplanted human astrocyte progenitors (Krencik *et al.*, 2011; Krencik and Zhang, 2011) and astrocytes (Shaltouki *et al.*, 2013) survived transplantation. Importantly, our preliminary studies have shown that transplanted astrocyte progenitors and astrocytes, generated by the Shaltouki protocols, were able to survive transplantation into the injured spinal cord, and support axonal growth and regeneration of sensory host axons into the graft (Haas/Ghobrial unpublished studies). These results are similar to previous reports utilizing GRP and astrocytes isolated from fetal tissue (Haas *et al.*, 2012; Haas and Fischer, 2013). The translation of astrocyte replacement strategies for SCI into the clinic requires the development of relevant protocols for their derivation from pluripotent cells and the generation of preclinical data for FDA approval. In the derivation of glial progenitors and astrocytes for transplantation particular attention must be paid to standardization of protocols to ensure minimal batch-to-batch variability and the removal of all pluripotent cells, which have the potential to form teratomas upon transplantation.

Endogenous Repair by Local Neural Stem Cells and Progenitors

Cell-based therapies for SCI have largely been focused on transplantation strategies, but the presence of NSC and progenitors in the adult spinal cord means an alternative approach that targets the mobilization of these endogenous cells and their repurposing for repair and for cell replacement, in particular. The use of endogenous cells for repair has several advantages over cell transplantation, including: immune compatibility, simplicity without the high cost associated with the isolation and preparation of cell stocks that need to receive FDA approval, and the lack of the serious safety issues inherent when dealing with ES/iPS-derived cells. The main challenge with the use of endogenous cell therapy is the poor understanding of the nature of NSC and progenitors in the adult spinal cord and their response not only to the primary injury, but also the inflammatory process that accompanies secondary injury. It is clear however, that the adult spinal cord contains NSC and progenitors, which have been shown *in vitro* to be multipotent, but are directed to a glial phenotype *in vivo* by the non-neurogenic environment

(Horner *et al.*, 2000; Cao *et al.*, 2001; McTigue and Sahinkaya, 2011). These cells reside predominantly in the white matter parenchyma or close to the central canal in the ependymal and subependymal regions (Horner *et al.*, 2000), and appear to be comprised of a heterogeneous population of multipotent ependymal cells, GFAP-positive cells, and OPC (Barnabe-Heider *et al.*, 2010; Fiorelli *et al.*, 2013). However, there are still unresolved questions regarding the locations, lineage diversity, and regulation of these cells with respect to their proliferation and differentiation properties. Nevertheless, the presence of self-renewing multipotent cells in the spinal cord, together with evidence for their proliferation following SCI, (Zai and Wrathall, 2005) support the possibility for their therapeutic potential by enhancing endogenous repair (McTigue *et al.*, 2001; Yang *et al.*, 2006). For example, intrathecal infusions of epidermal growth factor and fibroblast growth factor (Kojima and Tator, 2000) increased the numbers of proliferating cells, suggesting that it may be possible to modulate the endogenous pool available for repair. Other experimental approaches to modulate the properties of endogenous NSC and progenitors include the use of cytokines (e.g., TNF-α), growth factors (e.g., BMP), and transcription factors (e.g., Ngn2 and Mash1) and are well summarized in a review paper (Obermair *et al.*, 2008).

The presence of OPC in the adult spinal cord received considerable attention due to their potential contribution to the remyelination process following SCI. Adult OPC that are present throughout spared tissue proliferate and produce new oligodendrocytes, but the process is insufficient to restore the oligodendrocytes lost following injury and are unable to reverse the demyelination process. The limited remyelination that does occur after injury is characterized by thinner and shorter sheaths compared to those present before injury (Blakemore *et al.*, 1977). There are no definitive answers as to why endogenous OPC do not complete the remyelination process, but the failure is likely to be the result of the injury environment and astrogliosis, in particular, that inhibits the production of myelinating oligodendrocytes (Wang *et al.*, 2011), as well as the lack of growth factors that support full myelination (Mekhail *et al.*,

2012). Therapeutic strategies to improve myelination have therefore been focused on efforts to reduce oligodendrocyte cell death and the manipulation of the endogenous cell population to reduce astrogliosis and increase oligodendrocytes (Almad *et al.*, 2011).

Clinical Considerations

Current state of treatment

Although significant clinical improvements in the multidisciplinary care of a SCI patient from triage, acute surgical intervention, and rehabilitation have been made, there has been little progress in the translation of preclinical research into therapeutic intervention. The current state of treatment involves the transfer of patients to certified SCI center within 24 hours of SCI. In this setting, multidisciplinary care involves the coordinated efforts of an emergency room physician, trauma surgeon, neurological or orthopedic surgeon with training in spine surgery, and an ancillary team on-call for acute care needs. Initial patient evaluation encompasses an assessment of airway, breathing, and circulation, with continued support for these structures throughout the cycle of care. At this time, incoming patients receive a brief neurologic exam and assessment of the patient's Glascow Coma Score, as well as a preliminary evaluation for traumatic brain injury, given the relatively high concurrence with SCI. The extent of improvement remains largely dependent on the location and severity of SCI as well as the extent of neurological deficit below the level of injury.

There are currently two common treatments for acute SCI, both with limited efficacy: methylprednisolone (MP) and decompression surgery. MP is a corticosteroid is considered to be the only pharmacologic intervention capable of providing some benefit but has the risk of added medical comorbidity. MP is administered within 8 hours after injury as a 30mg/kg bolus with a subsequent maintenance dose of 5.4mg/kg for 24–48 hours (Bracken *et al.*, 1997). MP administration is highly controversial within the medical field due to criticism of the initial clinical trial design (and *post hoc* analyses), high rates of comorbidities, and questionable efficacy (Qian *et al.*, 2005). The only consensus regarding MP treatment is that better options are clearly needed (Bydon *et al.*, 2013).

More recently, a prospective cohort study demonstrated that surgical decompression and stabilization at the level of SCI improves functional outcomes when decompression occurs within 24 hours of injury (Fehlings *et al.*, 2012). The results are somewhat diminished by the lack of a randomized study, but the authors felt they could not ethically delay treatment to a trauma patient while neurological measures were worsening. Decompression surgery is the earliest time post-injury that patients could receive a NSC transplant in the clinical setting. The rationale for early decompression surgery is that removing pressure on the spinal cord limits the expansion of the *primary* injury. In contrast, the secondary injury will continue to develop after decompression. Theoretically, cells could be transplanted at the time of decompression to prophylactically treat secondary injury; however, cell transplantation within 24 hours of SCI may not be ideal, not only due to the potential increase in pressure within the spinal cord associated with the bolus delivery of cellular grafts, but also the microenvironment of the injured spinal cord contributing to decreased graft survival.

Consideration of preclinical data for safety and efficacy

Translating anatomical, neurological and behavioral data from animal models to the human condition presents several challenges. The vast majority of SCI research occurs in rodent models. While rodents are convenient models for a variety of lesions and transplant time points, they fail to adequately replicate the scale of human SCI. For example, anatomical features in the rat such as lesion and cavity size become a matter of tremendous concern in a human adult, as the volume of stem cells required to span large cavities may become impractical or unfeasible in terms of graft survival. Large animal models including pig (Zurita *et al.*, 2012; Lee *et al.*, 2013), and non-human primates (Iwanami *et al.*, 2005) are critical for the understanding of scale for NSC transplantation in SCI. In addition, specific animal species, such as non-human primates, more accurately model human recovery of function. Despite these features, uncertainty still exists regarding the extent that a cellular therapeutic must demonstrate efficacy in a preclinical setting in a particular injury and animal model prior to the initiation of clinical trials (Kwon *et al.*, 2013). As a result, there have been specific recommendations for the design and reporting of spinal cord injury experiments (Lemmon *et al.*, 2014), extensive discussions relating to the challenges of assessing functional recovery (Fouad *et al.*, 2013), new methods to integrate data from multiple preclinical studies across animal and injury models, and the provision of standardized guidelines for clinical translation (Ferguson *et al.*, 2013).

FDA regulation of cell production and clinical use

Good Laboratory Practice (GLP), Good Manufacturing Practice (GMP), and Good Clinical Practice (GCP) are standards established and enforced by the Food and Drug Administration (FDA) that guide experimental therapeutics through preclinical stages and clinical trials. GLP, GMP and GCP standards can be found in Title 21 of the Code of Federal Regulations (Good Laboratory Practice for Nonclinical Laboratory Studies, 21 C.F.R.). GLP standards are required to establish efficacy and safety in preclinical animal studies prior to approval for clinical trials. Despite the expected measure of control prior to human implementation, the GLP measures are vital in ensuring the integrity of preclinical conclusions. GMP standards establish the quality control for experimental therapeutics, including stem cell lines. This is extremely important as minor variations in laboratory conditions can influence the quality, reliability, reproducibility, and integrity of cellular stocks destined to be implanted in the human spinal cord. Prior to FDA approval of an investigational new drug (IND) application, a NSC line would have to be produced using GMP standards and deemed safe in a preclinical study using GLP standards. GCP standards establish practice for reporting of adverse events and efficacy in clinical trials. Taken together, GLP, GMP, and GCP standards provide a mechanism to minimize error in the reporting and evaluation of preclinical data and clinical trials.

Design of clinical trials

SCI is particularly difficult to treat experimentally given the heterogeneity of the spinal cord injured population, the location and severity of the lesion, neurological deficit, as well as the type of injury (contusion, laceration, or combination). Stem cell therapies offer unique hope for the treatment of acute and chronic SCI; however, SCI as a disorder and NSC as a treatment present unique challenges for the development of successful therapy and require well-designed and executed clinical trials. In the past decade, the International Society for Stem Cell Research (ISSCR) and the International Campaign for Cures of Spinal Cord Injury Paralysis (ICCP) have each gathered expert panels to develop guidelines for stem cell clinical trials and SCI clinical trials, respectively. These guidelines were developed to ensure patient safety and proper informed consent, while also delivering the greatest opportunity to produce clear, interpretable results. We will discuss the ISSCR and ICCP recommendations in detail, but other recommendations including the National Academy of Sciences (NAS, 2010) and the California Institute for Regenerative Medicine (CIRM, 2012) guidelines for human stem cell research may also be informative.

In 2009, ISSCR established guidelines for clinical trials using stem cells (ISSCR, 2009). This set of 40 recommendations covers a wide range of concepts for the development of clinical trials including informed consent (of donors *and* recipients), patient safety, the need for extensive post-transplantation follow-up, and the potential for post-mortem evaluation of stem cell grafts. The authors of the ISSCR guidelines make a well-reasoned and passionate plea for international regulatory agencies and governments to end the practice of stem cell tourism, where patients with little hope for treatment travel the world seeking expensive but unproven stem cell transplants. In 2006, the ICCP published a set of four papers that established guidelines for the conduct of SCI clinical trials, including stem cell trials. The four papers covered, clinical trial design (Lammertse *et al.*, 2007), inclusion and exclusion criteria (Tuszynski *et al.*, 2007), outcome measures (Steeves *et al.*, 2007), and the impact of spontaneous recovery on statistical power required for SCI trials (Fawcett *et al.*, 2007). These issues are interrelated and make SCI clinical trial design challenging. For example, the primary outcome measure of many SCI clinical trials is the ASIA score (particularly the motor score). Many SCI patients undergo spontaneous recovery and an ASIA neurological assessment can be unreliable, particularly within the first 24–48 hours after injury (Burns *et al.*, 2003). The reasons for this variability are many, and include co-morbidities and the administration of drugs for pain management that also effect cognitive ability. The ICCP makes many recommendations based on the predicted improvement, level and severity of injury, and the time since the injury. They recommend randomized clinical trials with a double-blind design (although an open label Phase I trial is acceptable). The power analysis reveals that time after injury, level of injury, ASIA score, and expected treatment effect all have large effects on the required number of patients. The enrollment figures are particularly severe for a therapy that must be administered acutely after injury. For example, a clinical trial that is conducted within 24 hours of the injury in a patient population that has ASIA A, thoracic injuries and has an expected treatment effect of 10 points on the ASIA motor score would require less than 50 patients per arm to determine efficacy. If that same trial was performed acutely in thoracic ASIA B patients (instead of ASIA A) and had a more modest expected effect (only 5 points on the ASIA motor score instead of 10), the trial would require a prohibitive 800 patients per arm to determine efficacy. This makes neuroprotective strategies particularly difficult to test in clinical trials because they would hypothetically work better for incomplete injuries (i.e. injuries with spared tissue to be protected from secondary injury) and would need to be administered as soon after injury as possible. Although these power analyses may seem discouraging, they truly call for the improvement of outcome measures that are more reliable, sensitive and predictive than the ASIA motor score. Such an outcome measure would have to be cheap and portable so it could be reliably administered within the first 24 hours after injury for use in a neuroprotective trial. Until such an outcome measure is available, ASIA A patients several weeks post-injury may be the best candidates for NSC clinical trials.

Other issues of timing must also be considered when transitioning from preclinical animal data to a clinical trial. The ideal time frame to administer a stem cell transplant in humans is not known; thus, care should be taken when comparing the results of animal studies and choosing a comparable timeframe in the human SCI population. Studies of postmortem human SCI tissue has shown that the cellular responses are similar in rodents and the human population (Norenberg *et al.*, 2004), indicating that reasonable comparisons between animal data and the human condition can be made. Many novel laboratory experiments are aimed at either cellular transplantation prior to the formation of the glial scar, or in a medium conducive to scar breakdown. Many prior SCI studies have transplanted in the first two weeks, due to concerns of peak inflammatory reactions at the site of injury limiting cell survival (Yoon *et al.*, 2007).

Given the propensity for patients with SCI to undergo anterior-posterior surgery for circumferential three-column decompression and stabilization, the delivery of stem cells would be ideally coordinated in the posterior surgery, to limit the number of spinal surgeries undergone by the patient. Since reliable clinical data shows the benefit to early spinal decompression at the site of SCI (Fehlings *et al.*, 2012) within 24 hours versus delayed, it would be prudent to have a viable cell stock capable of being implanted at the time of decompression within a 24-hour notice. Large quantities of hGRP can be banked for immediate use. Use of earlier embryonic or NSC in human populations are currently under investigation in the laboratory setting as xenografts, as well as in clinical use entering Phase I study this year (Table 1). Cells frozen up to three years can be utilized, although the tradeoff is the decreased cell viability after thawing, which they found to be close to 90%. In an acute setting of SCI, hGRP can be thawed in less than one hour. Viability will be of greater importance, as spanning a lesion cavity in an adult requires massive cell stocks, readily available for thawing.

Another final consideration would be the duration of immunosuppression for the purpose of restricting the host-response to donor cells. Since banked cells are not autologous, there is a need for immunosuppression. Since multisystem trauma patients are at an elevated risk for infection, this risk has to be weighed in. Furthermore, these patients are susceptible to infection from a number of routes depending on the extent of multisystem injury. Many trials underway at the present time use autologous mesenchymal cells with the hopes of eliminating the need for immunosuppression. Furthermore, the use of immunosuppression in high concentration for transplantation will risk impaired spine fusion. These risks of pseduoarthrosis are compounded in the elderly and point to the use of autologous, iPSC-derived cells or direct reprogramming of autologous cells.

The design of clinical trial should target very specific stages of injury, as the nature of the lesion and considerations for therapeutic efficacy may evolve over time, given the mechanism of the intervention. For example, in the acute stage, limiting secondary injury and cellular replacement may be likely therapeutic goals, whereas overcoming the glial scar may be less efficacious. In contrast, at the chronic stage, combining cellular grafts with strategies designed to digest the glial scar may be more promising in limiting secondary injury, a process that has already resolved. Preclinical data gathered from animal studies will be helpful in determining during which phase of SCI (acute, subchronic, chronic), treatment will be most useful (Steeves *et al.*, 2007). This is a particularly important consideration for stem cell transplantation strategies, not only due to the potential for these cells to prevent secondary injury and modify the injured environment, but also due to their sensitivity to lesion severity and inflammatory mediators. Conversely, an alternative consideration could be to design a trial with an even distribution of ASIA scales to see if any significantly different clinical outcomes are obtained as well as to maintain a timely enrollment of the patient population.

Furthermore, the initial care that a patient receives in the aftermath of SCI is also a critical factor that should be considered in the selection and design of clinical trials. For example, delayed transportation to a tertiary care facility offering early surgical intervention and therapy and limit secondary injury not only is injurious to the patient, but is also a limiting factor that may preclude enrollment into a clinical trial. Assessment of other comorbidities, such as concurrent TBI, should also be considered in clinical trial design. Unfortunately, given the inherent difficulties in clinical research and trial design for SCI, there is a lack of randomized, controlled trials.

Outcome measures

The establishment of reliable and quantitative outcome measures to assess functional recovery is a critical step in evaluation of the efficacy of treatments in animal models and the strongest element in translational considerations for clinical trials with patients. However, the complexity of lesions and animal models in SCI and the need to address motor, sensory, and autonomic functions have presented considerable challenges and pitfalls (Fouad *et al.*, 2013). As a result, there has been intense discussion about the level of evidence needed to demonstrate "relevant, meaningful efficacy" in preclinical studies for clinical translation (Kwon *et al.*, 2013). There has also been recent progress in the management of heterogeneous data from diverse preclinical models of SCI to discover "syndromic outcome metrics" for therapeutic testing using a multivariate, integrative approach (Ferguson *et al.*, 2013).

The same urgency exists in the clinic to classify the severity of the injury and to determine beneficial effects of treatment for patients by standardized measures. As a result, there have been various initiatives to produce accurate, sensitive, and reliable outcome tools for human SCI, which have recently been assessed in a set of recommendations by the spinal cord outcomes partnership endeavor, SCOPE (Alexander *et al.*, 2009). The growing experience with clinical trials has also generated important lessons as to which outcome measures have the greatest validity and reliability (Ditunno, 2010) and which detect not only neurological function, such as motor levels, sensory levels, and electrophysiology, but are also associated with a clear functional impact on individuals, such as self care and activities of daily living (Steeves *et al.*, 2012).

Finally, early prognosis in SCI is of importance not only at the patient level, as the ambulatory status greatly impacts direct clinical outcomes and associated morbidity (Curt and Dietz, 1997; Savic and Frankel, 1999) and serve as a reference for improvement associated with specific treatments. Clinical experience dictates that prognosis directly correlates with injury severity as graded by the ASIA Scale (American Spinal Cord Injury Association). However, many patients are unable to participate in this exam, either due to mental status fluctuations, sedatives, mechanical ventilation, or even medications that alter the sensorium. Others have attempted to provide additional prognosticating measurements (Curt and Dietz, 1997). Curt *et al.* utilized somatosensory evoked potentials (SSEP) in 104 consecutive SCI patients, measuring tibial or pudendal SSEP, ambulatory status (on a scale of 1 to 4, from non-ambulatory to no deficit), and ASIA score. They found that in acute tetraplegia, the presence of an SSEP signal was most predictive of partial recovery of ambulation, while in acute paraplegia, ASIA motor score was most predictive (Curt and Dietz, 1997).

Neural Stem Cell and Progenitor Cell-Based Clinical Trials for SCI

Human embryonic stem cells (hESC)

Geron introduced the use of hESC-derived cellular therapeutics for treatment of SCI to clinical trial in 2010 (www.clinicaltrials.gov). Their initial Phase I study enrolled 10 patients with a neurologically complete injury between T3 and T11. The enrolled subjects were transplanted with Geron's GRNOPC1 cell line, a hESC-derived OPC, 7–14 days after SCI. Only five patients were able to undergo treatment prior to the abrupt termination of the study due to a lack of financial resources. Nevertheless, of those patients that did receive transplants of GRNOPC1, no adverse effects were reported, marking a major milestone for the clinical feasibility of hESC-derived cellular therapies (McCusker, 2011). In 2013, Geron completed the divestiture of their hESC holdings, including the intellectual property covering the Phase I trial. Recently however, Asterias Biotherapeutics, a company founded by former Geron executives, acquired the intellectual property and has only recently begun enrolling for a phase I/II dose escalation trial after nearly two years (Akst, 2013) (clinicaltrials.org).

Human fetal neural stem cells

StemCells Inc. has an ongoing long-term observational Phase I/II trial following ASIA A, B, or C T2-T11 SCI patients transplanted with HuNSC-SC® (NSC derived from human fetal brain; gestational age 16–20 weeks), focusing on improvements in ASIA Impairment Scale (www.clinicaltrials.gov). StemCells Inc. has released a limited amount of data from the first three patients, all of whom have thoracic, complete, ASIA A SCI. Two of the three patients have reported changes in sensation within a few segments of the lesion, while the third has not demonstrated any changes (Schiffman, 2014). In addition, StemCells Inc. is currently recruiting ASIA A, B or C T2–T11 SCI subjects for a Phase I/II clinical trial to build upon the results of their initial trial and continue to evaluate the safety and efficacy of HuCNS-SC® (www.clinicaltrials.gov).

Neuralstem Inc. also has an ongoing Phase I clinical trial that is currently recruiting ASIA A, T2–T12 SCI subjects with chronic injuries to evaluate the safety of NSI-566 (NSC derived from the human spinal cord; gestational age 8 weeks) when transplanted into the injured cord (www.clinicaltrials.gov). In addition, a variety of secondary outcome measures will be used to evaluate functional improvement up to 60 months post-transplantation. Given that chronic SCI comprises the majority of SCI cases, this clinical trial represents an important step in evaluating therapeutics targeted at chronic injuries.

Olfactory mucosa

Olfactory mucosa has been evaluated as a source of cells for transplant therapy in SCI, serving as a convenient and autologous source of olfactory ensheathing cells (OECs) and NSCs (Lima *et al.*, 2010). These cells can be harvested from a SCI patient with only minimal morbidity, notably irreversible deficits in olfaction (Lima *et al.*, 2006; Chhabra *et al.*, 2009). A non-randomized human clinical trial demonstrated the safety of autologous OECs derived from the olfactory mucosa in ASIA A, C5–L5 SCI patients. Furthermore, some levels of neurologic improvement were noted but failed to reach statistical significance (Lima *et al.*, 2010).

Schwann cells

Although not a traditional NSC or progenitor cell therapy, Schwann cells are a promising cellular therapeutic with the potential to serve as an autologous therapy. Previous reports have demonstrated improvement in a set of non-consecutive patient case series (Rasouli *et al.*, 2006; Dinh *et al.*, 2007; Zhou *et al.*, 2012; Zaminy *et al.*, 2013). Currently, a Phase I clinical trial using autologous Schwann cells, isolated and expanded *in vitro* from the harvested sural nerve, and injected directly into the injured spinal cord of T3–T11 SCI subjects within seven days of injury, is ongoing (www.clinicaltrials.gov). In addition to examining the safety of transplanted cells, this study will also monitor the development of neuropathic pain and behavioral outcomes.

Conclusion

Spinal cord injury encompasses a complex series of events that culminate in neural cell loss and an inflammatory, inhibitory microenvironment that precludes axonal regeneration and functional recovery. Though endogenous cells mount a proliferative response in an attempt to replace lost cells and repair the injured cord, the endogenous repair mechanisms are limited and insufficient to promote anatomical and functional recovery. Cellular transplantation utilizing a variety of cell sources has been explored as a potential therapeutic strategy. Transplantation of neural-lineage cells, including NSC, neural progenitors (including neuronal and glial progenitors), olfactory ensheathing cells, and Schwann cells, isolated from a variety of sources, including the fetal central nervous system, derived from pluripotent cells, the adult central nervous system, or peripheral nerve, have been demonstrated to promote anatomical and functional recovery in animal models of spinal cord injury. A variety of these cells have progressed to clinical trials and have demonstrated safety and some evidence of neurological recovery. These results highlight the promising nature of cellular transplantation for treatment of human spinal cord injury and are encouraging for the design of future clinical trials.

References

Aguilar J, Humanes-Valera D, Alonso-Calvino E, Yague JG, Moxon KA, Oliviero A, Foffani G (2010) Spinal cord injury immediately changes the state of the brain. *J Neurosci* 30:7528–7537.

Akst J (2013) Geron's stem cell program sold. In: The Scientist.

Albin MS, Hung TK, Babinski M (1980) The patient with spinal cord injury. Epidemiology, emergency and acute care: advances in physiopathology and treatment. *Cur Prob Surg* 17:190–204.

Alexander MS, Anderson KD, Biering-Sorensen F, Blight AR, Brannon R, Bryce TN, Creasey G, Catz A, Curt A, Donovan W, Ditunno J, Ellaway P, Finnerup NB, Graves DE, Haynes BA, Heinemann AW, Jackson AB, Johnston MV, Kalpakjian CZ, Kleitman N, Krassioukov A, Krogh K, Lammertse D, Magasi S, Mulcahey MJ, Schurch B, Sherwood A, Steeves JD, Stiens S, Tulsky DS, van Hedel HJ, Whiteneck G. (2009) Outcome measures in spinal cord injury: recent assessments and recommendations for future directions. *Spinal Cord* 47:582–591.

Almad A, Sahinkaya FR, McTigue DM (2011) Oligodendrocyte fate after spinal cord injury. *Neurotherapeutics* 8:262–273.

Bareyre FM, Kerschensteiner M, Raineteau O, Mettenleiter TC, Weinmann O, Schwab ME (2004) The injured spinal cord spontaneously forms a new intraspinal circuit in adult rats. *Nat Neurosci* 7: 269–277.

Barnabe-Heider F, Goritz C, Sabelstrom H, Takebayashi H, Pfrieger FW, Meletis K, Frisen J (2010) Origin of new glial cells in intact and injured adult spinal cord. *Cell Stem Cell* 7:470–482.

Bernstein-Goral H, Bregman BS (1997) Axotomized rubrospinal neurons rescued by fetal spinal cord transplants maintain axon collaterals to rostral CNS targets. *Exp Neurol* 148:13–25.

Bithell A, Finch SE, Hornby MF, Williams BP (2008) Fibroblast growth factor 2 maintains the neurogenic capacity of embryonic neural progenitor cells in vitro but changes their neuronal subtype specification. *Stem Cells* 26:1565–1574.

Blakemore WF, Eames RA, Smith KJ, McDonald WI (1977) Remyelination in the spinal cord of the cat following intraspinal injections of lysolecithin. *J neurological Sci* 33:31–43.

Bonner JF, Blesch A, Neuhuber B, Fischer I (2010) Promoting directional axon growth from neural progenitors grafted into the injured spinal cord. *J Neurosci Res* 88:1182–1192.

Bonner JF, Connors TM, Silverman WF, Kowalski DP, Lemay MA, Fischer I (2011) Grafted neural progenitors integrate and restore synaptic connectivity across the injured spinal cord. *J Neurosci* 31:4675–4686.

Bracken MB, Shepard MJ, Holford TR, Leo-Summers L, Aldrich EF, Fazl M, Fehlings M, Herr DL, Hitchon PW, Marshall LF, Nockels RP, Pascale V, Perot PL, Jr., Piepmeier J, Sonntag VK, Wagner F, Wilberger JE, Winn HR, Young W (1997) Administration of methylprednisolone for 24 or 48 hours or tirilazad mesylate for 48 hours in the treatment of acute spinal cord injury. Results of the Third National Acute Spinal Cord Injury Randomized Controlled Trial. National Acute Spinal Cord Injury Study. *JAMA* 277:1597–1604.

Bregman BS, Reier PJ (1986) Neural tissue transplants rescue axotomized rubrospinal cells from retrograde death. *J Comp Neurol* 244: 86–95.

Burns AS, Lee BS, Ditunno JF, Jr., Tessler A (2003) Patient selection for clinical trials: the reliability of the early spinal cord injury examination. *J Neurotrauma* 20:477–482.

Bush TG, Puvanachandra N, Horner CH, Polito A, Ostenfeld T, Svendsen CN, Mucke L, Johnson MH, Sofroniew MV (1999) Leukocyte infiltration, neuronal degeneration, and neurite outgrowth after ablation of scar-forming, reactive astrocytes in adult transgenic mice. *Neuron* 23: 297–308.

Butt SJ, Kiehn O (2003) Functional identification of interneurons responsible for left-right coordination of hindlimbs in mammals. *Neuron* 38:953–963.

Bydon M, Lin J, Macki M, Gokaslan ZL, Bydon A (2013) The current role of steroids in acute spinal cord injury. *World Neurosurg.*

Cao Q, He Q, Wang Y, Cheng X, Howard RM, Zhang Y, DeVries WH, Shields CB, Magnuson DS, Xu XM, Kim DH, Whittemore SR (2010) Transplantation of ciliary neurotrophic factor-expressing adult oligodendrocyte precursor cells promotes remyelination and functional recovery after spinal cord injury. *J Neurosci* 30:2989–3001.

Cao Q, Xu XM, Devries WH, Enzmann GU, Ping P, Tsoulfas P, Wood PM, Bunge MB, Whittemore SR (2005a) Functional recovery in traumatic spinal cord injury after transplantation of multineurotrophin-expressing glial-restricted precursor cells. *J Neurosci* 25:6947–6957.

Cao Q, Xu XM, Devries WH, Enzmann GU, Ping P, Tsoulfas P, Wood PM, Bunge MB, Whittemore SR (2005b) Functional recovery in traumatic spinal cord injury after transplantation of multineurotrophin-expressing glial-restricted precursor cells. *J Neurosci* 25:6947–6957.

Cao QL, Zhang YP, Howard RM, Walters WM, Tsoulfas P, Whittemore SR (2001) Pluripotent stem cells engrafted into the normal or lesioned adult rat spinal cord are restricted to a glial lineage. *Exp Neurol* 167:48–58.

Chhabra HS, Lima C, Sachdeva S, Mittal A, Nigam V, Chaturvedi D, Arora M, Aggarwal A, Kapur R, Khan TA (2009) Autologous olfactory [corrected] mucosal transplant in chronic spinal cord injury: an Indian Pilot Study. *Spinal cord* 47:887–895.

Chipman PH, Toma JS, Rafuse VF (2012) Generation of motor neurons from pluripotent stem cells. *Prog Brain Res* 201:313–331.

CIRM (2012) The California Institute for Regenerative Medicine: Science, Governance, and the Pursuit of Cures: The National Academies Press.

Cummings BJ, Uchida N, Tamaki SJ, Salazar DL, Hooshmand M, Summers R, Gage FH, Anderson AJ (2005) Human neural stem cells differentiate and promote locomotor recovery in spinal cord-injured mice. *Proc Natl Acad Sci U S A* 102:14069–14074.

Curt A, Dietz V (1997) Ambulatory capacity in spinal cord injury: significance of somatosensory evoked potentials and ASIA protocol in predicting outcome. *Arch Physical Med Rehabilitation* 78:39–43.

Davies JE, Huang C, Proschel C, Noble M, Mayer-Proschel M, Davies SJ (2006) Astrocytes derived from glial-restricted precursors promote spinal cord repair. *J Biol* 5:7.

Davies JE, Proschel C, Zhang N, Noble M, Mayer-Proschel M, Davies SJ (2008) Transplanted astrocytes derived from BMP- or CNTF-treated glial-restricted precursors have opposite effects on recovery and allodynia after spinal cord injury. *J Biol* 7:24.

Davies SJ, Shih CH, Noble M, Mayer-Proschel M, Davies JE, Proschel C (2011) Transplantation of specific human astrocytes promotes functional recovery after spinal cord injury. *PLoS One* 6:e17328.

Dinh P, Bhatia N, Rasouli A, Suryadevara S, Cahill K, Gupta R (2007) Transplantation of preconditioned Schwann cells following hemisection spinal cord injury. *Spine* 32:943–949.

Ditunno JF (2010) Outcome measures: evolution in clinical trials of neurological/functional recovery in spinal cord injury. *Spinal Cord* 48:674–684.

Emdad L, D'Souza SL, Kothari HP, Qadeer ZA, Germano IM (2012) Efficient differentiation of human embryonic and induced pluripotent stem cells into functional astrocytes. *Stem Cells Dev* 21:404–410.

Fan C, Zheng Y, Cheng X, Qi X, Bu P, Luo X, Kim DH, Cao Q (2013) Transplantation of D15A-expressing glial-restricted-precursor-derived astrocytes improves anatomical and locomotor recovery after spinal cord injury. *Int J Biol Sci* 9:78–93.

Faulkner J, Keirstead HS (2005) Human embryonic stem cell-derived oligodendrocyte progenitors for the treatment of spinal cord injury. *Trans Immunol* 15:131–142.

Faulkner JR, Herrmann JE, Woo MJ, Tansey KE, Doan NB, Sofroniew MV (2004) Reactive astrocytes protect tissue and preserve function after spinal cord injury. *J Neurosci* 24:2143–2155.

Fawcett JW, Curt A, Steeves JD, Coleman WP, Tuszynski MH, Lammertse D, Bartlett PF, Blight AR, Dietz V, Ditunno J, Dobkin BH, Havton LA, Ellaway PH, Fehlings MG, Privat A, Grossman R, Guest JD, Kleitman N, Nakamura M, Gaviria M, Short D (2007) Guidelines for the conduct of clinical trials for spinal cord injury as developed by the ICCP panel: spontaneous recovery after spinal cord injury and statistical power needed for therapeutic clinical trials. *Spinal Cord* 45:190–205.

Fehlings MG, Vaccaro A, Wilson JR, Singh A, D WC, Harrop JS, Aarabi B, Shaffrey C, Dvorak M, Fisher C, Arnold P, Massicotte EM, Lewis S, Rampersaud R (2012) Early versus delayed decompression for traumatic cervical spinal cord injury: results of the Surgical Timing in Acute Spinal Cord Injury Study (STASCIS). *PloS One* 7:e32037.

Fehlings MG, Vawda R (2011) Cellular treatments for spinal cord injury: the time is right for clinical trials. *Neurotherapeutics* 8:704–720.

Ferguson AR, Irvine KA, Gensel JC, Nielson JL, Lin A, Ly J, Segal MR, Ratan RR, Bresnahan JC, Beattie MS (2013) Derivation of multivariate syndromic outcome metrics for consistent testing across multiple models of cervical spinal cord injury in rats. *PLoS One* 8:e59712.

Fiorelli R, Cebrian-Silla A, Garcia-Verdugo JM, Raineteau O (2013) The adult spinal cord harbors a population of GFAP-positive progenitors with limited self-renewal potential. *Glia* 61:2100–2113.

Fitch MT, Silver J (2008) CNS injury, glial scars, and inflammation: Inhibitory extracellular matrices and regeneration failure. *Exp Neurol* 209:294–301.

Fouad K, Hurd C, Magnuson DS (2013) Functional testing in animal models of spinal cord injury: not as straight forward as one would think. *Front Integrative Neurosci* 7:85.

Franklin RJ, Ffrench-Constant C (2008) Remyelination in the CNS: from biology to therapy. *Nat Rev Neurosci* 9:839–855.

Freeman MR (2010) Specification and morphogenesis of astrocytes. *Science* 330:774–778.

Garbossa D, Boido M, Fontanella M, Fronda C, Ducati A, Vercelli A (2012) Recent therapeutic strategies for spinal cord injury treatment: possible role of stem cells. *Neurosurg Rev* 35:293–311; discussion 311.

Good Laboratory Practice for Nonclinical Laboratory Studies (2014).

Graziano A, Foffani G, Knudsen EB, Shumsky J, Moxon KA (2013) Passive exercise of the hind limbs after complete thoracic transection of the spinal cord promotes cortical reorganization. *PLoS One* 8:e54350.

Gregori N, Proschel C, Noble M, Mayer-Proschel M (2002) The tripotential glial-restricted precursor (GRP) cell and glial development in the spinal cord: generation of bipotential oligodendrocyte-type-2 astrocyte progenitor cells and dorsal-ventral differences in GRP cell function. *J Neurosci* 22:248–256.

Grumbles RM, Almeida VW, Casella GT, Wood PM, Hemstapat K, Thomas CK (2012) Motoneuron replacement for reinnervation of skeletal muscle in adult rats. *J Neuropathol Exp Neurol* 71:921–930.

Haas C, Fischer I (2013) Human astrocytes derived from glial restricted progenitors support regeneration of the injured spinal cord. *J Neurotrauma* 30:1035–1052.

Haas C, Neuhuber B, Yamagami T, Rao M, Fischer I (2012) Phenotypic analysis of astrocytes derived from glial restricted precursors and their impact on axon regeneration. *Exp Neurol* 233:717–732.

Hadi B, Zhang YP, Burke DA, Shields CB, Magnuson DS (2000) Lasting paraplegia caused by loss of lumbar spinal cord interneurons in rats: no direct correlation with motor neuron loss. *J Neurosurg* 93: 266–275.

Han SS, Liu Y, Tyler-Polsz C, Rao MS, Fischer I (2004) Transplantation of glial-restricted precursor cells into the adult spinal cord: survival, glial-specific differentiation, and preferential migration in white matter. *Glia* 45:1–16.

Hefferan MP, Galik J, Kakinohana O, Sekerkova G, Santucci C, Marsala S, Navarro R, Hruska-Plochan M, Johe K, Feldman E, Cleveland DW, Marsala M (2012) Human neural stem cell replacement therapy for amyotrophic lateral sclerosis by spinal transplantation. *PLoS One* 7:e42614.

Herrera J, Yang H, Zhang SC, Proschel C, Tresco P, Duncan ID, Luskin M, Mayer-Proschel M (2001) Embryonic-derived glial-restricted precursor cells (GRP cells) can differentiate into astrocytes and oligodendrocytes in vivo. *Exp Neurol* 171:11–21.

Hester ME, Murtha MJ, Song S, Rao M, Miranda CJ, Meyer K, Tian J, Boulting G, Schaffer DV, Zhu MX, Pfaff SL, Gage FH, Kaspar BK (2011) Rapid and efficient generation of functional motor neurons from human pluripotent stem cells using gene delivered transcription factor codes. *Mol Ther* 19:1905–1912.

Hewett JA (2009) Determinants of regional and local diversity within the astroglial lineage of the normal central nervous system. *J Neurochem* 110:1717–1736.

Hill CE, Proschel C, Noble M, Mayer-Proschel M, Gensel JC, Beattie MS, Bresnahan JC (2004) Acute transplantation of glial-restricted precursor cells into spinal cord contusion injuries: survival, differentiation, and effects on lesion environment and axonal regeneration. *Exp Neurol* 190:289–310.

Hochstim C, Deneen B, Lukaszewicz A, Zhou Q, Anderson DJ (2008) Identification of positionally distinct astrocyte subtypes whose identities are specified by a homeodomain code. *Cell* 133:510–522.

Hofstetter CP, Holmstrom NA, Lilja JA, Schweinhardt P, Hao J, Spenger C, Wiesenfeld-Hallin Z, Kurpad SN, Frisen J, Olson L (2005) Allodynia limits the usefulness of intraspinal neural stem cell grafts; directed differentiation improves outcome. *Nat Neurosci* 8:346–353.

Horner PJ, Power AE, Kempermann G, Kuhn HG, Palmer TD, Winkler J, Thal LJ, Gage FH (2000) Proliferation and differentiation of progenitor cells throughout the intact adult rat spinal cord. *J Neurosci* 20: 2218–2228.

Houle JD, Cote MP (2013) Axon regeneration and exercise-dependent plasticity after spinal cord injury. *Ann N Y Acad Sci* 1279:154–163.

Houle JD, Reier PJ (1988) Transplantation of fetal spinal cord tissue into the chronically injured adult rat spinal cord. *J Comp Neurol* 269: 535–547.

Hu BY, Zhang SC (2010) Directed differentiation of neural-stem cells and subtype-specific neurons from hESCs. *Methods Mol Biol* 636: 123–137.

ISSCR (2009) ISSCR Guidelines for the Clinical Translation of Stem Cells. Curr Protoc *Stem Cell Biol* Appendix 1:Appendix 1B.

Iwanami A, Kaneko S, Nakamura M, Kanemura Y, Mori H, Kobayashi S, Yamasaki M, Momoshima S, Ishii H, Ando K, Tanioka Y, Tamaoki N, Nomura T, Toyama Y, Okano H (2005) Transplantation of human neural stem cells for spinal cord injury in primates. *J Neurosci Res* 80:182–190.

Jin Y, Neuhuber B, Singh A, Bouyer J, Lepore A, Bonner J, Himes T, Campanelli JT, Fischer I (2011) Transplantation of human glial restricted progenitors and derived astrocytes into a contusion model of spinal cord injury. *J Neurotrauma* 28:579–594.

Joosten EA, Veldhuis WB, Hamers FP (2004) Collagen containing neonatal astrocytes stimulates regrowth of injured fibers and promotes modest locomotor recovery after spinal cord injury. *J Neurosci Res* 77: 127–142.

Kalyani AJ, Piper D, Mujtaba T, Lucero MT, Rao MS (1998) Spinal cord neuronal precursors generate multiple neuronal phenotypes in culture. *J Neurosci* 18:7856–7868.

Kao T, Shumsky JS, Knudsen EB, Murray M, Moxon KA (2011) Functional role of exercise-induced cortical organization of sensorimotor cortex after spinal transection. *J Neurophysiol* 106:2662–2674.

Karimi-Abdolrezaee S, Eftekharpour E, Wang J, Morshead CM, Fehlings MG (2006) Delayed transplantation of adult neural precursor cells promotes remyelination and functional neurological recovery after spinal cord injury. *J Neurosci* 26:3377–3389.

Karimi-Abdolrezaee S, Eftekharpour E, Wang J, Schut D, Fehlings MG (2010) Synergistic effects of transplanted adult neural stem/progenitor cells, chondroitinase, and growth factors promote functional repair and plasticity of the chronically injured spinal cord. *J Neurosci* 30:1657–1676.

Keirstead HS, Nistor G, Bernal G, Totoiu M, Cloutier F, Sharp K, Steward O (2005) Human embryonic stem cell-derived oligodendrocyte progenitor cell transplants remyelinate and restore locomotion after spinal cord injury. *J Neurosci* 25:4694–4705.

Kim D, Kim CH, Moon JI, Chung YG, Chang MY, Han BS, Ko S, Yang E, Cha KY, Lanza R, Kim KS (2009) Generation of human induced pluripotent stem cells by direct delivery of reprogramming proteins. *Cell Stem Cell* 4:472–476.

Kliot M, Smith GM, Siegal JD, Silver J (1990) Astrocyte-polymer implants promote regeneration of dorsal root fibers into the adult mammalian spinal cord. *Exp Neurol* 109:57–69.

Kojima A, Tator CH (2000) Epidermal growth factor and fibroblast growth factor 2 cause proliferation of ependymal precursor cells in the adult rat spinal cord in vivo. *J Neuropathol Exp Neurol* 59:687–697.

Koliatsos VE, Xu L, Yan J (2008) Human stem cell grafts as therapies for motor neuron disease. Expert opinion on biological therapy 8: 137–141.

Krencik R, Weick JP, Liu Y, Zhang ZJ, Zhang SC (2011) Specification of transplantable astroglial subtypes from human pluripotent stem cells. *Nat Biotech* 29:528–534.

Krencik R, Zhang SC (2011) Directed differentiation of functional astroglial subtypes from human pluripotent stem cells. *Nat Protocols* 6:1710–1717.

Kwon BK, Soril LJ, Bacon M, Beattie MS, Blesch A, Bresnahan JC, Bunge MB, Dunlop SA, Fehlings MG, Ferguson AR, Hill CE, Karimi-Abdolrezaee S, Lu P, McDonald JW, Muller HW, Oudega M, Rosenzweig ES, Reier PJ, Silver J, Sykova E, Xu XM, Guest JD, Tetzlaff W (2013) Demonstrating efficacy in preclinical studies of cellular therapies for spinal cord injury — how much is enough? *Exp Neurol* 248:30–44.

Lammertse D, Tuszynski MH, Steeves JD, Curt A, Fawcett JW, Rask C, Ditunno JF, Fehlings MG, Guest JD, Ellaway PH, Kleitman N, Blight AR, Dobkin BH, Grossman R, Katoh H, Privat A, Kalichman M, International Campaign for Cures of Spinal Cord Injury P (2007) Guidelines for the conduct of clinical trials for spinal cord injury as developed by the ICCP panel: clinical trial design. *Spinal Cord* 45: 232–242.

Lee H, Shamy GA, Elkabetz Y, Schofield CM, Harrsion NL, Panagiotakos G, Socci ND, Tabar V, Studer L (2007) Directed differentiation and transplantation of human embryonic stem cell-derived motoneurons. *Stem Cells* 25:1931–1939.

Lee JH, Jones CF, Okon EB, Anderson L, Tigchelaar S, Kooner P, Godbey T, Chua B, Gray G, Hildebrandt R, Cripton P, Tetzlaff W, Kwon BK (2013) A novel porcine model of traumatic thoracic spinal cord injury. *J Neurotrauma* 30:142–159.

Lepore AC, Fischer I (2005) Lineage-restricted neural precursors survive, migrate, and differentiate following transplantation into the injured adult spinal cord. *Exp Neurol* 194:230–242.

Lepore AC, Maragakis NJ (2011) Stem cell transplantation for spinal cord neurodegeneration. *Methods Mol Biol* 793:479–493.

Lepore AC, O'Donnell J, Bonner JF, Paul C, Miller ME, Rauck B, Kushner RA, Rothstein JD, Fischer I, Maragakis NJ (2011) Spatial and temporal changes in promoter activity of the astrocyte glutamate transporter GLT1 following traumatic spinal cord injury. *J Neurosci Res* 89:1001–1017.

Li XJ, Hu BY, Jones SA, Zhang YS, Lavaute T, Du ZW, Zhang SC (2008) Directed differentiation of ventral spinal progenitors and motor neurons from human embryonic stem cells by small molecules. *Stem Cells* 26:886–893.

Lima C, Escada P, Pratas-Vital J, Branco C, Arcangeli CA, Lazzeri G, Maia CA, Capucho C, Hasse-Ferreira A, Peduzzi JD (2010) Olfactory mucosal autografts and rehabilitation for chronic traumatic spinal cord injury. *Neuroreha Neural Repair* 24:10–22.

Lima C, Pratas-Vital J, Escada P, Hasse-Ferreira A, Capucho C, Peduzzi JD (2006) Olfactory mucosa autografts in human spinal cord injury: a pilot clinical study. *J Spinal cord Med* 29:191–203; discussion 204–196.

Liu G, Detloff MR, Miller KN, Santi L, Houle JD (2012) Exercise modulates microRNAs that affect the PTEN/mTOR pathway in rats after spinal cord injury. *Exp Neurol* 233:447–456.

Lu P, Wang Y, Graham L, McHale K, Gao M, Wu D, Brock J, Blesch A, Rosenzweig ES, Havton LA, Zheng B, Conner JM, Marsala M, Tuszynski MH (2012) Long-distance growth and connectivity of neural stem cells after severe spinal cord injury. *Cell* 150:1264–1273.

Magnuson DS, Zhang YP, Cao QL, Han Y, Burke DA, Whittemore SR (2001) Embryonic brain precursors transplanted into kainate lesioned rat spinal cord. *Neuroreport* 12:1015–1019.

Marino RJ, Barros T, Biering-Sorensen F, Burns SP, Donovan WH, Graves DE, Haak M, Hudson LM, Priebe MM, Committee ANS (2003) International standards for neurological classification of spinal cord injury. *J Spinal cord Med* 26 Suppl 1:S50–56.

McCusker (2011) Geron updates Clinical Data from GRNOPC1. Spinal Cord Injury Trial 2014.

McDonald JW, Belegu V (2006) Demyelination and remyelination after spinal cord injury. *J Neurotrauma* 23:345–359.

McTigue DM, Sahinkaya FR (2011) The fate of proliferating cells in the injured adult spinal cord. *Stem Cell Res Ther* 2:7.

McTigue DM, Wei P, Stokes BT (2001) Proliferation of NG2-positive cells and altered oligodendrocyte numbers in the contused rat spinal cord. *J Neurosci* 21:3392–3400.

Medalha CC, Jin Y, Yamagami T, Haas C, Fischer I (2014) Transplanting neural progenitors into a complete transection model of spinal cord injury. *J Neurosci Res.*

Mekhail M, Almazan G, Tabrizian M (2012) Oligodendrocyte-protection and remyelination post-spinal cord injuries: a review. *Prog Neurobiol* 96:322–339.

Mothe AJ, Tator CH (2013) Review of transplantation of neural stem/progenitor cells for spinal cord injury. *Int J Dev Neurosci* 31:701–713.

Nag S (2011) Morphology and properties of astrocytes. *Methods Mol Biol* 686:69–100.

NAS (2010) Final Report of The National Academies' Human Embryonic Stem Cell Research Advisory Committee and 2010 Amendments to The National Academies' Guidelines for Human Embryonic Stem Cell Research: The National Academies Press.

Neuhuber B, Gallo G, Howard L, Kostura L, Mackay A, Fischer I (2004) Reevaluation of *in vitro* differentiation protocols for bone marrow stromal cells: disruption of actin cytoskeleton induces rapid morphological changes and mimics neuronal phenotype. *J Neurosci Res* 77:192–204.

Noble M (2006) Glial restricted precursors. In: Neural Development and Stem Cells (Rao, M., ed), pp 143–188 Totowa: Humana Press.

Norenberg MD, Smith J, Marcillo A (2004) The pathology of human spinal cord injury: defining the problems. *J Neurotrauma* 21:429–440.

Nout YS, Culp E, Schmidt MH, Tovar CA, Proschel C, Mayer-Proschel M, Noble MD, Beattie MS, Bresnahan JC (2011) Glial restricted precursor cell transplant with cyclic adenosine monophosphate improved some autonomic functions but resulted in a reduced graft size after spinal cord contusion injury in rats. *Exp Neurol* 227:159–171.

NSCISC (2013) Spinal Cord Injury Facts and Figures at a Glance, a publication of the National Spinal Cord Injury Statistical Center, Birmingham, Alabama.

Obermair FJ, Schroter A, Thallmair M (2008) Endogenous neural progenitor cells as therapeutic target after spinal cord injury. *Physiology (Bethesda)* 23:296–304.

Obokata H, Sasai Y, Niwa H, Kadota M, Andrabi M, Takata N, Tokoro M, Terashita Y, Yonemura S, Vacanti CA, Wakayama T (2014a) Bidirectional developmental potential in reprogrammed cells with acquired pluripotency. *Nature* 505:676–680.

Obokata H, Wakayama T, Sasai Y, Kojima K, Vacanti MP, Niwa H, Yamato M, Vacanti CA (2014b) Stimulus-triggered fate conversion of somatic cells into pluripotency. *Nature* 505:641–647.

Oka S, Honmou O, Akiyama Y, Sasaki M, Houkin K, Hashi K, Kocsis JD (2004) Autologous transplantation of expanded neural precursor cells into the demyelinated monkey spinal cord. *Brain Res* 1030:94–102.

Olby NJ, Blakemore WF (1996) Reconstruction of the glial environment of a photochemically induced lesion in the rat spinal cord by transplantation of mixed glial cells. *J Neurocytol* 25:481–498.

Oudega M, Xu XM (2006) Schwann cell transplantation for repair of the adult spinal cord. *J Neurotrauma* 23:453–467.

Pekny M, Nilsson M (2005) Astrocyte activation and reactive gliosis. *Glia* 50:427–434.

Qian T, Guo X, Levi AD, Vanni S, Shebert RT, Sipski ML (2005) High-dose methylprednisolone may cause myopathy in acute spinal cord injury patients. *Spinal Cord* 43:199–203.

Rao MS, Mayer-Proschel M (1997) Glial-restricted precursors are derived from multipotent neuroepithelial stem cells. *Dev Biol* 188:48–63.

Rao MS, Noble M, Mayer-Proschel M (1998) A tripotential glial precursor cell is present in the developing spinal cord. *Proc Natl Acad Sci U S A* 95:3996–4001.

Rasouli A, Bhatia N, Suryadevara S, Cahill K, Gupta R (2006) Transplantation of preconditioned schwann cells in peripheral nerve grafts after contusion in the adult spinal cord. Improvement of recovery in a rat model. *J Bone Joint Surg Am Vol* 88:2400–2410.

Reier PJ, Anderson DK, Thompson FJ, Stokes BT (1992) Neural tissue transplantation and CNS trauma: anatomical and functional repair of the injured spinal cord. *J Neurotrauma* 9 Suppl 1:S223–248.

Rolls A, Shechter R, Schwartz M (2009) The bright side of the glial scar in CNS repair. *Nat Rev Neurosci* 10:235–241.

Sahni V, Mukhopadhyay A, Tysseling V, Hebert A, Birch D, McGuire TL, Stupp SI, Kessler JA (2010) BMPR1a and BMPR1b signaling exert opposing effects on gliosis after spinal cord injury. *J Neurosci* 30:1839–1855.

Savic G, Frankel HL (1999) Prognosis and recovery in ischaemic and traumatic spinal cord injury. *J Neurol Neurosurg Psychiatry* 67:564–565.

Schiffman (2014) StemCells, Inc. Expands Phase I/II Spinal Cord Injury Trial to North America. vol. 2014.

See J FA, Fischer I, Neuhuber B. (2008) Preparing ventral spinal neurons from stem cells: setting the stage for therapeutic cell replacement in spinal cord injury. In: *Society for Neuroscience.*

See J FI, Neuhuber B. (2009) Repairing spinal cord circuitry after injury utilizing neural stem cells. In: *Internation Symposium on Neural Regeneration* Asilomar, CA.

Shaltouki A, Peng J, Liu Q, Rao MS, Zeng X (2013) Efficient generation of astrocytes from human pluripotent stem cells in defined conditions. *Stem Cells* 31:941–952.

Sharp J, Frame J, Siegenthaler M, Nistor G, Keirstead HS (2010) Human embryonic stem cell-derived oligodendrocyte progenitor cell transplants improve recovery after cervical spinal cord injury. *Stem Cells* 28:152–163.

Sharp KG, Yee KM, Steward O. (2014) A re-assessment of long distance growth and connectivity of neural stem cells after severe spinal. *Exp Neurol* 257:186–204.

Smith GM, Miller RH (1991) Immature type-1 astrocytes suppress glial scar formation, are motile and interact with blood vessels. *Brain Res* 543: 111–122.

Smith GM, Miller RH, Silver J (1986) Changing role of forebrain astrocytes during development, regenerative failure, and induced regeneration upon transplantation. *J Comp Neurol* 251:23–43.

Smith GM, Rutishauser U, Silver J, Miller RH (1990) Maturation of astrocytes in vitro alters the extent and molecular basis of neurite outgrowth. *Dev Biol* 138:377–390.

Smith GM, Silver J (1988) Transplantation of immature and mature astrocytes and their effect on scar formation in the lesioned central nervous system. *Prog Brain Res* 78:353–361.

Sofroniew MV (2009) Molecular dissection of reactive astrogliosis and glial scar formation. *Trends Neurosci* 32:638–647.

Sofroniew MV, Vinters HV (2010) Astrocytes: biology and pathology. *Acta Neuropathol* 119:7–35.

Son EY, Ichida JK, Wainger BJ, Toma JS, Rafuse VF, Woolf CJ, Eggan K (2011) Conversion of mouse and human fibroblasts into functional spinal motor neurons. *Cell Stem Cell* 9:205–218.

Soundararajan P, Lindsey BW, Leopold C, Rafuse VF (2007) Easy and rapid differentiation of embryonic stem cells into functional motoneurons using sonic hedgehog-producing cells. *Stem Cells* 25:1697–1706.

Stadtfeld M, Nagaya M, Utikal J, Weir G, Hochedlinger K (2008) Induced pluripotent stem cells generated without viral integration. *Science* 322:945–949.

Steeves JD, Lammertse D, Curt A, Fawcett JW, Tuszynski MH, Ditunno JF, Ellaway PH, Fehlings MG, Guest JD, Kleitman N, Bartlett PF, Blight AR, Dietz V, Dobkin BH, Grossman R, Short D, Nakamura M, Coleman WP, Gaviria M, Privat A, International Campaign for Cures of Spinal Cord Injury P (2007) Guidelines for the conduct of clinical trials for spinal cord injury (SCI) as developed by the ICCP panel: clinical trial outcome measures. *Spinal Cord* 45:206–221.

Takahashi K, Yamanaka S (2006) Induction of pluripotent stem cells from mouse embryonic and adult fibroblast cultures by defined factors. *Cell* 126:663–676.

Takazawa T, Croft GF, Amoroso MW, Studer L, Wichterle H, Macdermott AB (2012) Maturation of spinal motor neurons derived from human embryonic stem cells. *PLoS One* 7:e40154.

Tetzlaff W, Okon EB, Karimi-Abdolrezaee S, Hill CE, Sparling JS, Plemel JR, Plunet WT, Tsai EC, Baptiste D, Smithson LJ, Kawaja MD, Fehlings MG, Kwon BK (2011) A systematic review of cellular transplantation therapies for spinal cord injury. *J Neurotrauma* 28:1611–1682.

Tuszynski MH, Steeves JD, Fawcett JW, Lammertse D, Kalichman M, Rask C, Curt A, Ditunno JF, Fehlings MG, Guest JD, Ellaway PH, Kleitman N, Bartlett PF, Blight AR, Dietz V, Dobkin BH, Grossman R, Privat A, International Campaign for Cures of Spinal Cord Injury P (2007) Guidelines for the conduct of clinical trials for spinal cord injury as developed by the ICCP Panel: clinical trial inclusion/exclusion criteria and ethics. *Spinal Cord* 45:222–231.

Umbach JA, Adams KL, Gundersen CB, Novitch BG (2012) Functional neuromuscular junctions formed by embryonic stem cell-derived motor neurons. *PLoS One* 7:e36049.

Wang JJ, Chuah MI, Yew DT, Leung PC, Tsang DS (1995) Effects of astrocyte implantation into the hemisected adult rat spinal cord. *Neuroscience* 65:973–981.

Wang Y, Cheng X, He Q, Zheng Y, Kim DH, Whittemore SR, Cao QL (2011) Astrocytes from the contused spinal cord inhibit oligodendrocyte differentiation of adult oligodendrocyte precursor cells by increasing the expression of bone morphogenetic proteins. *J Neurosci* 31:6053–6058.

Warrington AE, Barbarese E, Pfeiffer SE (1993) Differential myelinogenic capacity of specific developmental stages of the oligodendrocyte lineage upon transplantation into hypomyelinating hosts. *J Neurosci Res* 34:1–13.

White RE, Jakeman LB (2008) Don't fence me in: harnessing the beneficial roles of astrocytes for spinal cord repair. *Restor Neurol Neurosci* 26: 197–214.

White TE, Lane MA, Sandhu MS, O'Steen BE, Fuller DD, Reier PJ (2010) Neuronal progenitor transplantation and respiratory outcomes following upper cervical spinal cord injury in adult rats. *Exp Neurol.*

Windrem MS, Nunes MC, Rashbaum WK, Schwartz TH, Goodman RA, McKhann G, 2nd, Roy NS, Goldman SA (2004) Fetal and adult human oligodendrocyte progenitor cell isolates myelinate the congenitally dysmyelinated brain. *Nat Med* 10:93–97.

Wu YY, Mujtaba T, Han SS, Fischer I, Rao MS (2002) Isolation of a glial-restricted tripotential cell line from embryonic spinal cord cultures. *Glia* 38:65–79.

Xu L, Ryugo DK, Pongstaporn T, Johe K, Koliatsos VE (2009) Human neural stem cell grafts in the spinal cord of SOD1 transgenic rats: differentiation and structural integration into the segmental motor circuitry. *J Comp Neurol* 514:297–309.

Yandava BD, Billinghurst LL, Snyder EY (1999) "Global" cell replacement is feasible via neural stem cell transplantation: evidence from the dysmyelinated shiverer mouse brain. *Proc Natl Acad Sci U S A* 96:7029–7034.

Yang H, Lu P, McKay HM, Bernot T, Keirstead H, Steward O, Gage FH, Edgerton VR, Tuszynski MH (2006) Endogenous neurogenesis replaces oligodendrocytes and astrocytes after primate spinal cord injury. *J Neurosci* 26:2157–2166.

Yang H, Mujtaba T, Venkatraman G, Wu YY, Rao MS, Luskin MB (2000) Region-specific differentiation of neural tube-derived neuronal restricted progenitor cells after heterotopic transplantation. *Proc Natl Acad Sci U S A* 97:13366–13371.

Yohn DC, Miles GB, Rafuse VF, Brownstone RM (2008) Transplanted mouse embryonic stem-cell-derived motoneurons form functional motor units and reduce muscle atrophy. *J Neurosci* 28:12409–12418.

Yoon SH, Shim YS, Park YH, Chung JK, Nam JH, Kim MO, Park HC, Park SR, Min BH, Kim EY, Choi BH, Park H, Ha Y (2007) Complete spinal cord injury treatment using autologous bone marrow cell transplantation and bone marrow stimulation with granulocyte macrophage-colony stimulating factor: Phase I/II clinical trial. *Stem Cells* 25:2066–2073.

Zai LJ, Wrathall JR (2005) Cell proliferation and replacement following contusive spinal cord injury. *Glia* 50:247–257.

Zaminy A, Shokrgozar MA, Sadeghi Y, Noroozian M, Heidari MH, Piryaei A (2013) Mesenchymal stem cells as an alternative for Schwann cells in rat spinal cord injury. *Iranian Biomedical J* 17:113–122.

Zhang Y, Barres BA (2010) Astrocyte heterogeneity: an underappreciated topic in neurobiology. *Curr Opin Neurobiol* 20:588–594.

Zhang YW, Denham J, Thies RS (2006) Oligodendrocyte progenitor cells derived from human embryonic stem cells express neurotrophic factors. *Stem Cells Dev* 15:943–952.

Zhou XH, Ning GZ, Feng SQ, Kong XH, Chen JT, Zheng YF, Ban DX, Liu T, Li H, Wang P (2012) Transplantation of autologous activated Schwann cells in the treatment of spinal cord injury: six cases, more than five years of follow-up. *Cell Trans* 21 Suppl 1:S39–47.

Zukor K, Belin S, Wang C, Keelan N, Wang X, He Z (2013) Short hairpin RNA against PTEN enhances regenerative growth of corticospinal tract axons after spinal cord injury. *J Neurosci* 33:15350–15361.

Zurita M, Aguayo C, Bonilla C, Otero L, Rico M, Rodriguez A, Vaquero J (2012) The pig model of chronic paraplegia: a challenge for experimental studies in spinal cord injury. *Prog Neurobiol* 97:288–303.

Chapter 18

Generating Different Neural Cell Types from iPSCs for Screening and Cell Therapy for CNS Disorders

Mohan C. Vemuri and Mahendra S. Rao

The discovery of pluripotent cells has changed how we view toxicology and discovery screening and has led to the development of novel strategies for the functional replacement of damaged cells. Progress in the field has been rapid but hampered by several critical roadblocks. These include the difficulty in making PSC, our ability to maintain them stably, the long process of differentiation, and the relative immaturity of the finally differentiated cells. Further progress will require developing highly reproducible processes that are scalable and economical enough to justify the transition to using PSC-derived cells in screening and therapy. This is particulalry true for the nervous system where access to primary neural cells was limited. In this chapter, we will review the advances made in manufacturing cells and the variety of human neural cell types that can be produced.

Human PSC Differentiation to CNS Neural Lineages

During normal human development, the fertilized egg passes through several stages of differentiation. These include germ layer formation by the process of gastrulation followed by epithelial differentiation followed by segregation of neural lineages from other ectodermal lineages. This segregation occurs early and leads to the appearance of a early neural precursor for the CNS and a stem cell for the PNS termed the neural crest stem cell. These lineages are still plastic and at least in rodents, some conversion between CNS stem cells and PNS stem cells is possible (Rao, 2004). Additional contribution to the the nervous system comes from cranial placodes that generate specific neurons or glia for the cranial nerves. The process of placode formation is akin to the neural tube formation, suggesting that epithelium in some regions retains its ability to differentiate into neural derivatives for some time during development (Liu *et al.*, 2012).

Developmental analysis performed in a variety of species has suggested that while it is overall similar there are several differences in the time of differentiation, the markers expressed, and the growth factor dependence at key stages of development. These are important to note as one applies learnings from one species in another. Perhaps the single most critical difference has been timing of differentiation. Early events take three times longer on average in human cell culture than they do in rodent cultures, with later maturation events taking even longer. Thus, embryoid body formation and germ layer segregation can be seen in as little as four days in rodent cultures while it takes 12 days or so to get germ layer differentiation with human cells. Developing oligodendrocytes in culture takes 100 days or so while obtaining (Shin *et al.*, 2007) mature dopaminergic neurons with their characteristic spiking activity takes 80 days or longer (Kriks *et al.*, 2011). This is in contrast with rodents where myelinating oligodendrocytes can be obtained in as little as three weeks while mature dopaminergic neurons may be obtained in less time. In the past decade, researchers for directed differentiation of PSCs into neural and glial lineages using specific growth factors have developed several protocols. Investigators have further refined protocols to not only develop a particular lineage but to directing expression of appropriate regional and positional markers for subtype specific lineages. For example, one can now not just make midbrain type of dopaminergic neurons but further direct differentiation to A9 dopaminergic neurons rather than neurons destined for the red nucleus or the A10 type of dopaminergic neurons (Ono *et al.*, 2007). Likewise it has been possible to generate striatal or forebrain or even hippocampal neurons (Muratore *et al.*, 2014). An abbreviated list of neural subtypes is provided in Table 1. Most of these methods have been developed by adapting protocols from rodent culture and evaluating rodent brain development in transgenic animals. These protocols vary considerably in terms of starting cell types, such as human iPSC or NSC using cells on feeder layers or co-culturing them with other cell types, and the overall degree of cell purity of the final cell population (Cai and Grabel, 2007). In the subsequent sections, we will discuss the advantages and disadvantages of some of the key protocols in more detail.

NSC Enrichment in Neural Rosettes — from Embryoid Bodies

In general, these methods involve human ESC or iPSC clumps that are first dissociated into near single cells (or very small clumps of 3–5 cells) and later aggregated into embryoid body (EB) suspension cultures. These embryoid bodies are subsequently attached to specific matrices such as poly-D-lysine or/and laminin coated culture dish surfaces for the generation of "neural rosettes." Neural rosettes are a radially organized columnar epithelial cell collection (Perrier *et al.*, 2004; Zhang *et al.*, 2001). The neural rosettes are comprised of cells expressing early neuroectodermal stem cell (NSC) markers such as Nestin, Pax6 and Sox1, and are capable of differentiating into various brain region specific neural and glial cell types in response to appropriate developmental cues (Li *et al.*, 2005; Perrier *et al.*, 2004). The broad neural and glial differentiation potential is unique to early rosette stage cells and is lost upon further *in vitro* maturation of NSCs. This observation is not surprising, and reflects *in vivo* CNS development. The ability of NSC to respond to patterning and specification signals at the neural plate stage is broad to begin with and much more restricted after neural tube closure (Jessell, 2000). A large

Table 1. Neural subtypes involved in specific neural disorders.

Neural disease	Experimental model	Cell type in disease	Progenitor cell	Growth factor	Progenitor cell markers	Mature differentiated markers	Tested in transplantation studies
Spinal cord Injury	Adult rat spinal cord injury models	Oligodendrocyte	Oligo progenitor cell	EGF, bFGF, RA	OLIG1, A2B5, SOX10, NG2	GalC, RIP, O4	Yes
Multiple Sclerosis	Treat demyelinated axons, in a coculture with rat hippocampal neurons	Oligodendrocyte	Oligo progenitor cell	EGF, bFGF, PDGF, RA	PDGFR, A2B5, NG2	O4, O1, MBP, PLP	No
Multiple Sclerosis	Remyelination models	Oligodendrocyte	Oligo progenitor cell	RA, EGF, bFGF, Noggin, Vitamin C, Mouse laminin	PDGFR, NG2, OLIG1/2, SOX10	O4, O1, MBP, PLP	Yes
Amyotrophic lateral sclerosis and spinal muscular atrophy	Transplantation of motoneuron progeny into the developing chick embryo	Motoneuron	Motoneuron Progenitor	BDNF, GDNF, AA, RA, SHH, Noggin	BF1, HOXB4, NKX6-1/6-2, OLIG1/2	NKX6.1, OLIG2, NGN2, ISL1, ChAT, VAChT, HB9, LHX3, HOX	Yes
Amyotrophic lateral sclerosis and spinal muscular atrophy	in vitro studies only	Motoneuron	Motoneuron Progenitor	bFGF, RA, SHH, BDNF, GDNF, IGF-1	OLIG1/2, NKX6-1/6-2, NGN2	NKX6.1, OLIG2, NGN2, ISL1, ChAT, VAChT, HB9, Synapsin	No
Parkinson's disease	Not applicable	DA neuron	DA precursor	SHH, FGF8, BDNF, AA, TGFβ / TGFβ	PAX2, PAX5, LMX, / EN1	MAP2, TH, AADC, VMAT, NURR 1, PTX3 / AADC, VMAT, NURR1, PTX3	No

(Continued)

Table 1. Neural subtypes involved in neural disorders (*Continued*)

Neural disease	Experimental model	Cell type in disease	Growth factor	Progenitor cell	Progenitor cell markers	Mature differentiated markers	Tested in transplantation studies
Parkinson's disease	*in vitro* drug screening	**DA neuron**	FGF2 or FGF8, SHH, BDNF, GDNF, cAMP, AA	DA precursor	EN1, OTX2, WNT1, PAX2, GBX2	TH, GABA, EN1, AADC	No
Parkinson's disease	Transplantation into the neostriataoffhydroxydopamine-lesioned parkinsonian rats	**DA neuron**	FGF2, FGF8, SHH, BDNF, GDNF, FBS BDNF, GDNF, FBS	DA precursor	EN1, PAX2, OTX2	TH, TUJ-1	Yes
Parkinson's disease	Transplantation into the striatum of hemi-parkinsonian rats	**DA neuron**	SHH, FGF8, BDNF, GDNF, AA, IGF-1	DA precursor	PAX2, EN1, NURR1, LMX1B	TH, EN1, AADC	Yes
Glial related diseases	Astrocyte related disease	**Astrocyte**	Cyclopamine, human astrocyte medium	—	—	GFAP, S100, GLAST, BDNF, GDNF	No
CNS/PNS diseases	Peripheral and Central Nervous System Neurons	**Peripheral Sensory Neurons**	Noggin, NGF	Neural precursor	NCAM, TUJ-1, SNAIL, dHAND, SOX9	Peripherin, BRN3, TH, TRkA	No
Macular Retinal Degeneration	Not applicable	**Retinal Pigmented Epithelium**	Noggin, Dickkopf-1,	Retinal progenitor	RX, PAX6, LHX2, SIX3	RPE-65	No

number of researchers have successfully used EB/rosette method to generate neural stem cells and subsequently differentiate NSCs to specific neural and glial lineages (Rao *et al.*, 2004). The readers are referred to an excellent review that depicts various methods of EB formation, neural rosette generation, isolation, and differentiation to down-stream neural subtypes using known conventional morphogens and growth factors. FGF8, SHH, Retinoic acid are used primarily to drive differentiation (Cai and Grabel, 2007) towards caudal phenotypes while Wnts and activin are used to drive differentiation to forebrain phenotypes. NSC, NEP or NPC as these cells have been varyingly named can be maintained in a proliferative state in culture using LIF, EGF, and FGF. More recent studies suggested that Wnts and BMPs inhibit neural stem cell induction by inhibiting the primitive neuro ectoderm formation, while LIF supports primitive neuro ectodermal formation from PSCs (Akamatsu *et al.*, 2009). These early studies provide an excellent framework to decipher the molecular chemokine and growth factor interplay in triggering select pathways to yield specific restricted lineage progenitors of nervous system.

Although the system appears to be straightforward, simple, and powerful to derive a single starting NSC population that will generate multiple sub-neural types along the rostro-caudal axis (Emborgh *et al.*, 2013), it is nevertheless, not without its complications. The same process with slight modifications can also yield PNS derivatives (Mica *et al.*, 2013) and such cells can be contaminating CNS cell preparation. The process is difficult to control and the number of rosettes formed is variable and can vary from cell line to cell line and experiment to experiment. Several investigators have therefore evaluated alternative protocols to reduce cell heterogeneity and improve efficiency. One such process of direct differentiation that skips the rosette stage is described below.

Enriched NSC Derivation in a Monolayer Culture Bypassing the Need for Embryoid Body Generation

Studer and his colleagues described an efficient way of neural conversion of PSC (Chambers *et al.*, 2009). They based their experiments on the observation that Wnt and TGF beta signaling inhibited neuroectoderm formation and reasoned that inhibiting these pathways may lead to default neural induction. This turned out to work effectively and they described a protocol of dual inhibition of SMAD signaling pathway, by using Noggin and a small molecule TGF beta inhibitor, SB431542 (Chambers *et al.*, 2009). The synergistic action of two inhibitors, Noggin and SB431542 of SMAD pathway, was sufficient for inducing rapid and complete neural induction in a monolayer adherent culture, bypassing the need for the embryoid body and rosette formation. While Noggin is known for BMP pathway inhibition, SB431542 is shown to inhibit Lefty/Activin/TGFβ pathways by blocking the phosphorylation of ALK4, ALK5, and ALK7 receptors. This study showed it is important to inhibit both of these pathways, since treatment with only one molecule is not sufficient enough to achieve full neural conversion. Further this study by Chamber's *et al.* also proved that the NSC population derived using this method of rosette/EB free dual SMAD inhibition, resulted in epiblast state of primitive NSC that retained positional (anterior-posterior and dorso-ventral) flexibility with the possibility of generating regional neural subtypes characteristic of different brain regions from the same starting population (Table 1).

The process was rapid and complete induction was achieved in as little as 11 days, with critical neural stem cell marker expression being observed as early as five days after initiation of the induction process. Their data suggested the presence of an intermediate cell type at day 5 of differentiation, as the cells were negative for OCT4 and PAX6 but showed peak expression of FGF5 along with OTX2, which are epiblast markers. Further in these cultures, an early expression of SOX1 was noticed, much earlier than other neuroepithelial markers such as PAX6 or ZIC1 or even the anterior CNS (FOXG1) and neural crest (p75) expression. Based on the expression of specific markers, it appears that SOX1 might likely be directly modulated by SMAD signaling in monolayer cultures, unlike PAX6 expression in Noggin/SB431542 treated cultures. This was the first report of highly efficient neural conversion of PSCs bypassing all the hurdles associated with EB/Rosette formation. In addition, this method also allowed further generation of neural subtypes from the NSCs derived using SMAD inhibition pathways, relatively in a much shorter period (~19 days) relative to 30–50-day protocols.

Although rapid and efficient, the process still did not achieve complete purity and the NSC population was heterogeneous. In addition, several investigators reported significant cell death during the process of cell culture. Another puzzling issue was the inability to passage the NSC derived by this process for longer time periods in culture as compared to the rosette derived NSC. Thus while this process has many advantages, it is often used when a stable intermediate is not required and one wished to directly proceed to further differentiated cells. Indeed, several investigators showed that terminally differentiated cells could be obtained from the dual SMAD inhibition process. Indeed, robust methods to derive, expand NSC and differentiate into all of the neuronal subtypes derived from neural tube, (such as midbrain dopaminergic neurons and hind brain motor neurons) and astrocytes, and oligodendrocytes have been reported (Table 1). Cell culture models in which NSCs are differentiated to astrocytes with subsequent global gene expression can help identify new genes that are pivotal for astrogenesis. Astrocytes are process-bearing cells distributed throughout the central nervous system and can comprise 20–25% or even up to 50% of the total volume in some brain regions. They play an integral role in normal homeostasis of the adult brain providing trophic support to both neurons and oligodendrocytes as well as degrading potential toxicants. Astrocytes are increasingly thought to play a role in multiple diseases including ALS and as such, techniques to generate astrocytes from IPSC have become important. Several groups have reported on the generation of astrocytes from fetal tissue and such commercial products are available (Figure 1). The readers are referred to more recent studies on the generation of astrocytes (Reinhardt *et al.*, 2013; Kondo *et al.*, 2014, Yuan *et al.*, 2013, Tang *et al.*, 2013, Shaltouki *et al.*, 2013) and oligodendrocytes (Wang *et al.*, 2013, Ogawa *et al.*, 2011, Emborgh *et al.*, 2013).

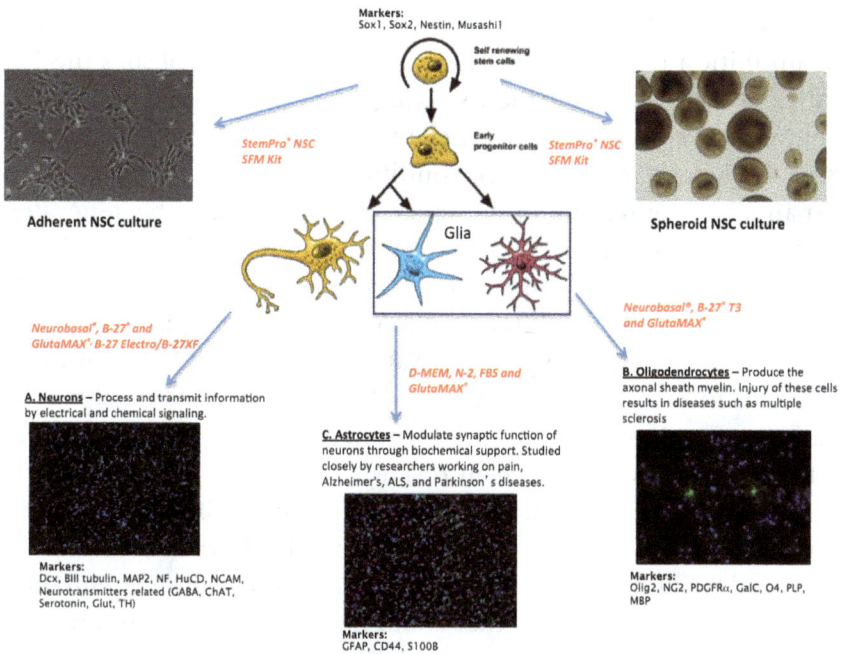

Figure 1. Human NSC Expansion in adherent monolayer cultures and as spheroids. Differentiation of human NSC to Neurons (bottom left panel), Oligodendrocytes (bottom right panel) and Astrocytes (bottom middle panel).

Developmental Pathways and Specification Signals for Neural Crest Cell Fate for PNS

The Neural Crest (NC) is a transient epithelium in vertebrates and is the source for stem and precursor populations of peripheral neurons and glial populations of sensory, autonomic and enteric nervous systems and pigmented cells in the skin such as melanocytes (Weston and Thiery, 2014). Post-neural induction (Groves and LaBonne, 2014; Harland, 1994), the embryonic ectoderm develops into two morphologically distinct epithelial domains: the thickened neural epithelium (the neural or medullary plate) and a thinner, non-neural epithelium. Specific signaling establishes NC potential within cells that exist at the boundary of the two epithelia (Aybar *et al.*, 2003). Recent work have identified the molecular components of signaling pathways involved in NC induction involving stochois-tic inhibition of BMP, TGF-β and Wnt pathways establishes the NC (Mica *et al.*, 2013;). Further, starting from pluripotent stem cells, neural crest cell fate can be efficiently induced by a combination of growth factors in a stromal conditioned culture media and an expandable population of neural crest stem cells can be generated that have characteristic NC expression markers, such as p75, Sox9, Sox10, CD44, HNK1. The expanded NC stem cells were further sub-jected to down-stream differentiation to myelinating Schwann cells of the PNS and Mesenchymal derivatives (Liu *et al.*, 2012). For more detailed information on NC, specification, induction, signaling pathways involved and the origin of mesectoderm, the readers are referred to an excellent recent review (Weston and Thiery, 2014).

In summary, the methods developed so far by different investiga-tors enable the generation of NSCs relevant for CNS or PNS popula-tions and facilitate the use of such NSC in down-stream differentiation of specific neural subtypes that could be relevant for neural disease modeling, phenotype screening as well as in early human brain devel-opment studies. Several gene expression studies of human fetal CNS development, along with differentiation of human neural stem cells to generic CNS neurons, made it possible to come up with a poten-tial panel of markers for each of the neural subtypes from different brain regions. In the following sections, some of the recent meth-ods developed and used to generate brain regional specific neural subtypes from pluripotent cells are described (Table 1, Figure 2).

Differentiation to Anterior Forebrain Neural Specification from Pluripotent Stem Cells via the Activation of SHH and Inhibition of Wnt Signaling

Forebrain cortical interneurons are thought to be affected in several complex CNS disorders such as schizophrenia, autism, epilepsy, Huntington's disease. Securing sufficient number of these cells from normal and affected individuals is important in disease modeling and for cell therapy approaches. However, this has been challeng-ing, as the cells undergo a protracted period of development *in vivo*.

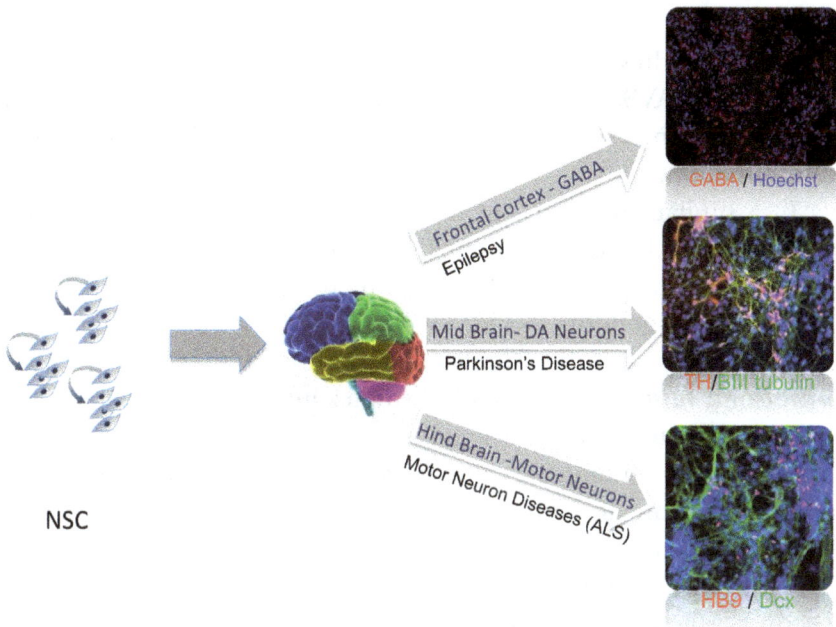

Figure 2. From primitive expandable population of human NSC, generation of front brain GABA neurons to model epilepsy, midbrain Dopaminergic neurons (DA) for Parkinson's disease and hindbrain motor neurons for motor neuron diseases such as ALS.

Recently, three different groups of researchers have identified small molecule, and growth factor-based strategies for efficient induction of human forebrain cortical interneurons. Lorenz Studer's group used an approach to inhibit the Wnt signaling at pharmacological doses, but simultaneously stimulate SHH pathway to effectively induce forebrain NKX2.1+ neural precursors (Maroof *et al*, 2013). They employed original dual SMAD inhibition protocol using Noggin and TGF Beta inhibitor SB431542 that robustly induced FOXG1/PAX6 precursors. Replacement of Noggin with ALK2/ALK3 inhibitor, LDN 193189 induced better PAX6 expression, but lowered the FOXG1 expression. To overcome this limitation, the authors used recombinant DKK1 or the tankyrase inhibitor XAV939, inhibitors of canonical Wnt signaling, that enhanced FOXG1 expression in a consistent manner, enabling a rapid and robust induction of forebrain fate across multiple iPSC donor lines (Maroof *et al.*, 2013). This is perhaps one of the earliest studies to show that the use of just three small molecules (XAV939, SB431542, LDN193189) at appropriate times in the differentiation process results in robust forebrain lineage differentiation.

In a similar approach but with emphasis on neural maturation, another group led by Kriegstein (Nicholas *et al.*, 2013) reported the direct differentiation of hPSC into median ganglionic eminence (MGE) like progenitors (NKX2-1+/FOXG1+) that were further taken through the process of maturation into forebrain interneurons. Both *in vitro* and *in vivo* transplantation studies into rodent brain showed that transplanted cells develop into GABAergic interneurons, but took a maturation time of ~ 7 months. These authors used embryoid body generation and by treating these EB's with a medium that contains B27 enriched with Y27632, Rho-associated kinase inhibitor; SB431542, TGFβ inhibitor; BMPR1A, bone morphogenetic protein receptor 1aFc chimera; DKK1, Dickkopf homolog 1; PM, Purmorphamine for a period of 25 days. The investigators then added BDNF; brain-derived neurotropic factor and DAPT, inhibitor of γ-secretase till day 35. The cells at this stage were either transplanted into animal models or co-cultured with cortical glial cells. Both in *in vitro* cultures as well as in transplantation experiments, they achieved maturation of hPSC-derived interneurons that exhibited GABA specific firing properties, formed synapses and exhibited functional GABAergic output. In the entire workflow, the authors could not collapse the developmental time for the generation of cortical interneurons; *in vitro* developmental times reflected the actual developmental time needed *in vivo* for the generation of front brain cortical neurons (Marin, 2013).

In a more recent paper, Su-Chun Zhang lab at University of Wisconsin developed a simpler and more efficient chemically defined system, in which PSCs are taken to embryoid body formation for the first seven days and then to primitive neuroepithelial cell fate for 10 days via EB attachment in neural induction media (DMEM/F12, NEAA, N-2 supplement and heparin). After which, the cells were patterned through NKX2.1 expressing MGE progenitors by treating with either sonic hedgehog or purmorphamine for two weeks (Liu *et al.*,

2013). The progenitors generated relatively pure population of fore-brain GABAergic interneurons by sixth week. This method relative to other two methods (Maroof *et al.*, 2013; Nicholas *et al.*, 2013) is much simpler, uses less number of small molecules or patterning factors reduces both cost and complexity, thereby eliminating variability. If, at all, there is any disadvantage, it is only with the formation of embry-oid bodies. However, the method appeared to be quite robust and has been tested on multiple human ESC and iPSC lines.

Neural Floor Plate Precursor Induction with SHH and a Simultaneous Inhibition of Dual SMAD Pathways can Generate Functional Midbrain Dopaminergic Neurons

Midbrain dopaminergic neurons are generated *in vivo* from the floor plate during embryonic development (Ono *et al.*, 2007) on exposure to sonic hedgehog (SHH), fibroblast growth factor 8a (FGF8a) and Wnt1 (Cooper *et al.*, 2010). Several *in vitro* culture pro-tocols have replicated the studies starting from PSC and deriving dopaminergic neurons (Kirkeby *et al.*, 2012; Kriks *et al.*, 2011; Xi *et al.*, 2012). These studies essentially converge on floor plate induction with SHH and neural induction with dual SMAD inhibition together with the activation of Wnt1 pathway by GSK3 inhibition. Recently, this method was further optimized for DA neuron patterning, signaling and generation from PSC (Sundberg *et al.*, 2013).

The investigators performed a systematic analysis of cell signal-ing pathways and cell lineage patterns using four different combi-natorial approaches with small molecules which primarily drove the dorsal ventral, frontal, middle and caudal patterning states. These studies suggested an efficient way to generate ventral mes-encephalic functional DA neurons with the following regimen for PSCs in a step-by-step detailed protocol:

Day 0–1: treat PSCs in culture with LDN193189 (LDN) (100nM), SB431542 (SB) (10µM).
Day 1–5: treat cultures with LDN193189 (LDN) (100nM), SB431542 (SB) (10µM), sonic hedgehog (SHH); purmorphomine; and FGF8a.

Day 5–7: treat cultures with LDN193189 (LDN)(100nM), sonic hedgehog (SHH); purmorphomine; and FGF8a.

Day 7–11: treat cultures only with LDN193189 (LDN)(100nM).

Day 4–13: Co-treat the cultures with CHIR99021 (CHIR) (Note this step overlaps with other treatments scheduled on days from 5–13).

Day 13–30: treat with maturation factors of BDNF (20ng/ml), cAMP (0.5mM), TGFβ(2ng/mL), GDNF(20ng/ml), Ascorbic Acid(200µM, and γ-secretase inhibitor DAPT(10nM).

In summary, though the method can still be simplified and optimized, this method efficiently supports the patterning of human pluripotent stem cells towards the ventral mesencephalic fate with FOXA2/OTX2 positive cellular phenotypes at 9 DIV of differentiation regimen. Further, this study also clearly suggests that GSK-3 inhibition leading to the activation of Wnt1 pathway during the days of 4–13 is critical for floor plate derived DA neural differentiation. The functional utility of human PSC-derived DA cells however would need to be evaluated in animal graft studies, although the authors mimicked this study with primate derived iPSC that showed transplantation tolerance in autologus graft studies (Sundberg *et al.*, 2013).

In a novel screening study, Gonzalez *et al.* (2013) reported a small molecule-based dopaminergic neural differentiation from pluripotent stem cells. This study used SB431542 and DMH1, a dorsomorphin analog to get human PSC-derived NSC in six days and NSCs were further expanded for four passages to get consistent NSC population with characteristic features of Nestin, mushashi and PAX6 positive cells that are greater than 90%. In a second step, the NSCs are primed towards dopaminergic differentiation with FGF8 (100ng/mL) and purmorphamine (2µM) for seven days, and then the cultures were subjected to select small molecule exposure towards terminal and mature dopaminergic differentiation. In such a screen, the investigators identified gugglesterone, a steroid that can effectively drive the maturation to dopaminergic neurons. The study showed that gugglesterone method is preferable over the conventional growth factors used such as BDNF,

GDNF, TGFb3, DAPT, dbcAMP, and ascorbic acid. Gene microarray study revealed an up-regulation of dopaminergic and neuronal associated markers such as MAPT, FOXA2, SYT4, FOXA1, DDC, ASCL1, and PINK1. Further validation with RT-PCR studies confirmed the DA neuron identity with markers such as PAX5, LMX1B, PITX3, NURR1, LMX1A, EN1, GIRK2, DDC, and VMAT2. Interestingly, compared to control cells (NSCs treated for one week with FGF8 and purmorphamine and two weeks with 0.1% DMSO instead of GS), GS-treated cells demonstrated a five-fold increase in dopamine secretion as determined by ELISA, indicating that by all means this could be an alternative approach, but needs a through reproducibility of its performance with various PSC lines.

A recent paper (Peng *et al.*, 2014) further reported the survival and engraftment of PSC-derived human dopaminergic neurons manufactured in GMP conditions, in rat Parkinson's disease model suggesting that dopaminergic precursors manufactured to scalability in GMP compatible process are engraftable and hence, have a direct relevance for drug discovery and cell therapy applications. The readers are directed to the following references for further details (Peng *et al.*, 2014; Momcilovic *et al.*, 2014).

Combination of Retinoic Acid or its Analogs for Caudal Specification and SHH for Ventralization can Generate Hind Brain Motor Neurons from Human Pluripotent Stem Cells

Motor neurons that innervate limb muscles are the critical neuron types that get affected early in amyotrophic lateral sclerosis (ALS). Over the past few years of development, simple protocols to differentiate human stem cells to motor neurons have become available (Amoroso *et al.*, 2013; Yang *et al.*, 2013; Jha *et al.*, 2014). Two of the most relevant methods are described here.

Amoroso *et al.* (Amoroso *et al.*, 2013) in a three-week protocol achieved the generation of motor neurons from pluripotent stem cells that uses only small molecules to induce neutralization, caudalization and ventralization features. Although the protocol steps involve an intermediary stage of embryoid body (EB) formation, there is no need for manual picking steps such as rosette picking. In brief, the protocol involves the following steps:

Day 0–3: Good quality hESCs were passaged [dispase (1mg/ml)] and plated as small, 50- to 100-cell clumps into ultralow adherent culture dishes. Cells were kept in suspension in hESC medium, supplemented with rock inhibitor Y27632 (10μM) to enhance single cell survival, bFGF (20ng/ml) to enhance growth, and SB435142 (10μM) and LDN193189(0.2μM) for neuralization.

Day 3: EBs were switched from hESC media to neural induction medium (DMEM/F: 12 with L-glutamine, NEAA, penicillin/streptomycin, heparin (2μg/ml); and N2 supplement) along with Y27632 (10μM), bFGF (20ng/ml), SB435142 (10μM) and LDN193189 (0.2μM).

Day 5: all-*trans* retinoic acid (RA: 0.1 or 1μM), ascorbic acid (0.4μg/ml), and brain-derived neurotrophic factor (10ng/ml) were added. Dual ALK inhibition (SB&LDN) was pursued until day 7.

Day 7: For ventralization, C25II modified Sonic hedgehog SHH (200ng/ml) or a human Smo agonist (HAG, 1μM) or mouse Smo agonist (SAG, 1μM) or Purmorphamine (1μM) was used.

Day 17: Culture medium was changed to Neurobasal and B27 with all previous factors plus and with the addition of insulin-like growth factor 1 (IGF-1:10ng/mL), glial cell line-derived neurotrophic factor (GDNF:10ng/mL), and ciliary neurotrophic factor (CNTF:10ng/mL).

Day 20: EBs were dissociated with 0.05% trypsin, plated onto poly-lysine/laminin-coated 8-well chamber slides at 0.2–0.5.10^6 cells/well. Plated neurons were cultured in the same medium with the addition of 25μM BME and 25μM glutamic acid (Sigma) and fixed 1 day later.

Following the expression of Hb9 and ISL1 as overlapping motor neuron markers followed the motor neuron identity. These studies show that Purmorphamine, SAG and Retinoic acid each at 1μM were more efficient in driving motor neuron differentiation. In the final population of motor neurons, RNA-seq analysis confirmed markers of spinal motor neurons (*ISL1, ISL2, HB9, RET*) as well as key cholinergic genes (*CHAT, CHT1, VACHT, CHRNA3, CHRNA4, CHRNB2*) were enriched in these cells. The cells seem to be functional based on unbiased gene ontology (GO) analysis and electrophysiology that revealed transmission of nerve impulses and, synaptic release of acetylcholine. Importantly, the cluster analysis of genes associated with neuronal development and differentiation contained key motor neuron markers [*MNX1 (HB9), RET, CHAT, ISL1*]. Based on their findings, the authors clearly suggest that a combination of HB9 and ISL1 is the most accurate measure of total motor neuron yield when reporter lines are unavailable.

More recently, a small molecule screen was developed for stem cell-derived motor neurons in order to find therapeutic interventions for ALS (Yang *et al.*, 2013). This method of screening for motor neurons appears to be fast, reproducible, and reliable which is similar to the method described by Amoroso *et al.*, but can be expanded for high throughput screening system. In brief, the steps are as follows:

Day 0–2: pluripotent cells were grown as embryoid bodies in DMEM/F12 containing 2% B27 and 1% N2.

Day 2: the embryoid bodies were treated with Dorsomorphin and SB 431542, (a TGF-B pathway inhibitor) to induce a neural lineage and, additionally, with retinoic acid and a smoothened agonist (smoothened agonist) at low dose on day 2.

Day 3: same as day 2 but with high dose smoothened agonist.

Day 7: EBs were dissociated and plated for motor neuron differentiation with RA and dorsomorphin.

Day 10: After a total of 10 days of embryoid body cultures, motor neuron specification factors were removed and motor neurons maturation factors such as BDNF, GDNF, CNTF (each at 20ng/mL) or a test compound, in this case Kenpaullone (up to 10μM) was added that gave best results with different human iPSC lines.

Day 18: Colonies were plated on poly-ornithine and laminin (PO/LAM)-coated plates to mature further to motor neurons in the same medium.

Day 30: Cultures were either dissociated to single cells with a papain solution and plated on PO/LAM-coated 384-well plates in Neurobasal-containing 2% B27 and 1% N2 in 10ng/mL of GDNF and BDNF or proBDNF for five days and subjected to staining for motor neuron markers such as Hb9, Isle1 etc.

This method appears to be relatively good and easy even to screen for drugs that could potentially be used in motor neuron diseases. Though the method was developed with mouse ESC, the authors further validated the process for use with hESC and iPSC lines in the study. Kenpaullone, a GSK-3 inhibitor, appears to be a better survival/ maturation enabling molecule, relative to GSK-3 inhibitors or to the compounds that recently failed in human clinical trials such as olesoxime or dexpramipexole. Hence, this method appears to be the most promising yet to obtain motor neurons from pluripotent stem cells. The work by Jha *et al.* (Jha *et al.*, 2014) in deriving inter-mediate proliferative precursors for spinal motor neurons offers an additional advantage of scalability, reporter line generation using intermediate motor neuron precursors — such as OLIG2 or HB9 — for mature motor neuron generation and facilitate the work flow involved in the study of motor neuron development in health and diseases paradigms.

Conclusions

This brief review describes the landscape of scientific progress that is driving successful differentiation of pluripotent stem cells towards multiple neural lineages. Important developments such as conventional rosette-based derivation of NSC with an intermediary state of embryoid formation, a rosette-free derivation of NSC from pluripotent cells in monolayer cultures are discussed. Further select current preferred and alternative methods starting from NSC or from PSC state, are presented showing how PSC can be coaxed towards forebrain (GABA, interneurons), midbrain (dopaminergic), and hind brain neurons (motor), relevant for stem cell mediated cell therapy and drug screening purposes for neurological diseases.

Acknowledgements

Author MV thanks Dr. Soojung Shin for the preparation and assistance with Figure 1.

References

Akamatsu W, DeVeale B, Okano H, Cooney AJ, van der Kooy D (2009) Suppression of Oct4 by germ cell nuclear factor restricts pluripotency and promotes neural stem cell development in the early neural lineage. *J Neurosci* 29:2113–2124.

Amoroso MW, Croft GF, Williams DJ, O'Keeffe S, Carrasco MA, Davis AR, Roybon L, Oakley DH, Maniatis T, Henderson CE *et al.* (2013) Accelerated high-yield generation of limb-innervating motor neurons from human stem cells. *J neurosci* 33:574–586.

Cai C, Grabel L (2007). Directing the differentiation of embryonic stem cells to neural stem cells. *Dev Dynamics* 236:3255–3266.

Chambers SM, Fasano CA, Papapetrou EP, Tomishima M, Sadelain M, Studer L (2009) Highly efficient neural conversion of human ES and iPS cells by dual inhibition of SMAD signaling. *Nat Biotech* 27:275–280.

Cooper O, Hargus G, Deleidi M, Blak A, Osborn T, Marlow E, Lee K, Levy A, Perez-Torres E, Yow A *et al.* (2010) Differentiation of human ES and Parkinson's disease iPS cells into ventral midbrain dopaminergic neurons requires a high activity form of SHH FGF8a and specific regionalization by retinoic acid. *Mol Cell Neurosci* 45:258–266.

Emborg ME, Liu Y, Xi J, Zhang X, Yin Y, Lu J, Joers V, Swanson C, Holden JE, Zhang SC (2013) Induced pluripotent stem cell-derived neural cells survive and mature in the nonhuman primate brain. *Cell Rep* 28: 646–650.

Jessell TM (2000) Neuronal specification in the spinal cord: inductive signals and transcriptional codes. *Nat Rev Genet* 1:20–29.

Jha BS, Rao M, Malik N (2014) Motor Neuron Differentiation from Pluripotent Stem Cells and Other Intermediate Proliferative Precursors that can be Discriminated by Lineage Specific Reporters. *Stem Cell Rev* **Aug** 5. [Epub ahead of print]

Kirkeby A, Grealish S, Wolf DA, Nelander J, Wood J, Lundblad M, Lindvall O, Parmar M (2012) Generation of regionally specified neural progenitors and functional neurons from human embryonic stem cells under defined conditions. *Cell Rep* 1:703–714.

Kondo T, Funayama M, Tsukita K, Hotta A, Yasuda A, Nori S, Kaneko S, Nakamura M, Takahashi R, Okano H, Yamanaka S, Inoue H (2014) Focal transplantation of human iPSC-derived glial-rich neural progenitors improves lifespan of ALS mice. *Stem Cell Rep* 12:242–249.

Kriks S, Shim JW, Piao J, Ganat YM, Wakeman DR, Xie Z, Carrillo-Reid L, Auyeung G, Antonacci C, Buch A *et al.* (2011) Dopamine neurons derived from human ES cells efficiently engraft in animal models of Parkinson's disease. *Nature* 480:547–551.

Liu Y, Liu H, Sauvery C, Yao L, Zarnowska ED, Zhang SC (2013) Directed differentiation of forebrain GABA interneurosn from human pluripotent stem cells. *Nat Protoc* 8:1670–1679.

Liu Q, Spusta SC, Mi R, Lassiter RN, Stark MR, Höke A, Rao MS, Zeng X (2012) Human neural crest stem cells derived from human ESCs and induced pluripotent stem cells: induction maintenance and differentiation into functional schwann cells. *Stem Cells Transl Med* 1:266–278.

Marin O (2013) Human cortical interneurons take their time. *Cell Stem Cell* 12:497–499.

Maroof AM, Keros S, Tyson JA, Ying SW, Ganat YM, Merkle FT, Liu B, Goulburn A, Stanley EG, Elefanty AG *et al.* (2013) Directed differentiation and functional maturation of cortical interneurons from human embryonic stem cells. *Cell Stem Cell* 12:559–572.

Mica Y, Lee G, Chambers SM, Tomishima MJ, Studer L (2013) Modeling neural crest induction melanocyte specification and disease-related pigmentation defects in hESCs and patient-specific iPSCs. *Cell Rep* 25:1140–1152.

Momčilović O, Liu Q, Swistowski A, Russo-Tait T, Zhao Y, Rao MS, Zeng X, (2014) Genome wide profiling of dopaminergic neurons derived from human embryonic and induced pluripotent stem cells. *Stem Cells Dev* 15:406–420.

Muratore CR, Srikanth P, Callahan DG, Young-Pearse TL (2014) Comparison and optimization of hiPSC forebrain cortical differentiation protocols. *PLoS One.* 28:e105807.

Nicholas CR, Chen J, Tang Y, Southwell DG, Chalmers N, Vogt D, Arnold CM, Chen YJ, Stanley EG, Elefanty AG *et al.* (2013) Functional maturation of hPSC-derived forebrain interneurons requires an extended timeline and mimics human neural development. *Cell Stem Cell* 12:573–586.

Ogawa S, Tokumoto Y, Miyake J, Nagamune T (2011) Induction of oligodendrocyte differentiation from adult human fibroblast-derived induced pluripotent stem cells. *In Vitro Cell Dev Biol Anim* 47:464–469

Ono Y, Nakatani T, Sakamoto Y, Mizuhara E, Minaki Y, Kumai M, Hamaguchi A, Nishimura M, Inoue Y, Hayashi H *et al.* (2007) Differences in neurogenic potential in floor plate cells along an anteroposterior location: midbrain dopaminergic neurons originate from mesencephalic floor plate cells. *Development* 134:3213–3225.

Peng J, Liu Q, Rao MS, Zeng X (2014) Survival and engraftment of dopaminergic neurons manufactured by a Good Manufacturing Practice-compatible process. *Cytotherapy* 16:1305–1312.

Perrier AL, Tabar V, Barberi T, Rubio ME, Bruses J, Topf N, Harrison NL, and Studer L (2004) Derivation of midbrain dopamine neurons from human embryonic stem cells. *Pro Nat Acad Sci U S A* 101:12543–12548.

Rao M (2004) Stem and precursor cells in the nervous system. *J Neurotrauma* 21:415–427.

Reinhardt P, Glatza M, Hemmer K, Tsytsyura Y, Thiel CS, Hoing S, Moritz S, Parga JA, Wagner L, Bruder JM *et al.* (2013) Derivation and expansion using only small molecules of human neural progenitors for neurodegenerative disease modeling. *PloS One* 8:e59252.

Shaltouki A, Peng J, Liu Q, Rao MS, Zeng X (2013) Efficient generation of astrocytes from human pluripotent stem cells in defined conditions. *Stem Cells* 31(5):941–952 *Stem Cell Res* 11:743–757.

Shin S, Sun Y, Liu Y, Khaner H, Svant S, Cai J, Xu QX, Davidson BP, Stice SL, Smith AK, Goldman SA, Reubinoff BE, Zhan M, Rao MS, Chesnut JD (2007) Whole genome analysis of human neural stem cells derived from embryonic stem cells and stem and progenitor cells isolated from fetal tissue. *Stem Cells* 25:1298–1306.

Sundberg M, Bogetofte H, Lawson T, Jansson J, Smith G, Astradsson A, Moore M, Osborn T, Cooper O, Spealman R *et al.* (2013) Improved cell therapy protocols for Parkinson's disease based on differentiation efficiency and safety of hESC- hiPSC- and non-human primate iPSC-derived dopaminergic neurons. *Stem Cells* 31:1548–1562.

Tang X, Zhou L, Wagner AM, Marchetto MC, Muotri AR, Gage FH, Chen G (2013) Astroglial cells regulate the developmental timeline of human neurons differentiated from induced pluripotent stem cells. *Stem Cell Res* 11:743–757.

Wang S, Bates J, Li X, Schanz S, Chandler-Militello D, Levine C, Maherali N, Studer L, Hochedlinger K, Windrem M, Goldman SA (2013) Human iPSC-derived oligodendrocyte progenitor cells can myelinate and rescue a mouse model of congenital hypomyelination. *Cell Stem Cell* 12: 252–264.

Weston JA, Thiery JP (2015) Pentimento: Neural Crest and the origin of mesectoderm. *Dev Biol* http://dx. doi.org/10.1016/j.ydbio. 2014.12.035i [Epub ahead of print].

Xi J, Liu Y, Liu H, Chen H, Emborg ME, Zhang SC (2012) Specification of midbrain dopamine neurons from primate pluripotent stem cells. *Stem Cells* 30:1655–1663.

Yang YM, Gupta SK, Kim K, Powers BE, Cerqueira A, Wainger BJ, Ngo HD, Rosowski KA, Schein PA, Ackeifi CA *et al.* (2013) A small molecule screen in stem-cell-derived motor neurons identifies a kinase inhibitor as a candidate therapeutic for ALS. *Cell Stem Cell* 12:713–726.

Yuan T, Liao W, Feng NH, Lou YL, Niu X, Zhang AJ, Wang Y, Deng ZF, (2013) Human induced pluripotent stem cell-derived neural stem cells survive migrate differentiate and improve neurologic function in a rat model of middle cerebral artery occlusion. *Stem Cell Res Ther* 14:73.

Zhang SC, Wernig M, Duncan ID, Brustle O, Thomson JA, (2001) *In vitro* differentiation of transplantable neural precursors from human embryonic stem cells. *Nat Biotech* 19:1129–1133.

Index